McGraw-Hill Education
SPECIALTY BOARD REVIEW

Anatomic Pathology

Primary Certification and Maintenance of Certification

D1612937

NOTICE

Medicine is an ever-changing science. As new research and clinical experience broaden our knowledge, changes in treatment and drug therapy are required. The authors and the publisher of this work have checked with sources believed to be reliable in their efforts to provide information that is complete and generally in accord with the standards accepted at the time of publication. However, in view of the possibility of human error or changes in medical sciences, neither the authors nor the publisher nor any other party who has been involved in the preparation or publication of this work warrants that the information contained herein is in every respect accurate or complete, and they disclaim all responsibility for any errors or omissions or for the results obtained from use of the information contained in this work. Readers are encouraged to confirm the information contained herein with other sources. For example, and in particular, readers are advised to check the product information sheet included in the package of each drug they plan to administer to be certain that the information contained in this work is accurate and that changes have not been made in the recommended dose or in the contraindications for administration. This recommendation is of particular importance in connection with new or infrequently used drugs.

McGraw-Hill Education
SPECIALTY BOARD REVIEW

Anatomic Pathology

Primary Certification and Maintenance of Certification

Deepa T. Patil, MD

Assistant Professor, Cleveland Clinic Lerner
  College of Medicine
Staff Pathologist, Cleveland Clinic
Department of Anatomic Pathology
Cleveland, Ohio

Deborah J. Chute, MD

Assistant Professor, Cleveland Clinic Lerner
  College of Medicine
Staff Pathologist, Cleveland Clinic
Department of Anatomic Pathology
Cleveland, Ohio

Richard A. Prayson, MD

Professor, Cleveland Clinic Lerner College
  of Medicine
Staff Pathologist, Cleveland Clinic
Department of Anatomic Pathology
Cleveland, Ohio

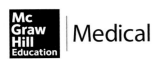 Medical

New York   Chicago   San Francisco   Athens   London   Madrid   Mexico City
Milan   New Delhi   Singapore   Sydney   Toronto

McGraw-Hill Education Specialty Board Review: Anatomic Pathology: Primary Certification and Maintenance of Certification

1 2 3 4 5 6 7 8 9 0   CTP/CTP   18 17 16 15 14 13

ISBN 978-0-07-179502-9
MHID 0-07-179502-2

This book was set in ITC Slimbach by Aptara, Inc.
The editors were Alyssa K. Fried and Christina M. Thomas.
The production supervisor was Catherine Saggese.
Project management was provided by Amit Kashyap, Aptara, Inc.
China Translation & Printing Services Ltd. was printer and binder.

This book is printed on acid-free paper.

Library of Congress Cataloging-in-Publication Data

Patil, Deepa T., author.
  Anatomic pathology / Deepa T. Patil, Deborah J. Chute, Richard A. Prayson.
        p. ; cm. — (McGraw-Hill specialty board review)
  Includes bibliographical references and index.
  ISBN 978-0-07-179502-9 (alk. paper) — ISBN 0-07-179502-2 (alk. paper)—
ISBN 978-0-07-179503-6 (ebook)
  I. Chute, Deborah J., author. II. Prayson, Richard A., author. III. Title.
IV. Series: McGraw-Hill specialty board review.
  [DNLM: 1. Pathology, Clinical—Examination Questions.
2. Anatomy—Examination Questions. QY 18.2]
  RB119
  616.07076—dc23
                                                      2013023701

CONTENTS

PREFACE

This book has been designed as a self-assessment guide for pathology residents and fellows preparing for the Anatomic Pathology Board Examination and for practicing pathologists who are preparing for the Anatomic Pathology Maintenance of Certification (MOC) examination to fulfill the cognitive expertise component (Part III) of MOC. The subject matter covered in this book includes a spectrum of topics that incorporate fundamental knowledge necessary for daily practice as well as information on the latest molecular and genetic techniques, which are an essential element of understanding the pathophysiology and therapeutics of disease processes. This book will improve content knowledge of the readers and allow them to test this knowledge with case-based scenarios.

The chapters have been categorized into topics that are similar to the modules outlined for the MOC examination. In addition, this book also includes some clinical pathology topics, such as lymph node and spleen, and laboratory management as applicable to the practice of anatomic pathology as well. This book has board-style multiple-choice questions in a one-best-answer format. The answers have been sequenced alphabetically and include a brief discussion about the salient features of the entity, diagnostic pitfalls, differential diagnosis, and provide an explanation for the incorrect choices. For additional reading, the most useful review articles and references have been provided at the end of each chapter. High-resolution gross and microscopic images have also been included to supplement the review process.

This book is certainly not meant to replace the regular reading and the invaluable practical knowledge gained from daily previewing and didactic sessions from experienced pathologists. The authors have been extremely fortunate to be taught by extraordinary and patient teachers. We share a common passion for teaching and are thankful to our residents and fellows who not only continue to enrich this interactive experience but also make learning fun. We hope that this volume will serve as a valuable supplementary resource for a succinct and organized approach toward successful board preparations.

ACKNOWLEDGMENT

We would like to express our gratitude to Ms. Shon Bryson for her contribution in organizing this book in a timely manner.

CHAPTER 1

CELL INJURY, INFLAMMATION, REPAIR, AND HEMODYNAMIC DISORDERS

1. A patient presents with liver failure and congestive heart failure, and a liver biopsy shows the following changes (see Figure 1-1—Prussian blue stain). What material's abnormal accumulation results in cellular injury and death in this disease?

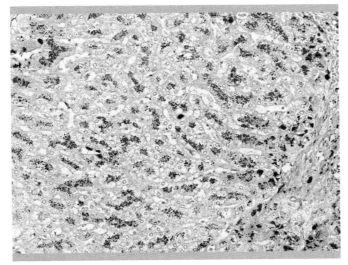

FIGURE 1-1

  (A) Bilirubin
  (B) Calcium
  (C) Iron
  (D) Lipofuscin
  (E) Melanin

2. Cells with irreversible injury undergoing cell death can show nuclear shrinkage, basophilia, and nuclear fragmentation (see Figure 1-2 cell at arrow). This process is called

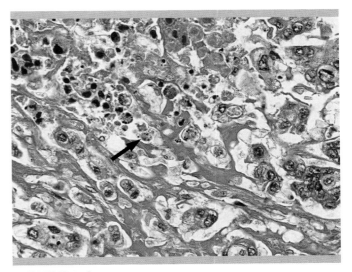

FIGURE 1-2

  (A) Balloon degeneration
  (B) Fatty change
  (C) Karyolysis
  (D) Karyorrhexis
  (E) Pyknosis

1

3. An atherosclerotic plaque ruptures and obstructs blood flow to a segment of kidney (see Figure 1-3). At 6 hours after the event, the involved kidney would show what pattern of necrosis on microscopic examination?

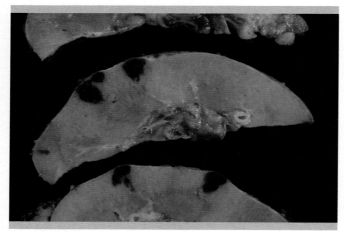

FIGURE 1-3

   (A) Caseous necrosis
   (B) Coagulative necrosis
   (C) Fibrinoid necrosis
   (D) Gangrenous necrosis
   (E) Liquefactive necrosis

4. A patient with renal failure on long-term dialysis and taking aluminum-based antacids presents with multiple lesions in the kidneys, lungs, and skin. A biopsy was performed (see Figure 1-4). This is an example of

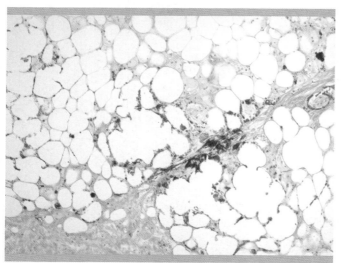

FIGURE 1-4

   (A) Dystrophic calcification
   (B) Fat necrosis

   (C) Heterotopic bone formation
   (D) Metastatic calcification
   (E) Metastatic carcinoma

5. The changes present in this skin biopsy (see Figure 1-5) are an example of which morphologic pattern of acute inflammation?

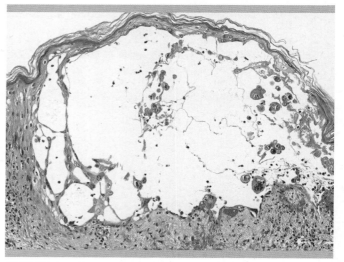

FIGURE 1-5

   (A) Abscess formation
   (B) Fibrinous inflammation
   (C) Serous inflammation
   (D) Suppurative inflammation
   (E) Ulcer formation

6. This pattern of inflammation (see Figure 1-6) is associated with which of the following diseases?

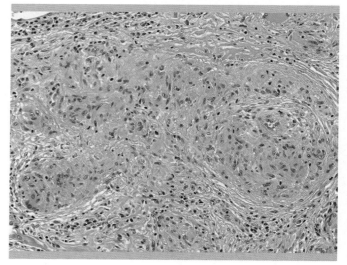

FIGURE 1-6

(A) Acute lung injury
(B) Nonspecific interstitial pneumonia
(C) Sarcoidosis
(D) *Staphylococcus aureus*
(E) Varicella virus

7. The thick pink material at the arrows in this photomicrograph (see Figure 1-7) is predominantly composed of what extracellular matrix protein?

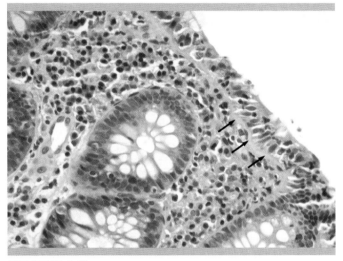

FIGURE 1-7

(A) Collagen type II
(B) Collagen type IV
(C) Elastin
(D) Fibrillin
(E) Hyaluronan

8. After a woman has her ear pierced, a keloid developed at the site of the piercing, which was subsequently excised (see Figure 1-8). Which of the following is incorrect about this abnormal repair response?

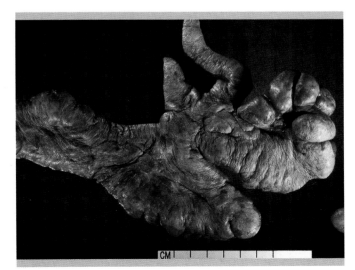

FIGURE 1-8

(A) Due to exuberant granulation tissue growth
(B) Fails to regress with normal remodeling
(C) May grow beyond the boundaries of the original wound
(D) Most common in African Americans
(E) Traumatic injury to the deep dermis is a typical inciting event

9. A patient with kidney disease (see Figure 1-9 electron micrograph of a typical glomerulus from this patient, CL = capillary lumen) and nephrotic syndrome has severe pitting edema in his lower legs. This edema is primarily caused by which of the following processes?

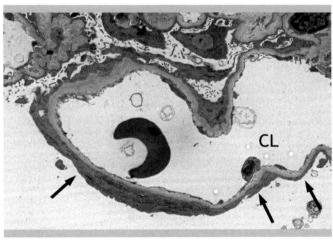

FIGURE 1-9

(A) Increased hydrostatic pressure due to arteriolar dilatation
(B) Increased hydrostatic pressure due to impaired venous return
(C) Increased vascular permeability
(D) Reduced plasma osmotic pressure
(E) Sodium retention

10. All of the following are examples of tissue hypertrophy except
(A) Biceps enlargement due to exercise
(B) Endometrial thickening due to excess estrogen
(C) Left ventricle enlargement due to high blood pressure
(D) Right ventricle enlargement due to pulmonary fibrosis
(E) Uterine enlargement during pregnancy

11. All of the following are examples of metaplasia except
(A) Apocrine change in the breast
(B) Barrett's esophagus
(C) Bronchial squamous mucosa in a smoker
(D) Myositis ossificans
(E) Notochord loss with development of the spinal cord

12. All of the following are true regarding ischemia except
    (A) Accumulation of toxic metabolites contributes to cell injury
    (B) Anaerobic glycolysis continues after the insult
    (C) Can be caused by reduced venous drainage
    (D) More rapid and severe than hypoxia alone
    (E) Most commonly due to blockage of arterial blood supply

13. Reversible cell injury is characterized by which of the following changes?
    (A) Apoptosis
    (B) Cell membrane disruption
    (C) Cellular swelling
    (D) Loss of mitochondrial function
    (E) Karyorrhexis

14. Which of the following situations would most likely result in liquefactive necrosis?
    (A) Acute pancreatitis
    (B) Pulmonary embolism
    (C) Pulmonary tuberculosis
    (D) Myocardial infarction
    (E) Stroke

15. A severely burned patient requires very high fluid replacement due to insensible losses from increased vascular permeability. All of the following are causes of increased vascular permeability and exudates in an inflammatory reaction except
    (A) Endothelial cell detachment
    (B) Endothelial cell necrosis
    (C) Leukocyte migration through vessel walls
    (D) Retraction of endothelial cells with gap formation
    (E) Transcytosis

16. During leukocyte recruitment to sites of cell injury, which of the following is not a phase of leukocyte recruitment?
    (A) Activation
    (B) Adhesion
    (C) Margination
    (D) Migration
    (E) Rolling

17. Which of the following is an example of chemotaxis?
    (A) Deposition of opsonins on target particles
    (B) Engulfment of microbes or dead cells by phagocytes
    (C) Expression of selectins on endothelial cell membranes
    (D) Increased vascular permeability due to cytokines
    (E) Movement of neutrophils along a gradient of bacterial products

18. Patients with chronic granulomatous disease suffer from recurrent bacterial infections that cannot be easily cleared despite normal numbers of leukocytes. This disease is an example of the importance of which function of leukocytes?
    (A) Engulfment of foreign particles
    (B) Oxidative burst
    (C) Production of cytokines
    (D) Recruitment to site of injury
    (E) Recognition of complement proteins

19. Nonsteroidal anti-inflammatory agents, such as aspirin, inhibit acute inflammatory reactions by what mechanism?
    (A) Down-regulating transcription of genes encoding cyclooxygenase 2 (COX)
    (B) Increasing vasoconstriction preventing leukocyte recruitment
    (C) Inhibiting conversion of cell membrane proteins to arachidonic acid
    (D) Preventing production of prostacyclin by COX1 and COX2
    (E) Reducing cell membrane expression of tumor necrosis factor (TNF) receptors

20. All of the following are true about chemokines except
    (A) Can be attached to cells or present in extracellular matrix
    (B) Different chemokines attract different leukocyte types
    (C) Function primarily as chemoattractants for leukocytes
    (D) Mediate the acute-phase systemic response
    (E) Some chemokine receptors mediate binding and entry of HIV into host cells

21. All of the following are true regarding the complement system except
    (A) Cleavage products of complement proteins are potent stimulators of other inflammatory responses
    (B) Does not interact with the coagulation cascade
    (C) Form the membrane attack complex (MAC)
    (D) Highly regulated system with many inhibitors
    (E) Present in the plasma in an inactive state

22. Acute-phase proteins, such as C-reactive protein (CRP), fibrinogen, and serum amyloid A (SAA), are up-regulated in acute inflammatory reactions. Which of the following is true regarding these proteins?

(A) Can bind to bacterial cells walls and act as opsonins
(B) CRP elevation is unreliable in predicting risk of myocardial infarction
(C) Not detectable in plasma in normal state
(D) Only certain acute inflammatory causes will result in up-regulation of these proteins
(E) Synthesized primarily by endothelial cells

23. All of the following tissues continuously proliferate throughout life, replacing destroyed cells except
(A) Bone marrow
(B) Duodenal mucosa
(C) Skeletal muscle
(D) Skin epithelium
(E) Uterine endometrium

24. A cell that retains the ability to continuously divide, but can only differentiate into one cell type (e.g., squamous epithelium) is called a(n)
(A) Embryonic stem cell
(B) Induced pluripotent stem cell
(C) Lineage-restricted stem cell
(D) Multipotent stem cell
(E) Pluripotent stem cell

25. Tyrosine kinase inhibitors, such as imatinib, most commonly act upon cell membrane receptors of growth factors, and prevent transduction of the signal across the cell membrane. Which of the following is true regarding cell membrane receptors with tyrosine kinase activity?
(A) Cyclic AMP pathway is the most common downstream effector molecule
(B) Ligand binding causes dimerization of the receptors, leading to tyrosine kinase activation
(C) Seven transmembrane alpha-helixes are almost always present
(D) Steroid hormones are ligands for receptors with tyrosine kinase activity
(E) The extracellular domain of the receptor has tyrosine kinase activity

26. The extracellular matrix of a tissue plays many important roles in tissue function and structure. Which of the following is not a function of the extracellular matrix?
(A) Creating a tissue microenvironment (e.g., barriers to solute diffusion in the kidney)
(B) Mechanical support of cells
(C) Production of signaling molecules
(D) Regulation of cell growth and proliferation
(E) Scaffolding for tissue renewal

27. All of the following are true about desmosomes except
(A) Are important in resisting shear forces
(B) Connect skeletal muscle cells to skeletal muscle cells
(C) Connect squamous cells to basement membrane
(D) Connect squamous cells to squamous cells
(E) Target of autoimmune antibodies in pemphigus vulgaris

28. Scar formation occurs when sufficient stromal framework damage prevents healing by cell regeneration alone. Which of the following is an example of scar formation?
(A) Abscess cavity filling and healing
(B) Bone marrow reconstitution after chemotherapy
(C) Epidermal repair after minor abrasions
(D) Liver hypertrophy after partial liver transplant
(E) Replacement of gut epithelium after an ischemic event

29. A surgeon performing a kidney transplant closes the skin incision with sutures, and the skin incision heals within a few weeks. This type of cutaneous wound healing is characterized by all of the following except
(A) Called healing by primary union
(B) Creation of a thin scar
(C) Limited cell death and connective tissue disruption
(D) Rapid re-epithelialization over the wound
(E) Significant wound contraction

30. A patient presents with unilateral pitting edema of the lower leg. An ultrasound shows a deep venous thrombosis. This edema is primarily caused by which of the following processes?
(A) Increased hydrostatic pressure due to arteriolar dilatation
(B) Increased hydrostatic pressure due to impaired venous return
(C) Increased vascular permeability
(D) Reduced plasma osmotic pressure
(E) Sodium retention

31. Primary hemostasis after trauma is achieved by which of the following processes?
(A) Arteriolar vasoconstriction
(B) Fibrin meshwork formation
(C) Increased vascular permeability
(D) Platelet plug formation
(E) Tissue plasminogen activity (t-PA)

32. Endothelial cells play an important role in the maintenance of normal hemostasis and clot formation after injury. Which of the following is not a function of endothelial cells in hemostasis?
    (A) Contain membrane-bound heparin-like molecules to inhibit thrombosis
    (B) Prevent platelet exposure to extracellular matrix proteins
    (C) Prostacyclin production to inhibit platelets
    (D) Secrete adenosine diphosphate (ADP), which promotes platelet inactivation
    (E) Synthesize tissue-type plasminogen activator (t-PA), which degrades clots

33. Platelets are critical in initially stopping tissue hemorrhage after injury. Which of the following is true regarding platelet function in hemostasis?
    (A) Alpha-granules contain ADP, calcium, and serotonin
    (B) Dense granules contain P-selectin, fibrinogen, and platelet factor 4
    (C) Platelet contraction is reversible
    (D) Platelets degrade thromboxane A2 to promote platelet aggregation
    (E) von Willebrand factor binding to glycoprotein Ib is primarily used for platelet adhesion

34. Excessive clot formation is prevented by activation of the fibrinolytic cascade. Which of the following is not true regarding fibrinolysis?
    (A) Fibrin degradation results in fibrin split products (FSP)
    (B) Plasmin is generated from plasminogen by tissue factor
    (C) Plasmin is the primary enzyme that breaks down fibrin
    (D) Streptokinase, produced by some bacteria, can also convert plasminogen to plasmin
    (E) Tissue plasminogen activator (t-PA) is most active when bound to fibrin

35. Abnormal blood flow (stasis and turbulence) promotes clot formation by which mechanism?
    (A) Exposure of extracellular matrix proteins to platelets
    (B) Increased activation of coagulation factors by shear forces
    (C) Increased production of t-PA by injured endothelial cells
    (D) Irregular flow presses platelets against endothelial cells
    (E) Laminar flow presses platelets against endothelial cells

36. Factor V Leiden is an inherited hypercoagulable state. Thrombosis in patients with Factor V Leiden is caused by what mechanism?
    (A) Absence of protein C, which cleaves factor V
    (B) Constitutive activation of factor V
    (C) Factor V resistance to cleavage by protein C
    (D) Factor V resistance to cleavage by protein S
    (E) Increased levels of factor V

37. A woman who was in a major motor vehicle accident has a femoral fracture. She develops shortness of breath, confusion, and thrombocytopenia shortly after arriving at the emergency room. What is the most likely cause of her symptoms?
    (A) Air embolism
    (B) Amniotic fluid embolism
    (C) Fat embolism syndrome
    (D) Pulmonary embolism
    (E) Sepsis

38. Shock is the final common, often fatal, pathway for many different disorders. All of the following are true about shock except
    (A) Compensatory mechanisms can initially maintain organ perfusion in shock
    (B) Peripheral vasoconstriction (cool, blue skin) is seen in all types of shock
    (C) Septic shock can occur even when the infection is localized
    (D) Shock results in impaired tissue perfusion and cellular hypoxia
    (E) Tissue hypoxia leads to cell death and release of toxins that accelerates shock

39. On routine serum chemistry testing, a patient is found to have elevated liver enzymes. A liver biopsy was performed and show chronic passive congestion (see Figure 1-10). What other pathologic process is this patient likely to have?

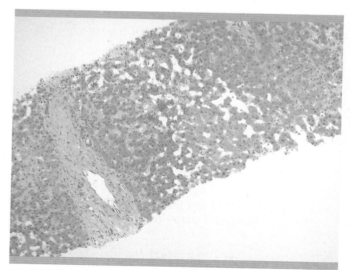

FIGURE 1-10

(A) Cirrhosis
(B) Congestive heart failure
(C) Hepatitis C
(D) Sepsis
(E) Thromboembolic disease

40. A patient with severe atherosclerosis presents with nausea, vomiting, and an elevated serum creatinine. A photomicrograph of what his kidney might look like is provided (see Figure 1-11). This macroscopic appearance is most consistent with which of the following processes?

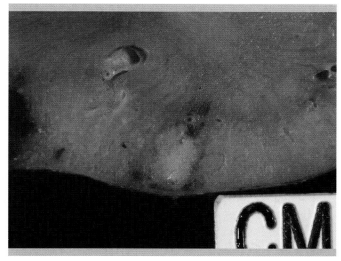

FIGURE 1-11

(A) Congestion
(B) Edema
(C) Hypertrophy
(D) Infarction
(E) Neoplasm

41. An important mechanism of cell injury is oxidative stress (often in the form of free radicals). An increase in free radicals would be seen in all of the following except
(A) Decreased glutathione peroxidase levels
(B) Elevated levels of vitamin E
(C) Ionizing radiation damage
(D) Leukocytes activated during inflammatory reactions
(E) Nitric oxide release

42. Most cells have a fixed number of divisions before becoming senescent. All of the following are causes of cellular aging except
(A) Calorie restriction
(B) Defective DNA replication
(C) Free radical generation
(D) Increasing cellular damage
(E) Telomere shortening

43. All of the following statements about apoptosis are true except
(A) Apoptosis is an integral part of embryogenesis
(B) Appears as cell fragments with intact cytoplasmic membranes
(C) Can be activated by FAS-FAS ligand binding
(D) Incites a brisk inflammatory response
(E) Occurs in normal germinal centers

44. All of the following are true about histamine except
(A) Histamine causes increased permeability of vessels
(B) Histamine is a plasma-derived protein
(C) Histamine release can be activated by C3a
(D) Histamine results in dilation of arterioles
(E) Histamine is stored in mast cell granules

45. A patient with a chronic autoimmune disease suffers from severe weight loss and anorexia, or cachexia. Which of the following inflammatory mediators is primarily responsible for this pathologic state?
(A) Complement proteins
(B) Histamine
(C) Nitric oxide
(D) Prostaglandin
(E) Tumor necrosis factor (TNF)

46. Macrophages are the main cellular component of chronic inflammatory processes. All of the following are true about macrophages except
(A) Able to ingest foreign particles
(B) Activated by interferon-gamma
(C) Derived from bone marrow stem cells
(D) Produce reactive oxygen species
(E) Short lived (6 hours or less)

47. Angiogenesis is a critically important part of all wound healing. All of the following are steps in angiogenesis except
(A) Basement membrane degradation
(B) Migration of endothelial cells
(C) Recruitment of peri-endothelial cells
(D) Vasodilation
(E) Wound contraction

48. Which is of the following is an example of autocrine signaling in cell growth?
    (A) Antigen presenting lymphocyte secretes cytokines that causes itself to proliferate
    (B) Injured hepatocyte releases cytokines, causing a nearby stem cell to proliferate
    (C) Macrophage secretes cytokines, causing a nearby fibroblast to proliferate
    (D) Pituitary cell secretes growth hormone, causing osteoblasts to proliferate
    (E) T-cell recognizing foreign viral particles induces a tissue cell to undergo apoptosis

49. At the end of 1 week, a healing skin wound has approximately 10% of the tensile strength of unwounded skin. At 3 months, what is the tensile strength of a healing skin wound (compared with unwounded skin)?
    (A) 20%
    (B) 40%
    (C) 50%
    (D) 80%
    (E) 100%

50. A patient with severe chronic renal failure goes out for dinner to a restaurant and eats a large amount of salted fish. The next day, he finds his legs are both swollen with edema. This edema is primarily caused by which of the following processes?
    (A) Increased hydrostatic pressure due to arteriolar dilatation
    (B) Increased hydrostatic pressure due to impaired venous return
    (C) Increased vascular permeability
    (D) Reduced plasma osmotic pressure
    (E) Sodium retention

51. Which of the following statements is incorrect regarding water as a component of the body?
    (A) Around 60% of lean body weight is water
    (B) Close to 25% of the body's water is in blood plasma
    (C) More than 50% of the body's water is within cells
    (D) Nearly 33% of the body's water is in extracellular spaces
    (E) The balance of intracellular and extracellular water is partially controlled by solutes

52. The coagulation cascade's primary purpose is to promote clot formation through thrombin generation. All of the following are true regarding the extrinsic pathway of the coagulation cascade except

(A) Includes factor XII (Hageman factor)
(B) Is identical to the intrinsic pathway from factor X onward
(C) Is the primary pathway for clotting in vivo after injury
(D) Prothrombin time (PT) primarily tests the extrinsic pathway
(E) Requires the addition of tissue lysates to promote clotting in vitro

53. Virchow's triad predicts that three abnormalities can result in abnormal thrombus formation. Virchow's triad includes
    (A) Endothelial injury, abnormal blood flow, and hypercoagulability
    (B) Endothelial injury, abnormal blood flow, and hypocoagulability
    (C) Endothelial injury, increased blood flow, and hypercoagulability
    (D) Endothelial secretion of prothrombotic products, abnormal blood flow, and hypercoagulability
    (E) Endothelial secretion of prothrombotic products, increased blood flow, and hypercoagulability

ANSWERS

1. **(C) Iron.**
   Accumulation of normal and abnormal intracellular proteins and materials can result in cell injury and death. The photomicrograph demonstrates abnormal accumulation of iron in the hepatocytes, which stains blue on Prussian blue stain. Patients with hemochromatosis have abnormal iron absorption regulation; systemic increased deposition of iron in otherwise normal tissues results in damage, and cell loss results in liver and heart failure. Abnormal calcium deposition can result in dystrophic and metastatic calcifications. Lipofuscin is composed of lipids and phospholipids, and is not injurious to cells, but is a common sign of other cellular injuries. Melanin deposition can rarely be abnormally deposited in the disorder ochronosis. Bilirubin is the main pigment of bile, and excess accumulation results in jaundice.

2. **(D) Karyorrhexis.**
   Karyorrhexis is a pattern of nuclear breakdown that shows pyknosis with subsequent nuclear fragmentation. Karyolysis occurs when nuclear DNA and chromatin are enzymatically degraded, resulting in faded nuclear staining. Pyknosis is characterized by nuclear shrinkage and increased basophilia without nuclear fragmentation. Balloon degeneration is a cytoplasmic change in hepatocytes characterized by cell swelling and vacuolation. Fatty change is

a cytoplasmic alteration seen in reversible cellular injury.

3. **(B) Coagulative necrosis.**
Coagulative necrosis most often occurs when an interruption in blood supply results in tissue ischemia and death. This pattern of necrosis preserves the tissue architecture for several days, but the cells are eosinophilic and lack nuclei. Liquefactive necrosis is characterized by digestion of the dead cells, resulting in a liquid, viscous mass; this pattern is frequently seen in bacterial infections and CNS infarction. Gangrenous necrosis refers to cell death, typically in a limb, which has superimposed infection. Caseous necrosis is most common in tuberculous infection, resulting in cheese-like white friable material. Fibrinoid necrosis is a special form of necrosis around vessels where immune complexes are deposited, resulting in a "bright pink" amorphous appearance.

4. **(D) Metastatic calcification.**
The photomicrograph demonstrates dark purple deposits of calcium within fibroadipose tissue, consistent with metastatic calcification. Metastatic calcification occurs in patients with severe hypercalcemia, and most commonly occurs in skin, mucosal sites, kidneys, lungs, systemic arteries, and pulmonary veins. Morphologically, the deposits resemble dystrophic calcification. However, dystrophic calcifications occur in the absence of hypercalcemia, and occur in sites of prior tissue injury, such as areas of necrosis or atherosclerotic plaques. Fat necrosis occurs in areas of fat destruction with saponification, most commonly in pancreatitis. Heterotopic bone formation can occur in areas of previous injury, and shows variably organized bone formation. Metastatic carcinoma would demonstrate neoplastic epithelial cells on biopsy.

5. **(C) Serous inflammation.**
The photomicrograph shows a skin blister caused by varicella virus (chicken pox) that resulted in an outpouring of thin fluid (serous fluid) due to vasodilation and increased vascular permeability. This is an example of serous inflammation, and is frequently seen in effusions from peritoneal, pleural, and pericardial cavities. Fibrinous inflammation occurs when even greater vascular permeability permits outpouring of both fluid and larger molecules, such as fibrin, which organize into a meshwork of eosinophilic threads (fibrinous material). Suppurative inflammation occurs when large numbers of neutrophils involve an area that often has undergone liquefactive necrosis; an abscess forms when this area forms a cavity trapped in a confined space or organ. Ulcer formation occurs when necrotic tissue close to

a surface (skin, mucosal, etc.) is sloughed, leaving a marked inflammatory response at the base of the defect.

6. **(C) Sarcoidosis.**
The photomicrograph depicts granulomatous inflammation, which is a distinctive pattern of chronic inflammation. Granulomatous inflammation is associated with *Mycobacterium tuberculosis* infection, sarcoidosis, syphilis, and many other processes. Acute lung injury is characterized by a serous or fibrinous inflammation, due to trauma of the lung microvasculature. Nonspecific interstitial pneumonia is characterized by a chronic inflammatory response composed predominantly of lymphocytes. *Staphylococcus aureus* usually incites a suppurative inflammatory response, and varicella infection leads to blisters, which are formed by a serous inflammatory response.

7. **(B) Collagen type IV.**
The structure at the arrows in the photomicrograph is basement membrane underlying epithelium. Basement membranes are predominantly composed of collagen type IV, along with laminin. Collagen type II is the predominant component of cartilage. Elastin fibers are an important component of large blood vessels, uterus, skin, and ligaments. Fibrillin is a glycoprotein that surrounds and supports elastin fibers, and alterations in this protein are the cause of Marfan syndrome. Hyaluronan is a glycosaminoglycan, which is abundant in many tissue types and provides lubrication for joints.

8. **(A) Due to exuberant granulation tissue growth.**
Keloid formation (hypertrophic scar formation) is caused by excessive collagen deposition, which persists and/or resists remodeling. This wound healing response can extend beyond the boundaries of the original wound, and is most commonly caused by a traumatic injury, which penetrates to the deep dermis. This aberration is more common in African Americans, for unknown reasons. Granulation tissue does not play a part in this abnormal wound healing response.

9. **(D) Reduced plasma osmotic pressure.**
Edema can be caused by an imbalance in solutes, plasma osmotic pressure, or hydrostatic pressure. Nephrotic syndrome can be caused by a variety of diseases; the photomicrograph in this example is suggestive of minimal change disease, with effacement of the normal podocyte foot structure (arrows) around capillary lumens (CL). In nephrotic syndrome, excessive albumin and protein are lost from the kidneys into the urine. This results in reduced plasma osmotic pressure, which results in movement of water from the plasma

into extracellular tissues. Reduced plasma osmotic pressure can also be caused by reduced synthesis of plasma proteins, which occurs in liver failure (cirrhosis) or starvation.

10. **(B) Endometrial thickening due to excess estrogen.**

Hypertrophy is a process of cellular adaptation to stress or injury, which results in enlargement of cells, without an increase in the number of cells. This adaptation most commonly occurs in tissues that cannot undergo cellular division, such as cardiac (answers C and D) and skeletal muscle (answer A). An increase in protein and myofilaments allows each muscle fiber to generate increased force. In pregnancy, the myometrial smooth muscle cells undergo significant hypertrophy in response to hormonal alterations (e.g., physiologic hypertrophy). In contrast, endometrium stimulated with estrogen demonstrates a marked increase in epithelial and stromal cells, which remain normal in size (hyperplasia).

11. **(E) Notochord loss with development of the spinal cord.**

Metaplasia is a reversible adaptive cellular response to injury where one cell type is replaced by another cell type without an overall change in tissue architecture. The most common metaplasia is conversion from columnar or respiratory epithelium to squamous epithelium, often in the trachea and bronchi in smokers. Other examples include Barrett's esophagus (squamous to glandular metaplasia), myositis ossificans (muscle to bone), and apocrine metaplasia of the breast (normal ductal epithelium to apocrine epithelium). In contrast, the notochord undergoes atrophy during fetal development to make room for later development of the spinal cord with a completely different architecture.

12. **(B) Anaerobic glycolysis continues after the insult.**

Ischemia is the most common type of cell injury and results in both hypoxia (reduction in oxygen supply to tissues), loss of nutrients, and loss of removal of toxic metabolites. Therefore, it results in more rapid and severe injury than hypoxia alone. It is most commonly caused by a blockage in arterial blood supply, but can be caused by reduced venous drainage that prevents adequate arterial perfusion. When hypoxia occurs in isolation, cells usually remain supplied with sufficient nutrients to continue anaerobic glycolysis for a period of time after the initial insult, but in ischemia, the nutrient supply is restricted, and cells rapidly exhaust glycolytic substrates.

13. **(C) Cellular swelling.**

Reversible injury to cells is characterized by a reduction in energy stores (ATP) and changes in ion concentrations, resulting in water influx. Morphologically, this is demonstrated by cellular swelling, microscopic vacuoles, and lipid vacuoles. Eventually, sufficient cellular injury occurs such that the damage becomes irreversible, resulting in cell death by either necrosis or apoptosis. Irreversible changes of injury resulting in necrosis are characterized by cell membrane disruption, lysosomal rupture, and severe mitochondrial damage. Apoptosis is a form of cell death that is more controlled and results in nuclear dissolution (karyorrhexis) and cell fragmentation without loss of membrane integrity.

14. **(E) Stroke.**

Liquefactive necrosis occurs when necrotic cells are digested, resulting in transformation of the dead cells into a liquid, viscous mass. This is most commonly seen in bacterial infections (abscess), but is also the pattern of CNS necrosis from ischemic events (e.g., stroke). Acute pancreatitis is an example of fat necrosis. Pulmonary tuberculosis is an example of caseous necrosis. Myocardial infarction is an example of coagulative necrosis. Pulmonary embolism does not typically result in necrosis due to the dual blood supply to the lungs.

15. **(C) Leukocyte migration through vessel walls.**

During acute inflammatory reactions, substantial fluid exudation occurs due to increased vascular permeability. This is accentuated in burned patients, who lose a substantial volume of exudate into the environment. The most common mechanisms of increased vascular permeability are formation of interendothelial spaces (through contraction and retraction of endothelial cells), endothelial injury (leading to necrosis or detachment), and transcytosis (transport of fluids and proteins across intact endothelial cells). While leukocyte migration is an important part of acute inflammatory responses, it does not contribute to fluid shifts.

16. **(A) Activation.**

The process of leukocyte recruitment to sites of cell injury is critically important in the inflammatory response. Leukocytes start this process by margination (moving to a peripheral location in the bloodstream along the vessel wall), and slow by rolling that is mediated by the selectin family of proteins. Once leukocytes come to rest, they adhere to the endothelium by integrin proteins, and then migrate through the endothelial wall. Activation does not occur until leukocytes have arrived at the site of cell injury and infection.

17. **(E) Movement of neutrophils along a gradient of bacterial products.**

    Chemotaxis is defined as cellular locomotion along a chemical gradient, which can be composed of bacterial products, cytokines, or complement proteins. While expression of selectins on endothelial cell membranes is important in the rolling phase of leukocyte recruitment, a gradient is not present. Opsonins are placed on target particles for engulfment, but this targeting for destruction does not necessarily result in cell locomotion. While cytokines can act as the chemical gradient for chemotaxis, their effect on vessel walls does not play a part in locomotion.

18. **(B) Oxidative burst.**

    In chronic granulomatous disease (CGD), an inherited defect in phagocyte oxidase reduces the amount of oxygen-free radicals that can be produced inside the leukocyte lysosome, which then combines with engulfed foreign particles (specifically bacteria) and destroys the foreign material. Patients with CGD have normal or increased numbers of leukocytes, which are appropriately recruited to sites of injury and engulf bacterial organisms, but are unable to kill them. They eventually develop a brisk macrophage infiltrate, which forms granulomas in an attempt to control the infection. While recognition of complement proteins, particularly C5a, is important in recognizing foreign particles by leukocytes, free radicals are still required for destruction.

19. **(D) Preventing production of prostacyclin by COX1 and COX2.**

    Nonsteroidal anti-inflammatory agents (NSAIDs), such as aspirin, block the activity of COX1 and COX2 enzymes, which convert arachidonic acid to prostaglandins, potent mediators of the inflammatory response. Steroids cause down-regulation in the transcription of COX genes, as well as many other inflammatory genes, and can also decrease the conversion of cell membrane lipids to arachidonic acid. Although reduction in TNF receptors would reduce the inflammatory response, this is not mediated by NSAIDS. NSAIDS do not play a direct role in vasoconstriction or vasodilation.

20. **(D) Mediate the acute-phase systemic response.**

    Chemokines are small proteins that function primarily as chemoattractants for various leukocytes. The CXC group attracts neutrophils; the CC group attracts monocytes, eosinophils, basophils, and lymphocytes; the C group attracts lymphocytes; and the CX3C group attracts monocytes and T-cells. The chemokine receptors CXCR4 and CCR5 have been implicated in the binding HIV-1 viral particles, and mediate viral entry into host cells. Chemokines can be present on cell membranes or in the extracellular matrix. The acute-phase systemic response is primarily mediated by TNF and IL-1, which are not classified as chemokines.

21. **(B) Does not interact with the coagulation cascade.**

    The complement system contains more than 20 proteins that function in a variety of ways: stimulate other inflammatory reactions (particularly C3a and C5a), act as opsonins to promote phagocytosis, and cause cell lysis when the MAC is formed. These proteins are synthesized by the liver, and are present ubiquitously in the plasma, in an inactivated state. Given the highly dangerous properties of an unchecked complement cascade, many potent inhibitors of this system exist in both the plasma and on the surface of healthy cells. This system is intimately connected with other plasma-derived systems; it can promote the coagulation cascade, and products of the coagulation cascade can initiate the complement cascade.

22. **(A) Can bind to bacterial cells walls and act as opsonins.**

    Acute-phase reaction proteins, the best known of which are CRP, fibrinogen, and SAA, are normally detected in plasma, but increase to more than 100x their normal plasma concentrations in the setting of an acute inflammatory reaction. The increase is regulated by several cytokines, including IL-1, IL-6, and TNF, which are common to nearly all acute inflammatory responses. These proteins can then bind to foreign materials and act as opsonins, help to clear chromatin debris, and alter normal lipid metabolism to help sustain inflammatory cells. Nearly all acute-phase proteins are produced by hepatocytes, not endothelial cells. CRP elevation has recently been found to be a sensitive marker of increased risk of myocardial infarction in patients with coronary artery disease.

23. **(C) Skeletal muscle.**

    The tissues of the body are generally classified into three groups: continually dividing, quiescent, and nondividing. Most mucosal sites of the body (gastrointestinal tract, oral cavity), skin, and bone marrow undergo continuous proliferation to replace cells that are lost on a daily basis. The endometrium of the uterus is another example of a continuously dividing tissue. In contrast, skeletal muscle, cardiac muscle, and nerves cannot undergo division to replace lost tissues except in limited circumstances. Quiescent tissues, such as liver, usually are not proliferating, but after injury can undergo significant proliferation to replace the lost tissue.

24. **(C) Lineage-restricted stem cell.**
    Stem cells are cells capable of continuously dividing and self-renewing, and have the capacity to give rise to cells that are highly differentiated. Embryonic stem cells or pluripotent stem cells are present in the early stages of embryogenesis, and are capable of differentiating into nearly all tissue cell types in the body. Induced pluripotent stem cells are adult somatic cells from a differentiated tissue (e.g., liver), which, when the nucleus is implanted into an enucleated oocyte, are then able to differentiate into any tissue type in the body, similar to embryonic stem cells. Multipotent stem cells are able to differentiate along a restricted set of divergent tissue types (e.g., marrow stem cells can become chondrocytes, osteoblasts, adipocytes, and endothelial cells). Lineage-restricted stem cells are most commonly found as reserve cells within a specific tissue type, and are only able to produce differentiated cells of that type.

25. **(B) Ligand binding causes dimerization of the receptors, leading to tyrosine kinase activation.**
    Many signaling molecules have receptors with tyrosine kinase activity, including epidermal growth factor, vascular endothelial growth factor, platelet-derived growth factor, c-KIT ligand, and insulin. These receptors are characterized by an intracytoplasmic domain that has tyrosine kinase activity. When ligand binds to the receptor it dimerizes, which activates the tyrosine kinase activity. Then, downstream effector molecules, such as MAP kinase, or phosphatidyl inositol-3 kinase (PI3), transmit the signal. G-protein-coupled receptors, which do not have tyrosine kinase activity, are characterized by seven transmembrane alpha-helixes coupled to the cyclic AMP pathway. Steroid hormones are unusual in that they diffuse through the cell membrane and bind to receptors in the nucleus that directly affect transcription.

26. **(C) Production of signaling molecules.**
    The extracellular matrix is composed of several macromolecules, such as collagen, which form a scaffolding on which tissue cells reside. It provides both structural support and cell anchorage, as well as mediating interactions between cells. Varied construction of the extracellular matrix can also result in different tissue microenvironments within the same organ (e.g., kidney compartments which concentrate urine in the nephron). Through interactions of extracellular matrix components and cell receptors (integrins), cellular growth and proliferation can be stimulated or suppressed. While signaling molecules can be stored in the extracellular matrix, they must be initially produced by a cell.

27. **(C) Connect squamous cells to basement membrane.**
    Desmosomes are part of the cadherin family of proteins that form junctions between cells of the same type. Desmosomes are important in connecting and holding together squamous cells and skeletal muscle cells and resisting shear forces. However, hemidesmosomes are responsible for binding squamous cells to the basement membrane underneath. In pemphigus vulgaris, autoantibodies against desmoglein 3, the major component of desmosomes, results in loss of keratinocyte to keratinocyte adhesion and blister formation.

28. **(A) Abscess cavity filling and healing.**
    When an abscess forms, extensive tissue damage and destruction of the extracellular matrix result in cavitation. The loss of stromal framework results in wound healing through scar formation, which involves deposition of collagen and other extracellular matrix components to fill the defect. Choices B, C, and E all are examples of tissue injury that do not affect the stromal framework and result in complete tissue restoration upon cellular regeneration. Choice D, liver hypertrophy after liver transplant, involves an increase in the number of hepatocytes within a normal tissue framework.

29. **(E) Significant wound contraction.**
    Cutaneous wound healing can occur by primary union or secondary union. Primary union occurs when sutures reapproximate thin wounds from clean surgical incisions. This type of healing involves very little cell death and tissue disruption, results in rapid re-epithelialization over the wound and ultimately a thin scar. In contrast, secondary union occurs when a large volume of tissue has been lost, resulting in significant cell death and connective tissue disruption. Secondary union is characterized by substantial collagen deposition that forms a large scar that over time will contract a substantial amount.

30. **(B) Increased hydrostatic pressure due to impaired venous return.**
    Edema can be caused by an imbalance in solutes, plasma osmotic pressure, or hydrostatic pressure. Deep venous thrombosis results in regional impaired venous return of blood to the heart, and the resultant increased hydrostatic pressure causes excess water to move into the extracellular tissues. An example of generalized impaired venous return is congestive right heart failure: the weakened pumping ability of the heart to return blood to the arterial system causes a buildup of blood within the venous system. This increase in hydrostatic venous pressure results in edema throughout the body, which is called anasarca.

31. **(D) Platelet plug formation.**
Hemostasis after injury proceeds through several distinct phases: initial vasoconstriction, primary hemostasis (platelet plug formation), secondary hemostasis (fibrin meshwork formation), and permanent plug formation with clot organization. Primary hemostasis is primarily driven by exposure of extracellular matrix proteins to the blood plasma, which promotes platelet adhesion and activation, ultimately forming a platelet plug that stops the extravasation of blood.

32. **(D) Secrete adenosine diphosphate (ADP), which promotes platelet inactivation.**
Endothelial cells are key players in the maintenance of normal hemostasis. Normal endothelial cells generally promote antithrombotic pathways, while injured endothelial cells promote thrombosis. Normal endothelial cells secrete several products that decrease thrombosis, including prostacyclin (an inhibitor of platelet activation), tissue-type plasminogen activator (which starts a cascade to degrade fibrin clots), and thrombomodulin (which binds thrombin and inactivates it). In addition, endothelial cells contain membrane-bound heparin-like molecules that help to inhibit thrombosis in the local environment. Finally, endothelial cells cover extracellular matrix proteins, which are potent stimulators of thrombosis. Endothelial cells also secrete adenosine diphosphatase, which degrades ADP, an essential molecule in platelet activation.

33. **(E) von Willebrand factor binding to glycoprotein Ib is primarily used for platelet adhesion.**
Platelets go through three phases during hemostatic plug formation. Initially, platelets adhere to the site of injury through binding of glycoprotein Ib (on platelet membranes) to von Willebrand factor (in the extracellular matrix). Then platelets secrete material stored in granules: alpha-granules contain P-selectin, fibrinogen, and platelet factor 4, while dense granules contain ADP, calcium, and serotonin. These products promote fibrin clot formation over the still-reversible platelet aggregate. Once a clot has formed, the platelets contract to form an irreversible mass that cements the clot in place. Platelets also synthesize thromboxane A2, which is a potent vasoconstrictor as a well as a promoter of platelet aggregation.

34. **(B) Plasmin is generated from plasminogen by tissue factor.**
The fibrinolytic cascade is initiated by the formation of fibrin clots in order to limit the extent of clot formation. Plasmin is the primary enzyme that breaks down fibrin, and is formed by the breakdown of plasminogen by either plasminogen activators or the coagulation factor XII pathway. t-PA, which is used as a clinical clot-busting drug, is most active when bound to fibrin, which is helpful in confining the activity to recent sites of thrombosis. Other enzymes can also activate plasmin, including urokinase-like PA and streptokinase (which is produced by some bacteria). When fibrin is broken down by plasmin, FSPs are released, which are elevated in states of high clot turnover, such as disseminated intravascular coagulation.

35. **(D) Irregular flow presses platelets against endothelial cells.**
Normal blood flow is laminar, which causes cellular products, including platelets, to flow in the central portion of the vessel, away from the endothelium, and pushes cell-poor plasma to the periphery of the vessel. Stasis and turbulence both result in platelets coming into contact with endothelium more easily, as well as preventing washing away of clotting factors. While over time endothelial cells may be damaged by turbulent blood flow, endothelial cells generally continue to prevent exposure of extracellular matrix proteins to blood plasma. t-PA increases fibrinolysis and destroys clots. It is generally produced by intact endothelial cells.

36. **(C) Factor V resistance to cleavage by protein C.**
Factor V Leiden is an inherited hypercoagulable state, which is caused by a mutation in factor V rendering it immune to cleavage by protein C. It results in a modest increase in hypercoagulability, and most commonly manifests by deep venous thrombosis. Protein C deficiency is the cause of another rare hypercoagulable state. The level of factor V is normal or slightly decreased in patients with Factor V Leiden, rather than increased. An increase in prothrombin is the cause of a different hypercoagulable state. Factor V Leiden still needs to be modified by thrombin to be activated (V to Va). Protein S is a cofactor for protein C, but is not the primary mechanism of inactivation of factor V in this disease.

37. **(C) Fat embolism syndrome.**
Embolisms occur when blood clots or other materials (air, amniotic fluid, or fat and bone marrow) are carried by the blood to distant sites in the body. The most common is embolism of a deep venous thrombosis to the pulmonary artery, termed a pulmonary embolism. This patient has had a recent major bone fracture, which predisposes her to fat and bone marrow embolism throughout the body. Patients who become symptomatic have fat embolism syndrome, which typically results in pulmonary problems, neurologic symptoms, anemia, and thrombocytopenia. This

syndrome is partly caused by vasculature occlusion by the embolized fat and partly due to toxic injury of the vessels from fatty acid release, and can be fatal in up to 15% of patients.

38. **(B) Peripheral vasoconstriction (cool, blue skin) is seen in all types of shock.**
Shock is a final pathway that results in decreased tissue perfusion, tissue hypoxia, and cell death, and can be fatal in over 20% of patients. Multiple different types of shock occur: cardiogenic (inability of the heart to maintain perfusion), hypovolemic (low blood volume due to fluid losses), septic shock (in the setting of infection), and neurogenic (anesthesia or neural injury). In the beginning, compensatory mechanisms can maintain tissue perfusion, such as vasoconstriction or catecholamine release. However, eventually this compensation will be inadequate and tissue hypoxia will result in cell death, which often accelerates the development of shock by releasing toxins and lysosomal enzymes. Septic shock can occur even when the infection is localized due to the cytokine release that results in a systemic response. Most patients with shock will have peripheral vasoconstriction (cool, blue extremities) in an attempt to maintain tissue perfusion, but in septic shock, patients will have peripheral vasodilation (warm, red extremities) due to vasodilation mediated by bacterial product release.

39. **(B) Congestive heart failure.**
Chronic congestion can result in tissue injury if longstanding in duration. Congestion is caused by a buildup of blood within vessels, causing dilatation and increased hydrostatic pressure. Tissues with congestion often appear cyanotic in color due to buildup of unoxygenated blood. In this example, congestive right heart failure resulted in chronic congestion of the liver. The biopsy demonstrates dilated central veins with deposition of hemosiderin and atrophy of hepatocytes around the central vein. Eventually, this process can lead to fibrosis and cirrhosis of the liver, imparting a "nutmeg" appearance on cut section. None of the other choices would result in this pattern of liver injury.

40. **(D) Infarction.**
Infarcts are areas of necrosis most commonly caused by interrupted blood supply from arteries or veins. Arterial infarcts are most commonly caused by either embolic material (e.g., atherosclerotic plaque) or local clot formation (e.g., from endothelial injury) that occludes blood flow. These infarcts appear wedge shaped as in this photomicrograph. In contrast, venous occlusions typically result in excess pooled blood that is unable to drain. Edema and hypertrophy would both result in increased

size of the organ, and edema would also cause the organ to look pale and wet. Congestion would result in a diffusely red organ. Neoplasms can have a variety of appearances, but most commonly would demonstrate expansile growth, irregular coloration, and an infiltrative border.

41. **(B) Elevated levels of vitamin E.**
Oxidative stress or generation of free radicals is an important mechanism of cell injury and death. Free radicals are chemical species that have a single unpaired electron in an outer orbit, and the unstable configuration can react with key components of the cell. The most common free radical is superoxide. Ionizing radiation, nitric oxide, and some chemicals can generate free radicals. Leukocytes produce free radicals in a carefully controlled reaction within lysosomes to destroy engulfed bacterial organisms. Glutathione peroxidase is an enzyme that breaks down free radicals. Vitamin E is a natural antioxidant that inactivates free radicals, and when increased, helps to reduce free radicals.

42. **(A) Calorie restriction.**
Cellular aging (senescence) is the result of progressive cellular functional decline and viability due to the accumulation of cellular damage. Multiple molecular mechanisms are responsible for this process, including free radical generation, which is a common cause of cellular injury. DNA repair mechanism failure also results in shortening of cellular longevity. Telomeres are short repeated DNA sequences (TTAGGG) at the end of chromosomes; during replication a short portion of the telomere is lost in most somatic tissues due to low-level expression of telomerase, with an eventual loss of cell replicative ability. In contrast, calorie restriction is one of the most effective ways of prolonging cell life span in vitro, and is mediated by proteins called sirtuins.

43. **(D) Incites a brisk inflammatory response.**
Apoptosis is a pathway of cell death caused by a tightly regulated cell suicide program, which can be mediated internally due to release of certain proteins, and externally through membrane receptors, most notably FAS and FAS-ligand. It is a normal component of many cellular processes, including germinal centers and embryogenesis. Morphologically, it is characterized by cell fragmentation but maintenance of cellular membranes prevents an inflammatory response.

44. **(B) Histamine is a plasma-derived protein.**
Histamine is a potent vasoactive amine, which is primarily stored in mast cells, basophils, and platelets. It is not a normal component of plasma due to its potent effects on blood vessels. Histamine

is believed to be the main effector of the initial increase in vasodilatation and increased vascular permeability in early acute inflammatory responses. Its release can be caused by physical injury (cold, heat), antibody binding to mast cells, or complement proteins such as C3a.

45. **(E) Tumor necrosis factor (TNF).**
TNF is believed to be the primary cytokine responsible for many of the systemic acute-phase responses in patients with an inflammatory process. Also involved in this response are IL-1 and IL-6. TNF has many proinflammatory effects, including endothelial activation, leukocyte recruitment, release of other cytokines, and matrix remodeling. However, it is the systemic effects of TNF that result in cachexia: fever, leukocytosis, increased acute-phase proteins, decreased appetite, and increased sleep. Histamine primarily results in vasodilation and increased vascular permeability. Complement proteins are involved in cell death and leukocyte chemotaxis and activation. Nitric oxide causes smooth muscle relaxation and can kill organisms through free radical generation. Prostaglandins are involved in vasodilatation, fever, and pain.

46. **(E) Short lived (6 hours or less).**
Macrophages derived from blood monocytes have a half-life of 1 day, while tissue macrophages can have life spans of months or years. Macrophages can be activated by a variety of stimuli, including INF-gamma, and are capable of ingesting foreign particles and destroying them using reactive oxygen species. All macrophages, including tissue macrophages, are believed to be derived from a bone marrow stem cell precursor.

47. **(E) Wound contraction.**
Most angiogenesis in wound healing occurs from preexisting vessels. To create a new vessel in this fashion, first the vessel dilates and has increased vascular permeability in response to vascular endothelial growth factor and nitric oxide. Then, the basement membrane surrounding the vessel must be removed, to allow migration of endothelial cells toward the site of the new vessel. Finally, peri-endothelial cells must be recruited to the area to support and sustain the new vessel. While wound contraction is an important part of wound healing, it does not play a role in angiogenesis.

48. **(A) Antigen presenting lymphocyte secretes cytokines that causes itself to proliferate.**
Autocrine signaling occurs when cells respond (usually by proliferating) to a signaling molecule they themselves secrete, such as a lymphocyte responding to a cytokine it secreted. Paracrine signaling occurs when cells respond to signaling molecules produced by other cells in a local microenvironment; answers B and C are examples of this. Endocrine signaling occurs when signaling molecules are released into the bloodstream to act on cells at distant sites; answer D is an example of this.

49. **(D) 80%.**
Tensile strength of wounds is largely dependent on collagen type I deposition; in the early stages of healing, there is net excess of collagen synthesis over collagen degradation as part of connective tissue remodeling. By 3 months, wounded skin typically has the tensile strength of 80% of unwounded skin. After 3 months, collagen synthesis rapidly decreases, and many wounds never recover 100% of unwounded skin strength.

50. **(E) Sodium retention.**
Edema can be caused by an imbalance in solutes, plasma osmotic pressure, or hydrostatic pressure. Patients with renal failure are unable to secrete sodium and water properly. When these patients consume a large dietary load of salt, the increased sodium will not be excreted normally, and diffuses into the extracellular tissues. With this movement of sodium (solute), water also moves, resulting in increased extracellular fluid (edema).

51. **(B) Close to 25% of the body's water is in blood plasma.**
Water is a very important component of almost all body tissues. By weight, water comprises 60% of the lean body tissues. Two-thirds of this (66%) is present within cells, and the other third (33%) is in extracellular spaces. However, most of the water in extracellular spaces is in the interstitial space of tissues; only 5% of the body's total water is present in blood plasma. A delicate balance between intracellular and extracellular water is largely controlled by solutes, vascular hydrostatic pressure, and plasma colloid osmotic pressure.

52. **(A) Includes factor XII (Hageman factor).**
Division of the coagulation cascade into intrinsic and extrinsic pathways is somewhat artifactual. These pathways were initially described this way because the extrinsic pathway required an exogenous trigger to initiate clotting in vitro; this turned out to be tissue factor present in tissue lysates. In contrast, the intrinsic pathway could be activated only by exposing factor XII (Hageman factor) to thrombogenic surfaces such as glass. Ironically, the extrinsic pathway is the most important in vivo for clotting after tissue injury, due to exposure of tissue factor to the clotting cascade. Both pathways are identical after activation of factor X. Prothrombin time (PT) tests the function of the external pathway, while partial

thromboplastin time (PTT) tests the function of the intrinsic pathway.

53. **(A) Endothelial injury, abnormal blood flow, and hypercoagulability.**
Virchow's triad includes endothelial injury, abnormal blood flow (stasis or turbulence), and hypercoagulability. Each of these processes, or a combination of them, can result in abnormal (non-physiologic) thrombosis. An increase in blood flow usually inhibits clot formation due to increased shear forces. Hypocoagulability usually results in a bleeding diathesis, rather than increased blood clot formation. Endothelial cells generally secrete anti-thrombotic products, and when endothelial cells are injured, the reduction in these products promotes clot formation.

SUGGESTED READING

1. Arnout J, Hoylaerts MF, Lijnen HR. Haemostasis. *Handb Exp Pharmacol.* 2006;176(Pt 2):1-41.
2. Cesarman-Maus G, Hajjar KA. Molecular mechanisms of fibrinolysis. *Br J Haematol.* 2005;129(3):307-321.
3. Diegelmann RF, Evans MC. Wound healing: an overview of acute, fibrotic and delayed healing. *Front Biosci.* 2004;9:283-289.
4. Edinger AL, Thompson CB. Death by design: apoptosis, necrosis and autophagy. *Curr Opin Cell Biol.* 2004;16(6):663-669.
5. Gabay C, Kushner I. Acute-phase proteins and other systemic responses to inflammation. *N Engl J Med.* 1999;340(6):448-454.
6. Heyworth PG, Cross AR, Curnutte JT. Chronic granulomatous disease. *Curr Opin Immunol* 2003;15(5):578-584.
7. Kroemer G, El-Deiry WS, Golstein P, et al. Classification of cell death: recommendations of the Nomenclature Committee on Cell Death. *Cell Death Differ.* 2005;12(2):1463-1467.
8. Kumar V, Abbas AK, Fausto N, Aster JC. Acute and chronic inflammation. In: Abbas AK, Kumar V, Fausto N, Aster JC, eds. *Robbins and Cotran Pathologic Basis of Disease.* 8th ed. Philadelphia, PA: Saunders Elsevier; 2010a:43-78.
9. Kumar V, Abbas AK, Fausto N, Aster JC. Cellular response to stress and toxic insults: adaptation, injury and death. In: Abbas AK, Kumar V, Fausto N, Aster JC, eds. *Robbins and Cotran Pathologic Basis of Disease.* 8th ed. Philadelphia, PA: Saunders Elsevier; 2010b:3-42.
10. Kumar V, Abbas AK, Fausto N, Aster JC. Hemodynamic disorders, thromboembolic disease, and shock. In: Abbas AK, Kumar V, Fausto N, Aster JC, eds. *Robbins and Cotran Pathologic Basis of Disease.* 8th ed. Philadelphia, PA: Saunders Elsevier; 2010c:111-134.
11. Kumar V, Abbas AK, Fausto N, Aster JC. Tissue renewal, repair and regeneration. In: Abbas AK, Kumar V, Fausto N, Aster JC, eds. *Robbins and Cotran Pathologic Basis of Disease.* 8th ed. Philadelphia, PA: Saunders Elsevier; 2010d:79-110).
12. Miller SB. Prostaglandins in health and disease: an overview. *Semin Arthritis Rheum.* 2006;36(1):37-49.
13. Moore KA, Lemischka IR. Stem cells and their niches. *Science.* 2006;311(5769):1880-1885.
14. Muller WA. Leukocyte-endothelial-cell interactions in leukocyte transmigration and the inflammatory response. *Trends Immunol.* 2003;24(6):327-334.
15. Parisi DM, Koval K, Egol K. Fat embolism syndrome. *Am J Orthop (Belle Mead NJ).* 2002;31(9):507-512.
16. Remick DG. Pathophysiology of sepsis. *Am J Pathol.* 2007;170(5):1435-1444.
17. Tosh D, Slack JM. How cells change their phenotype. *Nat Rev Mol Cell Biol.* 2002;3(3):187-194.
18. Van Haastert PJ, Devreotes PN. Chemotaxis: signalling the way forward. *Nat Rev Mol Cell Biol.* 2004;5(8):626-634.
19. Walport MJ. Complement. First of two parts. *N Engl J Med.* 2001a;344(14):1058-1066.
20. Walport MJ. Complement. Second of two parts. *N Engl J Med.* 2001b;344(15):1140-1144.

CHAPTER 2

ENVIRONMENTAL AND NUTRITIONAL DISEASES

1. An unconscious patient in the emergency room arrives after being rescued from a burning house. His skin has a cherry-red coloration similar to that seen in this medical examiner autopsy (see Figure 2-1). The most likely cause of his unconscious state is

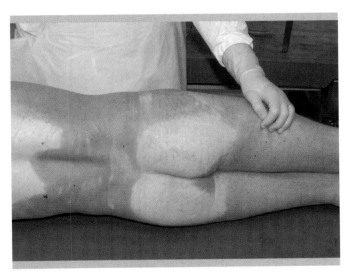

FIGURE 2-1

    (A) Acute carbon monoxide poisoning
    (B) Alcohol intoxication
    (C) Chronic carbon monoxide poisoning
    (D) Flame inhalation with resulting pulmonary injury
    (E) Oxygen deprivation

2. A 4-year-old child is anemic, and review of his blood smear demonstrates the following abnormality (see Figure 2-2). Which of the following is the most likely cause of his anemia?

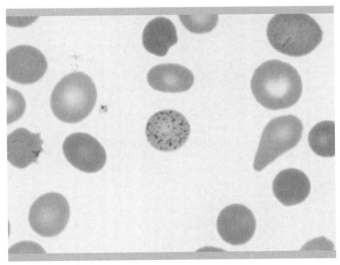

FIGURE 2-2

    (A) Acute lymphoblastic leukemia
    (B) Aplastic anemia
    (C) Hereditary spherocytosis
    (D) Lead toxicity
    (E) Sickle cell anemia

3. During a motor vehicle accident, a man sustains an injury that has the following appearance (see Figure 2-3); the tear in the skin demonstrates bridging strands of fibrous tissue. This type of injury is called a(n)

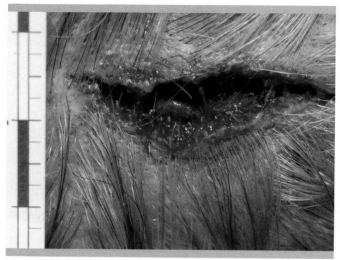

FIGURE 2-3

   (A) Abrasion
   (B) Contusion
   (C) Incised wound
   (D) Laceration
   (E) Puncture wound

4. The leading cause of morbidity and premature death globally is
   (A) Cardiovascular disease
   (B) Genetic disorders
   (C) Infectious disease
   (D) Toxin exposure
   (E) Undernutrition

5. One of the major components of smog is particulate matter, or "soot." Particulate matter pollution is most harmful when it is what size?
   (A) 10 µm or less
   (B) 20–40 µm
   (C) 50–100 µm
   (D) 100–150 µm
   (E) 150 µm or larger

6. All of the following are true regarding lead poisoning except
   (A) Gasoline is a major source of lead in the environment
   (B) Children absorb a greater percentage of ingested lead than adults

   (C) In adults, lead toxicity most commonly presents as a peripheral demyelinating neuropathy (wrist drop or foot drop)
   (D) Most absorbed lead is incorporated into teeth and bone
   (E) The maximum allowed lead blood level is 10 µg/dL

7. The most preventable cause of human death is
   (A) Asbestos exposure
   (B) Cardiovascular disease
   (C) Diphtheria
   (D) Hepatitis
   (E) Smoking

8. The effect of ionizing radiation on tissue is highly dependent on all of the following except
   (A) Field size
   (B) Tissue depth
   (C) Tissue type being irradiated
   (D) Total dose of radiation
   (E) Type of radiation (x-rays, gamma rays, neutrons, etc.)

9. A child with malnutrition has severe wasting, loss of muscle mass, growth retardation, and a head that appears too large for his body. He has had little to eat of any type of food. This type of malnutrition is called
   (A) Cachexia
   (B) Kwashiorkor
   (C) Marasmus
   (D) Secondary malnutrition
   (E) Wernicke–Korsakoff syndrome

10. Vitamin A is important in the function of all of the following except
   (A) Bone mineralization
   (B) Fatty acid metabolism
   (C) Mucus-secreting epithelium
   (D) Normal vision
   (E) Resistance to some infections

11. A 6-year-old child from rural Greenland has immigrated with her parents. At her initial checkup, her legs appeared "bowed" and a chest x-ray is notable for excess cartilage at the costochondral junction of the ribs. She is most likely suffering from which of the following disorders?
   (A) Achondroplasia
   (B) Osteomalacia
   (C) Osteoporosis
   (D) Rickets
   (E) Vitamin C deficiency

12. Leptin is a recently discovered regulatory protein involved in fat store regulation and obesity. Decreased leptin production in mice results in
    (A) Anorexia
    (B) Excessive overeating
    (C) Excessive weight loss
    (D) Increased heat production
    (E) Increased physical activity

13. Several environmental factors and chemicals have been found to be highly associated with specific cancers. Which of the following pairs is incorrectly matched?
    (A) Aflatoxin and hepatocellular carcinoma
    (B) High fiber intake and colon cancer
    (C) Nitrosamines and gastric cancer
    (D) Polycyclic hydrocarbons and bladder cancer
    (E) Vinyl chloride and hepatic angiosarcoma

14. All of the following are true regarding ethanol consumption except
    (A) Acetaldehyde is the major metabolite of alcohol, and is responsible for many of the toxic effects
    (B) Acute alcohol intoxication results in primarily CNS depressant effects
    (C) Alcohol dehydrogenase is the major enzyme responsible for metabolizing alcohol
    (D) Alcohol use results in more deaths than cocaine and heroin combined
    (E) Chronic alcoholism is associated with increased risk of cardiovascular disease and stroke

15. The leading cause of death in developed countries is
    (A) Cardiovascular disease
    (B) Genetic disorders
    (C) Infectious disease
    (D) Toxin exposure
    (E) Undernutrition

16. All of the following are true regarding the cytochrome P450 (CYP) enzyme system except
    (A) Activity can be increased or decreased depending on environmental exposures
    (B) CYP is located in the endoplasmic reticulum of the liver
    (C) Facilitates phase II reactions (glucuronidation, sulfation, methylation, and conjugation with glutathione)
    (D) Genetic polymorphisms in CYP can affect activity
    (E) Major metabolizer of many chemicals and drugs

ANSWERS

1. **(A) Acute carbon monoxide poisoning.**
   Carbon monoxide is an insidious component of air pollution, which in high levels can cause severe hypoxia and death. Hemoglobin binding to carbon monoxide is 200 times stronger than to oxygen; therefore, increased carboxyhemoglobin levels can result in hypoxia, even when adequate oxygen is present. Unconsciousness and death occur when carboxyhemoglobin levels rise above 60%. Acute carbon monoxide poisoning usually occurs in accidents and suicides with exposure to a high level of carbon monoxide; classic examples would include a smoldering fire in an enclosed space, or a suicide attempt by running a gasoline engine car in a closed garage. This classically results in a cherry-red coloration to the skin, due to the high carboxyhemoglobin levels. In contrast, chronic carbon monoxide poisoning is caused by persistent, low-level exposure to carbon monoxide, resulting in systemic hypoxia, classically affecting the central nervous system (impaired memory, vision, hearing, and speech). Patients with chronic carbon monoxide poisoning usually do not have sufficient levels of carboxyhemoglobin to have the classic cherry-red skin of an acute exposure.

2. **(D) Lead toxicity.**
   Children are the most susceptible group to environmental lead exposure. This most commonly occurs in older homes with chipping lead-based paint, which children ingest. The most severely injured systems are the central nervous system, hematopoietic system, gastrointestinal tract, and kidneys. In the blood, children most commonly have a microcytic, hypochromic anemia with punctate basophilic stippling or rare ring sideroblasts (seen on Prussian blue stain). This is due to the inhibition of two enzymes in heme synthesis, leading to insufficient hemoglobin.

3. **(D) Laceration.**
   Mechanical forces can cause various wounds. The classic appearance of a laceration is a jagged and irregular tear in the skin with bridging strands of fibrous tissue and vessels. This type of wound is caused by blunt force trauma with sufficient force to tear the soft tissues. In contrast, an incised wound is caused by a sharp object, like a knife, and leaves a smoother skin injury without bridging tissues (which were cut by the sharp edge). An abrasion occurs when blunt force trauma causes the superficial layers of skin to be lost but the remaining layers of the skin are intact. A contusion occurs when blunt force trauma injuries subcutaneous vessels, but does not tear the skin, leaving it intact. A puncture wound is

caused by a long narrow instrument that goes deeper into the tissue than the diameter of the cut.

4. **(E) Undernutrition.**
   The leading cause of global morbidity and premature death is undernutrition. When measured in terms of years of healthy life lost, more people suffer from poor nutrition, starvation, and poor development due to undernutrition than any other cause. This is primarily a cause of morbidity and mortality in underdeveloped countries. Infectious disease is another major cause of morbidity and mortality in underdeveloped countries, while cardiovascular disease is the primary source of morbidity and mortality in developed countries. Acute toxin exposure and genetic disorders represent a very small percentage of all deaths globally.

5. **(A) 10 μm or less.**
   Particulate matter is most harmful when it is able to deposit in the alveolar spaces of the lung, where it is engulfed by macrophages, inciting a brisk inflammatory reaction and tissue damage. Particulates in the air that are 10 μm or less in dimension are most likely to deposit in the lung alveoli, while larger particulates are more commonly cleared by nasal or upper respiratory mucosa and mucus.

6. **(A) Gasoline is a major source of lead in the environment.**
   Lead accumulates in the environment from a variety of sources, including mining, foundries, batteries, and older types of paint. Gasoline used to be a major contributor, but leaded gasoline has nearly vanished from the United States now. Children are particularly susceptible to lead poisoning, because they absorb 50% of ingested lead, compared with <15% absorbed by adults. In addition, children show greater neurotoxicity to lead, while adults most commonly present with a peripheral demyelinating neuropathy. About 80% or more of all absorbed lead is incorporated into teeth and bones, resulting in the so-called "lead lines" seen on x-rays of developing children's bones. In the United States, the maximum allowed blood level of lead for children is 10 μg/dL, but even at levels below this, subtle neurologic changes can be seen in affected children.

7. **(E) Smoking.**
   Smoking is the single most preventable cause of death. It results in an increase in cardiovascular disease, as well as pulmonary failure and increased risk of cancer in multiple organ systems. It results in nearly 5 million deaths worldwide, annually. Quitting smoking will reduce the overall mortality risk and the risk of death from cardiovascular disease within 5 years, and the risk of lung cancer

reduces by more than 20% after 5 years, but an increased risk of lung cancer persists for 30 years.

8. **(B) Tissue depth.**
   The effect of ionizing radiation is highly dependent on multiple factors. This includes field size (larger field size results in significantly more injury, even at lower doses), type of radiation (alpha particles do significantly more damage than x-rays or gamma rays), total dose (higher doses will result in more severe injury and toxicity), and tissue type being irradiated (testicular tissue is very sensitive to low doses, while skeletal muscle is relatively resistant). With the exception of alpha particles, most radiation types will pass through the body completely, and therefore the depth of the tissue is less important (e.g., superficial vs. deep thigh muscle).

9. **(C) Marasmus.**
   Severe protein-energy malnutrition in children typically takes two forms: marasmus (combined severe protein and energy deficiency) and kwashiorkor (severe protein deficiency with relatively spared calorie intake). Marasmus classically is depicted as children with growth retardation, loss of muscle mass, and a head too large for their body frame. In contrast, kwashiorkor is caused by a relative deficiency in protein intake, which leads to hypoalbuminemia with resulting edema, sparing of subcutaneous fat and muscle, and skin and hair discoloration. Cachexia is seen in patients with advanced cancer or AIDS, and is largely driven by cytokines rather than lack of protein and energy intake. Secondary malnutrition occurs in patients who are bedridden or ill and cannot feed themselves. Wernicke–Korsakoff syndrome is due to vitamin B1 (thiamine) deficiency.

10. **(A) Bone formation.**
    Vitamin A is vital to many different bodily functions, despite its association with vision and the eye. Its effect on the eye in deficiency is twofold; vitamin A deficient rod cells are less able to function leading to reduced vision, and loss of maintenance of the normal mucous-secreting epithelium of the cornea and lacrimal gland results in dry eye and eventually corneal destruction leading to complete loss of vision. In addition, vitamin A is important in maintenance of the immune system, and appears to play a role in fatty acid metabolism as well. Bone mineralization is primarily driven by vitamin D.

11. **(D) Rickets.**
    The clinical picture of this child with "bowing" legs and a "rachitic rosary" of the ribs on x-ray is classic for rickets in an ambulating child. Rickets is due to severe deficiency in vitamin D in a child with open epiphyseal plates, which results in unmineralized

bone that is weakened and deformed due to the body's attempts to reinforce the growing bone. This is most common in younger children from areas with limited sun exposure and lack of supplemented milk products. In adults, this disorder is called osteomalacia. Osteoporosis occurs when bone mineral density is decreased, but not to the extent seen in adults with severe vitamin D deficiency and osteomalacia. Achondroplasia is a genetic syndrome responsible for dwarfism. Vitamin C deficiency can result in scurvy, which is rare due to the abundance of ascorbic acid in many foods.

12. **(B) Excessive overeating.**
Leptin is synthesized by fat cells, and helps to provide a sense of "satiation" after eating, if fat stores are replenished. When leptin is decreased, mice act as if they are malnourished, and excessively overeat, gaining excessive weight. When leptin is increased, other effects (besides decreased consumption) are increased physical activity and increased heat production.

13. **(B) High fiber intake and colon cancer.**
All of the listed pairs have been shown to have significant associations except for high fiber intake and colon cancer. In fact, high fiber intake is protective from the development of colon cancer, but low fiber intake appears to have an increased risk of development of colon cancer, particularly when associated with high levels of consumption of animal fat.

14. **(E) Chronic alcoholism is associated with increased risk of cardiovascular disease and stroke.**
Ethanol consumption is widespread, and while moderate consumption is generally not toxic, nearly 100,000 deaths in the United States are attributable to alcohol use (50% related to drunken driving and alcohol-related homicides and suicides). This is more than the number of deaths due to heroin and cocaine combined per year. Ethanol is metabolized first to acetaldehyde by alcohol dehydrogenase, and acetaldehyde is responsible for most of the toxic

effects of ethanol. Acute alcohol intoxication results in CNS depressant effects. While chronic alcohol use can cause cardiomyopathy, it has a protective effect against atherosclerotic disease, with increased high-density lipoprotein (HDL) and decreased platelet function.

15. **(A) Cardiovascular disease.**
Ischemic heart disease and cerebrovascular disease are the leading causes of death in developed countries. In contrast, infectious disease and undernutrition are the leading causes of death in underdeveloped countries.

16. **(C) Facilitates phase II reactions (glucuronidation, sulfation, methylation, and conjugation with glutathione).**
The CYP enzyme system is one of the most important catalysts for phase I reactions (oxidation, reduction, hydrolysis) of chemicals and drugs in the body. These enzymes are located in the endoplasmic reticulum of the liver, and the activity can be increased or decreased by other environmental exposures (e.g., estrogen increases CYP activity), as well as be affected by genetic polymorphisms.

SUGGESTED READING

1. Badman MK, Flier JS. The adipocyte as an active participant in energy balance and metabolism. *Gastroenterology.* 2007;132(6):2103–2115.
2. Bellinger DC, Bellinger AM. Childhood lead poisoning: the torturous path from science to policy. *J Clin Invest.* 2006;116(4):853–857.
3. Holick MF. Resurrection of vitamin D deficiency and rickets. *J Clin Invest.* 2006;116(8):2062–2072.
4. Kumar V, Abbas AK, Fausto N, Aster JC. Environmental and nutritional diseases. In: Abbas AK, Kumar V, Fausto N, Aster JC, eds. *Robbins and Cotran Pathologic Basis of Disease.* 8th ed. Philadelphia, PA: Saunders Elsevier; 2010:399–445.
5. Schaible UE, Kaufmann SH. Malnutrition and infection: complex mechanisms and global impacts. *PLoS Med.* 2007; 4(5):e115.
6. Stone HB, Coleman CN, Anscher MS, McBride WH. Effects of radiation on normal tissue: consequences and mechanisms. *Lancet Oncol.* 2003;4(9):529–536.

CHAPTER 3

IMMUNOPATHOLOGY

1. Which of the following is not associated with innate immunity?
   (A) Antibodies
   (B) Antiviral defense
   (C) Complement system
   (D) Epithelial barriers
   (E) Initial response against infections

2. Which of the following is a feature of T-lymphocytes?
   (A) Constitute 60–70% of lymphocytes in peripheral blood
   (B) Develop from precursors in the bone marrow
   (C) Following antigenic stimulation, they develop into plasma cells that secrete antibodies
   (D) In a lymph node, they are localized to the follicles
   (E) Recognize antigen via receptors bound to CD20

3. The T-cell receptor (TCR) is characterized by all of the following features except
   (A) Each TCR gene rearrangement is antigen-specific
   (B) Each TCR gene is linked to CD3 complex and ζ proteins that facilitate signal transduction
   (C) It is a marker of T-cell lineage
   (D) TCR diversity is generated by germline rearrangement of TCRα and β genes
   (E) Unique rearrangement of TCR genes can be used as a molecular marker of T-cell clonality

4. Which of the following is a feature of major histocompatibility complex class I molecules?
   (A) They are expressed on all nucleated cells and platelets
   (B) They are encoded by a region called *HLA-D*
   (C) They form a complex with peptides that is recognized by CD4+ T-lymphocytes
   (D) They present molecules that are derived from extracellular microbes and soluble proteins
   (E) They are involved in eliminating bacteria and parasites

5. Immediate (type I) hypersensitivity is characterized by all of the following except
   (A) Develops within hours of exposure to previously sensitized antigen
   (B) Has two well-defined phases: immediate and late
   (C) Is mediated by the IgE class of immunoglobulins
   (D) Mast cells, basophils, and eosinophils are an important component of the inflammatory response
   (E) Susceptibility to immediate hypersensitivity is genetically determined

6. Which of the following is not a feature of mast cells?
   (A) Circulate in the peripheral blood in extremely small numbers
   (B) Contain metachromatic granules
   (C) Predominantly found near blood vessels, nerves, and subepithelial tissue
   (D) Release of granules can be triggered by codeine, morphine, adenosine, heat, and cold
   (E) Secrete primary mediators of immediate hypersensitivity such as biogenic amines, proteases, and heparin

7. Which of the following is an example of antibody-mediated (type II) hypersensitivity?
   (A) Arthus reaction
   (B) Autoimmune hemolytic anemia
   (C) Polyarteritis nodosa
   (D) Serum sickness
   (E) Systemic lupus erythematosus

8. Immune complex-mediated (type III) hypersensitivity is not associated with
   (A) Circulating and in situ immune complexes
   (B) IgM and IgG class of immunoglobulins
   (C) Immune attacks against exogenous and endogenous antigens
   (D) Opsonization and Fc receptor-mediated phagocytosis
   (E) Tissue damage as a result of inflammation at the site of immune complex deposition

9. Which is the following is not an example of type III hypersensitivity?
   (A) Goodpasture syndrome
   (B) Post-streptococcal glomerulonephritis
   (C) Reactive arthritis
   (D) Serum sickness
   (E) Systemic lupus erythematosus

10. A tuberculin reaction occurs as a result of all of the following except
    (A) Accumulation of mononuclear cells around small veins and venules
    (B) Delayed-type hypersensitivity reaction mediated by CD4+ T-lymphocytes
    (C) Dermal edema and deposition of fibrin in the interstitium
    (D) Immune complex deposition within vessel walls
    (E) Interferon-γ secreted by T-helper cells

11. Which of the following is not an example of type IV hypersensitivity?
    (A) Contact dermatitis
    (B) Multiple sclerosis
    (C) Myasthenia gravis
    (D) Rheumatoid arthritis
    (E) Type I diabetes mellitus

12. A 50-year-old woman presents with dry eyes, dry mouth, and enlargement of salivary glands. Which of the following antibodies is most likely to be associated with this condition?
    (A) Anti-double-stranded DNA
    (B) Anti-DNA topoisomerase I
    (C) Anti-histone
    (D) Anti-smooth muscle antigen
    (E) Anti-SS-A (Ro)

13. All the following patterns of indirect immuno-fluorescence correlate with a type of antibody encountered in autoimmune diseases except
    (A) Golgi
    (B) Homogeneous/diffuse
    (C) Nucleolar
    (D) Rim/peripheral
    (E) Speckled

14. A skin biopsy from a 53-year-old woman is shown below. All of the following features are associated with this condition except (Figure 3-1)

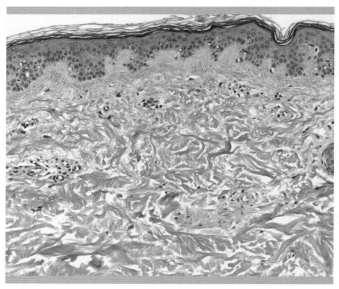

FIGURE 3-1

    (A) Endocarditis
    (B) Gastroesophageal reflux disease
    (C) Malabsorption syndrome
    (D) Pulmonary hypertension
    (E) Synovial hyperplasia

15. A 6-month-old baby boy presents with recurrent bacterial sinusitis, otitis media, and pneumonia. His workup reveals a marked decrease in peripheral B-lymphocytes, plasma cells, and serum immuno-globulins. The pediatrician suspects that this baby most likely has which of the following disorders?
    (A) Bruton agammaglobulinemia
    (B) Common variable immunodeficiency
    (C) DiGeorge syndrome
    (D) Hyper-IgM syndrome
    (E) Severe combined immunodeficiency

16. A 17-year-old female presents with chronic diar-rhea, malabsorption, and recurrent sinusitis. Based on the duodenal biopsy findings (see Figure 3-2), this patient most likely has

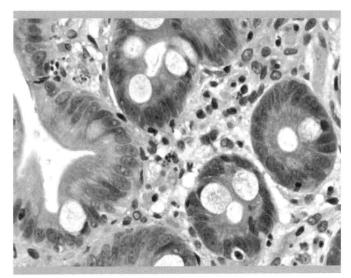

FIGURE 3-2

   (A) Adenosine deaminase deficiency
   (B) Complete absence of B-cells
   (C) Hypogammaglobulinemia
   (D) Low levels of circulating T-cells
   (E) Mutation in either CD40 or its ligand

17. DiGeorge syndrome is characterized by all of the
following except
   (A) Failure of development of the fourth and fifth
        pharyngeal pouches
   (B) Loss of cell-mediated immunity
   (C) Poor defense against fungal and viral infections
   (D) Tetany
   (E) 22q11 deletion

18. Which of the following disorders is characterized
by thrombocytopenia, eczema, and recurrent
infections, and follows an X-linked recessive pattern
of inheritance?
   (A) DiGeorge syndrome
   (B) Hyper-IgM syndrome
   (C) Severe combined immunodeficiency
   (D) Wiskott–Aldrich syndrome
   (E) X-linked agammaglobulinemia

19. The most commonly used enzyme-linked immuno-
sorbent assay (ELISA) targets which of the follow-
ing components of the human immunodeficiency
virus 1 (HIV-1) virion?
   (A) p7
   (B) p9
   (C) p17
   (D) p24
   (E) gp120

20. Which of the following antigens is involved in the
initial step of HIV infection?
   (A) p7
   (B) p9
   (C) p17
   (D) p24
   (E) gp120

21. A 25-year-old man develops cytomegalovirus
(CMV) retinitis. Which of these is the closest
estimate of his CD4+ T-lymphocytes cell count?
   (A) 40 cells/μL
   (B) 90 cells/μL
   (C) 200 cells/μL
   (D) 350 cells/μL
   (E) 600 cells/μL

22. A nodular skin lesion from a 25-year-old man with
history of intravenous drug abuse is shown in
Figure 3-3. This lesion is associated with which of
the following viral infection?

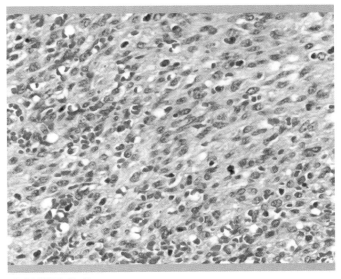

FIGURE 3-3

   (A) Epstein–Barr virus
   (B) Herpes simplex virus
   (C) Human herpesvirus 8
   (D) Human papilloma virus
   (E) JC virus

23. Which of the following lesions is not associated
with human herpes virus-8 (HHV-8) infection?
   (A) Kaposi's sarcoma
   (B) Multicentric Castleman's disease
   (C) Multiple myeloma
   (D) Nasopharyngeal carcinoma
   (E) Primary effusion lymphoma

24. A 65-year-old woman undergoes an endomyocardial biopsy that is shown in Figure 3-4. The histochemical stain of choice is

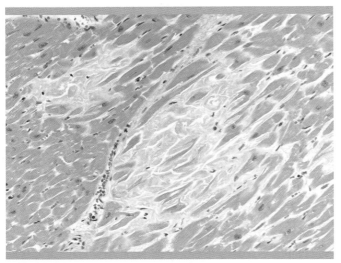

FIGURE 3-4

    (A) Congo red
    (B) Movat
    (C) Periodic acid-Schiff (PAS)
    (D) Reticulin
    (E) Trichrome

25. The hemodialysis-associated systemic form of amyloidosis is associated with which of the following amyloid proteins?
    (A) AA
    (B) Aβ
    (C) Aβ$_2$m
    (D) AL
    (E) ATTR

ANSWERS

1. **(A) Antibodies.**
   Innate immunity (also known as natural or native immunity) and adaptive immunity are the two broad categories of defense against infectious pathogens. The major components of innate immunity are epithelial barriers that block entry of microbes, phagocytic cells (including neutrophils, macrophages), dendritic cells, natural killer (NK) cells, and many plasma proteins including complement proteins. Inflammation is an important cellular reaction in which the phagocytic cells are recruited to recognize microbial components. The antiviral defense is mediated by dendritic cells and NK cells. In contrast, lymphocytes and their products, such as antibodies, are a major component of

adaptive immunity, which develops after exposure to microbes, and is more powerful than innate immunity.

2. **(A) Constitute 60–70% of lymphocytes in peripheral blood.**
   T-lymphocytes constitute the majority (60–70%) of the circulating peripheral lymphocyte population. They develop from precursors in the thymus (remember T = thymus, B = bone marrow). T-cells recognize specific cell-bound antigens via an antigen-specific T-cell receptor (TCR) that is noncovalently linked to CD3 complex and ζ chains that initiate activating signals. Following antigenic stimulation, it is the B-lymphocytes that develop into plasma cells, which secrete antibodies. Follicles within a lymph node are rich in B-lymphocytes, while T-lymphocytes are localized to the paracortical region.

3. **(D) TCR diversity is generated by germline rearrangement of TCRα and β genes.**
   TCR diversity is generated by somatic rearrangement, and not germline rearrangement of genes that encode TCRα and β chains. All cells in our body, including lymphocyte progenitors, contain TCR genes in a germline configuration, and it is only the T-cells that undergo TCR gene rearrangement during their development in thymus. Thus, presence of rearranged TCR genes serves as a marker of T-cell lineage. Furthermore, each T-cell and its progeny have a unique DNA rearrangement, which makes it possible to distinguish polyclonal (non-neoplastic) T-cell proliferations from monoclonal (neoplastic) proliferations.

4. **(A) They are expressed on all nucleated cells and platelets.**
   MHC class I molecules are encoded by three closely linked loci: HLA-A, HLA-B, and HLA-C. They bind to, and process molecules derived from viral antigens, and thus act as the primary defense against viral infections. As viruses may infect any nucleated cell in the body, MHC class I molecules are expressed in every nucleated cell as well as platelets. In contrast, MHC class II molecules can be induced on several cell types by the action of interferon-γ. Class I molecules interact with CD8+ T-lymphocytes, while class II molecules interact with CD4+ T-lymphocytes (remember the number 8—the product of numbers should be 8: class I and CD8 and class II and CD4).

5. **(A) Develops within hours of exposure to previously sensitized antigen.**
   Type I or immediate hypersensitivity develops within *minutes* of exposure to an antigen and is characterized by an immediate phase (vasodilation, smooth muscle spasm, glandular secretions) and

a late phase (tissue inflammatory infiltrate composed of eosinophils, basophils, mast cells, as well as CD4+ T-lymphocytes and tissue destruction). Mast cells and basophils have high-affinity receptors for the Fc portion of IgE class of antibodies, and this interaction leads to immediate release of primary and secondary mediators of hypersensitivity response. *Atopy* refers to predisposition of an individual to mount a hypersensitivity response to allergens. Nearly 50% of these individuals have a positive family history of allergy.

6. **(A) Circulate in the peripheral blood in extremely small numbers.**
Mast cells and basophils are similar in many respects, except that mast cells are localized to the tissue, while basophils are typically present in small numbers in the peripheral blood Mast cells contain a variety of cytoplasmic membrane-bound granules, such as biogenic amines (histamine), enzymes (neutral proteases, acid hydrolases), and proteoglycans (heparin, chondroitin sulfate). The acidic proteoglycan components bind to basic dyes such as toluidine blue, and generate a color (typically pink) that is different from the native color of the dye (typically blue; phenomenon know as metachromasia). In addition to allergens, various other stimuli such as drugs and physical stimuli may also activate mast cell degranulation.

7. **(B) Autoimmune hemolytic anemia.**
All the listed examples, except B, are immune complex-mediated (type III hypersensitivity) reactions. In type II hypersensitivity disorders (antibody-mediated diseases), the binding of antibodies to normal or altered cell-surface antigens leads to phagocytosis or lysis of the target cell by complement and Fc receptor-mediated activity. Some examples include transfusion reactions, erythroblastosis fetalis, autoimmune hemolytic anemia, and certain drug reactions, which occur due to antibody-mediated cell destruction and phagocytosis. In contrast, vasculitis, Goodpasture syndrome, and acute rheumatic fever, are caused by deposition of antibodies within the extracellular tissues. This triggers the complement system, which in turn leads to leukocyte recruitment and tissue damage. In some conditions such as myasthenia gravis, pemphigus vulgaris, Graves's disease, and pernicious anemia, type II hypersensitivity reaction is due to the production of antibodies that target cell-surface receptors. This interaction leads to impaired function *without* causing actual tissue damage.

8. **(D) Opsonization and Fc receptor-mediated phagocytosis.**
Type III hypersensitivity is characterized by deposition of antigen-antibody complexes within tissues, followed by activation of the complement system, recruitment of inflammatory cells, and tissue damage. Opsonization, and complement- and Fc receptor-mediated phagocytosis, are the mechanisms by which target cells are eliminated.

9. **(A) Goodpasture syndrome.**
Goodpasture syndrome is an example of type II hypersensitivity.

10. **(D) Immune complex deposition within vessel walls.**
Cell-mediated (type IV) hypersensitivity is initiated by sensitized T-lymphocytes and is composed of two subtypes: (1) delayed-type hypersensitivity reaction mediated by CD4+ T-lymphocytes and (2) direct cell cytotoxicity mediated by CD8+ T-cells. Tuberculin reaction is a classic example of delayed-type hypersensitivity reaction. Granulomatous inflammation is a pattern of inflammation usually associated with type IV hypersensitivity.

11. **(C) Myasthenia gravis.**
Myasthenia gravis is an example of type II hypersensitivity disease. Type IV (cell-mediated) hypersensitivity was originally described as an immunological response to a variety of organisms, including, *Mycobacterium tuberculosis*, fungi, protozoa, parasites, and viruses. In addition, skin sensitivity to chemicals, graft rejection as well as several autoimmune diseases listed above, are now known to be caused by T-cell-mediated hypersensitivity.

12. **(E) Anti-SS-A (Ro).**
The condition described above is Sjögren syndrome. It is a chronic autoimmune disease that commonly occurs in older women. It results from lymphocyte-mediated destruction of exocrine glands, such as lacrimal glands (dry eyes/keratoconjunctivitis sicca) and parotid glands (dry mouth/xerostomia). It may either occur in the primary form (sicca syndrome) or may be seen in association with other autoimmune conditions, such as rheumatoid arthritis, systemic lupus erythematosus, polymyositis, scleroderma, or mixed connective tissue disorders. Antibodies against two specific ribonucleoprotein antigens, SS-A (Ro) and SS-B (La), are detected in nearly 90% of patients with Sjögren syndrome.

13. **(A) Golgi.**
Indirect immunofluorescence is the most commonly used technique to demonstrate antibodies targeted against DNA, RNA, and nuclear proteins (generic antinuclear antibodies). Homogeneous/diffuse nuclear staining indicates the presence of anti-chromatin, anti-histones, and anti-double-stranded DNA antibodies. Rim/peripheral staining represents antibodies against double-stranded DNA. Speckled pattern is indicative of antibodies to non-DNA nuclear

constituents such as Sm antigen, ribonucleoprotein, SS-A, and SS-B reactive antigens. Golgi pattern of staining is usually encountered in immunohisto-chemistry as a perinuclear, dot-like immunoreactiv-ity. This pattern can be observed during immuno-histochemical staining performed for prolactin in pituitary adenomas, and CD117 in gastrointestinal stromal tumors.

14. **(A) Endocarditis.**
The image demonstrates deposition of dense colla-gen fibers within the dermis, along with thinning of the epidermis, loss of rete pegs, and atrophy of der-mal appendages. These features are characteristic of scleroderma (systemic sclerosis). Most patients have antibodies directed against DNA topoisom-erase-I (anti-Scl-70) antigen, and this subset of patients is more likely to have pulmonary fibrosis and peripheral vascular disease. The other anti-body found in patients with a limited form of the disease is anticentromere antibody (also found in primary biliary cirrhosis). Anticentromere antibody is largely restricted to patients with CREST syn-drome (calcinosis, Raynaud phenomenon, esopha-geal dysmotility, sclerodactyly, and telangiectasia). Gastroesophageal reflux results from dysfunctional lower esophageal sphincter, while malabsorption syndrome is a result of loss of intestinal villi and subepithelial fibrosis. In addition to inflammation of synovium and pulmonary involvement (pulmonary hypertension and interstitial fibrosis), patients may present with pericarditis, pericardial effusion, and myocardial fibrosis.

15. **(A) Bruton agammaglobulinemia.**
Bruton or X-linked agammaglobulinemia is one of the more common forms of primary immunodefi-ciency disorders. Mutations in a cytoplasmic tyro-sine kinase called B-cell tyrosine kinase (*Btk*) cause an arrest in B-cell maturation leading to an absence or marked decrease in peripheral B-cells, immuno-globulins, and plasma cells. The germinal centers in peripheral lymphoid organs are ill-formed. The T-cell function is completely normal. The *BTK* gene is located on long arm of the X chromosome at Xq.21.22. Hence, this disorder is almost entirely encountered in males.

16. **(C) Hypogammaglobulinemia.**
The figure shows complete lack of plasma cells, a feature associated with combined variable immu-nodeficiency (CVID, choice C), and X-linked agam-maglobulinemia (choice B). However, in contrast to X-linked agammaglobulinemia, patients with CVID have normal numbers of B-cells that are unable to differentiate into plasma cells, leading to hypogam-maglobulinemia. It affects both genders equally and

typically manifests in children and young adults. These patients have an increased risk for lymphoma and gastric cancer. Mutation in CD40 and/or its ligand is seen in hyper-IgM syndrome. DiGeorge syndrome is associated with low levels of T-lympho-cytes. Adenosine deaminase deficiency is the most common form of autosomal recessive severe com-bined immunodeficiency (SCID).

17. **(A) Failure of development of the fourth and fifth pharyngeal pouches.**
DiGeorge syndrome results from failure in the development of third and fourth pharyngeal pouches. Hypoplasia of thymus results in variable loss of cell-mediated immunity (T-cells), and thus leads to poor defense against fungal and viral infec-tions. Tetany results from hypocalcemia due to lack of parathyroids. The other clinical characteristics of this syndrome include congenital defects of the heart and great vessels and abnormal facies. This syndrome is now considered to be part of the 22q11 deletion syndrome, which also includes the velocar-diofacial syndrome.

18. **(D) Wiskott-Aldrich syndrome.**
Wiskott-Aldrich syndrome results from mutation in the *WAS* gene that maps to chromosome Xp11.23. Wiskott-Aldrich syndrome protein (WASP) is involved in maintaining the integrity of cytoskeleton and signal transduction. Patients have a variable loss of cell-mediated immunity, and are unable to produce antibodies against polysaccharide antigens. Serum IgG levels are usually normal, IgM levels are low, and IgA and IgE levels are usually elevated.

19. **(D) p24.**
HIV-1 is a retrovirus that belongs to the lentivirus family. The virus core is composed of major capsid protein p24, nucleocapsid protein p7/p9, two cop-ies of genomic RNA, and three enzymes: protease, reverse transcriptase, and integrase. p24 is the most readily detected antigen and is the target of the most commonly employed ELISA assay. A matrix protein called p17 surrounds the viral core. gp120 and gp41 are integral components of the viral enve-lope that play an important role in HIV infection.

20. **(E) gp120.**
CD4+ T lymphocytes bind to the gp120 envelope glycoprotein. This interaction leads to a conforma-tional change, and formation of a new recognition site for chemokine receptor CCR5 (expressed on both T-cells and macrophages)or CXCR4 (expressed on T-cells).

21. **(A) 40 cells/μL.**
As CD4+ T lymphocytes are primarily involved in the response against HIV infection, the peripheral CD4+ T-lymphocyte count is often used as a

surrogate for monitoring disease progression and response to treatment. Centers for Disease Control and Prevention (CDC) classifies HIV infection into three categories based on CD4+ T-lymphocyte count: ≥500 cells/μL, 200–499 cells/μL, and <200 cells/μL. The risk of developing *Pneumocystis jiroveci* infection is high in patients with acquired immunodeficiency syndrome (AIDS) with CD4+ T-lymphocyte count of <200 cells/μL. CMV retinitis develops in most patients when this counts drop below 50 cells/μL.

22. **(C) Human herpes virus-8.**

Kaposi sarcoma herpes virus (KSHV) or human herpes virus-8 (HHV-8) is a DNA virus that is causally linked to Kaposi's sarcoma. The lesion is characterized by proliferation of spindle cells that form slit-like vascular spaces. Extravasation of red cells, chronic inflammatory cells, and hyaline globules, are associated with this lesion. This proliferation is driven by a variety of cytokines produced by mesenchymal cells infected by KSHV or HIV-infected CD4+ T-lymphocytes. There are four subtypes of Kaposi's sarcoma: chronic/classic, transplant-associated, lymphadenopathic, and AIDS associated (epidemic). Grossly, the lesion progresses through three stages: early-macule/patch, intermediate-plaque, and late-nodule/tumor. The lesional cells often express the lymphatic marker D2-40 and vascular marker FLI-1.

23. **(D) Nasopharyngeal carcinoma.**

All of the above choices have been associated with HHV-8 infection, except nasopharyngeal carcinoma, which is associated with Epstein-Barr virus infection.

24. **(A) Congo red.**

The figure depicts amorphous, eosinophilic extracellular amyloid deposits. Although trichrome and PAS stain amyloid deposits gray-blue and magenta, respectively, Congo red stain imparts a characteristic orange-red color to the deposits. In addition, it has the unique ability to intercalate with the β-pleated structure, and produce an apple-green birefringence upon polarization. Cardiac amyloidosis (stiff heart syndrome) presents as restrictive cardiomyopathy and usually occurs as a complication of primary amyloidosis with AL (light chain) protein deposition.

25. **(C) Aβ₂m.**

β_2 microglobulin is a component of the MHC class I molecule that is deposited in patients undergoing long-term dialysis. AL (amyloid light chain) deposits are encountered in primary amyloidosis resulting from conditions such as multiple myeloma and other monoclonal B-cell proliferations. AA or serum amyloid-associated protein is produced in the liver and is associated with secondary amyloidosis. Secondary amyloidosis is associated with chronic inflammatory conditions such as rheumatoid arthritis, ankylosing spondylitis, inflammatory bowel disease, heroine abusers, as well as neoplasms such as renal cell carcinoma and Hodgkin disease. Transthyretin (TTR) is a protein that transports retinol and thyroxine. Its mutant form is deposited in familial amyloid polyneuropathies and senile systemic amyloidosis. Lastly, Aβ (β amyloid protein) forms the core of cerebral plaques found in Alzheimer's disease.

SUGGESTED READING

1. Falcone FH, Knol EF, Gibbs BF. The role of basophils in the pathogenesis of allergic disease. *Clin Exp Allergy.* 2011; 41:939-947.
2. Folpe AL, Chand EM, Goldblum JR, et al. Expression of Fli-1, a nuclear transcription factor, distinguishes vascular neoplasms from potential mimics. *Am J Surg Pathol.* 2001; 25:1061-1066.
3. Janeway CA Jr, Medzhitov R. Innate immune recognition. *Annu Rev Immunol.* 2002;20:197-216.
4. Kahn HJ, Bailey D, Marks A. Monoclonal antibody D2-40, a new marker of lymphatic endothelium, reacts with Kaposi's sarcoma and a subset of angiosarcomas. *Mod Pathol.* 2002;15:434-440.
5. Marrack P, Kappler J, Kotzin BL. Autoimmune disease: why and where it occurs. *Nat Med.* 2001;7:899-905.
6. Mebius RE. Organogenesis of lymphoid tissues. *Nat Rev Immunol.* 2003;3:292-303.
7. Notarangelo LD. Primary immunodeficiencies. *J Allergy Clin Immunol.* 2010;125:S182-S194.
8. Picken MM. Amyloidosis—where are we now and where are we heading? *Arch Pathol Lab Med.* 2010;134:545-551.
9. Schneider E, Whitmore S, Glynn KM, et al. Revised surveillance case definitions for HIV infection among adults, adolescents, and children aged <18 months and for HIV infection and AIDS among children aged 18 months to <13 years—United States, 2008. *MMWR Recomm Rep.* 2008;57: 1-12.
10. Stevenson M. HIV-1 pathogenesis. *Nat Med.* 2003;9:853-860.
11. Kumar V, Abbas AK, Fausto N, Aster JC. Diseases of the immune system. In: *Robbins and Cotran Pathologic Basis of Disease.* 8th ed. Philadelphia, PA: Saunders Elsevier; 2010: 183-258.

CHAPTER 4

NEOPLASIA

1. A 62-year-old male presents with a renal cyst. On examination, the cyst appears to be benign. A small ectopic rest of normal appearing adrenal cells is noted under the capsule of the kidney. The best designation for the latter lesion would be
   (A) Adenoma
   (B) Choristoma
   (C) Hamartoma
   (D) Hyperplasia
   (E) Teratoma

2. All of the following are considered morphologic changes associated with lack of differentiation or anaplasia in a tumor except
   (A) Abnormal nuclear morphology
   (B) Loss of polarity or orientation of cells
   (C) Mitosis
   (D) Nuclear to cytoplasm ratio of 1:5
   (E) Pleomorphism

3. Assuming that a transformed cell (cancer cell) is approximately 10 microns in diameter, how many population doublings must it undergo to produce 10^9 cells (weighing approximately 1 g)?
   (A) 10
   (B) 15
   (C) 20
   (D) 25
   (E) 30

4. Which of the following factors is least important in determining the rate of growth of a tumor?
   (A) Amount of collagen matrix in the environment
   (B) Doubling time of the tumor cells
   (C) Fraction of tumor cells in the replicative pool
   (D) Nutrient availability in the environment
   (E) Rate at which cells are lost

5. Which of the following tumors is least likely to metastasize?
   (A) Basal cell carcinoma of the skin
   (B) Cholangiocarcinoma of the liver
   (C) Endometrioid carcinoma of the ovary
   (D) Melanoma of the lung
   (E) Squamous cell carcinoma of the larynx

6. The pattern of lymph node involvement by metastatic tumor follows the natural routes of lymphatic drainage. Lymph node metastases in axillary lymph nodes would most likely result from dissemination of a breast cancer arising in which location?
   (A) Lower inner quadrant
   (B) Lower outer quadrant
   (C) Nipple region
   (D) Upper inner quadrant
   (E) Upper outer quadrant

7. Which of the following tumors has the greatest propensity for invasion of veins?
   (A) Adenocarcinoma of the lung
   (B) Adenocarcinoma of the colon
   (C) Basal cell carcinoma
   (D) Glioblastoma
   (E) Renal cell carcinoma

8. Cancer of which of the following organs is responsible for the greatest percentage of cancer deaths in males each year?
   (A) Colon/rectum
   (B) Leukemia
   (C) Lung
   (D) Pancreas
   (E) Prostate

9. Cancers of which of the following organs is responsible for the greatest percentage of cancer deaths in females each year?
   (A) Breast
   (B) Colon/rectum
   (C) Lung
   (D) Ovary
   (E) Pancreas

10. Increased risk of lung cancer is associated with all of the following occupational exposures except
    (A) Arsenic
    (B) Asbestos
    (C) Beryllium
    (D) Radon
    (E) Vinyl chloride

11. A relative of yours develops leukemia. You wonder if exposure to chemicals at his job may have contributed to cancer development. An increased risk of developing leukemia and lymphoma is associated with occupational exposure to which of the following agents?
    (A) Arsenic
    (B) Benzene
    (C) Cadmium
    (D) Chromium
    (E) Nickel compounds

12. All of the following are autosomal–dominant, inherited cancer syndromes except
    (A) Hereditary nonpolyposis colon cancer
    (B) Li–Fraumeni syndrome
    (C) Neurofibromatosis type 1
    (D) Neurofibromatosis type 2
    (E) Xeroderma pigmentosum

13. All of the following represent examples of defective DNA repair syndromes except
    (A) Ataxia-telangiectasia
    (B) Bloom syndrome
    (C) Hereditary nonpolyposis colon cancer
    (D) Li–Fraumeni syndrome
    (E) Xeroderma pigmentosum

14. A 52-year-old women presents with leukemia and a concern that her job may have exposed her to ethylene oxide. Ethylene oxide has been associated with an increased risk of developing leukemia. Ethylene oxide is used for all of the following except
    (A) Foodstuff fumigant
    (B) Hospital equipment sterilant
    (C) Paint
    (D) Ripening agent for fruits
    (E) Rocket propellant

15. The most common cause of cancer death in patients under 20 years of age is
    (A) Brain cancer
    (B) Bone cancer
    (C) Leukemia
    (D) Non-Hodgkin lymphoma
    (E) Thyroid cancer

16. A 34-year-old female is diagnosed with malignant melanoma of the skin. Mutations in which gene account for approximately 20% of familial melanoma kindreds?
    (A) BRCA-1
    (B) BRCA-2
    (C) p53
    (D) PATCH
    (E) p16INK4A

17. All of the following potentially form the molecular basis of cancer except
    (A) Activation of growth-promoting oncogenes
    (B) Activation of tumor suppressor genes
    (C) Alterations of apoptosis regulatory genes
    (D) Failure of DNA repair
    (E) Mutations in the somatic cell genome

18. Which of the following is not a function of cyclin D?
    (A) It is degraded through the ubiquitin-proteasome pathway
    (B) It is involved with activating CDK4
    (C) It is involved with phosphorylating the retinoblastoma-susceptibility protein
    (D) It is the first cyclin to increase in the cell cycle
    (E) Its level peaks during the M phase of the cell cycle

19. Progression through the S phase of the cell cycle and the initiation of DNA replication involves the formation of which complex?
    (A) Cyclin D–CDK4
    (B) Cyclin E–CDK2
    (C) Cyclin A–CDK4
    (D) Cyclin A–CDK2
    (E) Cyclin B–CDK1

20. All of the following are cell cycle inhibitors except
    (A) CDK1
    (B) p21
    (C) p27
    (D) p16INK4A
    (E) p14ARF

21. All of the following are true regarding p53 function except
    (A) It acts primarily through p21
    (B) It can promote apoptosis
    (C) It drives cell cycle progression
    (D) It functions as a tumor suppressor
    (E) Its levels are negatively regulated by MDM2

22. Epidermal growth factor receptor overexpression and/or amplification is least likely to be encountered with which of the following tumors?
    (A) Breast carcinoma
    (B) Glioblastoma
    (C) Leukemia
    (D) Ovarian carcinoma
    (E) Squamous carcinoma of the lung

23. A 64-year-old male presents with a stomach mass and is diagnosed with a gastrointestinal stromal tumor (GIST). Which of the following protooncogenes is most commonly associated with GIST?
    (A) ERB-B1
    (B) FMS
    (C) KIT
    (D) PDGF-R
    (E) RET

24. Testing for protooncogene H-RAS point mutations is most likely to be positive in which of the following cancers?
    (A) Bladder cancer
    (B) Colon cancer
    (C) Lung cancer
    (D) Melanoma
    (E) Pancreatic cancer

25. All of the following lesions of the gastrointestinal tract are associated with an increased risk of developing cancer except
    (A) Crohn disease
    (B) *Helicobacter pylori* gastritis
    (C) *Melanosis coli*
    (D) Tubular adenoma
    (E) Ulcerative colitis

26. A 6-year-old female is recently diagnosed with an adrenal neuroblastoma. Testing of which gene for evidence of amplification is warranted?
    (A) C-MYC
    (B) K-RAS
    (C) L-MYC
    (D) N-MYC
    (E) N-RAS

27. This tumor was discovered in a 7-year-old male. Mutations in which of the following genes is responsible for producing this neoplasm? (Figure 4-1)

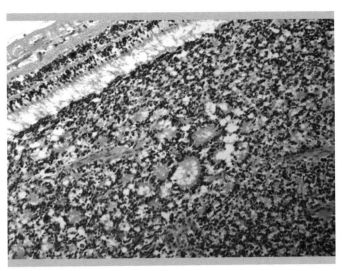

FIGURE 4-1

    (A) NF-1
    (B) NF-2
    (C) p53
    (D) PTEN
    (E) RB

28. The two-hit hypothesis of oncogenesis proposed by Knudson explains the inherited and sporadic occurrence of which of the following tumors?
    (A) Meningioma
    (B) Neuroblastoma
    (C) Retinoblastoma
    (D) Schwannoma
    (E) Wilms tumor

29. Inherited mutations in the APC/beta-catenin tumor suppression gene are associated with which of the following?
    (A) Familial adenomatous polyposis coli (APC)
    (B) Melanoma
    (C) Osteosarcoma
    (D) Ovarian carcinoma
    (E) Pancreatic carcinoma

30. All of the following are true regarding a breast cancer associated with BRCA-1 except
    (A) Along with BRCA-2 mutations, BRCA-1 mutations account for all cases of familial breast carcinoma
    (B) BRCA-1 gene mutations are also associated with the development of ovarian carcinoma
    (C) BRCA-1 gene mutations are not associated with development of sporadic breast carcinoma
    (D) BRCA-1 is involved in the regulation of estrogen receptor activity
    (E) The gene for BRCA-1 is located on chromosome 17

31. Many tumors stimulate the growth of host blood vessels (angiogenesis). All of the following are reasons why a tumor would promote angiogenesis except
(A) It facilitates metastasis
(B) It helps supply nutrients
(C) It helps supply oxygen
(D) It promotes apoptosis
(E) It stimulates the growth of the tumor with growth factor secretions

32. All of the following inhibit angiogenesis except
(A) Angiostatin
(B) Endostatin
(C) Thrombospondin-1
(D) Tumstatin
(E) Vascular endothelial growth factor (VEGF)

33. Invasion of the extracellular matrix by tumor cells is important in tumor infiltration and in gaining access to lymphatic and vascular spaces. All of the following are important steps in the process of tumor invasion of extracellular matrix except
(A) Attachment to matrix components
(B) Degradation of extracellular matrix
(C) Detachment of tumor cells from each other
(D) Migration of tumor cells
(E) Reaggregation of tumor cells

34. A tumor rich in matrix metalloproteinase 9 is best equipped to do which of the following
(A) Breakdown adipose tissue and cause fat necrosis
(B) Cleave type IV collagen
(C) Facilitate intravascular tumor aggregation
(D) Inactivate tumor cell mitochondria
(E) Loosen intercellular junctions

35. A 69-year-old woman presents with an elevated white blood cell count. Lymph node and bone marrow biopsies are performed. Genetic testing of the tumor demonstrates a t(9; 22) (q34; q11). The most likely diagnosis is
(A) Acute lymphocytic leukemia
(B) Burkitt lymphoma
(C) Chronic myeloid leukemia
(D) Follicular lymphoma
(E) Mantle cell lymphoma

36. Which of the following techniques allows one to obtain an expression profile of proteins contained in a particular tumor?
(A) DNA microarray
(B) Proteomics
(C) Pyrosequencing
(D) Reverse PCR
(E) Southern blotting

37. Loss of the p53 gene on chromosome 17p occurs at which stage of the adenoma–carcinoma sequence in colorectal cancer?
(A) Dysplastic foci → early adenoma
(B) Early adenoma → intermediate adenoma
(C) Intermediate adenoma → late adenoma
(D) Late adenoma → carcinoma
(E) Normal epithelium → carcinoma

38. The Ames test is used to test the mutagenic potential of a chemical carcinogen by examining the chemical's ability to induce mutations in what organism?
(A) Methicillin-resistant *Staphylococcus*
(B) *Salmonella typhi*
(C) *Salmonella typhimurium*
(D) *Staphylococcus aureus*
(E) *Staphylococcus epidermidis*

39. You are concerned that a patient's hepatic carcinoma might be related to an exposure to aflatoxin B1. This toxin is associated with which organism, which may grow on improperly stored rice, peanuts, or corn?
(A) *Aspergillus fumigatus*
(B) Hepatitis A virus
(C) *Salmonella typhi*
(D) *Shigella dysenteriae*
(E) *Shigella flexneri*

40. Exposure to UV rays of which wavelength are associated with the greatest risk of developing skin cancer?
(A) 200–240 nm
(B) 240–280 nm
(C) 280–320 nm
(D) 320–360 nm
(E) 360–400 nm

41. Which of the following cancers would most frequently be encountered in a person exposed to ionizing radiation?
(A) Bone cancer
(B) Gastrointestinal cancer
(C) Leukemia
(D) Lung cancer
(E) Thyroid cancer

42. A 38-year-old woman is diagnosed with invasive cervical squamous cell carcinoma. Which of the following human papilloma virus (HPV) types are least likely to be found in the tumor?
(A) 16
(B) 18
(C) 31
(D) 33
(E) 36

43. Which HPV proteins is involved with facilitating p53 degradation, resulting in a block in apoptosis and decreased p21 cell cycle inhibitor activity?
    (A) E1
    (B) E3
    (C) E5
    (D) E7
    (E) E9

44. Epstein–Barr virus (EBV) has been implicated in the development of all of the following cancers except
    (A) B cell lymphoma in HIV patients
    (B) Burkitt lymphoma, endemic type
    (C) Hodgkin lymphoma
    (D) Medullary breast carcinoma
    (E) Nasopharyngeal carcinoma

45. Which of the following molecules facilitates the entry of EBV in lymphoid cells?
    (A) CD3
    (B) CD4
    (C) CD19
    (D) CD20
    (E) CD21

46. All of the following are mechanisms of human infection or transmission of human T-cell leukemia virus type 1 (HTLV-1) except
    (A) Aerosolization
    (B) Blood products
    (C) Breast-feeding
    (D) Needle stick
    (E) Sexual intercourse

47. Which of the following mechanisms are employed by tumor cells to escape the host's immune system?
    (A) Antigen unmasking
    (B) Counteract immunosuppression
    (C) Decreased apoptosis of cytotoxic T-cells
    (D) Increased expression of major histocompatibility complex (MHC) molecules
    (E) Selective outgrowth of antigen-negative variants

48. All of the following may play a role in the development of cancer-related cachexia except
    (A) Androgen receptor
    (B) Interferon-gamma
    (C) Interleukin-1
    (D) Leukemia inhibitory factor
    (E) Tumor necrosis factor

49. Secondary polycythemia vera associated with increased production of erythropoietin is associated with which tumor?
    (A) Breast carcinoma
    (B) Gastric carcinoma
    (C) Hemangioblastoma
    (D) Thymoma
    (E) Uterine carcinosarcoma

50. A 46-year-old woman presents with metastatic carcinoma of unknown primary. On evaluation, she is noted to have elevated CA-15-3 level. The most likely site of origin of her cancer is
    (A) Breast
    (B) Colon
    (C) Liver
    (D) Pancreas
    (E) Ovary

51. Elevated carcinoembryonic antigen (CEA) levels may be encountered in all of the following settings except
    (A) Alcoholic cirrhosis
    (B) Colorectal carcinoma
    (C) Pituitary adenoma
    (D) Smoking
    (E) Ulcerative colitis

52. Hypertrophic osteoarthropathy and clubbing of the fingers is most likely to be associated with which malignancy?
    (A) Bronchogenic carcinoma
    (B) Melanoma
    (C) Pancreatic carcinoma
    (D) Renal carcinoma
    (E) Uterine sarcomas

ANSWERS

1. **(B) Choristoma.**
   Choristomas represent an ectopic rest of normal tissue. The presence of normal appearing adrenal cells in the capsule of the kidney would present an example of this entity. Hamartomas represent a mass of disorganized but mature specialized cells or tissue indigenous to a particular site. Adenoma is a term used to apply to benign epithelial neoplasms that form glandular patterns as well as benign tumors derived from glands that do not necessarily form glandular patterns, for example, parathyroid or pituitary adenoma. Hyperplasia represents an increase in the number of cells in an organ or tissue. Teratoma represents a benign tumor that is composed of a variety of parenchymal cell types representative of more than one germ layer and usually

of all three layers. Teratomas typically arise from totipotent cells and most commonly arise in the ovaries or testes.

2. **(D) Nuclear to cytoplasm ratio of 1:5.**
Lack of differentiation or anaplasia is characterized by a host of morphologic alterations including abnormal nuclear morphology with increased nuclear to cytoplasmic ratio typically approaching 1:1 or less than 1:1 versus the normal nuclear to cytoplasmic ratio of 1:4–1:6. Increased mitoses including atypical figures are associated with lack of differentiation and anaplasia. Cells typically lose their normal orientation or polarity with loss of differentiation. Nuclear pleomorphism, that is, a variation in cell and nuclear size and shape, is a common feature associated with anaplasia.

3. **(E) 30.**
In the parameters presented, the transformed cell must undergo at least 30 population doublings to produce 10^9 cells that would weigh approximately 1 g; this would result in a mass that could be grossly detected. Ten additional doublings would result in a mass that would be composed of 10^{12} cells which would translate into a 1 kg tumor.

4. **(A) Amount of collagen matrix in the environment.**
There are a variety of factors that play an important role in determining the rate of growth of a tumor. Doubling time of tumor cells, the percent of tumor cells that are in the replication pool, and the rate at which cells are lost or shed in the growing lesion are important determinant factors. Certainly, the available nutrients and oxygen in the environment of the tumor would also impact on a variety of these aforementioned factors. The amount of collagen matrix in the environment would not significantly impact the rate of growth of a tumor.

5. **(A) Basal cell carcinoma of the skin.**
As a general rule of thumb, the more aggressive and rapidly growing and larger a primary tumor is, the more likely it is to metastasize. Approximately 30% of newly diagnosed patients with solid tumors present with metastasis. Notable exceptions include certain skin cancers, like basal cell carcinoma, which commonly locally infiltrate rather than metastasize to distant sites. All of the other tumors listed as options for this question are well known to metastasize to distant sites.

6. **(E) Upper outer quadrant.**
Patterns of lymph node metastasis of tumors follow natural routes of lymphatic drainage. Carcinomas of the breast most commonly arise in the upper outer quadrant, which accounts for the common spread or metastasis of these tumors initially to the axillary lymph nodes. Breast cancers arising in the inner quadrants tend to drain to the lymph nodes within

the chest along the interior mammary arteries, resulting in initial metastases to infraclavicular and supraclavicular lymph nodes.

7. **(E) Renal cell carcinoma.**
Renal cell carcinoma is particularly well recognized as a tumor that has a tendency to invade veins; renal vein involvement with extension of a tumor into the inferior vena cava and sometimes all the way to the right heart have been well documented. Many hepatocellular carcinomas also show a tendency to penetrate veins in the portal triad and can spread in that fashion. The other tumor types listed as options less frequently directly invade blood vessels. Some tumors listed, such as basal cell carcinoma of the skin and glioblastoma tend to metastasize relatively infrequently.

8. **(C) Lung.**
Cancers arising in the lung are the most common cause of cancer death in males. Following lung, in descending order are, tumors arising in the colon/rectum, prostate gland, and pancreas. If one lists cancer incidence by site in males, the most commonly involved organs in order of involvement include the prostate gland, lung, and colon/rectum.

9. **(C) Lung.**
In women, the most common site of cancer resulting in cancer death is lung; this is followed in descending order by breast and colorectal tumors. In terms of estimated cancer incidence by site in women, the most commonly involved organs in order are breast, lung, and colon/rectum.

10. **(E) Vinyl chloride.**
An increased risk of developing lung cancers has been associated with occupational exposure to a variety of agents or groups of agents including arsenic and arsenic compounds, asbestos, beryllium and beryllium compounds, chromium, nickel, and radon and its decay products. Vinyl chloride is associated with angiosarcoma and tumors arising in the liver.

11. **(B) Benzene.**
Benzene has been associated with the development of leukemia and Hodgkin lymphoma. Arsenic compounds have been associated with the development of lung and skin cancers and hemangiosarcoma. Cadmium and cadmium compounds have been associated with the development of prostate cancer. Chromium compounds have been associated with the development of lung cancer. Nickel and nickel compounds have been associated with the development of nasal and lung cancer.

12. **(E) Xeroderma pigmentosum.**
Many of the common inherited cancer syndromes have an autosomal-dominant pattern of inheritance. This group includes retinoblastoma, Li–Fraumeni syndrome, melanoma syndrome, familial adenomatous

Chapter 4   NEOPLASIA

polyposis, colon cancer syndrome, neurofibromatosis types-1 and -2, breast and ovarian cancer syndromes, multiple endocrine neoplasia types 1 and 2, hereditary nonpolyposis colon cancer syndromes, and nevoid basal cell carcinoma syndrome. Examples of autosomal-recessive syndromes usually related to defects in DNA repair include xeroderma pigmentosum, ataxia-telangiectasia, Bloom syndrome, and Fanconi anemia.

13. **(D) Li–Fraumeni syndrome.**
Xeroderma pigmentosum, ataxia-telangiectasia, Bloom syndrome, and Fanconi anemia are all autosomal-recessive syndromes that are associated with defects in DNA repair mechanisms. Hereditary nonpolyposis colon cancer syndrome is associated with abnormalities in the MSH-2, MLH-1, and MSH-6 genes.

14. **(C) Paint.**
Ethylene oxide, which has been associated with the development of leukemia, is typically used as a ripening agent for fruits and nuts. It is also used in making rocket propellent, in fumigants for foodstuffs and textiles, and in sterilants for hospital equipment. Chromium compounds and benzene are potential agents that are used in paint manufacturing that may be associated with an increased risk of cancer.

15. **(C) Leukemia.**
The most common cause of cancer death in patients under the age of 20 years is leukemia followed by tumors of the central nervous system, tumors of bones and joints, and endocrine system tumors.

16. **(E) p16INK4A.**
In familial melanoma syndrome, mutations in the p16INK4A gene have been described. Mutations in this gene account for only about 20% of familial melanoma kindreds, suggesting that other factors may be involved in the familial predisposition in these cases. BRCA-1 and BRCA-2 are associated with breast and ovarian tumor development. p53 is associated with Li–Fraumeni syndrome. The PATCH gene is associated with the nevoid basal cell carcinoma syndrome.

17. **(B) Activation of tumor suppressor genes.**
There are a variety of factors that form the molecular basis of cancer development. Acquired environmental DNA damage is often the initial step in this process. Failure of repair mechanisms, which may involve inherited mutations in genes affecting DNA repair or genes affecting cell growth or apoptosis, may result in mutations in the genome of somatic cells. This, in turn, results in activation of growth-promoting oncogenes, inactivation of tumor suppressor genes, and alterations in genes that regulate apoptosis, culminating in unregulated cell proliferation and decreased apoptosis, which in turn yields a clonal expansion of cells.

18. **(E) Its level peaks during the M phase of the cell cycle.**
Cyclin D is the first cyclin to increase in the cell cycle. It appears in the mid G_1 phase and is no longer detectable in the S phase. During the G_1 phase of the cell cycle, cyclin D binds to and activates CDK4, forming a complex. The complex plays an important role in the cell cycle by phosphorylating the retinoblastoma-susceptibility protein. Phosphorylation of the retinoblastoma-susceptibility protein eliminates the main barrier to cell cycle progression and promotes replication. Cyclin D is degraded through the ubiquitin-proteasome pathway.

19. **(B) Cyclin E–CDK2.**
Progression through the S phase of the cell cycle and the initiation of DNA replication involves the formation of a complex with cyclin E and CDK2. The cyclin D and CDK4 complex is associated with the G_1 phase of the cell cycle. The cyclin A and CDK2 complex is associated with the G_2 phase of the cell cycle. The cyclin B and CDK1 complex is associated with the M phase of the cell cycle.

20. **(A) CDK1.**
The activity of the cyclin–CDK complexes is regulated by a variety of inhibitors. These CDK inhibitors are divided into the Cip/Kip and the INK4/ARF groups. p21 and p27 belong to the Cip/Kip family. CDK1 is a cyclin-dependent kinase that forms a complex with cyclin B and acts at the G_2/M transition.

21. **(C) It drives cell cycle progression.**
p53 acts as a tumor suppressor and is altered in the large number of different cancers. It is responsible for causing cell cycle arrest and apoptosis. It acts mainly via p21 to cause cycle arrest. Levels of p53 are negatively regulated by MDM2 through a feedback loop.

22. **(C) Leukemia.**
Epidermal growth factor receptor overexpression and/or amplification is associated with squamous cell carcinomas of the lung, gliomas (particularly glioblastoma), breast carcinomas, and certain ovarian carcinomas. Leukemia is more commonly associated with point mutations of the CSF-1 receptor.

23. **(C) KIT.**
GISTs are associated with point mutations on the KIT oncogene. ERB-B1 protooncogene abnormalities are associated with squamous cell carcinoma of the lung and gliomas. FMS abnormalities are associated with leukemia. PDGF-R abnormalities are associated with gliomas; only a small percentage of GISTs are associated with PDGF-R mutations. RET abnormalities are associated with multiple endocrine neoplasia types IIa and IIb, as well as familial medullary thyroid carcinomas.

24. **(A) Bladder cancer.**
    H-RAS point mutation is most commonly associated with bladder and renal tumors. K-RAS point mutations are noted in colon cancers and lung cancers. BRAF point mutations have been described in melanomas and thyroid cancers. Some pancreatic tumors are associated with K-RAS point mutations.

25. **(C) Melanosis coli.**
    There are a variety of inflammatory lesions of the gastrointestinal tract that have been described as increasing one's risk of developing cancer. These lesions include ulcerative colitis, Crohn disease, *Helicobacter pylori* gastritis, viral hepatitis, and chronic pancreatitis. Tubular and villous adenomas are also well-recognized as predisposing one to malignancy in the gastrointestinal tract. Melanosis coli is not known to be associated with an increased risk of developing cancer.

26. **(D) N-MYC.**
    N-MYC amplification has been associated with neuroblastomas and small cell carcinomas of the lung. C-MYC translocations are associated with Burkitt lymphoma. L-MYC amplification has been described in association with small cell carcinoma of the lung. K-RAS point mutations have been associated with colon, lung, and pancreatic tumors. N-RAS point mutations have been described with melanomas and certain hematologic malignancies.

27. **(E) RB.**
    The figure shows a retinoblastoma marked by normal retinal tissue and a tumor characterized by the presence of Flexner–Wintersteiner rosettes. This tumor is associated with mutations in the RB gene. The neurofibromatosis type 1 (NF-1) gene is associated with neurofibromas and NF-1 related sarcomas. NF-2 is associated with schwannomas and meningiomas. p53 is associated with many human cancers and is also particularly associated with Li–Fraumeni syndrome. PTEN gene abnormalities are associated with development of endometrial and prostate cancers and tumors associated with Cowden disease.

28. **(C) Retinoblastoma.**
    The two-hit hypothesis of oncogenesis proposed by Knudson explains the inherited and sporadic occurrence of retinoblastoma. The hypothesis suggests that in hereditary cases, one genetic change (or the first hit) is inherited from an affected parent and is therefore present in somatic cells in the body. The second mutation (or second hit) occurs in one of many retinal cells, which also carries the first mutation. In sporadic cases of retinoblastoma, either mutations or hits occur somatically within a single retinal cell. Normal alleles of the retinoblastoma locus must be inactivated by the two hits for the development of the tumor. The retinoblastoma gene is located on chromosome 13q14. Patients with familial retinoblastoma are also at increased risk for developing osteosarcoma and other soft tissue sarcomas.

29. **(A) Familial APC.**
    A mutation in the APC/beta-catenin tumor suppressor gene causes an inhibition of signal transduction, which results in an increased propensity to develop familial APC. Osteosarcoma is associated with a retinoblastoma (RB) gene abnormality. Carcinomas of the ovary and breast are associated with the BRCA-1 and the BRCA-2 gene abnormalities. Pancreatic cancer development is associated with somatic (not inherited) mutations of the APC/beta-catenin gene. Melanoma is likewise associated with somatic mutations of the APC/beta-catenin gene.

30. **(A) Along with BRCA-2 mutations, BRAC-1 mutations account for all cases of familial breast carcinoma.**
    BRCA-1 gene (chromosome 17) and BRCA-2 gene (chromosome 13) are associated with breast and ovarian cancers. Approximately 10–20% of breast carcinomas are familial. Mutations in BRCA-1 and BRCA-2 account for 80%, but not all of familial breast carcinoma cases. Mutations in BRCA-1 and BRCA-2 genes are associated with the development of nonfamilial or sporadic forms of breast carcinoma. BRCA-1 is involved in the regulation of estrogen receptor activity and is also a coactivator of the androgen receptor. Both genes participate in the process of homologous combination of DNA repair.

31. **(D) It promotes apoptosis.**
    Many tumors stimulate the growth of host blood vessels, a process known as angiogenesis. Tumor cells can generally not survive well when located beyond 1–2 mm from blood vessels. Neovascularization provides an opportunity to provide nutrients and oxygen to the growing tumor. Endothelial cells in areas of neovascularization may secrete a variety of grow factors including PDGF and insulin-like growth factor. Growth factors, in turn, can promote further tumor growth. The increased number of vessels also increases access to the vasculature by tumor cells, increasing the likelihood of metastasis. Angiogenesis does not promote apoptosis.

32. **(E) VEGF.**
    A variety of molecules can impede angiogenesis. Thrombospondin 1 can be produced by the tumor cells themselves and serve this function. Other anti-angiogenesis factors include angiostatin, which can be produced by the proteolytic cleavage of plasminogen, endostatin, and tumstatin. These latter

two molecules are derived by a cleavage of collagen material. VEGF or vascular endothelial growth factor along with basic fibroblast growth factor are pro-angiogenic factors.

33. **(E) Reaggregation of tumor cells.**
Invasion of extracellular matrix by tumor cells is important in tumor infiltration. This allows tumor cells to eventually gain access to lymphatic and vascular spaces for subsequent metastasis. There are a variety of important steps in the process of extracellular matrix invasion by tumor cells. These steps include detachment of the tumor cells from each other, attachment to matrix components, degradation of the extracellular matrix, and migration of the tumor cells through the matrix. Cell reaggregation is not part of this process.

34. **(B) Cleave type IV collagen.**
Matrix metalloproteinases 9 and 2 are collagenases that are involved with the cleavage of type IV collagen in epithelial and vascular-based membranes. This appears to play a role in allowing tumor cells to invade these structures. Metalloproteinases are not involved with loosening of intercellular junctions, inactivation of tumor cell mitochondria, breakdown of adipose tissue resulting in fat necrosis, or the facilitation of intravascular tumor aggregation.

35. **(C) Chronic myeloid leukemia.**
A t(9; 22) (q34; q11) is associated with chronic myeloid leukemia and involves the *ABL* gene on chromosome 9 and the *BCR* gene on chromosome 22. Acute leukemias are associated with t(4; 11) and t(6; 11). Burkitt lymphoma is associated with t(8; 14). Follicular lymphoma is associated with t(14; 18). Mantle cell lymphoma is associated with t(11; 14).

36. **(B) Proteomics.**
Proteomics is a technique that allows for protein expression profiling of tissues, body fluids, or serum. All of the other tests listed as options utilize DNA material and are not focused on protein expression.

37. **(D) Late adenoma → carcinoma.**
Loss of the p53 gene on chromosome 17p is a relatively late occurrence in the evolution of colorectal cancers and is associated with the development of carcinoma from late adenoma. The transformation of normal epithelium to dysplastic foci involves loss or mutation of the APC locus on chromosome 5q. Mutation of the RAS gene on chromosome 12p is associated with the early adenoma → intermediate adenoma lesions. Loss of a tumor suppressor on chromosome 18q is associated with the development of a late adenoma lesion from intermediate adenoma.

38. **(C) *Salmonella typhimurium*.**
The Ames test is one potential way of assessing the mutagenic potential of a chemical carcinogen. The test examines the ability of a chemical to induce mutations in the bacterial organism *Salmonella typhimurium*.

39. **(A) *Aspergillus fumigatus*.**
Aflatoxin B1 is a potent toxin that may result in the development of hepatic carcinoma. The toxin is produced by *Aspergillus fumigatus* and can grow on improperly stored corn, rice, or peanuts. The presence of hepatitis B virus infection can further facilitate the development of neoplasia in this setting.

40. **(C) 280–320 nm.**
Skin cancers are associated with light in the UVB spectrum (280–320 nm). Most of UVC light (200–280 nm) is filtered out by the ozone shield and mutagenic potential is significantly reduced. UV rays can result in inhibition of cell division and inactivation of enzymes, induction of mutations, and death of cells if the dosage is high enough.

41. **(C) Leukemia.**
Ionizing radiation, which is composed of electromagnetic rays (x-rays and gamma rays), and a particulate radiation including alpha particles, beta particles, protons, and neutrons are all potentially carcinogenic. Leukemias are the most frequently encountered tumors in human that have been exposed to radiation. Cancers of the breast, lung, salivary glands, and thyroid gland are in the next most frequently encountered group. Relatively uncommon in this setting are cancers of the skin, bone, and gastrointestinal tract.

42. **(E) 36.**
There are a variety of HPV types that have been documented to be particularly associated with the development of invasive squamous cell carcinoma. These types include HPV 16, 18, 31, 33, 35, and 51. The HPV types with a relatively low malignant potential are most commonly associated with HPV types 6 and 11.

43. **(D) E7.**
HPV-associated proteins E6 and E7 have a number of effects on the cell cycle. Both of these proteins enhance p53 degradation, resulting in a block in apoptosis and decreased activity of cell cycle inhibitor p21. E7 can associate with p21 and it can bind to RB. The overall effect of the proteins is to block apoptosis and remove the restraints to cell proliferation.

44. **(D) Medullary breast carcinoma.**
EBV is a member of the herpes virus family and has been associated with the development of a variety of cancers including B cell lymphomas in

immunocompromised patients, the endemic-type Burkitt lymphoma, Hodgkin lymphoma, and nasopharyngeal carcinoma. Medullary carcinoma of the breast is not known to be associated with EBV infection.

45. **(E) CD21.**
EBV can infect epithelial cells in the oropharynx and B lymphocytes. The virus gains access to the B cells via the CD21 molecule, which is expressed on all B cells.

46. **(A) Aerosolization.**
HTLV-1 is particularly common in certain parts of the world—Japan and the Caribbean basin. The virus particularly targets CD4-positive T lymphocytes. Mechanisms of human infection or transmission include sexual intercourse, blood products, and breast-feeding. The virus is not thought to be transmitted via aerosolization. Leukemia develops in only a small percentage of infected individuals (approximately 3–5%), often after a long latency period of up to six decades.

47. **(E) Selective outgrowth of antigen-negative variants.**
For tumor cells to take root and proliferate, they must develop mechanisms to evade the host immune system (in an immunocompetent host). Tumor cells can do this by a variety of mechanisms including a selected outgrowth of antigen-negative variants, a loss or reduced expression of MHC molecules, lack of costimulation, immunosuppression, antigen masking, and an apoptosis of cytotoxic T-cells.

48. **(A) Androgen receptor.**
Progressive loss of body fat and lean body mass usually accompanied by weakness, anemia, and anorexia is referred to as cachexia, a concomitant finding of many cancers. A variety of factors are thought to possibly play a role in this process, including tumor necrosis factor, interleukin-1, interferon-gamma, and leukemia inhibitory factor. Androgen receptor is not known to play a role in this process.

49. **(C) Hemangioblastoma.**
A variety of tumors have been known to be associated with the development of secondary polycythemia vera due to an increased production of erythropoietin. Included in this group of tumors are cerebellar hemangioblastomas, hepatocellular carcinomas, and renal cell carcinomas.

50. **(A) Breast.**
An elevated CA-15-3 level is most commonly associated with breast cancers. Colon and pancreatic cancers are associated with elevated CA-19-9 levels. Ovarian cancers are associated with elevated CA-125 levels. A subset of liver cancers may dem-onstrate increased alpha-fetoprotein levels. CEA levels may also be elevated in cancers of the colon and pancreas.

51. **(C) Pituitary adenoma.**
Elevated CEA levels may be encountered in a variety of neoplastic as well as nonneoplastic conditions. A significant percentage of colorectal, pancreatic, gastric, and breast carcinomas may demonstrate elevated CEA levels. A variety of benign conditions including hepatitis, inflammatory bowel disease, and alcoholic cirrhosis may result in elevated CEA levels. Small elevations have also been described in healthy smokers. Pituitary adenomas are not known to be particularly associated with elevated CEA.

52. **(A) Bronchogenic carcinoma.**
Hypertrophic osteoarthropathy and clubbing of the fingers is most commonly associated with bronchogenic carcinoma.

SUGGESTED READING

1. Bergers G, Benjamin L. Tumorigenesis and the angiogenic switch. *Nat Rev Cancer*. 2003;3:401-410.
2. Boon T, Van den Eynde B. Tumour immunology. *Curr Opin Immunol*. 2003;15:129-130.
3. Danial NN, Korsmeyer SJ. Cell death: critical control points. *Cell*. 2004;116:205-219.
4. Dunn GP, Bruce AT, Ikeda H, et al. Cancer immunoediting: from immunosurveillance to tumor escape. *Nat Immunol*. 2002;3:991-998.
5. Esteller M. Epigenetics in cancer. *N Engl J Med*. 2008;358: 1148-1159.
6. Evan GI, Vousden KH. Proliferation, cell cycle and apoptosis in cancer. *Nature*. 2001;411:342-348.
7. Jaffee EM, Hruban RH, Canto M, et al. Focus on pancreas cancer. *Cancer Cell*. 2002;2:25-28.
8. Kastan MB, Bartek J. Cell cycle checkpoints and cancer. *Nature*. 2004;432:316-323.
9. Knudson A. Two genetic hits (more or less) to cancer. *Nat Rev Cancer*. 2001;1:157-162.
10. Knudson AG. Cancer genetics. *Am J Med Genet*. 2002;111: 96-102.
11. Kutok J, Wang F. Spectrum of Epstein-Barr virus-associated diseases. *Annu Rev Pathol*. 2006;1:375-404.
12. Loeb LA, Loeb KR, Anderson JP. Multiple mutations and cancer. *Proc Natl Acad Sci USA*. 2003;100:776-781.
13. Lynch HT, de la Chapelle A. Hereditary colorectal cancer. *N Engl J Med*. 2003;348:919-932.
14. McLaughlin-Drubin ME, Munger K. Viruses associated with human cancer. *Biochim Biophys Acta*. 2008;1782:127-150.
15. Minna JD, Roth JA, Gazder AF. Focus on lung cancer. *Cancer Cell*. 2002;1:49-52.
16. Narod S. Modifiers of risk of hereditary colon cancer. *Oncogene*. 2005;25:5832-5836.

17. Pho L, Grossman D, Leachman SA. Melanoma genetics: a review of genetic factors and clinical phenotypes in familial melanoma. *Curr Opin Oncol.* 2006;18:173-179.

18. Radisky D, Muschler J, Bissell MJ. Order and disorder: the role of extracellular matrix in epithelial cancer. *Cancer Invest.* 2002;20:139-153.

19. Rustgi A. The genetics of hereditary colon cancer. *Genes Dev.* 2007;21:2525-2538.

20. Sahai E. Illuminating the metastatic cascade. *Nat Rev Cancer.* 2007;7:737-749.

21. Sherr CJ, McCormick F. The RB and p53 pathways in cancer. *Cancer Cell.* 2002;2:103-112.

22. Stricker TP, Kumar V. Neoplasia. In: Kumar V, Abbas AK, Fausto N, Aster JC, eds. *Robbins and Cotran Pathologic Basis of Disease.* 8th ed. Philadelphia, PA: Saunders Elsevier; 2010: 259-330.

23. Vousden K, Lane D. p53 in health and disease. *Nat Rev Mol Cell Biol.* 2007;8:275-283.

24. Ward R, Dirks P. Cancer stem cells: at the headwaters of tumor development. *Annu Rev Pathol.* 2007;2:175-189.

25. Weinberg RA, Hanahan D. The hallmarks of cancer. *Cell.* 2000;100:57-70.

26. zur Hausen H. Papillomaviruses and cancer: from basic studies to clinical application. *Nat Rev Cancer.* 2002;2:342-350.

CHAPTER 5

BONE AND SOFT TISSUE PATHOLOGY

1. Which of the following malignancies is least likely to develop bone metastasis?
   - (A) Breast carcinoma
   - (B) Colon carcinoma
   - (C) Lung carcinoma
   - (D) Prostate carcinoma
   - (E) Thyroid carcinoma

2. Patients with a mutation in the *retinoblastoma* gene are at risk for development of which type of bone tumor?
   - (A) Chondroblastoma
   - (B) Chondrosarcoma
   - (C) Ewing's sarcoma
   - (D) Giant cell tumor
   - (E) Osteosarcoma

3. All the following sarcomas can develop lymph node metastasis, except
   - (A) Alveolar soft part sarcoma
   - (B) Clear cell sarcoma
   - (C) Epithelioid sarcoma
   - (D) Rhabdomyosarcoma
   - (E) Synovial sarcoma

4. Which of the following tumors does not arise within the bony diaphysis?
   - (A) Adamantinoma
   - (B) Ewing's sarcoma
   - (C) Giant cell tumor
   - (D) Langerhans cell histiocytosis
   - (E) Lymphoma

5. The radiographic description of "permeative" and "moth-eaten" appearance is typically associated with an infiltrative, malignant process. Which of the following tumors is an exception to this rule and shows a well-circumscribed border?
   - (A) Chondrosarcoma
   - (B) Ewing's sarcoma
   - (C) Fibrosarcoma
   - (D) Multiple myeloma
   - (E) Osteosarcoma

6. The French Federation of Cancer Centers (FNCLCC) system is the most widely used system for grading soft tissue tumors. A score is generated based on tumor differentiation, mitotic activity, and presence of necrosis. Which of the following tumors would not be given a score of 3 for differentiation?
   - (A) Fibrosarcoma
   - (B) Mesenchymal chondrosarcoma
   - (C) Pleomorphic malignant fibrous histiocytoma
   - (D) Synovial sarcoma
   - (E) Well-differentiated liposarcoma

7. Which of the following tumors does not express CD34?
   - (A) Angiosarcoma
   - (B) Epithelioid sarcoma
   - (C) Dermatofibrosarcoma protuberans
   - (D) Hemangiopericytoma
   - (E) Rhabdomyosarcoma

8. Which of the following properties does not apply to neoplastic cells in a bone-forming tumor?
   - (A) The individual cells are large and polygonal with abundant cytoplasm
   - (B) Their eosinophilic cytoplasm is closely associated with newly formed matrix
   - (C) Their nuclei are polarized toward's the bone-forming surface
   - (D) Tumor cells resemble osteoblasts
   - (E) Tumor cells that are entrapped in the matrix often resemble non-neoplastic osteocytes

9. Which of the following types of collagen is most commonly found in skin, fascia, tendon, and bone?
   (A) Type I
   (B) Type II
   (C) Type III
   (D) Type IV
   (E) Type V

10. In a growing child, which part of the bone is responsible for increasing the diameter of the bone?
    (A) Cambium layer
    (B) Diaphysis
    (C) Epiphysis
    (D) Metaphysis
    (E) Sharpey's fibers

11. Following deposition of non-mineralized bone matrix (osteoid), how long does it take for the matrix to get mineralized?
    (A) 2 days
    (B) 7 days
    (C) 10 days
    (D) 15 days
    (E) 21 days

12. Which of the following markers is not considered to be a reliable biochemical marker of bone turnover?
    (A) Collagen N and C-telopeptides
    (B) Hydroxyproline and cross-linked collagen peptides
    (C) Serum alkaline phosphatase
    (D) Serum osteocalcin
    (E) Serum potassium

13. Which of the following features about woven bone is incorrect?
    (A) Associated with osteosarcoma and Paget's disease
    (B) Cells embedded within the matrix are typically large and closely packed
    (C) Contains haphazardly arranged collagen matrix
    (D) Polarized light microscopy highlights the presence of cement lines
    (E) Usually indicates a disease process

14. Histologic examination of tissue from fracture callus shows markedly cellular and hypervascular tissue with irregular islands of woven bone and cartilage. What is the approximate age of this fracture?
    (A) 2 days
    (B) 7 days
    (C) 15 days
    (D) 21 days
    (E) 30 days

15. Which of the following patient population is not at risk for developing osteomyelitis via hematogenous route?
    (A) Children
    (B) Diabetics
    (C) Intravenous drug users
    (D) Motor vehicle accident victims
    (E) Patients with peripheral vascular disease

16. In a case of osteomyelitis, the necrotic medullary bone that becomes isolated in a large cavity is referred to as
    (A) Brodie's abscess
    (B) Callus
    (C) Involucrum
    (D) Sequestrum
    (E) Sinus

17. A 5-year-old boy is admitted for a tibial fracture. Further investigation shows that he has blue sclera, poorly formed dentition, and hearing loss. The pediatrician suspects that he has a congenital disorder affecting collagen production. What is the most likely diagnosis?
    (A) Congenital hypophosphatasia
    (B) Ehlers–Danlos disease
    (C) Juvenile osteoporosis
    (D) Scurvy
    (E) Osteogenesis imperfecta

18. Which of the following clinical features is not associated with Ehlers-Danlos syndrome?
    (A) Blue sclera
    (B) Easy bruisability
    (C) Hearing loss
    (D) Hyperextensibility of the skin
    (E) Hypermobile joints

19. Erlenmeyer flask deformity of the bone is associated with which of the following bone conditions?
    (A) Osteitis deformans
    (B) Osteolysis
    (C) Osteopenia
    (D) Osteopetrosis
    (E) Osteoporosis

20. A 68-year-old man notices that he has been changing the size of his hat rather frequently to fit his enlarging head. Investigations reveal that he has a disorder that leads to an imbalance between activity of the osteoclasts and osteoblasts. Which of the following features is least likely to be associated with this condition?
    (A) Giant cell tumor arising in the facial bone
    (B) Increased numbers of cement lines

(C) Markedly elevated serum alkaline phosphatase activity

(D) Osteoporosis circumscripta affecting the skull

(E) Usually affects the peripheral skeleton

21. Which of the following findings favor a diagnosis of senile osteoporosis (type II osteoporosis) over post-menopausal osteoporosis (type I osteoporosis)?

(A) Decreased osteoblastic activity

(B) Increased urinary calcium levels

(C) Predominantly trabecular bone loss

(D) Rapid bone loss

(E) Tooth loss

22. An excision specimen from a patient with osteitis fibrosa cystica is shown here. Which of the following features is not associated with this condition? (Figure 5-1)

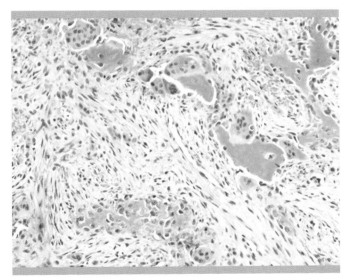

FIGURE 5-1

(A) Decreased parathyroid hormone

(B) Increased amount of woven bone

(C) Osteoclastic bone tunneling or dissecting bone resorption

(D) Peritrabecular marrow fibrosis

(E) Subperiosteal resorption on the radial side of middle phalanges

23. Which of the following conditions is associated with dystrophic calcification?

(A) Hyperparathyroidism

(B) Infarction

(C) Metastatic disease

(D) Myeloma

(E) Sarcoidosis

24. Which of the following pathologic features is not associated with osteoarthritis?

(A) Eburnated articular surface

(B) Osteophyte formation

(C) Rice bodies

(D) Subchondral cyst formation

(E) Surface fibrillation

25. A 25-year-old man presents with toe pain, and is found to have a lobulated, ossified mass in the soft tissue that does not seem to be attached to the distal phalanx. Histologically, the lesion is composed of lobulated, cellular cartilaginous tissue, with calcified fibrocartilagenous tissue toward's the periphery. What is the best diagnosis for this lesion?

(A) Florid reactive periostitis

(B) Nora's lesion

(C) Osteochondroma

(D) Osteoma

(E) Subungual exostosis

26. Which of the following clinicopathologic features is least likely to be associated with this painful lesion excised from the left leg of a 65-year-old man (see Figure 5-2)?

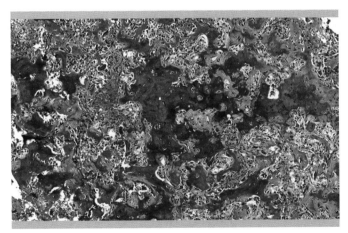

FIGURE 5-2

(A) Contains a central nidus

(B) Immature woven bone forms the major component of the lesion

(C) More than 50% cases occur in the lower extremities

(D) Painless lesion

(E) Usually measures <1 cm

27. A 40-year-old man is found to have an incidental, solitary, homogeneously dense intramedullary lesion in the left pelvic bone. The lesion has spiculated margins that blend with the adjacent cancellous bone. Histologically, it is composed entirely of lamellar bone with very minimal woven bone. What is the best diagnosis?
   (A) Enostosis (bone island)
   (B) Intramedullary osteosarcoma
   (C) Osteoblastic metastasis
   (D) Osteoblastoma
   (E) Osteoid osteoma

28. Which cortical surface-based bone-forming tumor grossly mimics a normal bone, and when multifocal, is associated with Gardner's syndrome?
   (A) Conventional osteosarcoma
   (B) Low-grade surface osteosarcoma
   (C) Osteoblastoma
   (D) Osteoid osteoma
   (E) Osteoma

29. Which of the listed features favors a diagnosis of osteosarcoma over aggressive osteoblastoma?
   (A) Coarse lace-like osteoid deposition
   (B) Distinct osteoblastic rimming
   (C) Epithelioid osteoblasts
   (D) Infiltrative borders
   (E) Lack of atypical mitoses

30. Which of the following clinicopathologic features is least likely to be associated with the bone tumor shown in Figure 5-3?

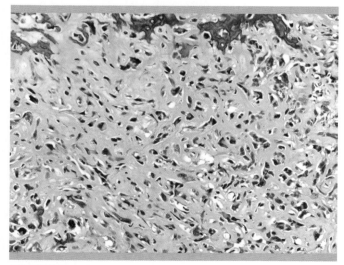

FIGURE 5-3

(A) A minimum of 10% malignant osteoid production is required for a diagnosis
(B) Bimodal age distribution
(C) Metaphysis is the most common location
(D) More common in males than in females
(E) Most common primary non-hematopoeitic malignancy of the skeletal system

31. Which of the following subtypes is the least common subtype of osteosarcoma?
   (A) Conventional high-grade osteosarcoma
   (B) High-grade secondary osteosarcoma
   (C) Intramedullary well-differentiated osteosarcoma
   (D) Parosteal osteosarcoma
   (E) Periosteal osteosarcoma

32. Which of the following features is helpful in classifying a surface osteosarcoma as a periosteal osteosarcoma as opposed to a parosteal osteosarcoma?
   (A) Broad-based, well-demarcated, solid, tan-white lesion
   (B) Cellular spindle cell proliferation with limited cytologic atypia
   (C) Minimal periosteal reaction on radiologic examination
   (D) Neoplastic cartilaginous areas admixed with severe cytologic atypia
   (E) Tumor located in the posterior aspect of proximal femur

33. Which of the following clinical conditions/syndromes is not considered to be a risk factor for the development of osteosarcoma?
   (A) Bilateral retinoblastomas
   (B) Chemotherapy
   (C) Chronic osteomyelitis
   (D) Li-Fraumeni syndrome
   (E) Paget's disease

34. Which of the following tumor is commonly associated with the formation of Codman triangle?
   (A) Aneurysmal bone cyst
   (B) Chondrosarcoma
   (C) Ewing sarcoma
   (D) Fibrous dysplasia
   (E) Osteogenic sarcoma

35. Which of the following cartilage-forming tumors is the best diagnosis for the lesion shown in this image? (see Figure 5-4)

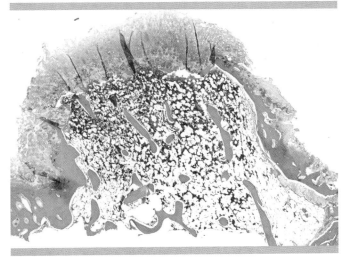

FIGURE 5-4

(A) Chondroblastoma
(B) Chondrosarcoma
(C) Enchondroma
(D) Osteochondroma
(E) Periosteal chondroma

36. A well-demarcated lytic lesion encountered in the epiphysis of a 20-year-old man is shown in Figure 5-5. Which of the following features is not typically related to this lesion?

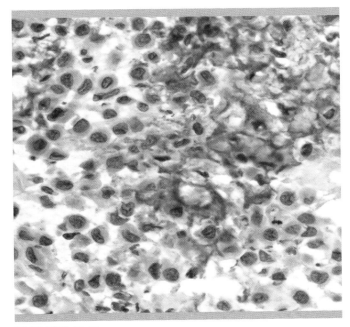

FIGURE 5-5

(A) Abundant blue hyaline cartilage
(B) Chicken wire calcifications
(C) Irregular distribution of osteoclastic giant cells
(D) Nuclear grooves
(E) Secondary aneurysmal bone cyst formation

37. An intramedullary tumor resected from a 35-year-old man is shown in Figure 5-6. All the following features are associated with this tumor, except

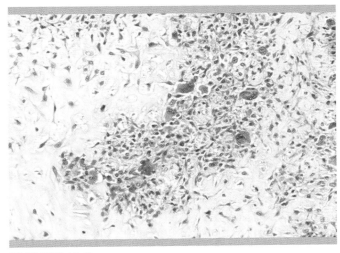

FIGURE 5-6

(A) Increased cellularity toward the periphery of the lobules
(B) Minimal cytologic atypia
(C) Nodules of hyaline cartilage
(D) Osteoclast-like giant cells
(E) Spindle or stellate cells with long cytoplasmic processes

38. Which of the following radiologic/pathologic feature, when present in a well-differentiated cartilage-forming lesion, warrants a diagnosis of a grade 1 chondrosarcoma?
(A) Dark nuclei with details visible at 400 × magnification
(B) Islands of cartilage permeating viable, lamellar bone
(C) Low cellularity with round chondrocytes within lacunae
(D) Ring calcifications
(E) Slow-growing mass

39. Based on the histologic features shown in Figure 5-7, which of these findings would be unusual for this lesion?

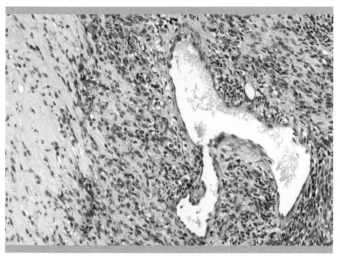

FIGURE 5-7

(A) Commonly occurs in the ribs, jaw, and pelvis
(B) Gritty calcifications, cystic change, hemorrhage, and necrosis, are common
(C) Hemangiopericytoma-like vascular pattern
(D) Peak age of occurrence is 70 years
(E) The smaller cells may express CD99

40. A 19-year-old teenager undergoes radiologic evaluation for knee pain and is found to have a 4.5-cm lytic lesion involving the metaphysis of the distal femur. It appears to be eccentrically located within the medullary cavity and is juxtaposed to the cortex. Based on the histologic findings shown in Figure 5-8, what is the best diagnosis?

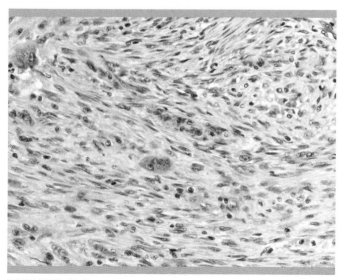

FIGURE 5-8

(A) Benign fibrous histiocytoma
(B) Desmoplastic fibroma
(C) Fibrous dysplasia
(D) Giant cell tumor
(E) Nonossifying fibroma

41. An 8-year-old boy presents with a tumor involving the diaphysis of femur (see Figure 5-9). Imaging studies reveal the presence of "onion skinning" and "sunburst" pattern of periosteal reaction. Which of the following genes is most frequently involved in the reciprocal translocation diagnostic of this tumor?

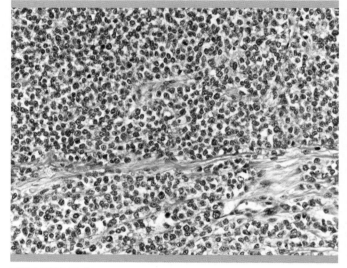

FIGURE 5-9

(A) *E1AF*, chromosome 2
(B) *ERG*, chromosome 21
(C) *ETV1*, chromosome 7
(D) *ETV4*, chromosome 17
(E) *FLI1*, chromosome 11

42. A 23-year-old woman undergoes curettage of a lytic lesion located in the distal femur. Which of the following features is not characteristic of this tumor? (See Figure 5-10.)

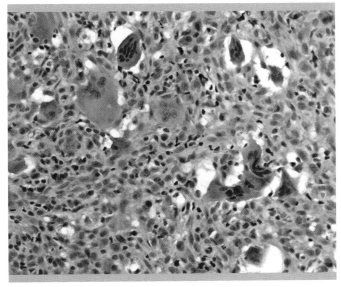

FIGURE 5-10

(A) Less than 2% of tumors may metastasize to the lung
(B) May show foci of osteoid deposition
(C) Nuclei of multinucleated giant cells are different from those of the mononuclear cell population
(D) Numerous mitotic figures may be found
(E) Tumor may demonstrate destruction of the cortex

43. A 60-year-old man presents with low back pain and is diagnosed with this sacrococcygeal tumor (see Figure 5-11). Which of the following immunohistochemical stains is not expressed by this tumor?

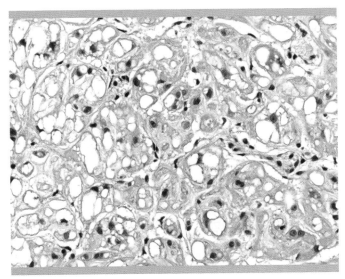

FIGURE 5-11

(A) Brachyury
(B) CDX-2
(C) Cytokeratin 8/18
(D) Epithelial membrane antigen (EMA)
(E) S-100

44. A 30-year-old man with history of trauma is found to have an expansile lytic lesion in the midshaft of right tibia. Imaging shows a "soap-bubble" appearance. Based on the image provided (see Figure 5-12), what is the best diagnosis?

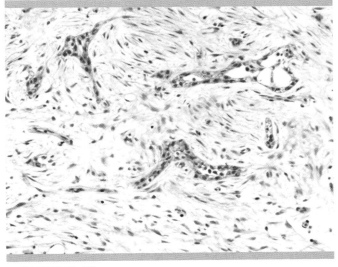

FIGURE 5-12

(A) Adamantinoma
(B) Benign fibrous histiocytoma
(C) Fibrous dysplasia
(D) Giant cell tumor
(E) Nonossifying fibroma

45. A rib tumor with sclerotic rind-like periphery and ground glass appearance resected from a 35-year-old man is shown in Figure 5-13. What is the best diagnosis for this lesion?

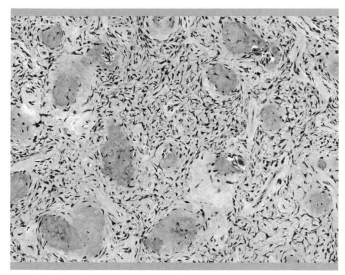

FIGURE 5-13

(A) Cemento-ossifying fibroma
(B) Desmoplastic fibroma
(C) Fibrous dysplasia
(D) Nonossifying fibroma
(E) Osteofibrous dysplasia

46. A 12-year-old boy undergoes resection of a rapidly growing forearm mass shown in Figure 5-14. Which of the following features is least likely to be associated with this lesion?

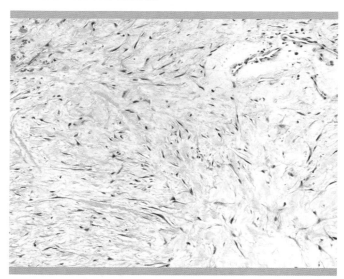

FIGURE 5-14

(A) Atypical mitotic activity can be seen
(B) Lesional cells are diffusely positive for smooth muscle actin

(C) Often contains extravasated red blood cells
(D) Often located in the deep subcutis
(E) Osteoclast-like giant cells are present in 10% of cases

47. A 60-year-old woman undergoes resection of a soft tissue mass located in the lower scapula (see Figure 5-15). What is the best diagnosis for this lesion?

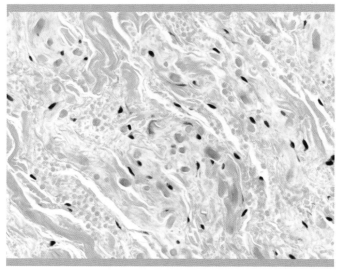

FIGURE 5-15

(A) Desmoplastic fibroblastoma
(B) Elastofibroma
(C) Fibroma of tendon sheath
(D) Keloid
(E) Spindle cell lipoma

48. What is the best diagnosis for this superficially located axillary mass excised from a 2-year-old infant (see Figure 5-16)?

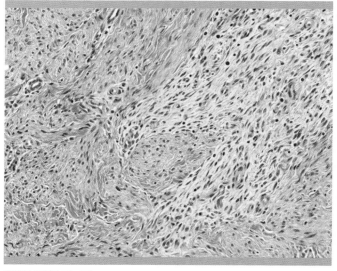

FIGURE 5-16

(A) Calcifying aponeurotic fibroma
(B) Fibrous hamartoma of infancy
(C) Giant cell fibroblastoma
(D) Myofibroma
(E) Lipofibromatosis

49. What percentage of cases of desmoid-type fibromatosis harbor mutations in the β-*catenin* gene ?
(A) 10%
(B) 15%
(C) 25%
(D) 50%
(E) 90%

50. A 45-year-old woman is diagnosed with myxoinflammatory fibroblastic sarcoma. Which of the following features is not typical of this tumor?
(A) Hyalinized and myxoid areas
(B) Lymphocytes and plasma cell-rich inflammation
(C) Pseudolipoblast-like cells
(D) Reed-Sternberg like cells
(E) Well-developed arborizing thick-walled vasculature

51. A 35-year-old man undergoes resection of this tumor located in upper thigh (see Figure 5-17). Which of the following molecular abnormalities is specific for this tumor?

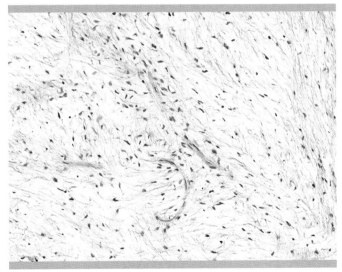

FIGURE 5-17

(A) t(2;13)
(B) t(7;16)
(C) t(12;15)
(D) t(12;22)
(E) t(17;22)

52. A 70-year-old man with a 1.5-cm superficial neck lesion is diagnosed with atypical fibroxanthoma. Which of the following features is associated with this tumor?

(A) Overlying epidermis is usually hyperplastic
(B) Patients have hyperlipidemia
(C) The lesional cells express CD68 and desmin
(D) Touton-type giant cells are diagnostic of this entity
(E) Usually occurs in sun-exposed areas

53. A 3.5-cm nodule excised from the trunk of a 40-year-old man shows a storiform arrangement of cells, with infiltration into the subcutaneous tissue in a honeycomb pattern. Which of immunohistochemical markers would be positive in the tumor cells?
(A) Caldesmon
(B) CD34
(C) Desmin
(D) S-100
(E) Smooth muscle actin

54. Angiomatoid fibrous histiocytoma is least likely to be associated with which of the following features?
(A) Cystic change
(B) Lesional cells that are positive for CD31 and CD34
(C) Occurs in children and young adults
(D) Shows molecular alterations similar to clear cell sarcoma of soft tissue
(E) Shows peripheral fibrous capsule with lymphocytic inflammation

55. A 52-year-old man undergoes excision of this poorly circumscribed mass located in the posterior aspect of neck (see Figure 5-18). What is the best diagnosis?

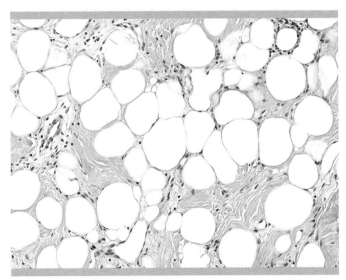

FIGURE 5-18

(A) Angiolipoma
(B) Elastofibroma
(C) Intramuscular lipoma
(D) Liposarcoma
(E) Spindle cell lipoma

56. Which of the following adipocytic lesions does not contain lipoblasts?
    (A) Angiolipoma
    (B) Chondroid lipoma
    (C) Lipoblastoma
    (D) Liposarcoma
    (E) Pleomorphic lipoma

57. All the listed features are characteristic of a dedifferentiated liposarcoma, except
    (A) Behaves less aggressively than other high-grade pleomorphic sarcomas
    (B) Can recur entirely as a well-differentiated liposarcoma
    (C) Dedifferentiated foci have to show high-grade morphology
    (D) Grossly presents as a distinct tan-white firm nodule in a background of adipose tissue
    (E) Retroperitoneum is the most common location

58. Which of the following genes is implicated in the karyotypic aberration found in this thigh mass resected from a 40-year-old man (see Figure 5-19)?

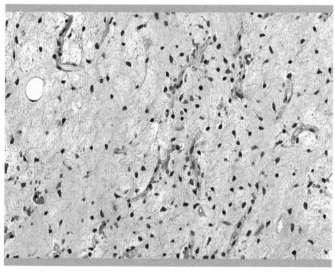

FIGURE 5-19

    (A) *CDK4*
    (B) *DDIT3*
    (C) *HMGA2*
    (D) *MDM2*
    (E) *OS1*

59. A 52-year-old woman undergoes excision of a left leg nodule that is shown in Figure 5-20. Which of the following clinicopathologic features is not typical of this lesion?

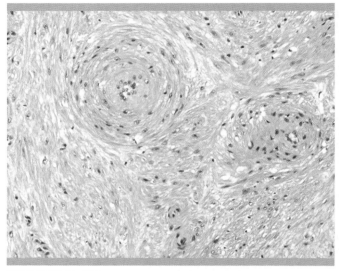

FIGURE 5-20

    (A) Degenerative atypia
    (B) Diffuse immunoreactivity with h-caldesmon
    (C) Extremities are commonly involved
    (D) Pain is a common presenting symptom
    (E) Venous subtype is most common histologic subtype

60. A 16-year-old teenager with history of renal transplant develops multiple liver nodules. A biopsy of one of these nodules shows Epstein–Barr virus (EBV)-associated smooth muscle tumor. Which of the following features is least likely to be associated with this entity?
    (A) Composed of well-differentiated and small, primitive smooth muscle cells
    (B) Lung and liver are commonly involved
    (C) Lymphocytic inflammatory infiltrate
    (D) Marked cytologic atypia
    (E) Usually arises approximately 3 years post-transplantation

61. A 4-year-old girl was found to have a polypoid soft tissue mass composed of bland spindle cells and myotubules arranged in a myxoid background. The lesion also shows occasional strap cells. What is the best classification for this lesion?
    (A) Adult rhabdomyoma
    (B) Botyroid rhabdomyosarcoma
    (C) Cellular rhabdomyoma
    (D) Fetal rhabdomyoma
    (E) Genital rhabdomyoma

62. A 7-year-old girl undergoes resection of a cervical polypoid tumor composed of small, undifferentiated spindle-to-epithelioid cells that are tightly packed

in a band-like arrangement beneath the epithelial surface. The cells are diffusely positive for MyoD1. What is the best diagnosis?
(A) Anaplastic rhabdomyosarcoma
(B) Alveolar rhabdomyosarcoma
(C) Botyroid rhabdomyosarcoma
(D) Embryonal rhabdomyosarcoma
(E) Spindle cell rhabdomyosarcoma

63. A 20-year-old man undergoes resection of a thigh mass shown in Figure 5-21. This lesion is diffusely positive for myogenin and negative for cytokeratin. Which of the following findings is not associated with this entity?

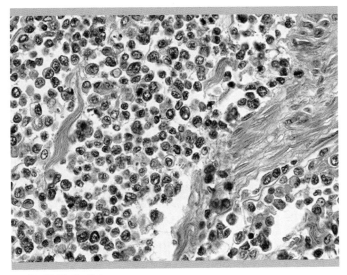

FIGURE 5-21

(A) Intracytoplasmic PAS-positive crystalline inclusions
(B) Multinucleated giant cells
(C) *PAX7/FKHR* translocation
(D) Poor clinical prognosis
(E) Rapidly growing mass

64. Which of the following vascular proliferations commonly occurs on the thumb, and shows an intravascular proliferation of bland endothelial cells within a thrombus?
(A) Bacillary angiomatosis
(B) Capillary hemangioma
(C) Glomeruloid hemangioma
(D) Spindle cell hemangioma
(E) Papillary endothelial hyperplasia

65. Bacillary angiomatosis is associated with all of the following features except
(A) Affects immunocompromised individuals
(B) Caused by infection with Human Herpes Virus-8
(C) Immunoreactivity with FLI-1 antibody
(D) Neutrophils and eosinophilic fibrin aggregates
(E) Visceral involvement is in the form of peliosis

66. Which of the following vascular lesions is associated with multisystem disease characterized by polyneuropathy, organomegaly, endocrinopathy, monoclonal gammopathy, and skin changes (POEMS syndrome)?
(A) Bacillary angiomatosis
(B) Capillary hemangioma
(C) Glomeruloid hemangioma
(D) Spindle cell hemangioma
(E) Papillary endothelial hyperplasia

67. Which of the following immunohistochemical markers is specifically expressed by juvenile capillary hemangioma and not by other vascular tumors?
(A) CD31
(B) CD34
(C) FLI-1
(D) GLUT1
(E) vWF

68. Which of the following vascular tumors is frequently found in patients with Maffucci syndrome and mimics Kaposi's sarcoma?
(A) Bacillary angiomatosis
(B) Capillary hemangioma
(C) Glomeruloid hemangioma
(D) Spindle cell hemangioma
(E) Papillary endothelial hyperplasia

69. Which of the following vascular lesions shows a central damaged vessel, an eosinophil-rich inflammatory infiltrate, and a characteristic "tombstone" pattern of endothelial cells?
(A) Deep hemangioma
(B) Epithelioid hemangioendothelioma
(C) Epithelioid hemangioma
(D) Glomeruloid hemangioma
(E) Kaposiform hemangioendothelioma

70. A 75-year-old man undergoes resection of this vascular tumor located in the liver. Which of the following markers is the least sensitive immunohistochemical marker of this lesion? (See Figure 5-22.)

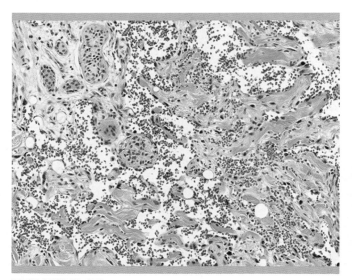

FIGURE 5-22

(A) CD31
(B) CD34
(C) ERG
(D) FLI1
(E) vWF

71. Which of the following parts of a nerve does neurofibroma arise from?
(A) Axon
(B) Endoneurium
(C) Fibroblasts
(D) Perineurium
(E) Schwann cell

72. Which of the following peripheral nerve sheath tumors has the highest risk for malignant transformation?
(A) Cutaneous NF1-associated neurofibroma
(B) Deep NF1-associated neurofibroma
(C) Non-NF1-associated neurofibroma
(D) Plexiform neurofibroma
(E) Solitary neurofibroma

73. Which of the following morphologic features is considered to be the diagnostic hallmark of diffuse neurofibroma?
(A) Hyalinization
(B) Multiple intraneural tumor nodules
(C) Myxoid change
(D) Wagner–Meissner bodies
(E) Storiform arrangement of cells

74. Which of the following findings is not associated with a neurofibroma undergoing malignant transformation?
(A) Cytologic atypia
(B) Increased cellularity
(C) Mitotic activity
(D) Necrosis
(E) Prominent S-100 immunoreactivity

75. Figure 5-23 shows a thigh mass that was resected from the peripheral aspect of a large nerve. Which of the following findings is not associated with this lesion?

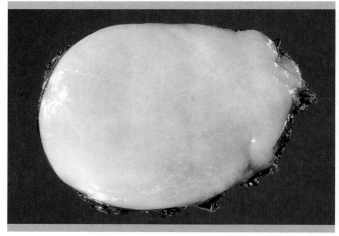

FIGURE 5-23

(A) Admixture of S-100, CD34, and EMA-positive cells
(B) Encapsulation
(C) Myxoid areas
(D) Perivascular hyalinization
(E) Verocay bodies

76. Which of the following clinical syndromes/complexes is observed in up to 50% of patients with psammomatous melanotic schwannoma?
(A) Carney complex
(B) Klippel-Trenaunay syndrome
(C) MEN-2
(D) NF1
(E) NF2

77. A 60-year-old man undergoes resection of a buttock mass composed of malignant spindle cells with geographic areas of necrosis and perivascular accentuation. They are weakly positive for S-100 and negative for cytokeratin. What is the best diagnosis?
(A) Fibrosarcoma
(B) Leiomyosarcoma
(C) Malignant peripheral nerve sheath tumor
(D) Malignant solitary fibrous tumor
(E) Monophasic synovial sarcoma

78. In a patient diagnosed with neuroblastoma, which of the following factors is associated with a good clinical prognosis?
    (A) Age at diagnosis <1 year
    (B) Deletion of chromosome 1p36
    (C) Higher stage
    (D) High mitosis–karyorrhexis index
    (E) Necrosis

79. A soft tissue mass resected from a 20-year-old man is shown in Figure 5-24. Molecular studies are positive for t(12;22). Which of these locations is the most common site of involvement by this tumor?

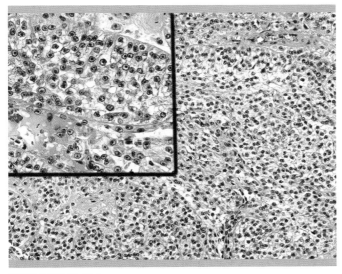

FIGURE 5-24

    (A) Ankle/foot
    (B) Hand
    (C) Knee
    (D) Neck
    (E) Retroperitoneum

80. Which of the following findings favors a diagnosis of giant cell tumor of tendon sheath over pigmented villonodular synovitis?
    (A) Extra-articular location
    (B) Hemosiderin
    (C) Mononuclear cells
    (D) Nodular growth pattern
    (E) Osteoclast-like giant cells

81. What percentage of epithelioid sarcomas shows loss of INI-1 expression?
    (A) 10%
    (B) 25%
    (C) 50%
    (D) 90%
    (E) 100%

ANSWERS

1. **(B) Colon carcinoma.**
   Of the listed tumors, colon cancer rarely metastasizes to the bone. Tumors that are at risk for metastatic bone disease include breast carcinoma, lung carcinoma, renal cell carcinoma, prostatic carcinoma, and thyroid carcinoma.

2. **(E) Osteosarcoma.**
   Nearly 40% of patients diagnosed with retinoblastoma demonstrate an autosomal-dominant pattern of inheritance. Patients with familial retinoblastomas are at risk for secondary malignancies that include osteosarcomas, rhabdomyosarcomas, and rhabdoid tumors.

3. **(A) Alveolar soft part sarcoma.**
   Sarcomas that have an ability to spread via lymphatics include clear cell sarcoma, epithelioid sarcoma, rhabdomyosarcoma, and synovial sarcoma. Alveolar soft part sarcoma usually spreads to the lungs via hematogenous route.

4. **(C) Giant cell tumor.**
   The knowledge about location of a bone tumor (epiphyseal, diaphyseal, or metaphyseal) is extremely helpful in diagnosing bone tumors. Tumors that arise in the epiphysis include giant cell tumor (choice C), chondroblastoma, and pigmented villonodular synovitis. Tumors arising in the metaphysis include osteosarcoma, nonossifying fibroma, osteochondroma, aneurysmal bone cyst, enchondroma, chondrosarcoma, and solitary bone cyst. Tumors arising in the diaphysis include all the listed choices, except choice C.

5. **(D) Multiple myeloma.**
   The radiographic descriptions "geographic" and "well-circumscribed" indicate that the tumor has well-defined borders and is most likely benign. As opposed to this, malignant tumors usually show "permeative" and "moth-eaten" appearance, and often show a distinct periosteal reaction. The only exception to this rule is multiple myeloma, which on radiographic evaluation, is characterized by well-defined punched-out lesions.

6. **(E) Well-differentiated liposarcoma.**
   Tumor differentiation is the most problematic aspect about grading soft tissue sarcomas using the FNCLCC system. The tumor differentiation is given a score of 1 if the sarcoma closely resembles normal adult mesenchymal tissue (choice E, well-differentiated liposarcoma). A differentiation score of 2 is given to sarcomas of certain histologic type (e.g., fibrosarcoma, myxoid liposarcoma, and conventional leiomyosarcoma), and a score of 3 is given to majority of the sarcomas such as synovial sarcoma,

embryonal sarcoma, mesenchymal chondrosarcoma, undifferentiated sarcoma, and sarcomas of doubtful tumor type.

7. **(E) Rhabdomyosarcoma.**
CD34 is typically considered to be a vascular marker and, therefore, is positive in both benign and malignant vascular neoplasms. In addition, it also stains dendritic interstitial and stromal cells. Other tumors that express CD34 include epithelioid sarcoma, gastrointestinal stromal tumor, dermatofibrosarcoma protuberans, solitary fibrous tumor, hemangiopericytoma, and blasts in myeloid leukemias.

8. **(C) Their nuclei are polarized toward the bone-forming surface.**
All the listed features are attributes of a neoplastic bone-forming tumor cell, except choice C. The nuclei of the tumor cells are often polarized away from the bone-forming surface, are eccentrically located, and show fine chromatin with prominent nucleoli. The resemblance of tumor cells to nonneoplastic osteocytes (choice E) is known as the normalization phenomenon.

9. **(A) Type I.**
Collagen accounts for nearly 70% of all body proteins and forms the major constituent of extracellular matrix. At least 29 different types of collagen have been recognized, and type I is the most common collagen among them. Type I collagen is commonly found in skin, fascia, tendon, and bone. Specific disorders are known to affect the synthesis of specific subtypes of collagen. For example, disorders of collagen type I include osteogenesis imperfecta and Ehlers-Danlos syndrome. Type II collagen is a major constituent of hyaline cartilage. Type IV collagen is present basement membranes, and the related disorders include Alport's syndrome, Goodpasture's syndrome, and porencephaly.

10. **(A) Cambium layer.**
The periosteum is composed of two layers: outer fibrous layer and inner cambium layer. The inner cambium layer has the potential for new bone formation. In children, this layer is responsible for increasing the width of the bone. In adults, the cambium layer gets activated by trauma, infection, or tumor, and results in periosteal reaction or periosteal new bone formation. Epiphysis is portion of the bone located between the articular surface and growth plate. Metaphysis is located immediately below the growth plate, and diaphysis is portion of the bone between the metaphyses. The periosteum is attached to the cortical surface of the bone by collagen fibers known as fibers of Sharpey.

11. **(C) 10 days.**
The time taken between the deposition of nonmineralized bone matrix (osteoid) by osteoblasts and mineralization of this matrix is known as the "mineralization lag." It usually takes about 10 days for this process to occur. Recognition of nonmineralized matrix is of importance in diagnosing certain metabolic disorders of the bone. This, however, depends on the morphologic variation introduced by the process of decalcification during histologic processing.

12. **(E) Serum potassium.**
Of the listed choices, serum phosphate and not serum potassium, is involved in bone metabolism. Compared to the other choices, cross-linked collagen peptides are considered to be relatively more specific indicators of bone turnover. They are only produced after bone synthesis is complete.

13. **(D) Polarized light microscopy highlights the presence of cement lines.**
Immature bone or woven bone, and mature or lamellar bone, are the two major types of mineralized bone tissues. Lamellar bone (or cortical bone) is characterized by layering of collagen around vascular channels (Haversian canals). The structural irregularities in this arrangement are seen as dark blue lines on H&E section, and these are called the *cement lines*. As opposed to this, woven bone is immature bone formed as a result of haphazard intertwining of collagen matrix. The recognition of this type of bone in a histologic section is important as it usually indicates the presence of a disease process. It may be associated with fracture callus, Paget's disease, bone-forming tumors, and hyperparathyroidism.

14. **(C) 15 days.**
The immature reparative tissue that develops at the site of fracture is referred to as fracture callus. Within a few days of injury, there is evidence of hemorrhage and bone marrow necrosis. Around 15 days, prominent vascularization and cellular proliferation occurs. If a biopsy is obtained during this time period, these changes can be misinterpreted as primary bone tumor or sarcoma.

15. **(D) Motor vehicle accident victims.**
Victims of motor vehicle accidents tend to acquire polymicrobial infections. These infections are usually a result of direct inoculation of bacteria. Hematogenous spread of osteomyelitis specifically occurs in the pediatric population, intravenous drug abusers, patients with peripheral vascular disease, and diabetes mellitus. The microorganisms that are isolated from pediatric patients include *Staphylococcus aureus*, *Hemophilus influenza*, *Streptococcus pyogenes*, and *Pseudomonas* species.

16. **(D) Sequestrum.**
    Sequestrum is the piece of devitalized medullary bone that gets separated from the surrounding bone. The extent of bone involvement may vary. If only a limited portion of bone is affected, a small abscess known as Brodie's abscess occurs. Radiographically, Brodie's abscess may mimic osteoid osteoma, eosinophilic granuloma, or small round blue cell tumor. Involucrum is the new bone formed by the cambium layer of periosteum.

17. **(E) Osteogenesis imperfecta.**
    Osteogenesis imperfecta (brittle bone disease) is the most commonly recognized congenital disorder affecting collagen production. Patients usually have a history of frequent fractures. The disorder consists of several distinct syndromes that may be inherited as an autosomal-dominant condition (most common), autosomal-recessive condition, or may arise as a result of spontaneous mutations. Most patients have poorly formed teeth and hearing loss. Thus far, eight distinct syndromes have been described; type I being the most common and mildest form of disease.

18. **(C) Hearing loss.**
    Ehlers-Danlos syndrome is a rare disorder of collagen synthesis. Six different subtypes have been identified. Most patients have osteopenia. Other classic clinical features include hyperextensible joints, easy bruisability, hyperextensibility of skin, dissecting aortic aneurysm (more common in type IV subtype), and arthritis. While blue sclera is a hallmark of osteogenesis imperfecta, it is not an uncommon finding in patients with Ehlers-Danlos syndrome.

19. **(D) Osteopetrosis.**
    Osteopetrosis (marble bone disease or Albers-Schönberg disease) is a rare disorder characterized by a marked increase in density of bones (osteosclerosis). The bones show loss of metaphyseal flare, and this results in typical Erlenmeyer flask deformity of extremities. This deformity commonly involves areas of rapid bone growth, such as lower femur, upper tibia, and upper humerus. This deformity can also be seen in patients with Gaucher's disease. Patients with osteopetrosis suffer from multiple fractures and anemia due to reduction in their marrow spaces. Radiographically, the bones show loss of demarcation between the cancellous and cortical bone.

20. **(E) Usually affects the peripheral skeleton.**
    The condition described here is Paget's disease (osteitis deformans). The most commonly affected bones include lumbar spine, skull, pelvis, femur, and tibia. Peripheral skeleton is rarely affected. In its early stage of prominent osteoclastic activity, the skull shows characteristic radiolucency due to bone resorption, without thickening of the bone, referred to as osteoporosis circumscripta. Histologically, this stage is characterized by increased numbers of osteoclasts, each with at least 10-20 nuclei. Simultaneously, there is osteoblastic activity with deposition of new bone on the opposite side. Radiologically, in the latter stage, there is an increase in bone density with loss of corticomedullary demarcation. During this stage, the bone resorption slows down, and the characteristic "mosaic" pattern is seen on histologic evaluation. The "mosaic" pattern represents exaggerated cement lines resulting from the increased rate of bone formation and bone resorption. Giant cell tumors may rarely complicate Paget's disease. In this setting, giant cell tumors typically involve unconventional areas such as skull, spine, and facial bones.

21. **(A) Decreased osteoblastic activity.**
    Osteopenia related to advancing age, that results in fractures, is known as osteoporosis. Based on clinical findings, Riggs and his colleagues classified osteoporosis into two types: type I or postmenopausal osteoporosis, and type II or senile osteoporosis. Postmenopausal osteoporosis results from rapid bone loss, and is associated with increased osteoclastic activity. It is believed that estrogen deficiency indirectly increases the sensitivity of osteoclasts to parathyroid hormone. This is usually associated with increased urinary calcium level and tooth loss. In contrast, senile osteoporosis is associated with slow bone loss (both cancellous and trabecular) as a result of both decreased osteoblastic activity and increased osteoclastic activity.

22. **(A) Decreased parathyroid hormone.**
    Osteitis fibrosa cystica or von Recklinghausen bone disease is a result of overproduction of parathyroid hormone. Increased levels of parathyroid hormone may be associated with parathyroid adenoma, hyperplasia, and rarely carcinoma (primary hyperparathyroidism), or chronic renal failure (secondary hyperparathyroidism). The radiologic features of osteitis fibrosa cystica include erosion of tufts of terminal phalanges and subperiosteal cortical resorption, especially on radial side of the middle phalanges. Histologically, there is marked osteoclastic bone resorption (tunneling), accompanied by peritrabecular fibrosis, and increased formation of woven bone.

23. **(B) Infarction.**
    Dystrophic calcification results from deposition of calcium hydroxyapatite in dead soft tissue. This type of calcification is observed in areas of coagulative

necrosis (infarction), caseous necrosis (tuberculosis), and fat necrosis. The type of calcification that occurs due to an increased calcium x phosphate product in blood (either due to hypercalcemia or hyperphosphatemia), is known as metastatic calcification. Choices A, C, D, and E, all cause metastatic calcification in areas that are subject to large pH changes, such as kidneys, alveoli, cornea, arterial media, and gastric mucosa.

24. **(C) Rice bodies.**
Changes of osteoarthritis begin at the articular surface and are characterized by erosion, cracking of the articular cartilage, and surface fibrillation (velvety appearance of the articular surface). Progressive joint damage causes complete denudation of the cartilage, exposure of polished subchondral bone (eburnation), and formation of subchondral cysts. Osteophyte formation is a unique feature of osteoarthritis. It occurs due to formation of new bone and cartilage. Loose bodies are free-floating fragments of damaged bone and cartilage present within joint spaces. Most often, they are composed of cartilage, which may occasionally get calcified. Rice bodies are fibrinous loose bodies associated with inflammatory rheumatoid arthritis.

25. **(B) Nora's lesion.**
The lesion described here is Nora's lesion or bizarre osteochondromatous proliferation. It is a rare, aggressive, tumorous lesion that involves hands and feet. Long tubular bones are rarely involved. It resembles osteochondroma radiologically. However, this lesion arises directly from the cortex, and lacks the characteristic continuity between lesional and cortical bone, seen in osteochondroma. Histologically, it can show a somewhat zonal proliferation of fibroblasts at the periphery, transitioning to cellular cartilage and immature bone adjacent to the cortex. Both florid reactive periostitis and subungual exostosis are in the differential. However, both these lesions are associated with trauma, while Nora's lesion is generally not related to trauma.

26. **(D) Painless lesion.**
The figure shows a tumor composed of immature woven bone with hypervascular stroma, characteristic of osteoid osteoma. Osteoid osteoma is benign bone-forming lesion that usually measures <1 cm. Nocturnal pain is a characteristic symptom, which is usually relieved by aspirin. It can occur in any bone; the majority of the cases arise in lower extremities. During surgery, the lesion may often be difficult to locate.

27. **(A) Enostosis (bone island).**
The lesion described in this question is best classified as enostosis or bone island. These are incidentally discovered lesions that may present with minimal pain. Because of the intramedullary location, the differential diagnosis includes intramedullary osteosarcoma, which is composed of trabecular bone (not lamellar bone) with infiltrative borders and malignant osteoid. Osteoblastic metastasis is composed of trabecular bone and is surrounded by nests of malignant epithelial cells. Osteoid osteoma and osteoblastic osteoma demonstrate trabecular bone with hypervascular stroma. Enostosis usually does not need to be treated. An autosomal-dominant form of this condition, known as osteopoikilosis, is characterized by multiple, bilateral, and symmetrical bone islands.

28. **(E) Osteoma.**
Osteoma is composed of woven and lamellar bone deposited in a cortical-type pattern rimmed with flat osteoblasts. All the features described in this question are characteristic of an osteoma, a benign bone-forming tumor that can mimic low-grade surface osteosarcoma (paraosteal osteosarcoma). The presence of flattened, bland osteoblasts and lack of cartilage helps in distinguishing these two entities. By definition, conventional osteosarcoma is composed of malignant osteoid. It shows infiltrative borders, and is usually located within medullary cavity of the bone. Osteoid osteoma and osteoblastoma, both characteristically demonstrate intertwining woven bone that is surrounded by cellular, richly vascularized stroma.

29. **(D) Infiltrative borders.**
Osteoblastoma is a benign bone-forming tumor that has several histologic variants that include cystic osteoblastoma, cartilage-forming osteoblastoma, aggressive osteoblastoma, and pseudomalignant osteoblastoma. Aggressive osteoblastoma is characterized by epithelioid osteoblasts that are 2–3 times the size of a normal osteoblast and show vesicular nuclei with prominent nucleoli. They can show coarse lace-like matrix deposition similar to an osteosarcoma. However, the presence of osteoblastic rimming and lack of significant cytologic atypia and atypical mitoses help in distinguishing this lesion from an osteosarcoma. Pseudomalignant osteoblastoma is another variant that may mimic an osteosarcoma. The osteoblasts in this variant are enlarged and have a degenerative/smudged appearance. Cystic osteoblastoma mimics an aneurysmal bone cyst, but lacks the organized pattern of bone deposition often seen in an aneurysmal bone cyst.

30. **(A) A minimum of 10% malignant osteoid production is required for diagnosis.**
The figure shows an example of an osteosarcoma, a tumor which is composed of bone matrix-producing

neoplastic cells. Any amount of neoplastic matrix, however minimal, is sufficient to categorize a tumor as an osteosarcoma. Osteosarcoma is the most common primary nonhematopoietic malignancy of the skeletal system. It primarily affects the metaphyseal region of distal femur, proximal tibia, and proximal humerus (foci of maximum bone growth). It has a bimodal peak age of presentation. Majority of the patients are adolescents and young adults.

31. **(C) Intramedullary well-differentiated osteosarcoma.**
The most common subtype of osteosarcoma is the conventional high-grade osteosarcoma (75–85%), followed by high-grade secondary osteosarcoma arising in a diseased bone (10%). The surface osteosarcomas comprise nearly 5–10% of osteosarcomas, and are further classified as well-differentiated juxtacortical osteosarcoma (parosteal osteosarcoma; 3–5%), juxtacortical intermediate-grade chondroblastic osteosarcoma (periosteal osteosarcoma; 2–4%), and high-grade surface osteosarcoma (1%). Of the given choices, intramedullary well-differentiated osteosarcoma is the least common subtype, and comprises 1% of all osteosarcomas.

32. **(D) Neoplastic cartilaginous areas admixed with severe cytologic atypia.**
Both parosteal and periosteal osteosarcomas are surface osteosarcomas that commonly occur in women. By definition, parosteal osteosarcomas are well-differentiated juxtacortical tumors that arise on the posterior aspect of the proximal femur. They are characterized by a fairly regular arrangement of woven bone surrounded by a cellular, bland-appearing, spindle cell proliferation. Hyaline cartilage, when present, is often seen in the form of a peripheral cap. The chondrocytes show mild to moderate cytologic atypia. Periosteal osteosarcomas usually affect the tibia, and by definition, are intermediate-grade chondroblastic osteosarcomas with lobules of cartilage containing severely atypical chondrocytes admixed with malignant osteoid. The tumor elicits a prominent periosteal reaction. Thus, all choices except D, are features associated with a parosteal osteosarcoma.

33. **(B) Chemotherapy.**
Osteosarcoma is associated with a variety of clinical conditions and syndromes. The best-known clinical association is radiation. Chemotherapy has not been associated with the development of osteosarcoma. Bloom, Rothmund-Thomson, Werner, Li-Fraumeni, and bilateral retinoblastoma syndrome, have been linked to development of osteosarcoma. In addition, osteosarcomas can also arise in the setting of preexisting bone diseases, such as Paget's disease, chronic osteomyelitis, and bone tumors, such as osteochondroma, enchondroma, fibrous dysplasia, osteoblastoma, giant cell tumor, unicameral bone cyst, and aneurysmal bone cyst.

34. **(E) Osteogenic sarcoma.**
Codman's triangle is commonly associated with osteogenic sarcoma. As the mass enlarges and invades beyond the cortex, layers of reactive new bone are deposited towards the proximal and distal aspect of the tumor. This increases the periosteal thickness and leads to the formation of Codman's triangle.

35. **(D) Osteochondroma.**
Osteochondroma is a benign, exophytic, cartilaginous tumor that occurs either in the sporadic (solitary) or syndromic (multiple) form. The common sites of involvement are distal femur, proximal tibia, and proximal humerus. Grossly, the medullary and cortical bony component of this lesion is in continuity with the underlying native bone. Histologically, the growth pattern resembles an epiphyseal growth plate. The tumor usually shows a thin (<1 cm) cartilaginous cap, below which are seen zones of endochondral ossification, regular trabecular bone, and fatty bone marrow. Malignant transformation is more common in the syndromic form of this tumor.

36. **(A) Abundant blue hyaline cartilage.**
The figure shows a chondroblastoma composed of uniform, oval, mononuclear cells, surrounded by amphophilic to eosinophilic fibrochondroid matrix. Although it is categorized as a cartilage-forming tumor, true hyaline cartilage is almost never seen in this tumor. Delicate pericellular calcification of the matrix is present in about 35% of cases. Secondary aneurysmal bone cyst formation has been documented in nearly 30% of cases.

37. **(C) Nodules of hyaline cartilage.**
The lesion shown in this figure is chondromyxoid fibroma, a benign tumor that typically arises in metaphysis of long bones. Proximal tibia is the most common location. Histologically, it is composed of nodules of myxoid matrix containing bland spindle-to-stellate cells. Increased cellularity with osteoclast-like giant cells is usually found towards the periphery of the nodules. Hyaline cartilage is almost never present in this tumor.

38. **(B) Islands of cartilage permeating viable, lamellar bone.**
The differential diagnosis of grade 1 chondrosarcoma is an enchondroma. Both the lesions are composed of nodules of hyaline cartilage. All the listed features (choices A, C, D, and E) are those of an enchondroma, except choice B, which is the best histologic criterion to diagnose a grade 1 chondrosarcoma.

Ring calcifications are due to mineralization of osteoid formed as a part of endochondral ossification in cartilaginous tumors. Nuclear atypia in a chondrocyte is typified by the ability to visualize nuclear details, such as vesicular chromatin, irregular nuclear membranes, and macronucleoli, at intermediate magnification (such as 200×). Radiologic findings of a pathologic fracture, periosteal reaction, cortical disruption, and soft tissue extension are features that are worrisome for a chondrosarcoma. While some degree of increased cellularity and cytologic atypia may be present in an enchondroma, the presence of permeation of viable, lamellar bone or infiltration of the Haversian canals warrants a diagnosis of a grade 1 chondrosarcoma. Binucleation can be present in benign as well as malignant tumors. Finally, the location of the lesion is also helpful. Enchondroma usually affects small tubular bones, while chondrosarcoma is a tumor of the pelvis, shoulder girdles, and ribs.

39. **(A) Commonly occurs in the ribs, jaw, and pelvis.**
The figure shows an example of a mesenchymal chondrosarcoma, a biphasic tumor that is composed of well-differentiated hyaline cartilage and a small round blue cell tumor. The small round blue cell component may show areas of spindling, hemorrhage, necrosis, and a hemangiopericytoma-like vascular pattern. As the small cell component may show immunoreactivity with CD99, Ewing's sarcoma needs to be excluded by other ancillary studies such as FISH. Unlike conventional chondrosarcoma, mesenchymal chondrosarcoma usually occurs in the second or third decade of life.

40. **(E) Nonossifying fibroma.**
The figure shows a benign tumor composed of spindle cell-rich stroma and multinucleated giant cells. The spindle cells show a storiform arrangement, and have uniform nuclei, changes diagnostic of nonossifying fibroma (metaphysical fibrous defect or fibrous cortical defect). The giant cells present in this lesion mimic a giant cell tumor. However, giant cell tumors involve both the epiphysis and metaphysis. Nonossifying fibromas are typically located in the metaphysis. Desmoplastic fibroma is composed of densely collagenized stroma admixed with bland spindle cells.

41. **(E) *FLI1*, chromosome 11.**
The clinical and pathologic features of this tumor are diagnostic of Ewing's sarcoma. It is composed of small cells with uniform round nuclei that show fine chromatin, inconspicuous nucleoli, and low mitotic activity. Spotty foci of necrosis and rosettes may be seen. The tumor usually demonstrates distinct types of periosteal reactions, such

as onion-skinning (layers of new bone formation), sunburst appearance (perpendicular orientation of new bone formation), Codman's triangle, and saucerization (concave pressure erosion of the cortex when bulk of the mass is confined between the periosteum and cortex). Membranous immunoreactivity with CD99 is often present. Cytogenetic analysis shows reciprocal translocation between the *EWS* gene located on chromosome 22 and rest of the genes listed in the question. The most frequent translocation involves the *FLI1* gene on chromosome 11.

42. **(C) Nuclei of multinucleated giant cells are different from those of the mononuclear cell population.**
The tumor depicted in this figure is giant cell tumor of the bone (also known as osteoclastoma). It commonly involves the metaphysis and epiphysis of long bones. It is a locally aggressive neoplasm, and <2% cases show evidence of distant metastasis. The multinucleated osteoclastic giant cells usually harbor several nuclei, and the nuclear features are identical to the mononuclear cell population present within the tumor (choice C is incorrect). The giant cells are uniformly distributed throughout the lesion. Abundant mitotic activity may be present; however, atypical mitotic figures are never seen. Osteoid deposition and spotty necrosis may be observed. The differential diagnosis of a giant cell-rich tumor includes aneurysmal bone cyst, benign fibrous histiocytoma, chondroblastoma, and giant cell-rich osteosarcoma.

43. **(B) CDX-2.**
The figure shows a lobulated neoplasm composed of cells with pale eosinophilic to bubbly cytoplasm (physaliphorous cells) and bland nuclei arranged in cords and clusters, embedded in a myxoid stroma. The chondroid variant almost exclusively occurs in the skull base. The tumor cells express brachyury, keratins 8/18, 19, epithelial membrane antigen, and S-100. Because of this patient's age, it is also important to exclude a metastatic carcinoma. CDX-2 is a marker of intestinal differentiation and would not be expected to be positive in this neoplasm.

44. **(A) Adamantinoma.**
The best diagnosis for this lytic lesion is adamantinoma. The figure shows epithelial cells surrounded by fibrous stroma. In some cases, the stroma may show woven bone rimmed by osteoblasts. Several histologic variants have been described: tubular, basaloid, squamous, spindle cell, osteofibrous dysplasia-like, and Ewing's sarcoma-like. Tubular variant (shown here) is the most common variant. The epithelial cells express pan-cytokeratin. Radiologically, the tumor shows multiple radiolucencies

surrounded by ring-shaped densities, giving rise to the typical "soap-bubble" appearance of this tumor.

45. **(C) Fibrous dysplasia.**
The lesion shown in this figure is composed of trabeculae of immature woven bone, without osteoblastic rimming, arranged in the form of Chinese characters or resembling the letters C, Y, and S. The rest of the choices are differentials for fibrous or fibro-osseous lesions. Desmoplastic fibroma (shows cortical destruction) and cemento-ossifying fibroma (usually can be shelled-out) can be differentiated on the basis of radiologic and clinical findings. Osteofibrous dysplasia is composed of woven bone and shows distinct osteoblastic rimming. Nonossifying fibroma lacks metaplastic bone formation. Fibrous dysplasia is now recognized as a non-neoplastic disorder resulting from a somatic mutation in the Gs alpha region of the *GNAS1* gene. McCune-Albright syndrome and Mazabraud syndrome are associated with this tumor.

46. **(A) Atypical mitotic activity can be seen.**
The lesion shown in this figure is diagnostic of nodular fasciitis, a variably cellular lesion composed of fibroblasts and myofibroblasts admixed with myxoid to collagenous stroma. The architecture is often referred to as "tissue-culture" pattern. The tumor shows delicate capillaries with extravasated red blood cells. Numerous mitotic figures may be seen; however, atypical mitoses are never present. The tumor cells express myofibroblastic markers, such as smooth muscle actin (tram-track pattern of staining), muscle-specific actin (clone HHF35), and calponin. Surgical resection is curative.

47. **(B) Elastofibroma.**
The lesion shown in this figure is an elastofibroma. The hallmark of this lesion is the presence of large, eosinophilic, fragmented elastic fibers, with a beaded appearance, embedded in a myxocollagenous and fatty stroma. The location of the lesion, and age of the patient, is quite typical of this lesion. None of the listed differentials contain elastic fibers diagnostic of this entity.

48. **(B) Fibrous hamartoma of infancy.**
The figure shows a lesion characterized by a triphasic pattern of mature fat, fascicles of fibroblastic proliferation, and myxoid areas of primitive mesenchymal cells, without evidence of mitotic activity or necrosis. These features are diagnostic of fibrous hamartoma of infancy. The lesional cells express CD34. The most common site of involvement is axilla and upper trunk. The lesion can recur locally. The hyalinized areas may resemble those seen in a giant cell fibroblastoma. Myofibroma usually shows a zonated growth pattern, with a peripheral myoid

appearance, and central hemangiopericytoma-like appearance. Lipofibromatosis (infantile fibromatosis) lacks the primitive mesenchymal elements seen in this lesion. Calcifying fibrotic aponeuroma is a fibroblastic lesion with abrupt foci of cartilaginous differentiation.

49. **(E) 90%.**
Desmoid-type fibromatosis usually occurs in distal extremities. It tends to be less cellular than superficial fibromatosis. About 90% of cases of desmoid-type fibromatosis show mutations in the *β-catenin* gene. This is reflected in the aberrant nuclear staining identified by immunohistochemistry.

50. **(E) Well-developed arborizing thick-walled vasculature.**
Myxoinflammatory fibroblastic sarcoma is a rare low-grade sarcoma arising in the distal extremities with a potential for local destruction. The lesion is characteristically composed of all the listed features, except for the presence of well-developed arborizing thick-walled vasculature, a feature typically associated with myxofibrosarcoma (myxoid malignant fibrous histiocytoma).

51. **(B) t(7;16).**
The figure shows an example of a low-grade fibromyxoid sarcoma (hyalinizing spindle cell tumor with giant rosettes) that is composed of spindle cells arranged in long sweeping fascicles in a myxoid and collagenous background. In myxoid areas, curvilinear or plexiform vessels can be seen. Occasionally, clusters of large rosettes with central hyalinized cores, surrounded by epithelioid cells, may also be seen in this lesion. The majority of these tumors show t(7;16) or supernumerary ring chromosomes composed of genetic material from chromosomes 7 and 16. Low-grade fibromyxoid sarcoma is considered to be one of the variants of adult fibrosarcoma; the other variants being conventional fibrosarcoma, sclerosing epithelioid fibrosarcoma, and myxofibrosarcoma. t(2;13) is associated with alveolar rhabdomyosarcoma, t(12;15) is found in infantile fibrosarcoma, t(12;22) is associated with angiomatoid fibrous histiocytoma, and t(17;22) is associated with dermatofibrosarcoma protuberans.

52. **(E) Usually occurs in sun-exposed areas.**
Atypical fibroxanthoma is a tumor composed of atypical spindle-to-pleomorphic cells with hyperchromatic nuclei in a fibrocollagenous background. These tumors tend to occur in sun-exposed areas, and affect older individuals. Radiation is considered to be another risk factor for this lesion. Numerous mitotic figures, including atypical mitoses, and multinucleated giant cells, are also seen. Touton-type giant cells may be present, but are not diagnostic of

this entity. The lesional cells express CD68, a histiocytic marker, but are negative for desmin and S-100. The differential diagnosis includes sarcomatoid carcinoma, melanoma, leiomyosarcoma, and malignant fibrous histiocytoma. It is distinguished from malignant fibrous histiocytoma by its size (usually <1.5 cm), dermal location, and lack of involvement of subcutaneous tissue.

53. **(B) CD34.**
Based on the clinical and pathologic features, the lesion described here is a dermatofibrosarcoma protuberans. It is a dermal-based proliferation of spindle cells arranged in a characteristic storiform pattern. The cells lack significant cytologic atypia or mitotic activity. They usually infiltrate the subcutaneous fat in a honeycomb or lace-like pattern. The lesional cells show strong immunoreactivity with CD34. Fibrosarcomatous transformation is characterized by increased cellularity, cytologic atypia, mitotic activity (>5 per 10 high-power fields), and less intense CD34 staining compared with the conventional tumor. The melanin-containing pigmented variant of this tumor is known as Bednar tumor. Giant cell fibroblastoma is the juvenile variant of this tumor that usually occurs in children younger than 5 years. All three lesions harbor t(17;22) translocation that fuses the *PDGF-β* gene with *COL1A1* gene.

54. **(B) Lesional cells that are positive for CD31 and CD34.**
Angiomatoid fibrous histiocytoma (AMFH) usually presents as a solitary subcutaneous mass involving the extremities. Other clinical symptoms that are associated with this lesion include fever, weight loss, anemia, and polyclonal gammopathy. All the listed findings, except choice B, are applicable to this entity. The tumor shows blood-filled cystic spaces that are lined by tumor cells, and not endothelial cells. Therefore, they do not express vascular markers CD31 and CD34. The cells have a unique immunophenotype in that they express desmin, epithelial membrane antigen, and CD68. The molecular alterations found in this tumor include t(12;22) (*FUS-ATF1*), t(11;22) (*EWS-ATF1*), and t(11;22) (*EWS-CREB1*); the latter two have also been described in clear cell sarcoma of soft tissue and gastrointestinal tract.

55. **(E) Spindle cell lipoma.**
The figure shows spindle cell lipoma that is marked by the presence of mature adipocytes and spindle cells admixed with ropey collagen fibers. Occasionally, hyperchromatic and multinucleated giant cells (floret cells) may also be seen, and represent the pleomorphic end of the spindle cell lipoma/

pleomorphic lipoma spectrum. Lipoblasts may also be seen. The lesional cells are diffusely positive for CD34.

56. **(A) Angiolipoma.**
Lipoblasts, once considered as a diagnostic hallmark of liposarcoma, are no longer a requisite criterion for diagnosing a liposarcoma. They may be present in many other benign adipocytic tumors, such as lipoblastoma, pleomorphic lipoma, chondroid lipoma, and spindle cell/pleomorphic lipoma.

57. **(C) Dedifferentiated foci have to show high-grade morphology.**
All the statements regarding dedifferentiated liposarcoma are true, except choice C. The dedifferentiated component does not have to show high-grade morphology. However, it does commonly occur in the form of an undifferentiated pleomorphic sarcoma or high-grade myxofibrosarcoma.

58. **(B) *DDIT3*.**
The figure shows a myxoid tumor with plexiform capillary network and rare monovacuolated lipoblasts, diagnostic of a myxoid liposarcoma. The lipoblasts usually tend to cluster around blood vessels. Within the spectrum of this lesion is round cell liposarcoma, which is composed of undifferentiated round hyperchromatic cells with increased mitotic activity and nuclear overlapping. The round cell component may constitute 5–80% of the lesion, and an increasing percentage of round cell component correlates with worse prognosis. Two distinct genetic events that have been documented in this entity include translocations involving the *DDIT3* gene on chromosome 12 and the *TLS* and *EWS* genes on chromosomes 16 and 22, respectively.

59. **(E) Venous subtype is most common histologic subtype.**
The lesion shown in this figure is an angioleiomyoma, which consists of fascicles of bland smooth muscle cells admixed with thin-walled vessels. Solid, venous, and cavernous, are the three histologic subtypes of this tumor. The solid variant shown in this figure is more common in women, involves the extremities, is very painful, and is the most common histologic subtype of angioleiomyoma. The cavernous and venous subtypes consist of smooth muscle bundles that are typically associated/merge with a vessel wall. Symplastic or degenerative nuclear changes can be rarely observed. However, any degree of true cytologic atypia should raise the suspicion for malignancy.

60. **(D) Marked cytologic atypia.**
All choices except D are typically associated with an EBV-associated smooth muscle tumor. A common clinical setting is that of multifocal lung and liver

lesions arising in immunocompromised patients (AIDS and post-transplantation). Histologically, the tumor shows a dual cell population composed of well-differentiated smooth muscle cells and small primitive cells. Admixed with the smooth muscle cells are small lymphocytes. Overall, the lesion resembles a well-differentiated smooth muscle neoplasm without significant cytologic atypia. Mitotic activity is variable. The tumor cells are positive for smooth muscle actin and express Epstein-Barr virus encoded early RNA (EBER).

61. **(D) Fetal rhabdomyoma.**
Depending on the age and location, mesenchymal tumors with skeletal muscle differentiation can be divided into adult, fetal, and genital rhabdomyomas. The tumor described in this question is the classic form of fetal rhabdomyoma. The immature form (cellular/intermediate rhabdomyoma) shows interlacing strap-like or ganglion-like cells. Lesions in the adults are typically composed of polygonal cells with eosinophilic granular or vacuolated cytoplasm. None of these tumors show cytologic atypia, mitotic activity, or necrosis. The fetal subtype can be difficult to distinguish from embryonal rhabdomyosarcoma; the latter characteristically shows prominent nuclear atypia.

62. **(C) Botyroid rhabdomyosarcoma.**
The age of the patient, and histologic and immunophenotypic findings, are those of a botyroid rhabdomyosarcoma. In addition to conventional rhabdomyosarcoma, choices A, C, and E, are the other subtypes of embryonal rhabdomyosarcoma. Thee botyroid variant characteristically shows a subepithelial, band-like condensation of primitive cells, known as the "cambium" layer. The tumor grossly presents as a polypoid lesion and typically involves hollow organs (gallbladder, cervix, etc.).

63. **(A) Intracytoplasmic PAS-positive crystalline inclusions.**
The tumor shown in this figure is an example of alveolar rhabdomyosarcoma. It usually affects extremities of young adults. The solid variant of this tumor is distinguished from alveolar soft part sarcoma by the lack of intracytoplasmic PAS-positive crystalline inclusions. The translocations associated with this tumor involve the *FKHR* gene on chromosome 13 and *PAX3* (chromosome 2) or *PAX7* (chromosome 1) genes. The t(1;13)-positive tumors have a less aggressive behavior compared with the t(2;13)-positive tumors. In general, alveolar rhabdomyosarcomas tend to have a poor prognosis.

64. **(E) Papillary endothelial hyperplasia.**
Papillary endothelial hyperplasia is a reactive vascular proliferation that usually occurs within a blood vessel and shows formation of pseudopapillary structures. In more developed lesions, the interanastomosing pattern can mimic an angiosarcoma. Papillary endothelial hyperplasia may involve a preexisting vascular neoplasm such as a hemangioma, especially in deeper locations.

65. **(B) Caused by infection with Human Herpes Virus-8.**
All the choices, except B, are associated with bacillary angiomatosis, which is a reactive vascular proliferation caused by infection with *Bartonella henselae* and *Bartonella quintana*. Histologically, the eosinophilic aggregates of fibrin often contain bacilli that can be highlighted by Warthin–Starry stain. In addition to FLI1, the lesional cells demonstrate immunoreactivity with other vascular markers, such as CD31, CD34, and factor VIII.

66. **(C) Glomeruloid hemangioma.**
Glomeruloid hemangioma is a rare vascular proliferation that occurs in nearly 25–45% of patients with POEMS syndrome (*p*olyneuropathy, *o*rganomegaly, *e*ndocrinopathy, *M*-protein, and *s*kin lesions). Histologically, this is a dermal lesion composed of ectatic blood vessels containing intraluminal nests of capillaries resembling glomeruli. In addition, the endothelial cells show large vacuoles that contain eosinophilic proteinaceous material (polytypic immunoglobulin).

67. **(D) GLUT1.**
While all the listed markers are positive in a variety of vascular neoplasms, GLUT1, or glucose transporter protein 1, expression is unique to juvenile capillary hemangioma. Juvenile capillary hemangioma usually shows more cellularity than a typical capillary hemangioma and contains large numbers of pericytic cells. Because of its solid growth pattern, the lesion may be confused with other round cell tumors.

68. **(D) Spindle cell hemangioma.**
Spindle cell hemangioma is a vascular proliferation that presents as a violaceous nodule involving the dermis/subcutaneous tissue. Histologically, this lesion shows dilated thin-walled vessels along with a zone of eosinophilic spindle cells that demonstrate slit-like spaces resembling Kaposi's sarcoma. Lack of mitotic activity, atypia, and inflammatory cells, is helpful in this distinction. The endothelial cells are epithelioid in appearance and contain vacuoles. Nearly 5% of cases are seen in association with Maffucci syndrome (hemangiomas and enchondromas).

69. **(C) Epithelioid hemangioma.**
Epithelioid hemangioma (angiolymphoid hyperplasia with eosinophilia) most commonly occurs as a small mass in the head and neck region. The

lesion commonly affects women and young adults. The endothelial cells protrude into the lumen (tombstone appearance) and show intracytoplasmic lumen formation, similar to epithelioid hemangioendothelioma. The accompanying inflammatory infiltrate is rich in eosinophils and lymphocytes.

70. **(E) vWF.**
CD31, FLI-1, and ERG are considered to have a >90% sensitivity for staining angiosarcoma compared to vWF. vWF is the least sensitive of all the listed markers and its sensitivity ranges from 50–75%.

71. **(A) Axon.**
A nerve is composed of axons surrounded by Schwann cells. Endoneurium is the connective tissue that surrounds axons, and is composed of Schwann cells, fibroblasts, collagen, capillaries, and mast cells. Groups of axons are, in turn, surrounded by perineurium and are referred to as a *fascicle*. As neurofibromas arise from the axon, they are composed of an admixture of several different cell types, including fibroblasts. In terms of treatment, due to their origin, the entire nerve must be removed in order to excise the lesion. In contrast, schwannomas are composed entirely of Schwann cells that encase the nerve and, thus, the tumor can be removed without disturbing the nerve.

72. **(D) Plexiform neurofibroma.**
Malignant transformation is most common in large, plexiform neurofibromas, followed by deep neurofibromas and cutaneous neurofibromas associated with NF1. Non-NF1-associated neurofibromas have a very low rate of malignant transformation. Plexiform neurofibroma is often associated with loose and hyperpigmented skin. Grossly, the enlarged and distorted nerve has a "bag of worms" appearance.

73. **(D) Wagner-Meissner bodies.**
Diffuse type neurofibroma usually presents as a plaque-like thickening of the dermis and infiltrates into the subcutaneous tissue in a honeycomb pattern, resembling dermatofibrosarcoma protuberans. Tactile corpuscle-like structures composed of elongated cells with eosinophilic cytoplasm, arranged in a whorled or lamellated configuration, referred to as Wagner-Meissner bodies, are characteristically associated with this entity.

74. **(E) Prominent S-100 immunoreactivity.**
Malignant transformation in a neurofibroma should be suspected when there is an increase in cellularity, particularly in areas with a fascicular growth pattern, uniform cytologic atypia, mitotic activity, and necrosis. The malignant foci usually show a reduction or complete loss of S-100 protein immunoreactivity.

75. **(A) Admixture of S-100, CD34, and EMA-positive cells.**
The figure shows a well-circumscribed tumor with a myxoid yellow cut surface. Given the close association with a nerve, these findings are suggestive of schwannoma. Neurofibromas usually arise in continuity with the main axis of the nerve. Immunohistochemically, schwannomas show uniform and diffuse immunoreactivity with S-100 protein that highlights Schwann cells. Occasionally, there may be rare foci of EMA-positive perineurial cells within the capsule or around vessels. Axons are never present. CD34 highlights intraneural fibroblasts, typically absent in schwannomas.

76. **(A) Carney complex.**
Psammomatous melanotic schwannoma is a melanin-containing tumor that arises from the sympathetic nervous system. As the name implies, the lesion is rich in psammomatous calcifications and melanin pigment-containing spindle cells with wavy nuclei. Up to 50% of patients with these tumors demonstrate other clinical findings of Carney's complex such as atrial myxomas, endocrine abnormalities, and pigment disorders. Klippel–Trenaunay syndrome is a congenital malformation associated with hemangiomas and varicose veins. MEN-2 is associated with mucosal neuromas. NF1 is associated with café-au-lait macules, neurofibromas, axillary freckling, optic glioma, Lisch nodules, and sphenoid dysplasia. NF2 is associated with bilateral acoustic schwannomas, meningiomas, gliomas, and lenticular opacities.

77. **(C) Malignant peripheral nerve sheath tumor.**
Based on the location, age, morphologic, and immunohistochemical features, the best diagnosis for this tumor is a malignant peripheral nerve sheath tumor (MPNST). The tumor occurs in older individuals and is composed of alternating hypocellular and hypercellular areas with foci of geographic necrosis. As opposed to the epithelioid variant, which shows diffuse, strong immunoreactivity with S-100 protein, the variant composed of spindle cells often shows weak staining with S-100. Monophasic synovial sarcoma is the closest differential; up to 20% of these tumors can also express S-100. Cytokeratin stain can be helpful, as monophasic synovial sarcomas usually show at least focal staining, while MPNSTs are generally negative. Additionally, monophasic synovial sarcomas are usually more eosinophilic in appearance while MPNSTs have a basophilic appearance.

78. **(A) Age at diagnosis <1 year.**
Low stage tumors, extra-adrenal location, lack of MYCN amplification, lack of 1p36 deletion, and low

mitosis-karyorrhexis index are associated with a better prognosis. Tumors that occur in children <1 year of age can undergo spontaneous involution. Tumors exhibiting differentiation and ganglion cells also have a relatively better prognosis.

79. **(A) Ankle/foot.**

The soft tissue tumor shown in this figure is a clear cell sarcoma characterized by the presence of epithelioid-to-spindled cells with clear-to-pale eosinophilic cytoplasm and prominent eosinophilic nucleoli (inset). It typically harbors the t(12;22) translocation involving the *EWS* and *ATF1* genes. It is the most common sarcoma of the foot and ankle. The tumor involves the tendon sheath, and is composed of nests of cells with prominent nucleoli. Multinucleate giant cells are fairly common. The cells express S-100 and a variety of melanocytic markers, and therefore, melanoma is an important differential diagnosis. Molecular testing and clinical information are important in this differential.

80. **(A) Extra-articular location.**

Giant cell tumor of tendon sheath (GCTTS) and pigmented villonodular synovitis (PVNS) represent the localized and diffuse forms of tenosynovial giant cell tumor. Both the tumors show overlapping histologic features and are composed of a nodular tumor with mononuclear cells and osteoclast-like giant cells. GCTTS usually presents as a single nodule and may involve extra-articular locations. Compared to PVNS, it is associated with sclerotic stroma, lesser hemosiderin, and more numerous giant cells.

81. **(D) 90%.**

Epithelioid sarcomas coexpress cytokeratin and vimentin. They do not express cytokeratin 5/6. Nearly 90% of tumors characteristically show loss of INI-1 protein expression. This finding helps in distinguishing them from carcinomas and other sarcomas. The tumor presents as an ulcerated nodule on the finger, hand, or arm. Histologically, it is composed of epithelioid cells, often surrounding a zone of necrosis. Proximal-type epithelioid sarcomas contain more pleomorphism and numerous rhabdoid cells.

SUGGESTED READING

1. Greenspan A, Steiner G, Knutzon R. Bone island (enostosis): clinical significance and radiologic and pathologic correlations. *Skeletal Radiol.* 1991;20(2):85-90.

2. Sundaram M, Falbo S, McDonald D, Janney C. Surface osteomas of the appendicular skeleton. *AJR Am J Roentgenol.* 1996 Dec;167(6):1529-1533.

3. Lucas DR, Unni KK, McLeod RA, O'Connor MI, Sim FH. Osteoblastoma: clinicopathologic study of 306 cases. *Hum Pathol.* 1994 Feb;25(2):117-134.

4. Unni KK, Dahlin DC. Osteosarcoma: pathology and classification. *Semin Roentgenol.* 1989 Jul;24(3):143-152.

5. Unni KK. Cartilaginous lesions of bone. *J Orthop Sci.* 2001; 6(5):457-472.

6. de Silva MV, Reid R. Chondroblastoma. *Ann Diagn Pathol.* 2003;7(4):205-213.

7. Wu CT, Inwards CY, O'Laughlin S, et al. Chondromyxoid fibroma. *Hum Pathol.* 1998;29:438-446.

8. Giudici MA, Moser RP Jr., Kransdorf MJ. Cartilaginous bone tumors. *Radiol Clin North Am.* 1993;31(2):237-259.

9. Murphey MD, Walker EA, Wilson AJ, et al. From the archives of the AFIP: imaging of primary chondrosarcoma: radiologic-pathologic correlation. *Radiographics.* 2003;23(5): 1245-1247.

10. Nakashima Y, Unni KK, Shives TC, Swee RG, Dahlin DC. Mesenchymal chondrosarcoma of bone and soft tissue. A review of 111 cases. *Cancer.* 1986 Jun 15;57(12):2444-2453.

11. Oliveira AM, Nascimento AG. Grading in soft tissue tumors: principles and problems. *Skeletal Radiol.* 2001;18;30:543-559.

12. Betsy M, Kupersmith LM, Springfield DS. Metaphyseal fibrous defects. *J Am Acad Orthop Surg.* 2004;12:89-95.

13. Folpe AL, Goldblum JR, Rubin BP, et al. Morphologic and immunophenotypic diversity in Ewing family tumors. A study of 66 genetically confirmed cases. *Am J Surg Pathol.* 2005;29:1025-1033.

14. Reid R, Banerjee SS, Sciot R. Giant cell tumor. *World Health Organization Classification of Tumors: Pathology and Genetics of Tumors of Soft tissue and Bone.* Lyon, France, IARC Press, 2002.

15. Yamaguchi T, Suzuki S, Ishiiwa H, et al. Benign notochordal cell tumors: a comparative histological study of benign notochordal cell tumors, classic chordomas, and notochordal vestiges of fetal intervertebral discs. *Am J Surg Pathol.* 2004;28:756-761.

16. Tirabosco R, Mangham DC, Rosenberg AE, et al. Brachyury expression in extra-axial skeletal and soft tissue chordomas: a marker that distinguishes chordoma from mixed tumor/myoepithelioma/parachordoma in soft tissue. *Am J Surg Pathol.* 2008;32(4):572-580.

17. Jain D, Jain VK, Vasishta RK, et al. Adamantinoma: a clinicopathological review and update. *Diagn Pathol.* 2008;3:8.

18. Riminucci M, Liu B, Corsi A, et al. Histopathology of fibrous dysplasia of bone in patients with activating mutations of the Gs alpha gene: sites-specific patterns and recurrent histological hallmarks. *J Pathol.* 1999;187:249-258.

19. Montgomery EA, Meis JM. Nodular fasciitis. Its morphologic spectrum and immunohistochemical profile. *Am J Surg Pathol.* 1991;15:942-948.

20. Miyoshi Y, Iwao K, Nawa G, et al. Frequent mutations in the beta-catenin gene in desmoid tumors from patients without familial adenomatous polyposis. *Oncol Res.* 1998; 10:591-594.

21. Montgomery EA, Devaney KO, Giordano TJ, et al. Inflammatory myxohyaline tumor of distal extremities with virocyte or Reed-Sternberg like cells: a distinctive lesion with

features simulating inflammatory conditions, Hodgkin's disease, and various sarcomas. *Mod Pathol*. 1998;11:384-391.

22. Evans H. Low-grade fibromyxoid sarcoma. A report of 12 cases. *Am J Surg Pathol*. 1993;17:595-600.

23. Guillou L, Benhattar J, Gengler C, et al. Translocation-positive low-grade fibromyxoid sarcoma: clinicopathologic and molecular analysis of a series expanding the morphologic spectrum and suggesting potential relationship to sclerosing epithelioid fibrosarcoma: a study from the French Sarcoma Group. *Am J Surg Pathol*. 2007;31:1387-1402.

24. Fletcher CDM. Benign fibrous histiocytoma of subcutaneous and deep soft tissue: a clinicopathologic analysis of 21 cases. *Am J Surg Pathol*. 1990;14:801-809.

25. Longacre TA, Smoller BR, Rouse RV. Atypical fibroxanthoma. Multiple immunohistologic profiles. *Am J Surg Pathol*. 1993;17:1199-1206.

26. Minoletti F, Miozzo M, Pedeutour F, et al. Involvement of chromosomes 17 and 22 in dermatofibrosarcoma protuberans. *Genes Chromosom Cancer*. 1995;13:62-65.

27. Fanburg-Smith JC, Miettinen M. Angiomatoid malignant fibrous histiocytoma: a clinicopathologic study of 158 cases and further exploration of the myoid phenotype. *Hum Pathol*. 1999;30:1336-1343.

28. Mentzel T, Calonje E, Fletcher CDM. Lipoblastoma and lipoblastomatosis: a clinicopathological study of 14 cases. *Histopathology*. 1993;23:527-533.

29. Henricks WH, Chu YC, Goldblum JR, et al. Dedifferentiated liposarcoma: a clinicopathologic analysis of 155 cases with proposal for an expanded definition of dedifferentiation. *Am J Surg Pathol*. 1997;21:271-281.

30. Orvieto E, Furlanetto A, Laurino L, et al. Myxoid and round cell liposarcoma: a spectrum of myxoid adipocytic neoplasia. *Semin Diagn Pathol*. 2001;18:267-273.

31. Deyrup AT, Lee VK, Hill CE, et al. Epstein-Barr virus-associated smooth muscle tumors are distinctive mesenchymal tumors reflecting multiple infection events: a clinicopathologic and molecular analysis of 29 tumors from 19 patients. *Am J Surg Pathol*. 2006 Jan;30(1):75-82.

32. Sorensen PHB, Lynch JC, Qualman SJ, et al. PAX3-FKHR and PAX-7FKHR gene fusions are prognostic indicators in alveolar rhabdomyosarcoma: a report from the children s oncology group. *J Clin Oncol*. 2002;11:2672-2679.

33. Perkins P, Weiss SW. Spindle cell hemangioendothelioma. An analysis of 78 cases with reassessment of its pathogenesis and biologic behavior. *Am J Surg Pathol*. 1996;20:1196-1204.

34. Fetsch JF, Weiss SW. Observations concerning the pathogenesis of epithelioid hemangioma (angiolymphoid hyperplasia) *Mod Pathol*. 1991;4:449-455.

35. Ferner RE, O'Doherty MJ. Neurofibroma and schwannoma. *Curr Opin Neurol*. 2002;15:679-684.

36. Utiger CA, Headington JT. Psammomatous melanotic schwannoma. A new cutaneous marker for Carney's complex. *Arch Dermatol*. 1993;129:202-204.

37. Zhou H, Coffin CM, Perkins SL, et al. Malignant peripheral nerve sheath tumor: a comparison of grade, immunophenotype, and cell cycle/growth activation marker expression in sporadic and neurofibromatosis 1-related lesions. *Am J Surg Pathol*. 2003;27:1337-1345.

38. Shimada H, Ambros IM, Dehner LP, et al. Terminology and morphologic criteria of neuroblastic tumors. Recommendations by the International Neuroblastoma Pathology Committee. *Cancer*. 1999;86:349-363.

39. Antonescu CR, Tschernyavsky SJ, Woodruff JM, et al. Molecular diagnosis of clear cell sarcoma: detection of EWS-ATF1 and MITF-M transcripts and histopathological and ultrastructural analysis of 12 cases. *J Mol Diagn*. 2002;4:44-52.

40. Folpe AL. Tenosynovial giant cell tumor and pigmented villonodular synovitis. *Skeletal Radiol*. 2007;36:899-900.

41. Laskin WB, Miettinen M. Epithelioid sarcoma: new insights based on an extended immunohistochemical analysis. *Arch Pathol Lab Med*. 2003;127:1161-1168.

CHAPTER 6

BREAST PATHOLOGY

1. A 45-year-old woman has a screening mammogram, and a stellate lesion is identified. An excisional biopsy was performed (see Figure 6-1). Which of the following features is characteristic of this lesion?

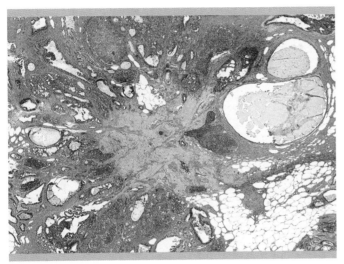

FIGURE 6-1

(A) Absence of myoepithelial cells on immunohistochemical staining
(B) Angular-shaped glands with open lumens
(C) Desmoplastic, cellular stroma
(D) Minimal cytologic atypia
(E) Peripheral lobular architecture around a central scar

2. A 47-year-old woman has a breast biopsy, which shows the following change within a large duct (see Figure 6-2). Which of the following statements regarding this process is accurate?

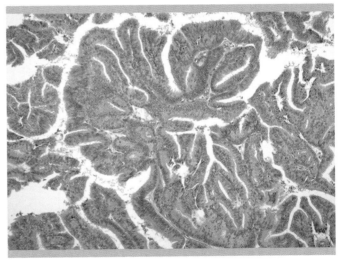

FIGURE 6-2

(A) Excision is not required
(B) Fibrovascular cores are well developed and thick
(C) Immunohistochemical staining for myoepithelial cells will be negative
(D) Most patients present with a nipple discharge
(E) Usual-type epithelial hyperplasia is common

3. A 61-year-old woman has a breast biopsy (see Figure 6-3). Which of the following features would favor an interpretation of usual ductal hyperplasia rather than low-grade ductal carcinoma in situ?

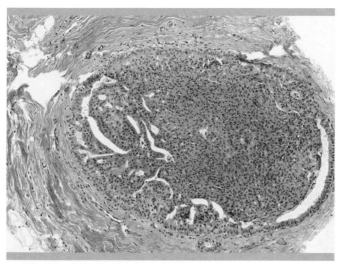

FIGURE 6-3

(A) Attenuated or incomplete myoepithelial layer
(B) Distinct epithelial cell margins
(C) Nuclei parallel to the direction of the epithelial bridge
(D) Rounded spaces within the epithelial proliferation
(E) Spaces evenly distributed throughout the epithelial proliferation

4. A 43-year-old woman has a right breast biopsy (see Figure 6-4). What is her lifetime risk of developing invasive carcinoma in the contralateral (left) breast?

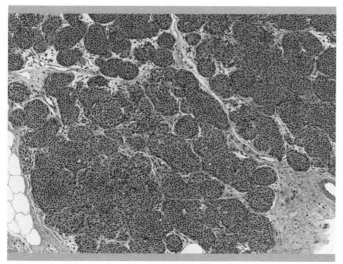

FIGURE 6-4

(A) She is not at risk for developing breast cancer
(B) The risk is identical to her right breast
(C) The risk is 20% higher compared with her right breast
(D) The risk is 20% less compared with her right breast
(E) The risk is 40% less compared with her right breast

5. A 57-year-old woman presents to her physician for a unilateral red nipple with a scale crust. A biopsy of the nipple is performed (see Figure 6-5). Which of the following is accurate regarding this process?

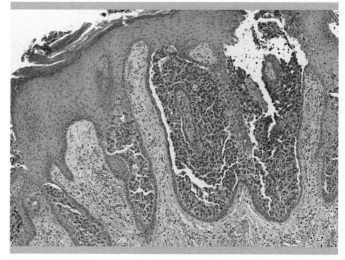

FIGURE 6-5

(A) A patient with ductal carcinoma in situ and this finding is staged as pT4 disease due to skin involvement
(B) Less than 50% of cases are associated with an underlying invasive or in situ mammary carcinoma
(C) Melanocytic markers are usually positive in these lesions
(D) Occurs in approximately 10% of patients with breast cancer
(E) The neoplastic cells are positive for HER2 immunohistochemical expression

6. A 53-year-old woman has a breast biopsy performed (see Figure 6-6). At local excision, which of the following features is most important in predicting recurrence in this breast?

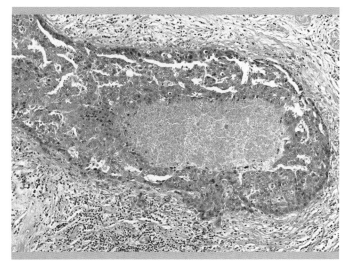

FIGURE 6-6

(A) Distance to margin <1 mm
(B) Estrogen receptor positivity
(C) Greatest dimension of the lesion
(D) High nuclear grade
(E) Necrosis

7. A 61-year-old woman has a punch biopsy of the skin of her breast performed, which shows the following change (see Figure 6-7). What clinical exam finding is typical in patients with this process?

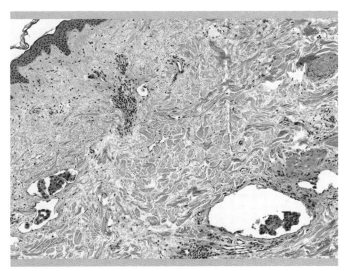

FIGURE 6-7

(A) Bilateral milky nipple discharge
(B) Black-brown nodule with irregular borders
(C) Puckered skin involved by a firm exophytic mass
(D) Red swollen breast that has an irregular surface, resembling the surface of an orange
(E) Scaly white plaques and patches

8. A woman undergoes a breast excision (see Figure 6-8). Which of the following findings would favor an interpretation of lobular carcinoma in situ (LCIS) over cancerization of the lobules by ductal carcinoma in situ (DCIS)?

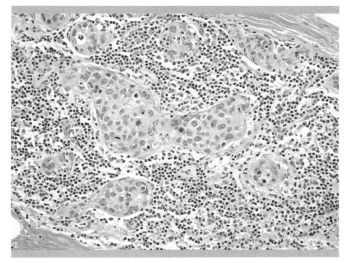

FIGURE 6-8

(A) Fibroplasia in the surrounding stroma
(B) Large pleomorphic cells with significant atypia
(C) No staining for high-molecular weight cytokeratin
(D) Presence of DCIS in surrounding ducts
(E) Strong staining for E-cadherin

9. A 58-year-old woman undergoes a modified radi-
    cal mastectomy for breast cancer (see Figure 6-9).
    Which of the following features, if present, would
    likely mitigate the more favorable prognosis
    typically associated with this lesion?

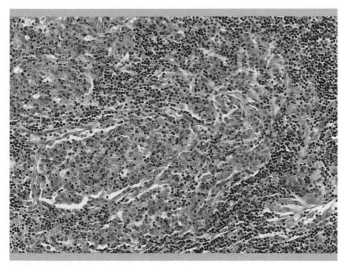

FIGURE 6-9

(A) Absent lymphoplasmacytic infiltrate
(B) >75% syncytial growth pattern
(C) High mitotic rate
(D) Pleomorphic (high grade) nuclei
(E) Well-circumscribed microscopically

10. A 67-year-old woman has a breast biopsy (see
    Figure 6-10). All of the following statements
    regarding this lesion are true except

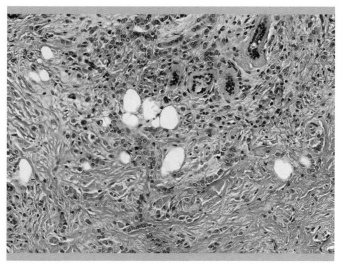

FIGURE 6-10

(A) E-cadherin immunohistochemistry is negative
(B) Intracytoplasmic mucin droplets are
    characteristic
(C) Margin assessment is problematic due to "skip"
    lesions
(D) Retained normal breast structures is common
(E) Typically presents as microcalcifications on
    mammography

11. A 56-year-old woman undergoes local excision of a
    breast lesion (see Figure 6-11). All of the following
    statements regarding this lesion are true except

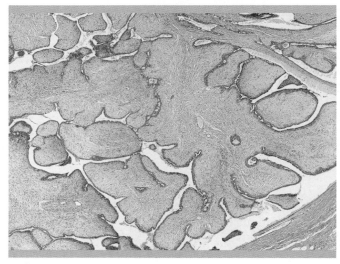

FIGURE 6-11

(A) Absence of epithelial elements in a low-power
    field is a worrisome feature for malignancy
(B) Heterologous elements (liposarcoma) can be
    seen
(C) Hypercellular stroma is a worrisome feature for
    malignancy
(D) Metastases are most commonly composed of
    the stromal component
(E) Surgical excision with wide margins is required

12. A 41-year-old woman undergoes excisional biopsy
    of a breast mass (see Figure 6-12). What immuno-
    histochemical staining profile will the lesional cells
    demonstrate?

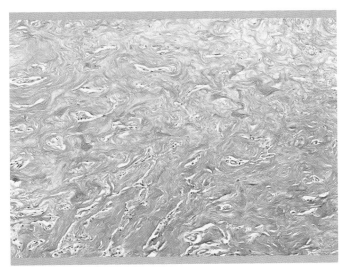

FIGURE 6-12

(A) Positive for CD31 and factor VIII; negative for smooth muscle actin, cytokeratin
(B) Positive for cytokeratin and E-cadherin; negative for CD31, smooth muscle actin, factor VIII
(C) Positive for cytokeratin; negative for CD31, E-cadherin, smooth muscle actin, factor VIII
(D) Positive for S-100; negative for CD31 and cytokeratin
(E) Positive for smooth muscle actin; negative for CD31, factor VIII, cytokeratin

13. A breast biopsy shows the following features (see Figure 6-13). What is the most likely clinical history associated with this process?

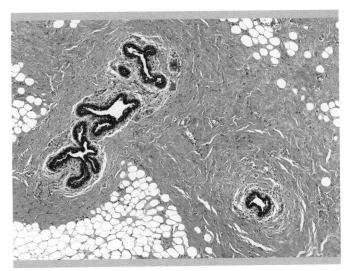

FIGURE 6-13

(A) A 13-year-old boy with breast enlargement
(B) A 23-year-old woman with a rubbery well-circumscribed mass
(C) A 45-year-old woman with bloody nipple discharge
(D) A 54-year-old woman with microcalcifications on mammography
(E) A 71-year-old woman with a spiculated mass on magnetic resonance imaging

14. A 36-year-old woman presents with a palpable breast lump. A biopsy is performed (see Figure 6-14). What clinical history is she most likely to provide upon additional questioning?

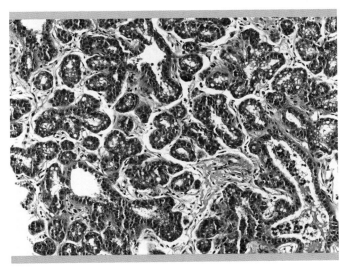

FIGURE 6-14

(A) Family history of early breast cancer and uterine cancer
(B) Recent pregnancy and breastfeeding
(C) Recent trauma to the breast
(D) Swollen red breast with peau d'orange-like texture
(E) Variable breast tenderness that follows her menstrual cycle

15. A 58-year-old woman has a breast biopsy performed (see Figure 6-15). Which of the following statements is true regarding this lesion?

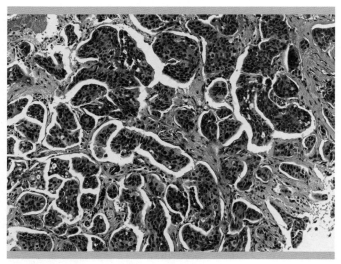

FIGURE 6-15

(A) Almost always a "pure" tumor morphology
(B) Better prognosis than invasive ductal carcinoma, no specific type
(C) Epithelial membrane antigen immunohistochemical staining shows "inside out" apical staining
(D) Less than 40% of cases have lymph node metastasis at presentation
(E) Majority of cases are negative for estrogen receptor immunohistochemistry

16. A 66-year-old woman undergoes biopsy of a breast mass (see Figure 6-16). What is the most appropriate management of this tumor?

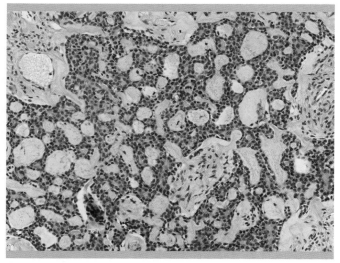

FIGURE 6-16

(A) Complete excision with axillary lymph node dissection
(B) Complete excision with optional sentinel lymph node biopsy
(C) Complete excision with subsequent estrogen receptor-antagonist therapy (e.g., tamoxifen)
(D) Modified radical mastectomy with adjuvant chemotherapy
(E) No excision is necessary due to the benign natural history of this disease

17. A 14-year-old girl presents with a breast mass near the areola. A biopsy is performed (see Figure 6-17). What genetic abnormality is associated with this lesion?

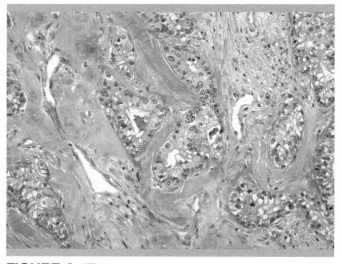

FIGURE 6-17

(A) *BRCA1* mutation
(B) *HER2* amplification
(C) *TP53* mutation
(D) t(X;18) *SYT–SSX* translocation
(E) t(12;15) *ETV6–NTRK3* translocation

18. A 75-year-old woman presents with red nodules on the skin of her breast. A biopsy was performed (see Figure 6-18). What clinical history is most likely to be associated with this lesion?

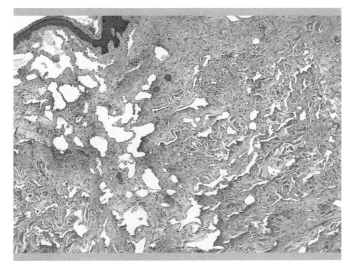

FIGURE 6-18

   (A) Chronic sun damage and atypical nevus
   (B) Swelling and enlargement of the breast with a deep ill-defined mass
   (C) Previous contralateral invasive lobular carcinoma and mastectomy
   (D) Previous ipsilateral invasive ductal carcinoma and lumpectomy
   (E) Weeping, crusted nipple and underlying spiculated lesion on mammography

19. A 36-year-old woman is found to have a well-circumscribed lesion involving the nipple (see Figure 6-19). All of the following statements regarding this process are true except

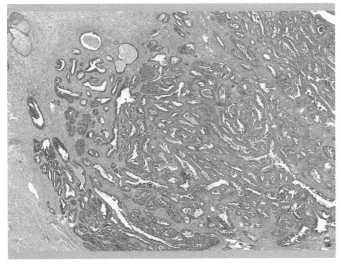

FIGURE 6-19

   (A) Complete excision is recommended to prevent recurrence
   (B) Haphazard architecture can mimic infiltrating carcinoma
   (C) Highly associated with an underlying breast carcinoma
   (D) Often associated with papillary proliferations in adjacent ducts
   (E) The glands are lined by two cell layers (epithelial and myoepithelial)

20. A 41-year-old woman undergoes breast reduction surgery, and the following finding is present in one duct profile (see Figure 6-20). What is the origin of the eosinophilic hyaline material present?

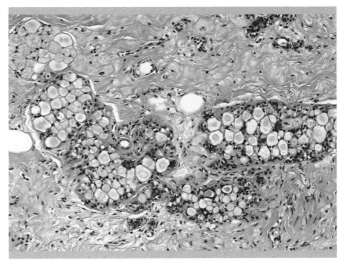

FIGURE 6-20

   (A) Basement membrane proteins produced by myoepithelial cells
   (B) Foreign material secondary to prior surgery
   (C) Mucin produced by signet ring carcinoma
   (D) Organizing fibrin formed secondary to intra-ductal hemorrhage
   (E) Secretory product produced by apocrine epithelial cells

21. A 52-year-old woman undergoes breast core biopsy
    that shows several dilated ducts lined by the follow-
    ing epithelium (see Figure 6-21). What is the most
    appropriate management based on the findings
    present in this core biopsy?

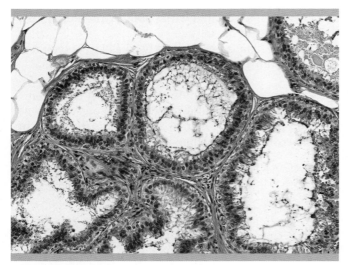

FIGURE 6-21

   (A) Local excision of this area to exclude malignancy
   (B) Repeat core biopsy
   (C) Return to routine screening
   (D) Sentinel lymph node biopsy and wide local
       excision
   (E) Simple mastectomy

22. A 53-year-old woman undergoes breast excision
    (see Figure 6-22). What is the expected estrogen
    receptor (ER), progesterone receptor (PR), and
    E-cadherin immunohistochemical profile of this
    proliferation?

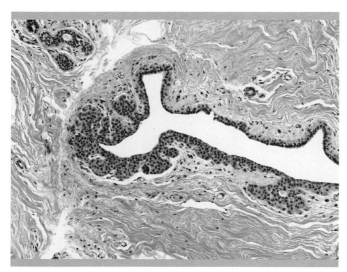

FIGURE 6-22

   (A) Negative for ER, PR, and E-cadherin
   (B) Positive for E-cadherin and negative for ER and
       PR
   (C) Positive for ER and negative for PR and
       E-cadherin
   (D) Positive for ER and PR and negative for
       E-cadherin
   (E) Positive for ER, PR, and E-cadherin

23. A 49-year-old woman has a palpable mass in the
    subareolar region. A biopsy is performed (see
    Figure 6-23). What the best interpretation?

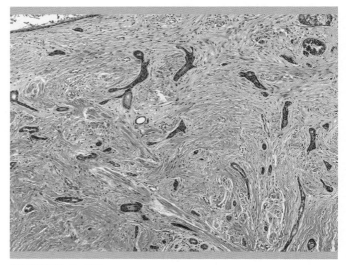

FIGURE 6-23

   (A) Nipple adenoma
   (B) Solitary intraductal papilloma
   (C) Syringomatous adenoma
   (D) Subareolar mastitis
   (E) Tubular carcinoma

24. A 47-year-old woman is found to have a discrete,
    well-circumscribed radiodensity on mammography,
    which the surgeon enucleates easily at local exci-
    sion. However, on histopathologic examination,
    the lesion has the following appearance (see
    Figure 6-24). What is the best interpretation
    based on the clinical findings?

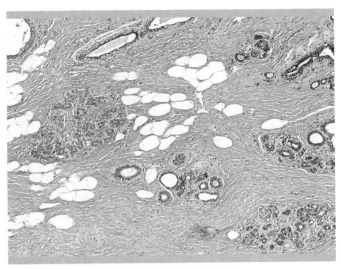

FIGURE 6-24

   (A) Fibroadenoma
   (B) Invasive ductal carcinoma
   (C) Mammary hamartoma
   (D) Normal breast
   (E) Phyllodes tumor

25. A 53-year-old woman undergoes a breast biopsy, which demonstrates microglandular adenosis. All of the following are true regarding this lesion except
   (A) Complete excision is recommended to exclude malignancy
   (B) Luminal material is periodic acid Schiff positive, diastase resistant
   (C) Solitary glands within fibroadipose tissue are indicative of invasion
   (D) Strong S-100 staining is typical
   (E) The gland profiles lack myoepithelial cells

26. What is the current recommended handling protocol for the evaluation of clinically negative sentinel lymph nodes in the workup of invasive breast cancer according to the College of American Pathologists?
   (A) Section at 1-mm intervals and submit every other section
   (B) Section at 1-mm intervals and submit the entire node
   (C) Section at 2-mm intervals and submit every other section
   (D) Section at 2-mm intervals and submit the entire node
   (E) Section at 5-mm intervals and submit the entire node

27. A 72-year-old woman presents with a breast mass. On core biopsy, abundant mucinous material is seen. Which of the following features would favor a diagnosis of mucocele-like lesion over mucinous (colloid) carcinoma?
   (A) Adjacent ducts containing ductal carcinoma in situ
   (B) Cribriform clusters of epithelial cells lacking calponin staining
   (C) Immunohistochemical staining for synaptophysin
   (D) Rare epithelial cells present within the mucin
   (E) Strips of epithelial cells positive for p63

28. A woman undergoes breast biopsy and is found to have ductal carcinoma in situ (DCIS). A small focus of invasion is identified along the profile of one large duct. What size must this area be in order to qualify as microinvasion?
   (A) ≤0.5 mm
   (B) ≤1.0 mm
   (C) ≤3.0 mm
   (D) ≤5.0 mm
   (E) There is no definition for microinvasion in the breast

29. Which of the following lesions, if present on a breast biopsy, is associated with a mildly increased risk of developing invasive carcinoma over a woman's lifetime when compared with a woman without any other risk factors?
   (A) Apocrine metaplasia
   (B) Duct ectasia
   (C) Fibroadenoma
   (D) Nonproliferative fibrocystic change
   (E) Sclerosing adenosis

30. A 35-year-old woman has a strong family history of breast cancer, and genetic testing demonstrates a *BRCA1* gene mutation. All of the following statements regarding this genetic alteration are true except
   (A) Associated with poorly differentiated breast cancers
   (B) Between 20% and 40% of women with this mutation will develop ovarian cancer
   (C) High association with HER2 positive breast cancers
   (D) Lifetime risk of breast cancer is 40–90%
   (E) Prevalence is higher in Ashkenazi Jewish women

31. Which of the following is not associated with an increased risk of developing breast cancer?
    (A) First-degree relative with breast cancer
    (B) Non-Hispanic white ethnicity
    (C) Postmenopausal hormone replacement therapy
    (D) Younger age at first live birth (20 years or younger)
    (E) Younger age at menarche (11 years or younger)

32. A 39-year-old woman is diagnosed with bilateral invasive ductal carcinomas. Her history is notable for a previous osteosarcoma of the humerus at age 23 years. What genetic syndrome and mutation are most likely present in this woman?
    (A) Cowden syndrome, *PTEN* mutation
    (B) Hereditary breast and ovarian carcinoma syndrome, *BRCA1* mutation
    (C) Li–Fraumeni syndrome, *TP53* mutation
    (D) Lynch syndrome, *MLH1* mutation
    (E) von Hippel–Lindau syndrome, *VHL* mutation

33. Recent studies using gene expression profiling of breast carcinomas have identified five major patterns of gene expression, the most common of which is "luminal A." Which of the following best describes luminal A type breast cancers' morphologic appearance and immunohistochemical staining pattern for estrogen receptor (ER), progesterone receptor (PR), and HER2?
    (A) Moderately differentiated HER2 positive invasive ductal carcinoma
    (B) Poorly differentiated triple negative (ER, PR, HER2) invasive ductal carcinoma
    (C) Poorly differentiated triple positive (ER, PR, HER2) invasive ductal carcinoma
    (D) Well-differentiated ER-positive invasive ductal carcinoma
    (E) Well-differentiated ER-positive invasive lobular carcinoma

34. Which of the following special types of invasive breast carcinoma is associated with a worse prognosis than infiltrating ductal carcinoma, not otherwise specified?
    (A) Adenoid cystic carcinoma
    (B) Basal-like carcinoma
    (C) Colloid carcinoma
    (D) Medullary carcinoma
    (E) Tubular carcinoma

35. Which of the following findings on breast needle core biopsy can be followed without surgical excision?
    (A) Acellular stromal mucin pools
    (B) Atypical lobular hyperplasia in a woman with a mass

    (C) Columnar cell lesion with atypia (flat epithelial atypia)
    (D) Fibroadenoma without atypia and with an appropriate clinical exam
    (E) Papillary lesion

36. Which of the following factors is the most important predictor of death in women with invasive carcinoma of the breast?
    (A) Estrogen receptor status
    (B) Histologic grade
    (C) Mitotic rate
    (D) Sentinel lymph node status
    (E) Tumor size

37. The Nottingham Grading System (NGS) is used to determine the grade of invasive carcinomas of the breast and is an important independent prognostic factor. Which of the following tumor descriptions is appropriately graded [assume a high-power field (HPF) diameter of 0.50 mm]?
    (A) Invasive ductal carcinoma with 20% tubule formation, marked pleomorphism, and 25 mitotic figures per 10 HPF—grade 2
    (B) Invasive ductal carcinoma with 50% tubule formation, moderate nuclear atypia, and 11 mitotic figures per 10 HPF—grade 3
    (C) Invasive ductal carcinoma with 90% tubule formation, marked pleomorphism, and 2 mitotic figures per 10 HPF—grade 1
    (D) Invasive lobular carcinoma with 5% tubule formation, marked pleomorphism, and 3 mitotic figures per 10 HPF—grade 1
    (E) Invasive lobular carcinoma with 5% tubule formation, minimal atypia, and 1 mitotic figure per 10 HPF—grade 2

38. A woman has a breast biopsy that shows a marked epithelial proliferation within a duct profile. The differential diagnosis includes low-grade ductal carcinoma in situ (DCIS), lobular carcinoma in situ involving a duct, or usual ductal hyperplasia. Which immunohistochemical staining profile would favor an interpretation of low-grade DCIS?
    (A) 34BE12 (cytokeratin 903) and cytokeratin 5/6 (CK5/6) cannot distinguish between usual ductal hyperplasia and in situ carcinoma
    (B) Negative for 34BE12 (cytokeratin 903) and CK5/6
    (C) Positive for 34BE12 (cytokeratin 903) and CK5/6
    (D) Positive for 34BE12 (cytokeratin 903), negative for CK5/6
    (E) Positive for CK5/6 and negative for 34BE12 (cytokeratin 903)

39. A 43-year-old woman who has a germline *BRCA1* gene mutation presents with pulmonary insufficiency and is found to have a large pleural effusion. Her history is significant for an invasive ductal carcinoma of the breast and high-grade ovarian serous carcinoma. Which panel of immunohistochemical stains would be most useful in determining the site of origin of her pleural metastasis?
    (A) Cytokeratin 7 and cytokeratin 20
    (B) Cytokeratin 20 and estrogen receptor
    (C) Estrogen receptor and progesterone receptor
    (D) Gross cystic disease fluid protein (GCDFP) and TTF-1
    (E) Gross cystic disease fluid protein (GCDFP) and WT1

40. A woman with invasive ductal carcinoma of the breast undergoes sentinel lymph node biopsy, and after careful hematoxylin and eosin examination, no tumor cells are seen. Immunohistochemical staining with cytokeratin is performed. All of the following statements regarding immunohistochemical staining of sentinel lymph nodes for breast cancer are true except
    (A) Benign nodal reticulum cells can be positive for cytokeratin
    (B) Immunohistochemistry for the detection of metastatic breast carcinoma in sentinel lymph nodes is controversial
    (C) Morphology and location of cytokeratin positive cells are important in final evaluation
    (D) Rare single cells identified by immunohistochemistry alone are classified as pN0(i+)
    (E) Tumor cells measuring 1.0 mm identified by IHC alone are classified as pN1mi(i+)

41. A woman undergoes breast core biopsy for microcalcifications on mammogram, and an interpretation of flat epithelial atypia (columnar cell lesion with atypia) is rendered. What is the most likely neoplasm to be present in association with this process?
    (A) Apocrine carcinoma
    (B) High-grade ductal carcinoma in situ
    (C) Invasive ductal carcinoma, grade 3
    (D) Invasive tubular carcinoma
    (E) Medullary carcinoma

42. A breast biopsy shows an atypical epithelial cell proliferation forming small nests in a background of radial-scar-like fibrosis. Which of the following immunohistochemical stains would be most helpful in determining the presence or absence of invasion?
    (A) Cytokeratin 903 (34BE12)
    (B) E-cadherin
    (C) Estrogen receptor
    (D) Smooth muscle myosin heavy chain
    (E) S-100

43. According to the American Society of Clinical Oncology and the College of American Pathologists, standard fixation and tissue handling are needed to optimize HER2 status evaluation in breast cancer tissue. Which of the following scenarios is optimal for HER2 evaluation by immunohistochemistry?
    (A) Core biopsy of ductal carcinoma in situ fixed in 10% neutral buffered formalin for 10 hours
    (B) Core biopsy of invasive ductal carcinoma fixed in 10% neutral buffered formalin for 8 hours
    (C) Core biopsy of invasive ductal carcinoma fixed in 10% neutral buffered formalin for 41 minutes
    (D) Excisional biopsy of invasive ductal carcinoma fixed in 10% neutral buffered formalin for 50 hours
    (E) Excisional biopsy of invasive ductal carcinoma fixed in Carnoy's solution for 15 hours

44. HER2 testing in breast cancer can be performed using either immunohistochemistry (IHC) or fluorescence in situ hybridization (FISH). Which of the following would be considered a positive result for the purposes of trastuzumab therapy?
    (A) FISH HER2 average copy number of 5 signals per nucleus
    (B) FISH HER2/CEP17 ratio of 3.1
    (C) FISH polysomy of chromosome 17 (5 copies)
    (D) IHC staining for HER2 with continuous membranous staining of 10% of cells
    (E) IHC staining for HER2 with incomplete weak membranous staining in 80% of cells

45. A woman with clinical stage I invasive ductal carcinoma is given options of mastectomy, wide local excision (WLE) with postoperative radiation, or WLE without postoperative radiation to the ipsilateral breast. She asks her oncologist for more information regarding the difference in overall survival and local recurrence between these two options. Assuming her lymph nodes and margins will be negative, what do you tell her?
    (A) Mastectomy has a significantly higher risk of local recurrence than WLE with or without radiation
    (B) Mastectomy has a significantly lower risk of death than WLE with or without radiation
    (C) There is no significant difference in overall survival and local recurrence between these three therapies
    (D) WLE without radiation has a significantly higher risk of local recurrence than WLE with radiation
    (E) WLE with radiation has a significantly higher risk of local recurrence than WLE without radiation

46. A woman undergoes breast core biopsy for suspicious microcalcifications identified on mammography. However, the core biopsy shows only normal breast tissue without calcifications. All of the following are appropriate next steps except
    (A) Clinical and radiologic correlation of the mammogram and specimen radiograph
    (B) Deeper levels to examine for a lesion
    (C) Polarization of the slides for calcium oxalate crystals
    (D) Radiologic examination of the tissue block for residual calcifications
    (E) Repeat core biopsy, since the lesion was missed on first biopsy

47. A woman undergoes an excisional biopsy of a breast lesion (see Figure 6-25). What is the most likely clinical presentation of this lesion?

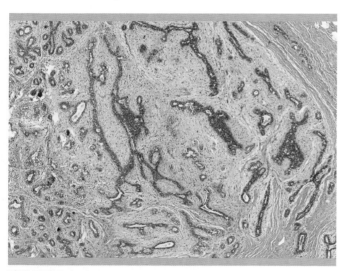

FIGURE 6-25

    (A) Bloody nipple discharge
    (B) Complex cystic lesion on ultrasound
    (C) Ill-defined subareolar mass
    (D) Microcalcifications on mammography
    (E) Mobile well-circumscribed mass

48. A 42-year-old woman undergoes mammography and a stellate mass-like abnormality is found that has calcifications. An excisional biopsy is performed (see Figure 6-26). What clinical history is most likely associated with this process?

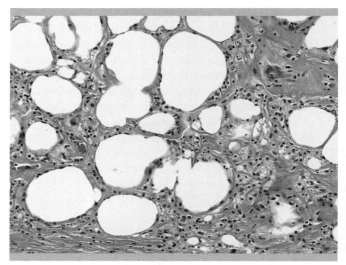

FIGURE 6-26

    (A) Family history of early breast cancer and uterine cancer
    (B) Recent pregnancy and breastfeeding
    (C) Recent trauma to the breast
    (D) Swollen red breast with peau d'orange-like texture
    (E) Variable breast tenderness that follows her menstrual cycle

49. A 41-year-old woman undergoes breast biopsy, and the histology shows a poorly differentiated carcinoma with solid nests, marked stromal lymphocytic infiltration, an infiltrative border, high mitotic rate, and necrosis. Genetic testing is positive for a *BRCA1* mutation. What immunohistochemical staining profile is most likely to be present in this tumor?
    (A) Positive for epidermal growth factor receptor (EGFR) and cytokeratin 5/6 (CK5/6); negative for estrogen receptor (ER), progesterone receptor (PR), and HER2/nu
    (B) Positive for ER, EGFR, and CK5/6; negative for PR and HER2/nu
    (C) Positive for ER, PR, and HER2/nu; negative for EGFR and CK5/6
    (D) Positive for ER, PR; negative for HER2/nu, EGFR, and CK5/6
    (E) Positive for HER2/nu; negative for ER, PR, EGFR, and CK5/6

50. Which of the following findings, if present on mammography, would be suspicious for an underlying malignancy?
    (A) Asymmetry in breast density
    (B) Clustered pleomorphic microcalcifications
    (C) Cup-shaped calcifications
    (D) Density with well-defined borders
    (E) "Tramline" or tubular microcalcifications

51. Which of the following lesions is not believed to arise from the terminal duct lobular unit (TDLU) of the breast?
    (A) Fibroadenoma
    (B) Fibrocystic change
    (C) Infiltrating ductal carcinoma
    (D) Infiltrating lobular carcinoma
    (E) Solitary papilloma

ANSWERS

1. **(E) Peripheral lobular architecture around a central scar.**
   The photomicrograph demonstrates a radial scar, or complex sclerosing lesion, which is considered a benign reactive process. Radial scars can mimic invasive carcinoma both on radiography and gross examination, due to formation of a stellate lesion with a central scar and radiating fibrosis. In contrast to infiltrating carcinoma, radial scars classically have dense fibrous stroma, often with elastosis, and retain a myoepithelial cell layer in each gland profile. In addition, the glands are often compressed and irregular, particularly in the center of the lesion, while in the periphery, a retained lobular architecture imparts a "flower-head-like" appearance at low power. Tubular carcinoma can be difficult to distinguish from radial scars, but tubular carcinomas classically have angular-shaped glands with open lumens and lack myoepithelial cells. In general, minimal cytologic atypia is present, but this does not distinguish radial scar from low-grade ductal carcinoma and tubular carcinoma. Also, radial scars can have epithelial atypia, particularly when apocrine metaplasia is present.

2. **(C) Immunohistochemical staining for myoepithelial cells will be negative.**
   The photomicrograph shows a papillary proliferation within a large duct, which is characterized by thin, delicate to absent fibrovascular cores, lined by an atypical epithelial proliferation of tall cells without an underlying myoepithelial cell layer. These features are diagnostic of papillary ductal carcinoma in situ (DCIS). It can be confused with intraductal papillomas, which, in contrast, typically have well-developed broad fibrovascular cores lined by two cell populations. Papillary DCIS most commonly presents as a mass, rather than nipple discharge, and nearby DCIS is common, but usual-type epithelial hyperplasia is uncommon and should raise the possibility of an intraductal papilloma involved by DCIS. Complete excision of this lesion is recommended due to the risk of developing subsequent invasive carcinoma.

3. **(C) Nuclei parallel to the direction of the epithelial bridge.**
   The photomicrograph shows a duct filled with a usual-type ductal hyperplasia. Usual ductal hyperplasia is characterized by an epithelial proliferation, which can range from mild thickening to bridging and filling the duct lumen. Features that favor usual ductal hyperplasia are minimal atypia, unevenly arranged cells that often appear "streaming," formation of irregular, slit-like spaces that are haphazardly arranged and accentuated at the periphery of the duct lumen, and indistinct cell borders. The myoepithelial layer in usual ductal hyperplasia is typically intact, and can be accentuated. When epithelial bridges form, the oval nuclei of the epithelial cells are arranged parallel to the direction of the bridge. In contrast, low-grade ductal carcinoma in situ is characterized by a monotonous population of epithelial cells that form rounded rigid spaces, typically evenly distributed throughout the proliferation, distinct cell borders, and minimal-to-mild atypia. The myoepithelial cell layer is often absent or attenuated in carcinoma in situ. When epithelial bridges form, the oval nuclei are often at right angles (perpendicular) to the direction of the bridge.

4. **(B) The risk is identical to her right breast.**
   The photomicrograph demonstrates lobular carcinoma in situ, characterized by expansion of more than 50% of the acini in the lobule by a monotonous population of atypical epithelial cells, which often appear to lack cellular cohesion. The presence of lobular carcinoma in situ is a marker of significant risk for the development of subsequent breast carcinoma. Follow-up studies suggest that invasive carcinoma will develop in 25–35% of women over their lifetime, after a biopsy showing lobular carcinoma in situ. The invasive carcinoma can be ductal or lobular type, although the proportion of invasive lobular carcinomas is higher in this group compared with the average population. The risk of developing invasive carcinoma is the same for both breasts; in contrast, after an interpretation of ductal carcinoma in situ, the invasive carcinoma is almost always in the ipsilateral breast.

5. **(E) The neoplastic cells are positive for HER2 immunohistochemical expression.**

   The photomicrograph demonstrates an example of Paget disease of the nipple. This is a rare manifestation of breast cancer, and occurs in <5% of all patients. Patients present with a red, scaly nipple, which is itchy, mimicking eczema. Malignant cells from an underlying mammary carcinoma (in nearly 100% of patients, an underlying ductal carcinoma in situ (DCIS) or invasive ductal carcinoma can be demonstrated) extend through the ductal system to involve the epidermis of the skin of the nipple. These infiltrate as single cells or small clusters, showing large nuclei, prominent nuclei, and abundant pale cytoplasm that often mimics neoplastic melanocytes. Immunohistochemical staining of Paget disease is positive for HER2 and negative for estrogen receptor (ER), progesterone receptor (PR), and melanocytic markers; this is also the typical profile of the underlying carcinoma, which is usually high-grade and poorly differentiated. The presence of Paget disease of the nipple does not count as skin invasion for the purposes of staging; in fact, when a woman is found to have DCIS with Paget disease, but no invasive carcinoma, the tumor is staged as pTis (Paget).

6. **(A) Distance to margin <1 mm.**

   The photomicrograph demonstrates high-grade ductal carcinoma in situ (DCIS), characterized by markedly atypical ductal cells with central comedonecrosis. The Van Nuys prognostic index is used to predict the likelihood of recurrence when evaluating women with DCIS (without invasive carcinoma), and uses the lesion size, distance to margin, and histology (high grade, low grade with necrosis, or low grade without necrosis). Subsequent studies have shown that the single most important predictor of recurrence in women with conservative breast therapy after DCIS is margin status; almost no women have been found to have recurrence after excision with a margin >10 mm (1.0 cm), while women with a margin of <1 mm had a significant increase in local recurrence. Estrogen receptor immunohistochemistry is often performed on DCIS for therapeutic decisions, but does not play a role in the prediction of recurrence risk.

7. **(D) Red swollen breast that has an irregular surface, resembling the surface of an orange.**

   The photomicrograph demonstrates multiple dermal lymphatic spaces filled with malignant cells, consistent with an inflammatory breast carcinoma. This diagnosis requires clinical correlation and demonstration of a unilateral large, red, swollen breast with an irregular surface, resembling the surface of an orange, called peau d'orange. The observed changes are secondary to an invasive carcinoma, which usually shows extensive involvement of the underlying breast, and extensive involvement and obstruction of the dermal lymphatics of the skin. This obstruction results in edema and fibrosis of the skin, causing the coarse, swollen texture of the breast. Bilateral milky discharge would be associated with lactational changes or galactorrhea. A black-brown nodule with irregular borders would be suspicious for malignant melanoma. Puckered skin, involved by a firm, exophytic mass, is highly suspicious for direct skin involvement by an invasive breast carcinoma, but this finding is not sufficient for a diagnosis of inflammatory breast carcinoma. Scaly white plaques and patches are suggestive of eczema or psoriasis.

8. **(C) No staining for high-molecular weight cytokeratin.**

   The photomicrograph demonstrates ductal carcinoma in situ (DCIS) extending into the lobules, so-called "cancerization of the lobules." It can be difficult to distinguish this process from lobular carcinoma in situ (LCIS), but is important because of the risk of developing subsequent carcinoma in the opposite breast. Morphologic features that favor an interpretation of cancerization of the lobules by DCIS include DCIS in surrounding ducts, marked nuclear atypia, necrosis, marked inflammation surrounding the lobule, and a fibroplastic desmoplasia surrounding the lobule. In contrast, morphologic features that favor an interpretation of LCIS include recognized patterns of LCIS in the surrounding breast, small monotonous cells with less atypia, intracytoplasmic lumens within the cell, and lack of inflammation or fibroplasia in the surrounding stroma. Immunohistochemical stains can be helpful in confirming the morphologic appearance; LCIS should be negative for E-cadherin and high-molecular weight cytokeratins, while DCIS in the lobule should be strongly positive for both stains.

9. **(A) Absent lymphoplasmacytic infiltrate.**

   The photomicrograph shows a classic example of a medullary carcinoma of the breast. A diagnosis of medullary carcinoma requires a predominant (>75%) syncytial growth pattern. Other classic features of this diagnosis include a brisk stromal lymphoplasmacytic response, large pleomorphic nuclei, a high mitotic rate, and a well-circumscribed border. Classic, or pure, medullary carcinomas of the breast have a significantly better prognosis than the typical invasive ductal carcinoma, despite a high-grade appearance and an absence of immunohistochemical staining for estrogen receptor or progesterone receptor. Tumors that have some, but not all, features of medullary carcinoma are called "atypical medullary carcinoma of the breast"; examples of atypical features would include absence of a lymphoplasmacytic infiltrate, low mitotic rate, and an infiltrative tumor edge. Most studies have shown that there is no survival advantage for patients with atypical medullary carcinoma compared with invasive ductal carcinoma, not otherwise specified. Therefore, strict criteria should be used before making a diagnosis of medullary carcinoma, and the phrase "invasive carcinoma with medullary features" may be appropriate for tumors that do not fulfill all criteria.

10. **(E) Typically presents as microcalcifications on mammography.**
The photomicrograph demonstrates an example of classical invasive lobular carcinoma of the breast, characterized by discohesive malignant cells infiltrating the stroma in a linear or "Indian-file" arrangement. Classical lobular carcinoma is almost always well differentiated with minimal nuclear atypia, and these tumors are usually estrogen receptor-positive and HER2-negative. The absence of staining for E-cadherin is distinctive, and over half of invasive lobular carcinomas have truncating mutations in the *E-cadherin* gene. The presence of intracytoplasmic mucin droplets, which are periodic acid Schiff or mucin positive, is also distinctive, although other tumors can show similar changes. Other features distinctive of invasive lobular carcinoma include preservation of residual normal breast tumors in the center of the lesion (often with a targetoid arrangement of tumor cells around them) and skip lesions, which make evaluation of the margins particularly challenging on local excision. Invasive lobular carcinomas very rarely present with calcifications; instead, most present as a palpable mass, although some cases present with diffuse infiltration of the breast, which is very difficult to detect clinically.

11. **(C) Hypercellular stroma is a worrisome feature for malignancy.**
The photomicrograph demonstrates a phyllodes tumor, which is characterized by a leaf-like arrangement of epithelium (containing myoepithelial cells) lining a cellular stroma, which increases in density just under the epithelial surface. Phyllodes tumors are differentiated from fibroadenomas by the presence of a hypercellular stroma and the leaf-like architecture. Therefore, hypercellular stroma is seen in both benign and malignant phyllodes tumors. Some phyllodes tumors have an increased risk of recurrence and metastasis and are called

"malignant" phyllodes tumors. Features that distinguish malignant from benign phyllodes tumors include an infiltrative margin, marked atypia, high mitotic activity (>10 mitotic figures per 10 high-power fields), necrosis, and stromal overgrowth (the absence of any epithelial elements in one low-power field). Heterologous stromal elements (liposarcoma, osteosarcoma, etc.) can be seen in these tumors. Wide surgical excision is the treatment of choice to reduce the risk of local recurrence. When metastasis occurs, it is almost always the stromal component that is present.

12. **(E) Positive for smooth muscle actin; negative for CD31, factor VIII, cytokeratin.**
The photomicrograph demonstrates an example of pseudoangiomatous hyperplasia (PASH) of the breast. PASH is characterized by anastomosing, angulated, and slit-like spaces lined by thin spindle cells within a background of dense keloid-like collagenous tissue. PASH can form a solid mass or can be part of other benign processes. It usually occurs in young women associated with hormonal stimulation. These spindle cells are myofibroblastic but can be easily mistaken for endothelial cells from a low-grade angiosarcoma. Immunohistochemical staining can be helpful in identification this lesion; the spindle cells are positive for smooth muscle actin and vimentin, and negative for CD31, factor VIII, and cytokeratin. Of note, PASH spindle cells can be positive for CD34, which should not be mistaken as evidence of a vascular tumor.

13. **(A) A 13-year-old boy with breast enlargement.**
The photomicrograph shows breast tissue with an increased number of large ducts and lacking lobules, associated with mild epithelial hyperplasia and fibrosis, consistent with gynecomastia. Gynecomastia is most common in young boys at the start of puberty and typically is unilateral. A second peak occurs in men older than 50, and can be associated with increased estrogen due to liver disease or obesity. Epithelial hyperplasia is common, but atypical ductal hyperplasia or carcinoma in situ is extremely rare. A rubbery, well-circumscribed mass in a young woman would most likely be a fibroadenoma. A 45-year-old woman with bloody nipple discharge is the most common presentation of intraductal papilloma. An older woman with microcalcifications or a spiculated mass on imaging is highly concerning for in situ or invasive carcinoma.

14. **(B) Recent pregnancy and breastfeeding.**
The photomicrograph demonstrates lactational change in the breast, characterized by closely packed, dilated acini with little intervening stroma, and epithelium showing cytoplasmic vacuolization.

In a woman who is not currently pregnant or breastfeeding, these changes are called a residual lactating lobule, particularly when isolated to a single lobule. While the most common history in this setting is prior pregnancy, occasionally nulliparous women can have this change. In contrast, a history of recent trauma to the breast should raise concern for fat necrosis, while variable breast tenderness that follows the menstrual cycle in association with a lump is most commonly due to fibrocystic change. A woman with a swollen red breast that has a peu d'orange-like texture is concerning for an inflammatory breast carcinoma. Finally, women who have an invasive breast carcinoma in their 30s most commonly have *BRCA1* or *BRCA2* mutations, which are associated with early onset of breast and gynecologic neoplasms, often in several family members.

15. **(C) Epithelial membrane antigen immunohistochemical staining shows "inside out" apical staining.**

The photomicrograph demonstrates an example of invasive micropapillary carcinoma of the breast. Micropapillary carcinoma is characterized by nests of carcinoma that appear to be present within clear spaces, mimicking lymphovascular invasion. A true fibrovascular core is not appreciated in the center of the nests, but the cells are oriented with the apical surface outward; this can be highlighted on epithelial membrane antigen immunohistochemical staining, which shows an "inside out" pattern. Invasive micropapillary carcinoma almost always is found admixed with more conventional invasive ductal carcinoma, and the presence of this pattern is associated with a significantly worse prognosis compared with invasive ductal carcinoma of no specific type. These tumors have a high rate of lymph node metastasis at presentation (over 70%). Over 60% of cases are positive for estrogen and progesterone receptors.

16. **(B) Complete excision with optional sentinel lymph node biopsy.**

The photomicrograph shows an example of adenoid cystic carcinoma of the breast, characterized by epithelial and basal/myoepithelial cells with associated cyst-like eosinophilic basement membrane material showing cribriform, tubular, or solid growth. Unlike adenoid cystic carcinomas of salivary glands, this entity in the breast has a very favorable prognosis, and is usually amenable to complete excision with negative margins. Lymph node metastasis is uncommon (<7% of patients), and therefore sentinel lymph node biopsy is optional, although usually performed in current management trends. Chemotherapy (conventional or antiestrogenic) is not usually indicated nor is complete axillary lymph node dissection in the absence of sentinel lymph node metastasis. These tumors can rarely behave in a malignant fashion, and therefore excision is required.

17. **(E) t(12;15) *ETV6–NTRK3* translocation.**

The photomicrograph demonstrates an example of secretory carcinoma of the breast, characterized by a microcystic or tubular growth pattern of low-grade cells with abundant granular-to-foamy cytoplasm with prominent intracellular and extracellular eosinophilic secretions in a background of dense hyalinized stroma. Originally termed "juvenile carcinoma," these tumors are the most common form of breast cancer in children and young adults, and have a very favorable prognosis with only rare reports of recurrence and metastasis. Simple mastectomy is considered curative in most cases. Recently, the majority of these tumors have been found to harbor a t(12;15) translocation that creates a fusion protein from ETV6 and NTRK3. This translocation is not seen in any other breast carcinomas but is seen rarely in other tumors at other sites. These tumors are most commonly negative for estrogen receptor, progesterone receptor, and HER2. The t(X;18) *SYT–SSX* is the translocation associated with synovial sarcoma. *TP53* mutations are seen in many sporadic tumors and in patients with Li–Fraumeni syndrome, and *BRCA1* mutations account for a large proportion of hereditary breast carcinomas in young women, which often have a triple-negative or medullary-like appearance.

18. **(D) Previous ipsilateral invasive ductal carcinoma and lumpectomy.**

The photomicrograph demonstrates an angiosarcoma of the breast involving the dermis of the skin. Angiosarcomas of the breast occur in two forms: (1) primary angiosarcoma usually occurs in middle-aged women and presents with a deep mass or swelling/enlargement of the breast without involvement of the skin and (2) postradiation angiosarcoma usually occurs in women over 60 years with a prior history of breast cancer treated with lumpectomy and radiation to the ipsilateral breast, and arise in the dermis of the skin with or without extension into the underlying breast parenchyma. In this case, the involvement of the skin in an older woman is highly suggestive of a postirradiation angiosarcoma. Chronic sun damage and atypical nevi would suggest a malignant melanoma of the skin of the breast, and a weeping crusted nipple with an underling spiculated lesion is suggestive of Paget disease of the nipple related to an underlying invasive ductal carcinoma.

19. **(C) Highly associated with an underlying breast carcinoma.**

    The photomicrograph demonstrates an example of a nipple adenoma; these lesions occur in the subareolar region and may involve the nipple surface. They are composed of a haphazard arrangement of ducts, which are lined by two cell layers. The periphery of the lesion is well circumscribed, although nearby ducts may have papillomas or papillary epithelial hyperplasia. These lesions are considered benign, and local excision alone is recommended to prevent local recurrence. Nipple adenomas are almost never associated with an underlying carcinoma; only rarely have coexistent or subsequent carcinomas been reported.

20. **(A) Basement membrane proteins produced by myoepithelial cells.**

    The photomicrograph demonstrates collagenous spherulosis of the breast, a benign incidental finding that occurs in small ducts and lobules. It is characterized by rounded eosinophilic fibrillar or hyaline material filling the lumen of the duct and surrounded by small elongated bland myoepithelial cells. On electron microscopy and immunohistochemical studies, the rounded material is composed of basement membrane proteins, predominantly collagen IV, which are believed to be produced by the surrounding myoepithelial cells. Recognition of this process is important to prevent misdiagnosis as adenoid cystic carcinoma of the breast (which should be infiltrative and form a mass), signet ring carcinoma, or ductal carcinoma in situ.

21. **(A) Local excision of this area to exclude malignancy.**

    The photomicrograph shows dilated ducts lined by cells with columnar cell change with atypia, characterized by 1–2 cell layers of columnar epithelium with prominent apical snouts and low-grade cytologic atypia (rounded nuclei, increased nuclear-to-cytoplasmic ratio, prominent nucleoli, appearance similar to the cells of tubular carcinoma). Also called *flat epithelial atypia* by some authors, this change is considered benign, but has been associated with an increased risk of malignancy in the nearby breast tissue, particularly invasive tubular carcinoma and invasive lobular carcinoma. Therefore, excisional biopsy from this area is recommended to exclude malignancy.

22. **(D) Positive for ER and PR, and negative for E-cadherin.**

    The photomicrograph demonstrates a large duct with pagetoid spread of lobular neoplasia underneath the ductal epithelium. E-cadherin is helpful in distinguishing lobular from ductal epithelial proliferations: lobular neoplasia is negative for E-cadherin, while ductal neoplasia is positive for E-cadherin. Lobular neoplasia (lobular carcinoma in situ and invasive lobular carcinoma) are almost always ER and PR-positive and negative for HER2 amplification. In contrast, the ER, PR, and HER2 profile of ductal carcinoma in situ is more variable, particularly in high-grade lesions.

23. **(C) Syringomatous adenoma.**

    The photomicrograph demonstrates an example of a syringomatous adenoma of the nipple. This is a very rare tumor that occurs exclusively in the subareolar region and is composed of many epithelial-lined tubular structures within a fibrous stroma, which often has a myxoid or hyaline change. The tubular structures are classically "comma" shaped. Infiltration between muscle fibers, other glandular structures, and around nerves can be seen. Most of the epithelial-lined structures have two cell layers, although some may be lined by squamous epithelium. These tumors appear very similar to other syringomatous tumors at other sites, but in the nipple they behave in a benign fashion. Complete excision with clear margins is recommended to prevent recurrence. In contrast, a nipple adenoma also occurs in the subareolar region, but is well circumscribed, associated with papillary proliferation in adjacent ducts, and does not have "comma" shaped structures. Subareolar mastitis occurs in the subareolar region, but is an inflammatory process associated with acute and chronic inflammation and keratinizing squamous metaplasia of large ducts. Solitary intraductal papillomas can occur in the subareolar region, but are entirely intraductal with no infiltration into the surrounding tissues. Finally, tubular carcinoma has some similarities to syringomatous adenoma of the nipple (both have angular glands with infiltration into surrounding structures), but tubular carcinoma lacks a second cell layer (no myoepithelial cells) and does not occur in a subareolar location.

24. **(C) Mammary hamartoma.**

    The photomicrograph demonstrates normal breast tissue interspersed with fibroadipose tissue. No significant pathologic abnormality is present. In the presence of a clinically recognized, distinct, well-circumscribed lesion, which on examination mimics a fibroadenoma, but histologically is composed of essentially normal breast elements, a diagnosis of mammary hamartoma is most appropriate. Mammary hamartomas can contain disorganized ductal and lobular structures, an increase in hyalinized stroma, intermixed fibroadipose tissue, and occasionally increased smooth muscle tissue and heterologous elements. Mammary hamartomas are most commonly mistaken for fibroadenomas and phyllodes tumors, but in general, show less organization and less cellular stroma than these tumors. These lesions are benign, and excision is curative. Good clinical correlation is required to make this diagnosis, as otherwise normal breast can have a similar morphologic appearance.

25. **(C) Solitary glands within fibroadipose tissue are indicative of invasion.**
Microglandular adenosis is an unusual lesion generally considered to be benign, but rarely can be associated with carcinoma. Therefore, complete excision is recommended, when found on a breast biopsy sample. Microglandular adenosis is characterized by small round gland profiles lined by a single cell layer of flat epithelial cells without atypia or apical snouts. Most glands contain eosinophilic secretions, which are periodic acid Schiff positive, diastase resistant. The arrangement of the glands is unusual; typically the glands are arranged in a haphazard pattern, with glands embedded within otherwise normal fibroadipose tissue. Immunohistochemical staining for myoepithelial cells is negative, but the epithelial cells are strongly positive for S-100.

26. **(D) Section at 2-mm intervals and submit the entire node.**
The use of sentinel lymph node biopsy in the evaluation of women with invasive breast cancer has significantly increased in the last 10 years, due to the reduced rates of complications (compared with full axillary lymph node dissections) and a similar detection of clinically relevant metastatic disease. The false negative rate of sentinel lymph node evaluation for the presence of axillary lymph node metastasis varies from 0% to 28% but, on average is <10%, particularly in women with more than one sentinel node biopsied. A nodal metastasis larger than 2 mm is considered a macrometastasis and is considered clinically relevant by all groups. In order to maximize detection of clinically relevant malignancy in the sentinel node, special handling protocols are recommended to increase sensitivity. This includes serially sectioning the lymph node at 2-mm intervals and submitting the entire node for histopathologic examination, with at least 1 hematoxylin and eosin section per slice evaluated. Some authors advocate sectioning perpendicular to the long axis of the node to increase the percentage of subcapsular sinus examined. Some authors advocate the use of immunohistochemical stains to detect of very small (micrometastasis or isolated tumor

cells) lesions, but others contend this is not cost-effective, and the clinical significance of metastases <2 mm (particularly under 0.2 mm) continues to be uncertain.

27. **(E) Strips of epithelial cells positive for p63.**
The presence of abundant mucinous material on core biopsy raises a differential diagnosis of mucinous carcinoma, mucocele-like lesion, and myxoid fibroadenoma. Mucocele-like lesions occur when large ducts fill with mucinous material, and undergo duct rupture with subsequent extravasation of mucinous material into the surrounding stroma. Within the duct, the mucin typically compresses the ductal epithelium, but occasionally epithelial hyperplasia can be present. The extravasated mucin is usually acellular, but occasional strips of benign epithelium with an intact myoepithelial layer (positive for p63 or calponin) can be seen. In contrast, mucinous carcinoma of the breast is characterized by abundant extracellular mucin that contains floating, mildly atypical cells, which lack a myoepithelial layer. Mucinous carcinomas can be hypocellular or hypercellular; on core biopsy of a hypocellular carcinoma, no epithelial cells may be seen in the mucin. Therefore, complete excision of any mucinous lesion on breast biopsy is required to exclude neoplasia. Mucinous carcinomas will have neuroendocrine differentiation in up to 20% of cases (staining positive for synaptophysin), but this is not seen in mucocele-like lesions. The presence of DCIS in adjacent ducts should raise concern for a mucinous carcinoma, as most tumors are mixed mucinous and ductal carcinoma, not otherwise specified.

28. **(B) ≤1.0 mm.**
Microinvasion in a breast lesion that is predominantly composed of DCIS must be no larger than 1.0 mm in greatest dimension. There can be more than one focus of microinvasion, but no single focus can measure >1.0 mm. Helpful features to identify microinvasion are the presence of stromal desmoplasia and the absence of myoepithelial cells (best demonstrated by immunohistochemical stains). Microinvasion is most commonly seen in association with high-grade DCIS, usually comedo necrosis type.

29. **(E) Sclerosing adenosis.**
Many epidemiological studies have examined the lifetime risk of developing invasive breast carcinoma for women with benign breast disease. For the most part, nonproliferative breast disease does not increase the risk of subsequent invasive carcinoma. This includes nonproliferative fibrocystic change, fibroadenomas, large duct ectasia, and apocrine metaplasia. Proliferative disease without

atypia is associated with a mild risk of cancer (~1.5- to 2-fold increase), which includes florid usual ductal hyperplasia, sclerosing adenosis, intraductal papillomas, and complex sclerosing lesions (radial scar). Proliferative disease with atypia is associated with a moderate risk of cancer (4- to 5-fold increase), which includes atypical ductal hyperplasia and ALH. Carcinoma in situ (lobular or ductal) is associated with a 8- to 10- fold increased risk of cancer.

30. **(C) High association with HER2-positive breast cancers.**
Mutation in *BRCA1* accounts for over 50% of all hereditary forms of breast cancer. *BRCA1* is on chromosome 17q21, and a variety of mutations can occur in this gene; the specific mutation present affects the overall risk of developing carcinoma for these women. Depending on the mutation type, the lifetime risk of developing breast cancer in these women is between 40% and 90%. These women are also at significantly increased risk of developing ovarian carcinoma (20–40% lifetime risk). The breast carcinomas that develop in association with *BRCA1* are more likely to be poorly differentiated, many of which have a medullary-like appearance. In addition, these tumors commonly appear "basal-like" type on gene profiling studies and are most commonly of the triple negative immunophenotype (negative for ER, PR, and HER2). The prevalence of *BRCA1* gene mutations is <1% in the general population but is nearly 3% within the Ashkenazi Jewish population.

31. **(D) Younger age at first live birth (20 years or younger).**
Epidemiological studies have demonstrated a variety of risk factors that increase the risk of development of subsequent breast carcinoma. The strongest epidemiological risk factors include female gender and older age (breast cancer prevalence peaks at 75–80 years, with the average age at diagnosis between 46 and 61 years). Other risk factors that are incorporated into the Breast Cancer Risk Assessment Tool (BCRAT) include age at menarche (younger than 11 years leads to increased risk), age at first live birth (older than 35 years leads to increased risk, younger than 20 years leads to reduced risk), first-degree relatives with breast cancer, race/ethnicity (non-Hispanic white women are more likely to develop breast cancer), and the presence of an atypical breast biopsy previously. Additional risk factors include postmenopausal hormone replacement therapy, high breast density, and prior radiation exposure.

32. **(C) Li–Fraumeni syndrome, *TP53* mutation.**
The most common hereditary cause of breast carcinoma is the hereditary breast and ovarian carcinoma syndrome, which involves mutations of *BRCA1* or *BRCA2*. This syndrome is associated with the early development of breast and ovarian carcinomas, but not sarcomas. Li–Fraumeni syndrome, which is caused by mutations of the *TP53* gene, is the second leading cause of inherited breast carcinoma, and is also associated with the development of sarcomas, brain tumors, and leukemia, often at a young age. While Cowden syndrome (*PTEN* mutation) is also associated with breast cancer, it is more often associated with benign hamartomatous growths and uterine and thyroid cancers rather than sarcomas. Lynch syndrome (*MLH1*, *MSH2*, *MSH6*, or *PMS2* mutation) is associated with colorectal and endometrial carcinomas, while von Hippel–Lindau syndrome (*VHL* mutation) is associated with hemangioblastomas (particularly of the central nervous system) and kidney carcinomas.

33. **(D) Well-differentiated ER-positive invasive ductal carcinoma.**
Recent studies using gene profiling of invasive ductal carcinomas have identified five major patterns of gene expression. The most common pattern is "luminal A," which comprises over 40% of invasive ductal carcinomas of no special type, and classically occurs in postmenopausal women who have well-differentiated ER-positive invasive ductal carcinomas. The gene profiling of this type is dominated by genes regulated by ER. The next most common pattern is "luminal B," which classically is a moderately to poorly differentiated invasive ductal carcinoma that is "triple positive" for ER, PR, and HER2. This group contains those ER-positive tumors that are most likely to present with lymph node metastasis. The third most common type is "basal-like," which is typically a poorly differentiated ductal carcinoma that is "triple negative" for ER, PR, and HER2, and is unique in the expression of markers typical of myoepithelial or basal cells (p63, CK5/6, etc.). The fourth most common type is "HER2 positive" that comprises ER-negative HER2-positive invasive ductal carcinomas. The final group is called "normal breast-like" and is classically well-differentiated invasive ductal carcinomas that are ER positive, but have a gene expression profile very similar to normal breast.

34. **(B) Basal-like carcinoma.**
Many different special types of infiltrating carcinoma of the breast have been reported, both

because of the unique morphologic appearance of these tumors and for important prognostic information. Several types of carcinoma have been found to have a better prognosis than infiltrating ductal carcinoma, not otherwise specified; these include tubular carcinoma, medullary carcinoma, colloid carcinoma, adenoid cystic carcinoma, and secretory carcinoma. On the other hand, subtypes that are associated with a worse prognosis include invasive micropapillary carcinoma, basal-like carcinoma, metaplastic carcinoma, and HER2-positive carcinomas.

35. **(D) Fibroadenoma without atypia and with an appropriate clinical exam.**
When women have a breast core biopsy result that is not malignant, sometimes it can be difficult to know in what situations clinical follow-up is appropriate and when excision is still required to exclude malignancy. Current recommendations include excisional biopsy of the following processes on core biopsy: atypical ductal hyperplasia, papillary lesions (including intraductal papilloma), radial scars, columnar cell lesions with atypia (flat epithelial atypia), mucocele-like lesions (including acellular stromal mucin), and fibroepithelial lesions that are not readily diagnosed as fibroadenoma, have atypia, or in which the clinical setting is not appropriate for fibroadenoma. The decision of when to excise ALH and LCIS is more complex; excision is recommended in women where DCIS involving lobules cannot be excluded, another lesion is present that requires excision is present, or if there is radiologic–pathologic discordance (e.g., spiculated mass or microcalcifications and only ALH on biopsy). However, when ALH is present as an incidental finding, clinical follow-up can be appropriate.

36. **(D) Sentinel lymph node status.**
The single most important predictor of death for women with invasive carcinoma of the breast is the presence or absence of distant metastasis. The second most important predictor is the presence or absence of axillary lymph node metastasis, which for most current breast surgeons is approached by sentinel lymph node biopsy. The presence of lymph node metastasis results in a significant reduction in overall survival at 5 years (92% vs. 75% or less). The third most important predictor of survival is tumor size; tumors over 2 cm and over 5 cm have an increasingly poor prognosis. Other minor predictors of survival include histologic grade and mitotic rate. ER status is primarily used to determine therapeutic options.

37. **(C) Invasive ductal carcinoma with 90% tubule formation, marked pleomorphism, and 2 mitotic figures per 10 HPF—grade 1.**
The NGS uses a combination of gland/tubule formation, nuclear atypia, and mitotic atypia to determine the overall grade of the tumor. Each component is scored from 1 to 3, and a total score of 3–5 is grade 1, score of 6–7 is grade 2, and score of 8–9 is grade 3. Tubule formation is scored as follows: score 3—<10%, score 2—10–75%, and score 1—>75% tubule formation. Nuclear atypia is scored as follows: score 3—marked pleomorphism, score 2—moderate atypia, and score 1—minimal atypia. Mitotic activity is highly dependent on HPF diameter; a HPF diameter of 0.50 mm is scored as follows: score 3—more than 15 mitotic figures per 10 HPFs, score 2—8–14 mitotic figures per 10 HPFs, and score 1—<7 mitotic figures per 10 HPFs. Therefore, answer A is grade 3, answer B is grade 2, answer C is grade 1, answer D is grade 2, and answer E is grade 1.

38. **(B) Negative for 34BE12 (cytokeratin 903) and CK5/6.**
While morphology is considered the gold standard in distinguishing usual ductal hyperplasia from an in situ carcinoma of the breast, sometimes the area involved is too small for definitive morphologic interpretation, or artifact makes interpretation difficult. Immunohistochemical stains for 34BE12 (cytokeratin 903) and CK5/6 have been used to help distinguish between usual ductal hyperplasia and DCIS, and can also be used in the distinction of LCIS from DCIS, although E-cadherin loss is considered the most specific marker of lobular neoplasia. Usual ductal hyperplasia typically shows strong and diffuse staining for both 34BE12 and CK5/6, while DCIS is most often negative for both markers. In contrast, LCIS remains strongly positive for 34BE12, but is negative for CK5/6, and will also show loss of E-cadherin.

39. **(E) Gross cystic disease fluid protein (GCDFP) and WT1.**
The most useful way to distinguish the site of origin of a metastatic tumor is to compare the morphology of the metastasis with the prior tumor morphology. However, when this is not possible, immunohistochemical stains can be helpful in distinguishing the site of origin of metastasis. Between 60% and 77% of breast cancers are positive for GCDFP15, which is highly specific for breast origin. Almost all breast cancers are positive for cytokeratin 7 and negative for cytokeratin 20, but this immunoprofile is not specific to breast cancer, and can be seen in lung and female genital

tract adenocarcinomas. ER and PR staining can be helpful if the prior breast carcinoma's receptor status is known, but ER can also be positive in ovarian tumors and occasionally in other sites including lung. In the discrimination of breast carcinoma from ovarian carcinoma, both tumors will most commonly be positive for cytokeratin 7 and ER; therefore GCDFP15 and WT1 are the most likely panel to distinguish breast from ovarian origin (GCDFP positive in breast, WT1 positive in ovarian), although rarely this panel will be noninformative.

40. **(E) Tumor cells measuring 1.0 mm identified by IHC alone are classified as pN1mi(i+).**
The use of IHC for the evaluation of sentinel lymph nodes in patients with invasive breast carcinoma remains controversial. While many groups consider IHC more sensitive for the detection of small lesions, other groups believe that the use of IHC increases the identification of rare tumor cells, which are not clinically relevant, and that close sectioning of nodes and careful histopathologic examination are sufficient to detect almost all clinically relevant disease. Regardless, the use of IHC in this fashion does introduce the risk of false positive results; benign reticulum cells of a node, plasma cells, and rarely histiocytes can show focal staining for cytokeratin. When isolated cytokeratin-positive cells are present, careful evaluation of the morphology of these cells (atypical nuclei, abundant cytoplasm) and location (clustering, subcapsular or intra-follicular sinus) is helpful in excluding benign mimics. When isolated tumor cells are identified by IHC alone, the appropriate nodal staging is pN0(i+). However, once a tumor focus is identified as >0.2 mm, it is classified as pN1mi, regardless of whether it is detected on hematoxylin and eosin stain or IHC alone.

41. **(D) Invasive tubular carcinoma.**
Flat epithelial atypia, or columnar cell lesion with atypia, is a relatively recently recognized pathologic pattern seen in breast pathology. Characterized by dilated terminal ducts lined by 1–2 cell layers of columnar epithelium with prominent apical snouts and low-grade cytologic atypia (rounded nuclei, increased nuclear to cytoplasmic ratio, prominent nucleoli, appearance similar to the cells of tubular carcinoma), this process is considered benign, but has been associated with an increased risk of nearby malignancy. The most common malignancy to be associated with flat epithelial atypia is invasive tubular carcinoma. In one study, 95% of pure tubular carcinomas were associated with nearby columnar cell lesions, most of which showed

atypia. Other tumors associated with flat epithelial atypia include low-grade DCIS and lobular neoplasia.

42. **(D) Smooth muscle myosin heavy chain.**
Determining the presence or absence of invasion in breast lesions can be difficult, particularly when the nests of epithelial cells are small, irregular, and the myoepithelial layer is attenuated. This is a particular problem when DCIS involves a radial scar. Immunohistochemical staining for myoepithelial cells can be very helpful in confirming the presence or absence of invasion. Currently, the most sensitive and specific immunohistochemical markers of myoepithelial differentiation in the breast include p63, calponin, and smooth muscle myosin heavy chain. Other markers that are less specific but still have a high sensitivity include smooth muscle actin and high-molecular weight keratin (CK5). Older markers of myoepithelial cells, such as S-100 and CD10, have largely fallen out of favor due to the very low specificity and low sensitivity. Cytokeratin 903 (34BE12) can be used to distinguish DCIS from LCIS and usual ductal hyperplasia from DCIS. Loss of E-cadherin is the most sensitive marker of lobular neoplasia. ER is largely used as a prognostic marker for subsequent therapy.

43. **(B) Core biopsy of invasive ductal carcinoma fixed in 10% neutral buffered formalin for 8 hours.**
The American Society of Cancer Oncology and College of American Pathologists recommend tissue fixation in 10% neutral buffered formalin for 6–48 hours for excisional biopsies, and >1 hour for core biopsies, for the optimal evaluation of HER2 IHC. HER2 should only be assessed on invasive carcinoma, and not on in situ processes. If a laboratory uses an alternative fixative (such as Carnoy's solution), it must validate the performance characteristics of the assay to show that they are concordant with results using buffered formalin in the same samples. Tissue fixed longer than 48 hours in formalin or shorter than 6 hours in formalin for excisional biopsies may alter immunohistochemical staining, and the report should qualify any negative result with this information.

44. **(B) FISH HER2/CEP17 ratio of 3.1.**
According to the American Society of Clinical Pathology and the College of American Pathologists guidelines for HER2 testing in breast cancer, either IHC or florescence in situ hybridization (FISH) can be used to determine the HER2 status for the purposes of trastuzumab therapy. When using FISH, a positive result consists of either a

HER2/CEP17 ratio of >2.2 (CEP17 is the centromeric signal for chromosome 17), or an average of more than 6 HER2 signals per nucleus for assays without an internal CEP17 probe. A negative result with FISH consists of a HER2/CEP17 ratio of <1.8, or an average of <4 copies of HER2 per nucleus. An equivocal result is defined as a FISH HER2/CEP17 ratio of 1.8–2.2, or an average copy number of HER2 signals of 4–6. When using IHC, 3+ is considered positive, 0–1+ is considered negative, and 2+ is considered equivocal. A 3+ result is defined as strong continuous membranous staining of >30% of tumor cells. A 2+ result is defined as strong continuous staining of <30% of tumor cells, or weak or nonuniform complete membrane staining in at least 10% of cells. A 1+ result is defined as weak, incomplete membrane staining in any proportion of cells, and 0 is defined as no staining. Polysomy of chromosome 17 is not generally associated with response to trastuzumab, and should be considered a negative result. When an equivocal result occurs, reflex testing by another modality is recommended for further stratification.

45. **(D) WLE without radiation has a significantly higher risk of local recurrence than WLE with radiation.**
Multiple prospective, randomized clinical trials have compared mastectomy to WLE or lumpectomy for the treatment of invasive breast cancer. Most studies have shown that when WLE is performed with negative margins and postoperative radiation therapy to the breast is performed, there is no difference in overall survival or local recurrence compared with women treated with mastectomy. Women who are treated with WLE without radiation therapy have a significantly increased risk of local recurrence compared with women who undergo WLE with radiation. However, it is still somewhat uncertain whether there is a difference in overall survival for women who do not undergo radiation versus those who do undergo radiation after WLE. Several studies have suggested that there is a small decrease in death due to breast cancer after radiation, but this is offset by a small increase in deaths due to other causes than breast cancer in the irradiated group. WLE with radiation therapy is recommended for women for whom the tumor is unifocal, the tumor is small and margins or resection can be reasonably free of cancer, and a good cosmetic result is achievable.

46. **(E) Repeat core biopsy, since the lesion was missed on first biopsy.**
Clinical and radiologic correlation is essential when evaluating any core biopsy of the breast. Particularly when a core biopsy is performed for suspicious mammographic calcifications, a careful examination of the specimen for calcification is essential. In most cases, stereotactic core biopsies performed for calcifications will have a postbiopsy mammogram performed to ensure that the calcifications were removed. Rarely, a breast core biopsy for calcifications will show benign breast tissue without calcification on the hematoxylin and eosin (H&E) slide. When this occurs, it is the responsibility of the breast pathologist to ensure that all possible sources of missed calcifications are evaluated prior to the performance of a repeat core biopsy. This includes deeper sections in the block, polarization of the tissue for calcium oxalate crystals (which are clear on H&E staining), radiologic examination of the tissue block for residual calcifications, and close correlation with the radiologist and clinician.

47. **(E) Mobile well-circumscribed mass.**
The photomicrograph demonstrates an example of a fibroadenoma, characterized by an epithelial proliferation lined by ductal and myoepithelial cells within a stromal proliferation that is hypocellular and can be hyaline or myxoid. Occasional epithelial hyperplasia, cystic change, and sclerosis can occur. Fibroadenomas most commonly present as a well-circumscribed mobile mass in young women and are often multiple and bilateral. In older women, fibroadenomas most commonly present as a density on mammography, usually without calcifications.

48. **(C) Recent trauma to the breast.**
The photomicrograph demonstrates fat necrosis, characterized by foreign body giant cells, foamy macrophages, and chronic inflammation surrounding injured fat cells. The most common history provided for a woman with these changes is either recent trauma to the breast or recent surgical biopsy of the breast. A woman who was recently pregnant and/or breastfeeding in association with a mass may show residual lactational change or acute mastitis. Variable breast tenderness that follows the menstrual cycle in association with a lump is most commonly due to fibrocystic change. A woman with a swollen red breast that has a orange peel-like texture is concerning for an inflammatory breast carcinoma. Finally, women who have an invasive breast carcinoma in their 30s most commonly have *BRCA1* or *BRCA2* mutations, which are associated with early onset of breast and gynecologic neoplasms, often in several family members.

49. **(A) Positive for epidermal growth factor receptor (EGFR) and cytokeratin 5/6 (CK5/6); negative for estrogen receptor (ER), progesterone receptor (PR), and HER2/nu.**
Patients with *BRCA1* germline mutation are at high risk of developing breast carcinoma throughout their lifetime. In addition, these patients are more likely to present with grade 3 tumors that behave aggressively. Recently, molecular analysis has identified a subset of breast tumors that are highly associated with *BRCA1* mutation and have a unique gene expression profile notable for upregulation of several myoepithelial and basal cell-like markers. These tumors have been termed "basal-like" tumors, and morphologically are almost always high-grade tumors with solid cell nests, atypical medullary features (including marked stromal lymphocyte infiltration and syncytial growth), geographic necrosis, and very high mitotic activity. Immunohistochemical evaluation of these "basal-like" tumors shows strong staining for vimentin, EGFR, CK5/6 and CK18, variable staining for p63 and S-100, and no staining for ER, PR, and HER2/nu.

50. **(B) Clustered pleomorphic microcalcifications.**
A majority of women over the age of 50 years will undergo routine screening by mammography. The features associated with benign and malignant processes in the breast have been well studied. General features that are highly associated with malignancy include ill defined and/or spiculated densities within the breast and the presence of parenchymal distortion. In contrast, densities with a well-defined border are almost always benign. The presence of breast density asymmetry is very nonspecific; it is very common for women to have asymmetric breast density on mammography. Only when asymmetry in breast density is a change from prior imaging studies does asymmetry become worrisome for malignancy. Calcifications are an important part of mammographic evaluation of the breast and can occur in both benign and neoplastic processes. Features that favor neoplastic calcification include clustering, pleomorphism (of size and shape), branching, and ductal distribution. Features that favor a benign calcification include tubular or "tramline" calcifications (due to vascular calcification), teacup calcification (due to calcification settling to the bottom of cysts), and broken-needle linear calcifications (due to duct ectasia). However, biopsy may be required in many cases to confirm the nature of the calcifications.

51. **(E) Solitary papilloma.**
The TDLU is believed to be the source or area of involvement of the majority of pathologic processes in the breast. The TDLU is composed of the acinus, intralobular terminal duct, and extralobular terminal duct. Most ductal carcinomas, lobular carcinomas, in-situ carcinomas, epithelial hyperplasias, fibroadenomas, and fibrocystic change are believed to arise in the TDLU. In contrast, only a few lesions are believed to arise from other structures in the breast; this would include solitary intraductal papilloma (arising from medium sized ducts), nipple adenoma, large duct ectasia, and Paget disease of the breast.

SUGGESTED READING

1. Abdel-Fatah TM, Powe DG, Hodi Z, Lee AH, Reis-Filho JS, Ellis IO. High frequency of coexistence of columnar cell lesions, lobular neoplasia, and low grade ductal carcinoma in situ with invasive tubular carcinoma and invasive lobular carcinoma. *Am J Surg Pathol.* 2007;31(3):417-426.

2. Arber DA. Effect of prolonged formalin fixation on the immunohistochemical reactivity of breast markers. *Appl Immunohistochem Mol Morphol.* 2002;10(2):183-186.

3. Edge SB, BD, Carducci MA, Compton CC (eds.). *AJCC Cancer Staging Manual.* 7th ed. New York, NY: Springer; 2009.

4. Fisher B, Anderson S, Bryant J, et al. Twenty-year follow-up of a randomized trial comparing total mastectomy, lumpectomy, and lumpectomy plus irradiation for the treatment of invasive breast cancer. *N Engl J Med.* 2002;347(16):1233-1241.

5. Frances P, O'Malley SEP, Anna Marie Mulligan (eds.). *Breast Pathology.* 2nd ed. Philadelphia PA: Elsevier; 2011.

6. Giri D. Recurrent challenges in the evaluation of fibroepithelial lesions. *Arch Pathol Lab Med.* 2009;133(5):713-721.

7. Jacobs TW, Connolly JL Schnitt SJ. Nonmalignant lesions in breast core needle biopsies: to excise or not to excise? *Am J Surg Pathol.* 2002;26(9):1095-1110.

8. Lerwill MF. Current practical applications of diagnostic immunohistochemistry in breast pathology. *Am J Surg Pathol.* 2004;28(8):1076-1091.

9. Lester SC, Bose S, Chen YY, et al. Protocol for the examination of specimens from patients with invasive carcinoma of the breast. *Arch Pathol Lab Med.* 2009;133(10):1515-1538.

10. Livasy CA, Karaca G, Nanda R, et al. Phenotypic evaluation of the basal-like subtype of invasive breast carcinoma. *Mod Pathol.* 2006;19(2):264-271.

11. Lloyd J, Flanagan AM. Mammary and extramammary Paget's disease. *J Clin Pathol.* 2000;53(10):742-749.

12. O'Malley FP, Mohsin SK, Badve S, et al. Interobserver reproducibility in the diagnosis of flat epithelial atypia of the breast. *Mod Pathol.* 2006;19(2):172-179.

13. Querci Della Rovere G, Benson JR. A critique of the sentinel node concept. *Breast.* 2006;15(6):693-697.

14. Ross JS, Fletcher JA. HER-2/neu (c-erb-B2) gene and protein in breast cancer. *Am J Clin Pathol.* 1999;112(1 suppl 1): S53-S67.

15. Schnitt SJ, Vincent-Salomon A. Columnar cell lesions of the breast. *Adv Anat Pathol.* 2003;10(3):113-124.

16. Singletary SE, Greene FL, Sobin LH. Classification of isolated tumor cells: clarification of the 6th edition of the American Joint Committee on Cancer Staging Manual. *Cancer.* 2003;98(12):2740-2741.

17. Tavassoli FA, Peter D (eds.). *World Health Organization Classification of Tumours: Pathology and Genetics of Tumours of the Breast and Female Genital Organs.* Lyon, France: IARC Press; 2003.

18. Vasudev P, Onuma K. Secretory breast carcinoma: unique, triple-negative carcinoma with a favorable prognosis and characteristic molecular expression. *Arch Pathol Lab Med.* 2011;135(12):1606-1610.

19. Yaziji H, Taylor CR, Goldstein NS, et al. Consensus recommendations on estrogen receptor testing in breast cancer by immunohistochemistry. *Appl Immunohistochem Mol Morphol.* 2008;16(6):513-520.

CHAPTER 7

CARDIOVASCULAR PATHOLOGY

1. Atrial myocytes contain electron-dense granules in their cytoplasm referred to as *specific atrial granules*. What do these "granules" represent?
   (A) Alpha-actinin protein
   (B) Gap junctions
   (C) Golgi apparatus
   (D) Lysosomes
   (E) Storage site for atrial natriuretic peptide

2. All of the following are normal components of a heart valve except
   (A) Dense collagenous core
   (B) Elastin rich layer
   (C) Endothelial covering
   (D) Loose connective tissue
   (E) Macrophages

3. All of the following are important components of the heart's conduction system except
   (A) AV node
   (B) Bundle of His
   (C) Right bundle branch
   (D) Sinoatrial node
   (E) Spongiosa

4. You are performing an autopsy on a "healthy" 79-year-old male. In examining the heart, all of the following are considered aging changes except
   (A) Brown atrophy
   (B) Increased epicardial fat
   (C) Increased left atrial cavity
   (D) Increased left ventricular cavity
   (E) Lipofuscin deposition

5. In a patient with congestive heart failure, all of the following mechanisms help maintain arterial pressure and perfusion of organs except

   (A) Activation of the renin-angiotensin-aldosterone system
   (B) Increased filling volumes dilating the heart
   (C) Inhibition of atrial natriuretic peptide release
   (D) Release of norepinephrine
   (E) Ventricular remodeling

6. Which of the following is least associated with the development of cardiac hypertrophy?
   (A) Increased basophilic degeneration
   (B) Increased mitochondrial number
   (C) Increased number of sarcomeres
   (D) Increased protein synthesis
   (E) Increased size of nuclei

7. Alterations in the expression of miRNAs (miR-208 downregulation and miR-195 upregulation) have been associated with which pathologic process?
   (A) Atrial septal defects
   (B) Cardiac amyloid accumulation
   (C) Cardiac dilatation
   (D) Cardiac hypertrophy
   (E) Myxoid mitral value disease

8. Which of the following is the least likely cause of left-sided heart failure?
   (A) Hypertension
   (B) Ischemic heart disease
   (C) Mitral stenosis
   (D) Patent foramen ovale
   (E) Restrictive cardiomyopathy

9. All of the following are likely morphologic findings in the lung of a patient with left-sided heart failure except
   (A) Edematous widening of alveolar septa
   (B) Heart failure cells
   (C) Interstitial fibrosis
   (D) Intraalveolar edema
   (E) Perivascular and interstitial edema

10. At autopsy, you note the presence of hepatospleno-megaly, peripheral edema, a pleural effusion, and ascites in a 36-year-old woman. The findings in the heart are shown in Figure 7-1. The most likely underlying etiology is which of the following?

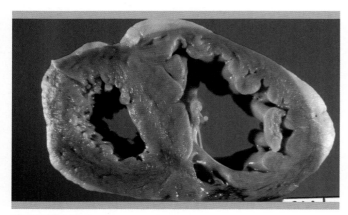

FIGURE 7-1

   (A) Cardiac amyloidosis
   (B) Diabetes
   (C) Primary pulmonary hypertension
   (D) Renal artery stenosis
   (E) Systemic hypertension

11. The most commonly encountered congenital heart defect is which of the following?
   (A) Atrial septal defect
   (B) Patent ductus arteriosus
   (C) Pulmonary stenosis
   (D) Tetralogy of Fallot
   (E) Ventricular septal defect

12. Which of the following cardiac defects is associated with fibrillin mutations (Marfan syndrome)?
   (A) Atrial septal defect
   (B) Pulmonary stenosis
   (C) Tetralogy of Fallot
   (D) Truncus arteriosus
   (E) Valvular abnormalities

13. The most common genetic cause of congenital heart disease is which of the following?
   (A) Klinefelter syndrome
   (B) Trisomy 13
   (C) Trisomy 18
   (D) Trisomy 21
   (E) Turner syndrome

14. Evidence of paradoxical embolism is most likely to be encountered with which of the following?
   (A) Atrial septal defect
   (B) Atrioventricular septal defect
   (C) Patent ductus arteriosus
   (D) Tetralogy of Fallot
   (E) Ventricular septal defect

15. In the fetal circulation, the ductus arteriosus shunts blood from the
   (A) Aorta to the pulmonary artery
   (B) Aorta to the pulmonary vein
   (C) Pulmonary artery to the aorta
   (D) Pulmonary artery to the pulmonary vein
   (E) Pulmonary vein to the aorta

16. A 2-day-old newborn is autopsied and a complex cardiac malformation is discovered at autopsy. You suspect a tetralogy of Fallot. All of the following are features you expect to find except
   (A) Overriding aorta
   (B) Right ventricular hypertrophy
   (C) Subpulmonary stenosis
   (D) Tricuspid atresia
   (E) Ventricular septal defect

17. Which of the following cardiac malformations is likely to present with cyanosis early in life?
   (A) Atrial septal defect
   (B) Patent ductus arteriosus
   (C) Patent foramen ovale
   (D) Tetralogy of Fallot
   (E) Ventricular septal defect

18. Which of the following is not a usual feature of a total anomalous pulmonary venous connection?
   (A) Hypertrophic left ventricle
   (B) Hypoplastic left atrium
   (C) Pulmonary trunk dilation
   (D) Right ventricular dilation
   (E) Right ventricular hypertrophy

19. A 42-year-old woman has a history of hypertension in the upper extremities and hypotension in the lower extremities. She has radiographic evidence of erosions of the undersurfaces of the ribs. A holosystolic murmur was noted on physical exam. Which of the following autopsy findings would best explain her presentation?
    (A) Coarctation of the aorta
    (B) Patent ductus arteriosus
    (C) Persistent truncus arteriosus
    (D) Pulmonary stenosis
    (E) Transportation of the great arteries

20. A 12-year-old suspected of having Williams–Beuren syndrome is being autopsied. She has an "elfin" facial appearance with hypercalcemia, cognitive impairment, widely spaced teeth, and colic and nocturnal enuresis. Which of the following findings would most likely be encountered in the heart?
    (A) Myxoid mitral valve
    (B) Patent ductus arteriosus
    (C) Pulmonary atresia
    (D) Supraclavicular aortic stenosis
    (E) Tricuspid stenosis

21. In examining coronary arteries, a fixed lesion obstructing what percent of the vessel lumen is generally required to cause ischemia precipitated by exercise?
    (A) 25%
    (B) 40%
    (C) 50%
    (D) 60%
    (E) 75%

22. Which of the following represents episodic myocardial ischemia caused by coronary artery spasm?
    (A) Crescendo angina
    (B) Prinzmetal angina
    (C) Stable angina
    (D) Typical angina
    (E) Unstable angina

23. In the absence of significant coronary artery disease, all of the following should be looked for at autopsy as potential explanations for an acute transmural myocardial infarct except
    (A) Basilar artery aneurysm
    (B) Evidence of cocaine use
    (C) Infective endocarditis
    (D) Vascular dissection
    (E) Vasculitis

24. Which of the following best explains the pathologic finding illustrated (Figure 7-2) in a 62-year-old male?

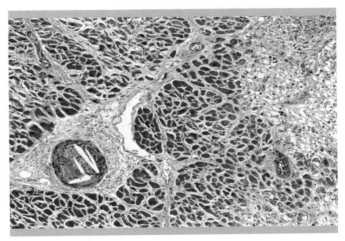

FIGURE 7-2

    (A) Cardiopulmonary resuscitation
    (B) Fat emboli
    (C) Multiple myeloma
    (D) Renal cell carcinoma
    (E) Sickle cell disease

25. Which of the following is least important in determining the location, size, and morphology of a myocardial infarct?
    (A) Duration of occlusion
    (B) Heart rate
    (C) Metabolic needs
    (D) Rate of coronary artery thrombus development
    (E) Size of the coronary artery

26. This lesion seen (Figure 7-3) in the heart of a 47-year-old male represents which of the following?

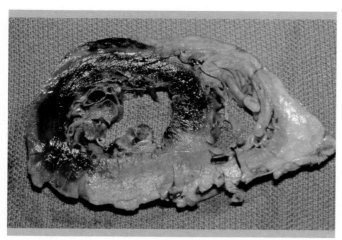

FIGURE 7-3

(A) Myocardial infarct—2 hours
(B) Myocardial infarct—24 hours
(C) Myocardial infarct—5 days
(D) Myocardial infarct—>1 week
(E) Postmortem artifact

27. A myocardial infarct marked by a prominent neutrophilic component and coagulative necrosis with loss of myocyte nuclei and striation is approximately how old?
(A) 12 hours
(B) 1 day
(C) 2 days
(D) 5 days
(E) 1 week

28. In acute myocardial infarcts (2–3 hours old), immersing tissue sections in which solution can be helpful in identifying the lesion?
(A) Luxol fast blue
(B) Methylene blue
(C) Periodic acid Schiff
(D) Sulfated alcian blue
(E) Triphenyltetrazolium chloride

29. Which of the following findings is most suggestive of reperfusion injury in an ischemic myocardium?
(A) Granulation tissue
(B) Increased eosinophils
(C) Myocardial necrosis with hemorrhage and contraction bands
(D) There are no morphologic correlates
(E) Yellow-white gross appearance

30. Which of the following is the least likely finding in a 72-year-old male who sustained a myocardial infarct with subsequent myocardial rupture?
(A) Acute ventriculoseptal defect
(B) Cardiac tamponade
(C) Fibrinous pericarditis
(D) Hemopericardium
(E) New onset mitral regurgitation

31. Which of the following would be the least likely to be encountered in a 62-year-old male who had a left ventricular aneurysm at autopsy secondary to a myocardial infarct?
(A) History of arrhythmia
(B) History of dyspnea on exertion
(C) Mural thrombus
(D) Pedal edema
(E) Rupture of the aneurysm wall

32. The most common cause of a fatal arrhythmia resulting in sudden cardiac death is which of the following?
(A) Acute myocardial ischemia
(B) Aortic stenosis
(C) Illicit drug use
(D) Mitral valve prolapse
(E) Myocarditis

33. A 42-year-old male, at autopsy, is noted to have a dilated and hypertrophic right ventricle with mild fibrous thickening of the tricuspid valve. All of the following are possible explanations for these findings except
(A) Chronic obstructive pulmonary disease
(B) Diffuse pulmonary interstitial fibrosis
(C) Marked obesity
(D) Massive pulmonary embolus
(E) Primary pulmonary hypertension

34. All of the following are true regarding bicuspid aortic valves except
(A) Increased risk of developing aortic dilation
(B) May cause regurgitation
(C) Mitral valve is usually normal in congenital bicuspid aortic valve cases
(D) Prevalence of approximately 5–10%
(E) Responsible for about half of all aortic stenosis cases in adults

35. The changes shown (Figure 7-4) in this mitral valve of a 50-year-old male are secondary to which of the following?

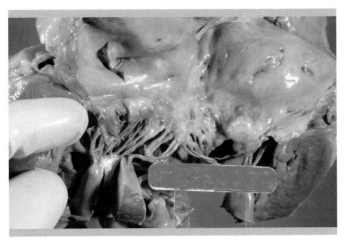

FIGURE 7-4

(A) Congenital abnormality
(B) Infective endocarditis
(C) Marfan syndrome
(D) Myxomatous degeneration
(E) Rheumatic fever

36. Which of the following is not a finding associated with rheumatic heart disease?
    (A) Fibrinoid necrosis of heart valves
    (B) Foci of lymphocytes, macrophages, and plasma cells
    (C) Left atrial thickenings
    (D) Pancarditis
    (E) The aortic valve is the most frequently involved heart valve.

37. A 60-year-old woman dies of septicemia and multifocal brain infarcts. Needle track marks are found on the legs and forearms. The most likely etiologic agent is which of the following?
    (A) *Aspergillus fumigatus*
    (B) *Haemophilus* species
    (C) *Kingella* species
    (D) *Staphylococcus aureus*
    (E) *Streptococcus viridans*

38. At autopsy, all of the following findings are suggestive of bacterial endocarditis except
    (A) Janeway lesions
    (B) Osler nodes
    (C) Roth spots
    (D) Splinter hemorrhages
    (E) Trousseau syndrome

39. A 36-year-old woman has multiple small, sterile pink vegetations with a warty appearance on the undersurface of the atrioventricular valves microscopically. The involved heart valves show focal valvulitis with fibrinoid necrosis. The underlying etiology of these vegetations is which of the following?
    (A) Ankylosing spondylitis
    (B) Rheumatic fever
    (C) Sarcoid
    (D) Syphilis
    (E) Systemic lupus erythematosus

40. A 49-year-old male is diagnosed with a carcinoid tumor of the lung. Which of the following cardiac manifestations is most likely to develop as part of carcinoid heart disease?
    (A) Aortic valve insufficiency
    (B) Aortic valve stenosis
    (C) Mitral valve stenosis
    (D) Pulmonary valve insufficiency
    (E) Tricuspid valve insufficiency

41. Which of the following complications of a prosthetic mitral valve is best illustrated (Figure 7-5) in this 38-year-old male?

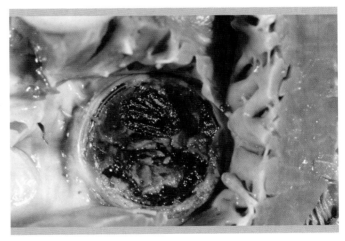

FIGURE 7-5

(A) Infective endocarditis
(B) Metastatic carcinoma embolus adherence
(C) Myxoma
(D) Thrombosis
(E) Valve dehiscence

42. A 42-year-old male presents with a dilated cardiomyopathy at autopsy. Which of the following conditions would least likely explain this presentation?
    (A) Alcohol use
    (B) Doxorubicin use
    (C) Glycogen storage disease
    (D) Hemochromatosis
    (E) Myocarditis

43. A 46-year-old male presents with systolic dysfunction and a dilated cardiomyopathy. A biopsy of the heart is taken, and the pathology is shown in Figure 7-6. The most likely etiology of the cardiomyopathy is which of the following?

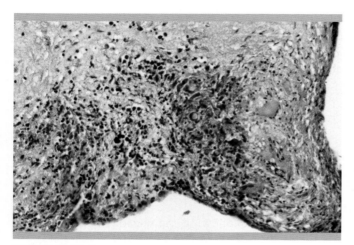

FIGURE 7-6

(A) Alcohol
(B) Amyloidosis
(C) Fabry disease
(D) Radiation
(E) Sarcoidosis

44. A variety of cytoskeletal protein abnormalities have been described as genetic causes of dilated cardiomyopathy including all of the following proteins except
(A) Desmin
(B) Dystrophin
(C) Myosin-binding protein C
(D) Sarcoglycan
(E) Titin

45. A patient presents with Naxos syndrome, characterized by planter and palmer hyperkeratosis of the skin and a mutation in the *plakoglobin* gene. Which of the following cardiac abnormalities is likely to be encountered in this patient?
(A) Amyloid accumulation
(B) Hypersensitivity myocarditis
(C) Loeffler endomyocarditis
(D) Mitral valve prolapse
(E) Right ventricular cardiomyopathy

46. A 24-year-old male is diagnosed with a hypertrophic cardiomyopathy. All of the following are expected pathologic findings in the heart except

(A) Endocardial thickening of the left ventricular outflow tract
(B) Interstitial fibrosis
(C) Myofiber disarray
(D) Thickening of the aortic valve leaflets
(E) Ventricular septal thickening

47. A 46-year-old female presents with a myeloproliferative disorder, a large cardiac mural thrombus, and eosinophilia. This patient is at risk for developing which of the following?
(A) Endocardial fibroelastosis
(B) Hypersensitivity myocarditis
(C) Loeffler endomyocarditis
(D) Parasitic infection
(E) Systemic lupus erythematosus

48. The finding shown in (Figure 7-7) this heart biopsy from a 38-year-old male is most consistent with an infection by which organism?

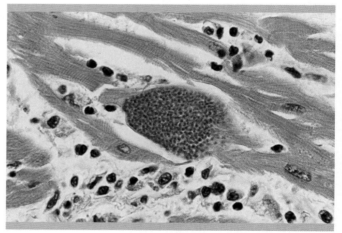

FIGURE 7-7

(A) *Borrelia*
(B) *Candida*
(C) *Neisseria*
(D) *Toxoplasma*
(E) *Trichinella*

49. A 72-year-old male with a history of restrictive cardiomyopathy is autopsied. The heart is shown in cross section (Figure 7-8). There is no evidence of significant disease in the other organs examined. The findings are most consistent with which of the following diagnoses?

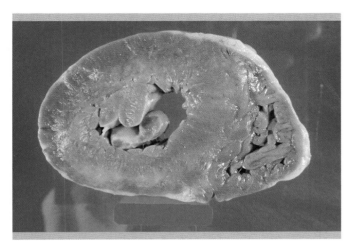

FIGURE 7-8

(A) Chagas disease
(B) Coxsackie virus B myocarditis
(C) Hemochromatosis
(D) Hypothyroidism
(E) Senile cardiac amyloidosis

50. The heart shown here is from a 48-year-old female. Which of the following would least likely explain the finding illustrated in Figure 7-9?

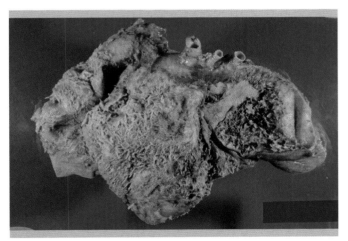

FIGURE 7-9

(A) Hyperthyroidism
(B) Postoperative trauma
(C) Rheumatic fever
(D) Systemic lupus erythematosus
(E) Uremia

51. The most common site of origin of the mass seen in a 52-year-old female is (Figure 7-10)

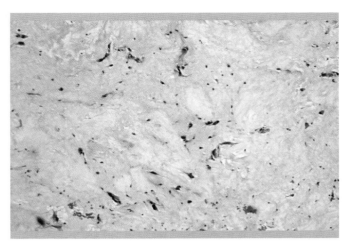

FIGURE 7-10

(A) Left atrium
(B) Left ventricle
(C) Proximal aorta
(D) Right atrium
(E) Right ventricle

52. The lesion shown in Question 51 is associated with which of the following syndromes?
(A) Carney complex
(B) MEN type IIA
(C) Neurofibromatosis type I
(D) Tuberous sclerosis
(E) von Hippel–Lindau

53. The lesion illustrated in Figure 7-11 arising in the left ventricle of a 12-year-old with seizures is associated with which of the following?

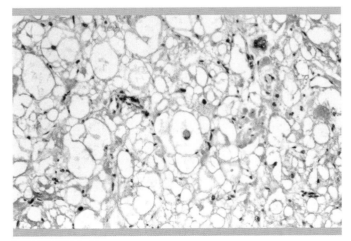

FIGURE 7-11

(A) Carney complex
(B) MEN type IIA
(C) Neurofibromatosis type I
(D) Tuberous sclerosis
(E) von Hippel–Lindau

54. The lesion shown in Figure 7-12 attached to the mitral valve of a 56-year-old male represents which of the following?

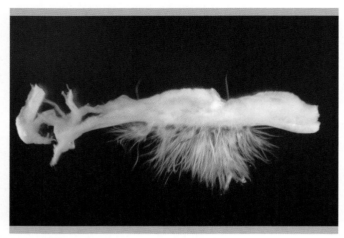

FIGURE 7-12

(A) Metastatic renal cell carcinoma
(B) Myxoma
(C) Noninfective endocarditis
(D) Papillary fibroelastoma
(E) Parasitic infection

55. Multifocal metastatic tumors are discovered at autopsy in the heart of a 72-year-old female. The most likely site of origin for these tumors would be which of the following?
(A) Colon
(B) Lung
(C) Lymph node
(D) Ovary
(E) Skin

56. Which of the following factors is least likely to result in endothelial cell dysfunction?
(A) Bacterial products
(B) Cigarette smoke
(C) Complement
(D) Hypoxia
(E) Laminar flow

57. All of the following serve as promotors of vascular smooth muscle cell migratory and proliferative activities except
(A) Endothelin-I
(B) Interferon-γ
(C) Interleukin-1
(D) Nitric oxide
(E) Thrombin

58. Which of the following endocrine lesions are least likely to present with hypertension?
(A) Aldosteronoma
(B) Congenital adrenal hyperplasia
(C) Growth hormone secreting pituitary adenoma
(D) Pancreatic glucagonoma
(E) Pheochromocytomas

59. All of the following are well-established environmental factors that can be related to hypertension except
(A) Increased salt intake
(B) Obesity
(C) Physical activity
(D) Smoking
(E) Stress

60. All of the following are true statements regarding Mönckeberg medial sclerosis except which of the following?
(A) It affects muscular arteries
(B) Calcific deposits common
(C) Metaplastic osseous metaplasia may develop
(D) Often clinically asymptomatic
(E) Patients typically young and female

61. All of the following are true regarding C-reactive protein except
(A) Activates complement
(B) Exercise increases levels
(C) Induces a prothrombotic state
(D) Opsonizes bacteria
(E) Synthesized primarily by the liver

62. All of the following pathogenic events are associated with the development of atherosclerosis except
(A) Endothelial cell injury
(B) Lipoprotein depletion
(C) Monocyte adhesion to the endothelium
(D) Platelet adhesion
(E) Smooth muscle proliferation

63. All of the following may result in dyslipoproteinemia by affecting the circulating levels of lipids except
(A) Alcoholism
(B) Chronic obstructive pulmonary disease
(C) Diabetes mellitus
(D) Hypothyroidism
(E) Nephrotic syndrome

64. Which of the following blood vessels is/are the most extensively involved by atherosclerosis?
    (A) Basilar artery
    (B) Coronary arteries
    (C) Internal carotid arteries
    (D) Popliteal arteries
    (E) Renal arteries

65. All of the following are histologic components of the typical atherosclerotic plaque except
    (A) B lymphocytes
    (B) Collagen
    (C) Macrophages
    (D) Smooth muscle cells
    (E) T lymphocytes

66. All of the following are factors that may be associated with abrupt changes in atherosclerotic plaque configuration and superimposed thrombosis except
    (A) Blood pressure
    (B) LDL level
    (C) Plaque composition
    (D) Plaque structure
    (E) Platelet reactivity

67. A 39-year-old malnourished woman presents with a coronary artery aneurysm. An underlying vitamin deficiency is suspected as the possible etiology. Which vitamin deficiency can cause alterations of collagen cross linking, predisposing one to aneurysm development?
    (A) Vitamin A
    (B) Vitamin B6
    (C) Vitamin C
    (D) Vitamin D
    (E) Vitamin E

68. All of the following are pathologic changes associated with the development of cystic medial degeneration except
    (A) Decreased extracellular matrix synthesis
    (B) Increased glycosaminoglycan
    (C) Increased scar tissue
    (D) Loss of elastic fibers
    (E) Smooth muscle proliferation

69. A 72-year-old male was noted to have extensive hemorrhage at the time of autopsy. The etiology of the hemorrhage is shown in Figure 7-13. In addition to hemorrhage, all of the following are potential complications of this lesion except

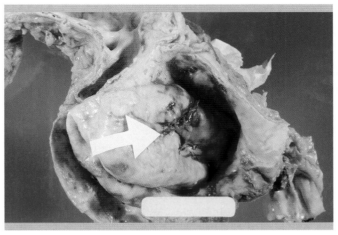

FIGURE 7-13

    (A) Embolism
    (B) Impingement on adjacent structures
    (C) Obstruction of a blood vessel
    (D) Thrombosis
    (E) Vasculitis

70. A 69-year-old male presents with an aortic aneurysm dissection confined to the ascending aorta. This lesion would be classified as which of the following?
    (A) DeBakey type I
    (B) DeBakey type II
    (C) DeBakey type III
    (D) DeBakey type IV
    (E) DeBakey type V

71. Which of the following is considered primarily a large vessel vasculitis?
    (A) Churg–Strauss disease
    (B) Giant cell arteritis
    (C) Kawasaki disease
    (D) Polyarteritis nodosa
    (E) Wegener granulomatosis (granulomatosis with polyangiitis)

72. A 29-year-old woman is diagnosed with hepatitis B infection. She is at the greatest risk for developing which of the following?
    (A) Churg–Strauss disease
    (B) Hypersensitivity vasculitis
    (C) Polyarteritis nodosa
    (D) Takayasu arteritis
    (E) Wegener granulomatosis (granulomatosis with polyangiitis)

73. A 42-year-old woman presents with necrotizing vasculitis. Laboratory testing reveals that she has anti-proteinase-3 antineutrophil cytoplasmic antibodies. Which of the following is most consistent with her diagnosis?
    (A) Churg–Strauss vasculitis
    (B) Giant cell arteritis
    (C) Microscopic polyangiitis
    (D) Polyarteritis nodosa
    (E) Wegener granulomatosis (granulomatosis with polyangiitis)

74. A 38-year-old woman presents with decreased pulses in the upper extremities and aortic changes shown in Figure 7-14. All of the following are true regarding the disease she has except

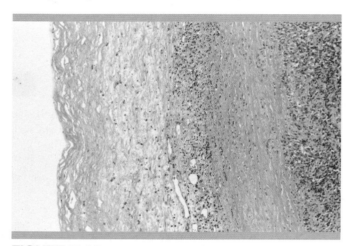

FIGURE 7-14

    (A) Granulomatous inflammation is commonly observed
    (B) Intimal thickening of involved vessels is a common finding
    (C) May also present with ocular disturbances
    (D) Patients are typically over 50 years of age
    (E) The disease shows a predilection for involving the aortic arch

75. The findings observed on this sural nerve biopsy shown in Figure 7-15 are most consistent with which of the following?

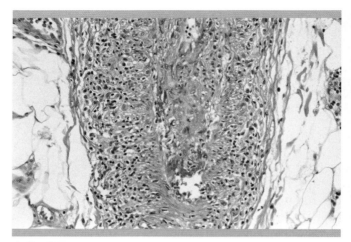

FIGURE 7-15

    (A) Chronic inflammatory demyelinating polyneuropathy
    (B) Cytomegalovirus neuritis
    (C) Microscopic polyangiitis
    (D) Polyarteritis nodosa
    (E) Thromboangiitis obliterans

76. A 62-year-old male presents with necrotizing glomerulonephritis, pulmonary capillaritis, and several skin lesions. A skin lesion is biopsied and shows small venules infiltrated by neutrophils accompanied by fragmented neutrophils. The diagnosis in this case is which of the following?
    (A) Churg–Strauss syndrome
    (B) Kawasaki disease
    (C) Leukocytoclastic vasculitis
    (D) Polyarteritis nodosa
    (E) Wegener granulomatosis (granulomatosis with polyangiitis)

77. All of the following are true regarding Buerger disease except
    (A) Affects large- and medium-sized arteries
    (B) Increased prevalence among Japanese and inhabitants of the Indian subcontinent
    (C) Luminal thrombosis with microabscesses common
    (D) Most patients have a history of heavy smoking
    (E) Pain at rest with ulceration on the fingers and toes

78. A 72-year-old woman with a history of hypertension, diabetes, Raynaud, phenomenon, lymphedema of the lower extremities, and recently diagnosed adenocarcinoma of the lung, now presents with Trousseau phenomenon. Which of the following is most closely related to the cause of her new presentation?
    (A) Diabetes
    (B) Hypertension
    (C) Lung adenocarcinoma
    (D) Lymphedema
    (E) Raynaud phenomenon

79. Which of the following is least likely to result in secondary lymphedema?
    (A) *Aspergillus* infection
    (B) Axillary lymph node dissection
    (C) Filariasis
    (D) Radiation
    (E) Renal cell carcinoma

80. Over 90% of internal mammary artery vascular grafts are patent at 10 years; only 50% of saphenous veins grafts are patent at 10 years. All of the following may account for vein graft occlusion except
    (A) Aneurysm
    (B) Atherosclerosis
    (C) Intimal thickening
    (D) Thrombosis
    (E) Blood vessel collapse

81. All of the following are evidence of myocyte hypertrophy except
    (A) Coarse nuclear chromatin pattern
    (B) Irregularity of the nuclear membrane
    (C) Multiple nuclei
    (D) Size greater than a 3000X field
    (E) Two or more nucleoli

82. Of patients with unexplained cardiomyopathy evaluated by an endomyocardial biopsy, the most common identifiable etiology is which of the following?
    (A) Amyloid
    (B) Ischemic cardiomyopathy
    (C) Myocarditis
    (D) Sarcoid
    (E) Substance abuse

83. All of the following are true regarding the entity illustrated in Figure 7-16, which is arising in the heart of a 1-year-old female, except

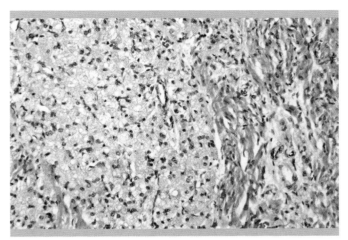

FIGURE 7-16

    (A) Heart valves may be involved.
    (B) More common in females.
    (C) Patients may present with sudden death.
    (D) Represents a premalignant lesion.
    (E) The cells are cardiac myocytic in origin.

84. The most common tumor of the heart presenting in childhood is which of the following?
    (A) Fibroma
    (B) Hemangioma
    (C) Lipoma
    (D) Paraganglioma
    (E) Rhabdomyoma

85. A 62-year-old male presents with dyspnea and right atrial mass. The lesion is resected and shown in Figure 7-17. Which of the following is the best diagnosis of this lesion?

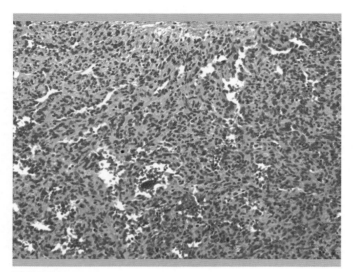

FIGURE 7-17

    (A) Angiosarcoma
    (B) Malignant fibrous histiocytoma
    (C) Metastatic melanoma
    (D) Rhabdomyoma
    (E) Rhabdomyosarcoma

ANSWERS

1. **(E) Storage site for atrial natriuretic peptide.**
   Atrial myocytes are generally smaller than ventricular myocytes and more haphazardly arranged than myocytes in the ventricles. Some of these cells contain electron-dense granules in the cytoplasm known as specific atrial granules. These granules are storage sites for atrial natriuretic peptide. This peptide is responsible for causing vasodilation, natriuresis, and diuresis.

2. **(E) Macrophages.**
   All four heart valves contain a dense collagenous core (fibrosa) near the outflow surface, a central core of loose connective tissue (spongiosa), and a layer rich in elastin. The outside of the heart valve is covered by endothelial cells. Macrophages within the heart-valve leaflets are an abnormal finding.

3. **(E) Spongiosa.**
   Spongiosa refers to the loose connective tissue core that comprises a heart valve. The heart's conduction system includes the SA node, which is located near the junction of the right atrial appendage and the superior vena cava; the AV node located in the

right atrium along the atrial septum; the bundle of His, which runs from the right atrium to the top of the ventricular septum; and the right and left bundle branches.

4. **(D) Increased left ventricular cavity.**
   There are a variety of changes that occur in the heart as a result of increasing age. Increased epicardial fat, increased brown atrophy, lipofuscin deposition, basophilic degeneration, and amyloid deposits are all such changes that affect the myocardium. Increased left atrial cavity size and decreased left ventricular cavity size are also aging changes that affect the chambers of the heart. Calcification of the aortic and mitral valves and fibrous thickening of valve leaflets accompanied by Lambl excrescences (small processes that develop on the closure line of the aortic and mitral valves probably resulting from the organization of small thrombi) are valvular changes that may be seen with increasing age.

5. **(C) Inhibition of atrial natriuretic peptide release.**
   There are a variety of mechanisms that allow the body to maintain arterial pressure in the perfusion of organs in the setting of congestive heart failure. Among these findings are increasing functional cross-bridge formations within the sarcomeres resulting from increased filling volumes with heart dilatation, hypertrophy without chamber dilatation, release of norepinephrine, activation of the renin-angiotensin-aldosterone system, and release of (not inhibition) of atrial natriuretic peptide.

6. **(A) Increased basophilic degeneration.**
   Increased basophilic degeneration is a finding associated with increased aging and is marked by an accumulation of a gray-blue by-product of glycogen metabolism. Increased protein synthesis, increased mitochondrial number, increased numbers of sarcomeres, and an increased size of myocyte nuclei are all findings associated with cardiac hypertrophy.

7. **(D) Cardiac hypertrophy.**
   Alterations in the expression of miRNAs have been associated with cardiac hypertrophy. miRNAs are small noncoding RNAs that inhibit the expression of proteins at the level of mRNA.

8. **(D) Patent foramen ovale.**
   The most common causes of left-sided heart failure include ischemic heart disease, hypertension, aortic and mitral valvular diseases, and a variety of myocardial diseases including restrictive cardiomyopathy. A patent foramen ovale is not typically associated with left-sided heart failure.

9. **(C) Interstitial fibrosis.**
   Common findings in lungs of a patient with left-sided heart failure include perivascular and inter-

stitial edema that usually accounts for the Kerley B-lines observed on chest films and accumulation of edema within intraalveolar spaces and alveolar septa. Hemosiderin-laden macrophages within alveolar spaces, known as heart failure cells, are also a common feature. Pulmonary interstitial fibrosis is typically not a finding associated with left-sided heart failure.

10. **(C) Primary pulmonary hypertension.**
    The findings described in this case are associated with right-sided heart failure. Primary pulmonary hypertension may result in right-sided failure or cor pulmonale. The other findings listed in the question are more typically associated with left-sided heart failure.

11. **(E) Ventricular septal defect.**
    The most commonly encountered congenital heart malformation is ventricular septal defect followed by atrial septal defect and pulmonary stenosis.

12. **(E) Valvular abnormalities.**
    The underlying defects in Marfan syndrome result from mutations in the *fibrillin* gene, which can be associated with valvular defects and aortic aneurysms.

13. **(D) Trisomy 21.**
    A variety of genetic abnormalities are associated with congenital heart disease. The most common of these is trisomy 21 or Down syndrome. Trisomy 13, 18, and Turner syndrome also carry an increased risk of cardiac congenital disease.

14. **(D) Tetralogy of Fallot.**
    Paradoxical embolism refers to conditions in which there is a right-to-left shunt, allowing emboli arising in peripheral veins to bypass the lungs and directly enter the systemic circulation. Of the cardiac malformations listed as options for this question, the tetralogy of Fallot is characterized by a right-to-left shunt, which may predispose one to development of paradoxical embolism.

15. **(C) Pulmonary artery to the aorta.**
    The ductus arteriosus normally shunts blood from the pulmonary artery to the aorta, which serves to bypass the lungs.

16. **(D) Tricuspid atresia.**
    The tetralogy of Fallot is marked by a ventricular septal defect accompanied by an obstruction of the right ventricular outflow track known as subpulmonary stenosis, an overriding aorta, and right ventricular hypertrophy. Tricuspid atresia is not typically a part of the tetralogy of Fallot.

17. **(D) Tetralogy of Fallot.**
    Of the cardiac malformations that can present with cyanosis early in life, the tetralogy of Fallot is the most common. Generally, these are the conditions

that result in a right-to-left shunt. Other abnormalities that less commonly present in this fashion include a persistent truncus arteriosus, tricuspid valve atresia, and a total anomalous pulmonary venous connection.

18. **(A) Hypertrophic left ventricle.**
    The total anomalous pulmonary venous connection is a condition in which the pulmonary veins do not directly join the left atrium. A patent foramen ovale or atrial septal defect is usually present. The result of this malformation is hypertrophy and dilation of the right side of the heart and dilation of the pulmonary trunk. The left atrium is hypoplastic; the left ventricle is usually normal in size.

19. **(A) Coarctation of the aorta.**
    The findings present in this patient are typical of those encountered with coarctation of the aorta, which represents a narrowing or constriction of the aorta.

20. **(D) Supraclavicular aortic stenosis.**
    Supraclavicular aortic stenosis has been associated with Williams–Beuren syndrome. The ascending aortic wall is abnormally thickened, which results in luminal constriction. The defect for disorder has been located to a deletion on chromosome 7, which may interfere with the interaction between elastin and the smooth muscle cell during arterial development.

21. **(E) 75%.**
    In examining coronary arteries, 75% fixed lesional obstruction is generally required to cause ischemia precipitated by exercise (angina).

22. **(B) Prinzmetal angina.**
    Prinzmetal angina is a form of episodic myocardial ischemia that is due to a spasm of the coronary arteries. Angina encountered in this setting is usually not related to heart rate, blood pressure, or physical activity and responds to vasodilating agents. Stable or typical angina is caused by an imbalance in coronary perfusion, usually due to coronary atherosclerosis. This is produced by physical activity or emotional excitement that increases cardiac workload. Angina is usually relieved by rest or administration of a vasodilating agent. Crescendo or unstable angina refers to increasingly frequent pain for prolonged duration that is precipitated by progressively lower levels of physically activities. This angina may even occur at rest and is often caused by a disruption of an atherosclerotic plaque with formation of a mural thrombus, embolization, or vasospasm.

23. **(A) Basilar artery aneurysm.**
    In the absence of significant coronary artery disease, a variety of other conditions and causes

should be entertained. Coronary artery spasm, induced by cocaine use, can provide a potential explanation. Embolism from the left atrium associated with atrial fibrillation, left-sided mural thrombus, infective endocarditis, or paradoxical emboli (in patients with a patent foramen ovale) may also provide explanations. Less commonly, disorders affecting the blood vessels including vasculitis, sickle cell disease, amyloid deposition in blood vessel walls, low systemic pressure, and vascular dissection may provide explanations. Aneurysm of the basilar artery in the head is not responsible for the development of acute myocardial infarction.

24. **(A) Cardiopulmonary resuscitation.**
A small atheroembolus is observed in one of the blood vessels situated in the myocardium. This may have originated from a cardiopulmonary resuscitation, which dislodged atherosclerotic material that subsequently embolized to the heart.

25. **(E) Size of the coronary artery.**
There are a variety of factors, which may impact location, size, and the morphologic features of an acute myocardial infarct. Among these many factors include the location, severity, and rate of development of the coronary artery obstruction; the duration of the obstruction; the size of the vascular bed being profused by the obstructed vessel; the metabolic needs of the myocardium; the presence of collateral blood vessels; the specifics of coronary arterial spasm including site and severity; and other factors such as heart rate, oxygenation, and cardiac rhythm. The size of the coronary artery, by itself, is not intrinsically important.

26. **(B) Myocardial infarct—24 hours.**
The hyperemic, darkly mottled myocardium, as seen in this picture, is most consistent with an infarct that is 12–24 hours old. Infarcts less than 4 hours typically may not be evident on routine gross inspection. An infarct of 5 days age would have a central yellow-tan softening surrounded by hyperemic border. Infarcts that are older than 1 week may show depressed infarct margins and eventually the development of scar tissue.

27. **(C) 2 days.**
Coagulation necrosis with loss of myocyte nuclei and striations and a prominent neutrophilic interstitial infiltrate is generally encountered in a myocardial infarct of 1–3 days age. At 12 hours, early evidence of coagulation necrosis with edema and hemorrhage may be seen. At 24 hours, pyknosis with myocyte hypereosinophilia, marginal contraction band necrosis, and early neutrophilic infiltrate may be evident. At 5 days, early disintegration of dead muscle fibers with dying neutrophils and early

macrophage infiltrate may be evident. At 7 days, macrophages predominate and the early development of granulation tissue at the margin of the infarct may be evident.

28. **(E) Triphenyltetrazolium chloride.**
Triphenyltetrazolium chloride may be useful in delineating infarcts of 2–3 hours age, which may otherwise not be readily discernible on gross inspection. The staining relies on the ability of dehydrogenase enzymes and cofactors in the tissue to react with tetrazolium salts to form a red formazan dye.

29. **(C) Myocardial necrosis with hemorrhage and contraction bands.**
Perfusion injury is usually marked grossly by evidence of hemorrhage and microscopically by the presence of hemorrhage, myocardial necrosis, and contraction bands.

30. **(C) Fibrinous pericarditis.**
Myocardial rupture is one of the well-recognized complications of a myocardial infarct. Rupture of the ventricular free wall, which is the most common scenario, may result in a hemopericardium and cardiac tamponade. Rupture of the ventricular septum may create an acute ventricular septal defect. Rupture of the papillary muscle may result in an acute severe mitral regurgitation. The greatest risk for a myocardial wall rupture is at 3–7 days after myocardial infarct. Fibrinous pericarditis, although a complication of myocardial infarct, is not typically a complication of myocardial rupture.

31. **(E) Rupture of the aneurysm wall.**
A true ventricular aneurysm is bounded by the myocardium that has become scarred. This is in contrast to a false aneurysm, which represents a localized hematoma communicating with the ventricular cavity. The complications of a ventricular aneurysm include a mural thrombus formation, history of arrhythmias, and findings related to heart failure such as a history of dyspnea on exertion and pedal edema. Rupture of the wall of the ventricular aneurysm is not common.

32. **(A) Acute myocardial ischemia.**
The most common trigger for a fatal arrhythmia is acute myocardial ischemia. A fatal arrhythmia may be a cause of sudden cardiac death. The other conditions listed as options are also known causes of cardiac sudden death. Sudden cardiac death is defined by an unexpected death from cardiac causes in individuals without symptomatic heart disease or early after symptom onset.

33. **(D) Massive pulmonary embolus.**
The findings described in this case are consistent with those of cor pulmonale. These cases are

marked by right ventricular hypertrophy and dilatation. Thickening of the muscle bundles in the outflow tract immediately below the pulmonary valve and thickening of the moderator band, which is a muscle bundle that connects the ventricular septum to the anterior right ventricular papillary muscle, may be seen. Hypertrophy of the right ventricle may cause some compression of the left ventricular chamber, resulting in regurgitation and fibrous thickening of the tricuspid valve. Cor pulmonale is associated with a variety of disorders of the pulmonary parenchyma, pulmonary vessels, pulmonary arterial constrictions, and disorders affecting chest wall movement. A massive pulmonary embolus may result in acute cor pulmonale, which would not manifest with the changes seen in the heart as described in this scenario. The other entities listed as options in this question are all possible causes of chronic cor pulmonale, which better fits with the gross appearance of the heart.

34. **(D) Prevalence of approximately 5–10%.**
Bicuspid aortic valve has a prevalence of approximately 1% (not 5–10%). It is the most common congenital cardiovascular malformation in humans. Clinically, it may result in aortic stenosis or regurgitation. It is associated with an increase risk of infective endocarditis and aortic dilation. Over half of aortic stenosis cases in adults are due to bicuspid aortic valves. The mitral valve is often normal in appearance in such cases.

35. **(E) Rheumatic fever.**
Changes seen in this mitral valve are most consistent with that of rheumatic fever. The major findings encountered in rheumatic valvulitis include leaflet thickening, fusion and shortening of the commissures, and thickening and fusion of the chordae tendineae.

36. **(E) The aortic valve is the most frequently involved heart valve.**
The most frequent heart valve in case of chronic rheumatic heart disease is the mitral valve, which is affected in approximately 2/3 of cases. The aortic valve is involved in approximately 25% of cases. Aschoff bodies are encountered in acute rheumatic fever and are marked by a foci of T lymphocytes, macrophages, and plasma cells. Inflammation may be found in any other the layers of the heart (pancarditis). Left atrial thickenings may be observed in rheumatic fever (MacCallum plaques). Fibrinoid necrosis of heart valve may also be encountered in association with rheumatic heart disease.

37. **(D) *Staphylococcus aureus.***
Changes seen in this valve are consistent with infective endocarditis. Infective endocarditis is marked by large irregular vegetations on the valve cuffs that can extend onto the chordae. The history in this patient suggests intravenous drug use; *Staphylococcus aureus* is the most common organism associated with the development of infective endocarditis in this clinical setting. *Streptococcus viridans* is commonly encountered in patients who have had previously damaged or otherwise abnormal valves and recent dental work. Prosthetic valve endocarditis is most commonly caused by coagulase-negative *Staphylococcus*.

38. **(E) Trousseau syndrome.**
Trousseau syndrome represents a migratory thrombophlebitis, typically associated with malignancies. The other findings listed here including splinter hemorrhages, Janeway lesions (erythematous or hemorrhagic, nontender lesions on the palms or soles), Osler nodes (subcutaneous nodules in the fingers), and Roth spots (retinal hemorrhages in the eye) are all findings that may be seen in longstanding infective endocarditis.

39. **(E) Systemic lupus erythematosus.**
The findings described here are most consistent with those seen in association with systemic lupus erythematosus (also know as Libman–Sacks endocarditis). The lesions are typically small, multiple, and sterile. They may be located on the undersurfaces of the atrioventricular valves, the valvular endocardium, chords, or on the mural endocardium of the ventricles or atria. Microscopically, the vegetations are made up of fibrous eosinophilic material and may show remnants of nuclei damaged by antinuclear antigen bodies. Focally prominent inflammation with fibrinoid necrosis of the valve may also be evident.

40. **(E) Tricuspid valve insufficiency.**
Carcinoid heart disease is a result of the effect of carcinoid tumors on the heart. The changes are best seen in the endocardium and right heart valves. These lesions are marked by a plaque-like endocardial fibrous thickenings on the inside surfaces of the cardiac chambers and the tricuspid and pulmonic valves. These thickenings are composed of smooth muscle cells in collagen fibers admixed with an acid mucopolysaccharide matrix. The most common cardiac manifestation is tricuspid valve insufficiency, followed by pulmonic valve insufficiency.

41. **(D) Thrombosis.**
The prosthetic heart valve shown in figure shows evidence of thrombosis on the surface of the valve. Complications of artificial valves include thromboembolic events, infective endocarditis, structural deterioration of the valve, intravascular hemolysis due to shearing forces, leakage around the valve, or obstruc-

tion due to fibrosis of the valve. Hemorrhages related to anticoagulant therapy may also be encountered.

42. **(C) Glycogen storage disease.**
    Glycogen storage disease is more typically associated with hypertrophic cardiomyopathy. All of the other entities listed as options result in a dilated cardiomyopathy, which is marked by an impairment of contractility, resulting in systolic disfunction.

43. **(E) Sarcoidosis.**
    The presentation of systolic dysfunction suggests a dilated cardiomyopathy. Of the entities listed, sarcoidosis is known to be associated with dilated cardiomyopathy. Amyloid and radiation usually result in a restrictive cardiomyopathy; Fabry disease is associated with hypertrophic cardiomyopathy. Alcohol can also result in a dilated cardiomyopathy. The presence of a non-necrotizing granuloma on the biopsy supports the sarcoidosis diagnosis.

44. **(C) Myosin-binding protein C.**
    There are a variety of cytoskeletal protein abnormalities that have been described as genetic causes of dilated cardiomyopathy. This includes abnormalities of sarcoglycan, dystrophin, desmin, titin, and mitochondrial proteins. Myosin-binding protein C abnormalities are associated with the development of genetic cases of hypertrophic cardiomyopathy.

45. **(E) Right ventricular cardiomyopathy.**
    Naxos syndrome is a rare disorder marked by arrhythmogenic right ventricular cardiomyopathy and hyperkeratosis of the palmer and plantar skin surfaces. The abnormality is associated with a mutation in the gene encoding for plakoglobin.

46. **(D) Thickening of the aortic valve leaflets.**
    Hypertrophic cardiomyopathy is marked by an impairment of compliance, resulting in diastolic disfunction. These hearts are marked by prominent hypertrophy, asymmetrical septal hypertrophy, myofiber disarray, fibrosis of the heart wall, left ventricular outflow tract obstruction, and thickened septal vessels. Thickening of the aortic valve leaflets is not generally a feature of hypertrophic cardiomyopathy.

47. **(C) Loeffler endomyocarditis.**
    Loeffler endomyocarditis is marked by endomyocardial fibrosis often accompanied by large mural thrombi and peripheral eosinophilia. There is an association of Loeffler endomyocarditis with a myeloproliferate disorder marked by chromosomal arrangements involving platelet-derived growth factor alpha and beta genes. Eosinophilia may also be encountered in hypersensitivity myocarditis and parasitic infections.

48. **(D)** *Toxoplasma.*
    Toxoplasma, which is shown in figure, may be a cause of myocarditis.

49. **(E) Senile cardiac amyloidosis.**
    Amyloid deposition is one of several potential causes of a restrictive endocarditis in which there is an impairment of cardiac wall compliance, resulting in diastolic disfunction. The hearts in these patients may range from normal to firm and rubbery and often have a pale coloration, as shown in figure. Hemochromatosis and myocarditis are most commonly associated with dilated cardiomyopathies. In hemochromatosis, the iron deposition gives the heart a rust-brown coloration.

50. **(A) Hyperthyroidism.**
    The changes shown in figure grossly are consistent with a fibrinous pericarditis. Fibrinous pericarditis may be seen in association with a variety of conditions including postinfarction (Dressler syndrome), uremia, following radiation, rheumatic fever, lupus, and trauma such as one might sustain from surgery. Hyperthyroidism is not known to be commonly associated with the development of fibrinous pericarditis.

51. **(A) Left atrium.**
    The mass shown in figure is consistent with an atrial myxoma and is marked by abundant amorphus extracellular matrix in which there are small blood vessel formations and small collections of myxoma cells. Myxomas represent the most common primary tumor of the heart and can arise in any of the four chambers and in association with heart valves, although the majority of them (90%) arise in the atria (left > right).

52. **(A) Carney complex.**
    The lesion shown in Question 51 represents an atrial myxoma. Atrial myxomas are known to be associated with Carney complex (10% of myxomas), which is an autosomal-dominant disorder marked by cardiac and extracardiac myomas, pigmented skin lesions, and endocrine overactivity. Many of these cases are associated with mutations on the *PRKAR1* gene on chromosome 17.

53. **(D) Tuberous sclerosis.**
    The lesion shown in figure represents a left ventricular mass in a child and is consistent with a rhabdomyoma arising in the heart. Cardiac rhabdomyomas are associated with tuberous sclerosis.

54. **(D) Papillary fibroelastoma.**
    The lesion shown in figure grossly is consistent with a papillary fibroelastoma. These are typically located on heart valves and consist of hair-like projections. Microscopically, these projections are composed of a core of myxoid connective tissue and elastic fibers that is covered by a surface endothelium. Small pieces of the lesion may break off and embolize.

55. **(B) Lung.**
    The most frequent tumors to metastasize to the heart are carcinomas of the lung, carcinomas of the

breast, melanomas, leukemias, and lymphomas. The most common sites of metastasis are the right ventricle and right atrium. Involvement by the right atrium from the tumor directly extending from the inferior vena cava should raise the possibilities of renal cell carcinoma and hepatocellular carcinoma.

56. **(E) Laminar flow.**
A variety of factors may result in the development of endothelial cell dysfunction including turbulent blood flow, hypertension, increased cytokines, activated complement, bacterial products, lipid products, advanced glycation products, hypoxia, acidosis, viruses, and cigarette smoke. Laminar flow is encountered in normal situations and does not cause endothelial dysfunction.

57. **(D) Nitric oxide.**
All of the factors listed here serve as promoters of vascular smooth muscle cell migration and proliferative activities except nitric oxide, which serves as an inhibitor. Other inhibitors include heparan sulfate and TGF-beta.

58. **(D) Pancreatic glucagonoma.**
A variety of endocrine conditions are known to be associated with the development of hypertension, including adrenal cortical hyperfunction (Cushing syndrome, primary aldosteronism, congenital adrenal hyperplasia, and licorice toxicity), pheochromocytoma, acromegaly from a pituitary adenoma, hypothyroidism, hyperthyroidism, pregnancy induced changes, and consumption of exogenous hormones including oral contraceptives and glucocorticoids. Pancreatic glucagonoma is not known to be associated with hypertension.

59. **(C) Physical activity.**
A variety of environmental factors that can promote hypertension include stress, obesity, smoking, heavy consumption of salt, and physical inactivity.

60. **(E) Patients typically young and female.**
Mönckeberg medial sclerosis is characterized by calcific deposits involving muscular arteries, typically in patients over the age of 50. Metaplastic bone formation may be seen in the vessel wall. Most patients are typically asymptomatic clinically.

61. **(B) Exercise increases levels.**
C-reactive protein in an acute phase is a reactant, which is generated primarily in the liver. It plays a role in the innate immune response by opsonizing bacteria and activating complement. When it is secreted by cells within an atherosclerotic plaque, it can activate local endothelial cells and induce a prothrombotic state. Exercise, weight loss, and smoking cessation all have been documented to reduce, not increase, C-reactive protein levels.

62. **(B) Lipoprotein depletion.**
A variety of pathogenic events are associated with the development of atherosclerosis in blood vessels. These events include endothelial cell injury, accumulation of lipoproteins, adhesion of monocytes to the endothelium, adhesion of platelets to the endothelium, release of a variety of factors (from activated platelets, macrophages, and vascular wall cells), smooth muscle cell proliferation, increased production of extracellular matrix, and lipid accumulation.

63. **(B) Chronic obstructive pulmonary disease.**
There are a variety of abnormalities that can result in a dyslipoproteinemia. Some of these may result from mutations that alter apoproteins or lipoprotein receptors. Abnormalities that affect circulating levels of lipids, including nephrotic syndrome, alcoholism, diabetes, and hypothyroidism, may also result in dyslipoproteinemia. Chronic obstructive pulmonary disease is not known to be associated with dyslipoproteinemia.

64. **(B) Coronary arteries.**
Of the vessels listed as options to the question, the coronary arteries are most extensively involved by atherosclerosis.

65. **(A) B lymphocytes.**
Major components of an atherosclerotic plaque include smooth muscle cells, macrophages, predominantly T lymphocytes, extracellular matrix (including collagen, elastic fibers, and proteoglycans), and lipid material. B lymphocytes are not a major component of atherosclerotic plaques.

66. **(B) LDL level.**
Atherosclerotic plaque changes can have significant clinical consequences. These changes may include intimal surface rupture or erosion of the plaque, resulting in increased thrombogenesis or hemorrhage into the plaque expanding its volume. A variety of factors may play a role in the development of these complications including plaque structure and composition, blood pressure, and platelet reactivity. LDL levels do not directly impact on the development of abrupt atherosclerotic plaque changes.

67. **(C) Vitamin C.**
Vitamin C or ascorbic acid deficiency interferes with collagen cross-linking, resulting in a weakened blood vessel wall and an increased risk of developing an aneurysm.

68. **(E) Smooth muscle proliferation.**
Cystic medial degeneration is marked by a loss, not proliferation, of smooth muscle cells and is also characterized by increased glycosaminoglycan, decreased extracellular matrix synthesis, loss of elastic fibers, and increased scar tissue.

69. **(E) Vasculitis.**
The pathology illustrated here represents as aortic aneurysm with a tear and focal dissection. Potential complications of aneurysms include rupture and hemorrhage, obstruction of a branch vessel resulting in ischemic injury downstream of that vessel, embolism from atheroma or mural thrombi, impingement of a large aneurysm on adjacent structures, or presentation as an abdominal mass resembling a tumor. Vasculitis is generally not thought of as a complication of aneurysms.

70. **(B) DeBakey type II.**
The aneurysm confined to the ascending aorta is consistent with a DeBakey type II aneurysm. DeBakey type I aneurysms involve both the ascending and descending aorta. The DeBakey type III aneurysms involve the descending aorta. There are no DeBakey type IV or V aneurysms. Aneurysms are alternatively classified as type A (involving the proximal or ascending aorta) or type B (exclusively involving the descending aorta). The more serious complications are associated with the dissections involving the type A lesions.

71. **(B) Giant cell arteritis.**
Giant cell or temporal arteritis and Takayasu arteritis are vasculitic conditions that target large blood vessels. Polyarteritis nodosa and Kawasaki disease involve medium-sized vessels. Small vessel vasculitis conditions include Wegener granulomatosis, Churg–Strauss syndrome, and microscopic polyangiitis.

72. **(C) Polyarteritis nodosa.**
In hepatitis B infection, viral proteins can form immune complexes that can be found in the serum and contribute to the development of vascular lesions. Almost 1/3 of patients with polyarteritis nodosa have an underlying hepatitis B infection, related to complexes of hepatitis B antibody to the surface antigen.

73. **(E) Wegener granulomatosis (granulomatosis with polyangiitis).**
Wegener granulomatosis is associated with the presence of antiproteinase-3 antineutrophil cytoplasmic antibodies (c-ANCA). Antimyeloperoxidase antineutrophil cytoplasmic antibodies (p-ANCA) are associated with Churg–Strauss syndrome and microscopic polyangiitis.

74. **(D) Patients are typically over 50 years of age.**
The clinical presentation and pathologic findings showing vasculitis involving the aorta are most consistent with Takayasu vasculitis. This condition involves medium- and large-sized vessels and often presents with ocular disturbances and weaknesses in the pulses of the upper extremities, due to involvement of branch vessels coming off the aortic arch. The disorder typically affects younger patients (less than 50 years) with increased risk in the Japanese population. Pathologically, the vasculitis is marked by an irregular thickening of the vessel wall with intimal hyperplasia. This thickening results in a narrowing of the vessel lumen, resulting in the decreased peripheral pulses. Chronic inflammation sometimes accompanied by granulomas and patchy necrosis is also evident.

75. **(D) Polyarteritis nodosa.**
The sural nerve biopsy shown in figure shows a medium-sized artery with infiltration of the blood vessel wall by inflammatory cells and necrosis consistent with polyarteritis nodosa.

76. **(C) Leukocytoclastic vasculitis.**
Microscopic polyangiitis represents a necrotizing vasculitis that typically affects smaller-size blood vessels. Patients most commonly present with necrotizing glomerulonephritis and pulmonary capillaritis. Skin lesions are also fairly common and are marked by infiltrating and fragmented neutrophils. The findings in the skin are often referred to as leukocytoclastic vasculitis.

77. **(A) Affects large- and medium-sized arteries.**
Buerger disease or thromboangiitis obliterans is classically a segmental thrombosing acute and chronic inflammatory condition involving medium- and small-sized arteries. Patients are usually heavy smokers and are young (typically less than 35 years of age). There is an increased risk of developing this disorder in certain ethnic groups including Israelis, Japanese, and inhabitants of the Indian subcontinent. Luminal thromboses with microabscesses are a common histologic finding. Clinically, patients may initially present with phlebitis and Raynaud symptoms. These often progress to severe pain at rest, due to neural involvement and the eventual development of chronic ulcerations on the fingers and toes.

78. **(C) Lung adenocarcinoma.**
Of the patients presenting findings, the one most likely for the Trousseau sign is lung adenocarcinoma. The Trousseau phenomenon represents a migratory thrombophlebitis.

79. **(A)** *Aspergillus* **infection.**
A variety of causes of secondary lymphedema include malignant tumors obstructing the lymphatic channels, surgical procedures resulting in a removal of a group of lymph nodes (such as axillary lymph node dissection), postradiation-associated scarring, certain migratory parasitic organisms such as filariasis, and postinflammatory thrombosis and scarring. *Aspergillus* infection is usually not responsible for the development of lymphedema.

80. **(E) Blood vessel collapse.**
Blood vessel collapse is usually not responsible for vein graft occlusions. All of the other findings listed may be responsible for vein graft occlusion.

81. **(A) Coarse nuclear chromatin pattern.**
Histologic evidence of myocyte hypertrophy includes irregularity of the nuclear contour, increased muscle fiber size greater than a 3000X field, multinucleation, and multiple nuclei. A coarse nuclear chromatin pattern does not seem to correlate reliably with myocyte hypertrophy.

82. **(C) Myocarditis.**
Studies that have examined clinical pathologic diagnoses in patient with unexplained cardiomyopathy evaluated by endomyocardial biopsy have shown that approximately half of the patients have an idiopathic cardiomyopathy. Of patients with an identifiable etiology that can be established on the biopsy, myocarditis is the most common culprit.

83. **(D) Represents a premalignant lesion.**
The pathology illustrated in figure represents a histocytoid cardiomyopathy. This condition represents a congenital hamartoma marked by multiple microscopic clusters of myocytes showing cleared cytoplasm, resembling histocytes. The condition typically presents in infancy or childhood with a female predominance. Symptoms may include sudden death, congestive heart failure, and arrhythmias. Almost any part of the heart, including the heart valves, may be involved by the process. The lesion is not felt to represent a premalignant condition.

84. **(E) Rhabdomyoma.**
The most common tumor of the heart presenting in childhood is a rhabdomyoma. This lesion is most notable for its association with tuberous sclerosis. Histologically, the cells making up the rhabdomyoma are often diffusely vacuolated and marked by strands of myofiber cytoplasm, so-called "spider cells."

85. **(A) Angiosarcoma.**
Angiosarcoma represents the most common cardiac sarcoma. Typically, angiosarcomas are right-sided tumors that infiltrate the pericardium and can metastasize to the lungs. Most other sarcomas more commonly arise in the left atrium. The figure shows a cellular lesion marked by vascular lumina lined by atypical appearing epithelioid cells, characteristic of angiosarcoma.

SUGGESTED READING

1. Abril A, Calamia KT, Cohen MD. The Churg-Strauss syndrome (allergic granulomatous angiitis): review and update. *Semin Arthritis Rheum.* 2003;33:106-114.
2. Angelini A, Calzolari V, Thiene G, et al. Morphologic spectrum of primary restrictive cardiomyopathy. *Am J Cardiol.* 1997;80:1046-1050.
3. Amano J, Kono T, Wada Y, et al. Cardiac myxoma: its origin and tumor characteristics. *Ann Thorac Cardiovasc Surg.* 2003;9:215-221.
4. Aretz H, Billingham ME, Edwards WD, et al. Myocarditis: a histologic definition and classification. *Am J Cardiovasc Pathol.* 1987;1:3-14.
5. Bonsib SM. Polyarteritis nodosa. *Semin Diag Pathol.* 2001;18:14-23.
6. Bruneau BG. The developmental genetics of congenital heart disease. *Nature.* 2008;451:943-948.
7. Burke AP, Virmani R. Cardiac myxomas: a clinicopathologic study. *Am J Clin Pathol.* 1994;100:671-680.
8. Burke AP, Virmani R. Cardiac rhabdomyoma, a clinicopathologic study. *Mod Pathol.* 1991;4:70-74.
9. Burke A, Virmani R. The cardiovascular system. In: Silverberg SG, DeLallis RA, Frable WJ, LiVolsi VA, Wick MR, eds. *Silverberg's Principles and Practice of Surgical Pathology and Cytopathology.* 4th ed. Philadelphia, PA: Churchill Livingstone Elsevier; 2006:1041-1089.
10. Charles AK, Gresham GA. Histopathological changes in venous grafts and in varicose and non-varicose veins. *J Clin Pathol.* 1993;46:603-606.
11. Cooper LT Jr. Giant cell myocarditis: diagnosis and treatment. *Herz.* 2000;25:291-298.
12. Crotty TB, Li C-Y, Edwards WD, et al. Amyloidosis and endomyocardial biopsy: correlation of extent and pattern of deposition with amyloid immunophenotype in 100 cases. *Cardiovasc Pathol.* 1995;4:39-42.
13. Dare A, Veinot JT, Edwards WD, et al. New observations on the etiology of aortic valve disease: a surgical pathologic study of 236 cases from 1990. *Hum Pathol.* 1993;24:1330-1338.
14. Dare AJ, Harrity PF, Tazelaar HD, et al. Evaluation of surgically excised mitral valves: revised recommendations based on changing operative procedures in the 1990s. *Hum Pathol.* 1993;24:1286-1293.
15. Donsbeck AB, Ranchere D, Coindre JM, et al. Primary cardiac sarcomas: an immunohistochemical and grading study with long-term follow-up of 24 cases. *Histopathology.* 1999;34:295-304.
16. Edwards A, Bermudez C, Piwonka G, et al. Carney's syndrome: complex myxomas. Report of four cases and review of the literature. *Cardiovasc Surg.* 2002;10:264-275.
17. Eiken PW, Edwards WD, Tazelaar DH, et al. Surgical pathology of nonbacterial thrombotic endocarditis in 30 patients, 1985–2000. *Mayo Clin Proc.* 301;76:1204-1212.
18. Falk E, Shah PK, Fuster V. Coronary plaque disruption. *Circulation.* 1995;92:657-671.
19. Felker GM, Hu W, Hare JM, et al. The spectrum of dilated cardiomyopathy. The Johns Hopkins experience with 1278 patients. *Medicine (Baltimore).* 1999;78:270-283.
20. Frances RJ. Arrhythmogenic right ventricular dysplasia/cardiomyopathy. A review and update. *Int J Cardiol.* 2006;110:279-287.
21. Hall S, Barr W, Lie JT, et al. Takayasu's arteritis. A study of 32 North American patients. *Medicine.* 1985;64:89-99.
22. Hansson G, Robertson AK, Söderberg-Nauelér C. Inflammation and atherosclerosis. *Annu Rev Pathol.* 2006;1:297-329.
23. Janssen HL, Van Zonneveld M, Van Nunen AB, et al. Polyarteritis nodosa associated with hepatitis B virus infection. The role of antiviral treatment and mutations in the hepatitis B virus genome. *Eur J Gastroenterol Hepatol.* 2004;16:801-807.

24. Jennette JC, Falk RJ. Anti-neutrophil cytoplasmic autoantibodies: discovery, specificity, disease associations and pathogenic potential. *Adv Pathol Lab Med.* 1995;8:363-377.

25. Jennette JC, Thomas DB, Falk RJ. Microscopic polyangiitis (microscopic polyarteritis). *Semin Diag Pathol.* 2001;18:3-13.

26. Kamalakannan D, Rosman HS, Eagle KA. Acute aortic dissection. *Crit Care Clin.* 2007;23:779-800.

27. Kurup AN, Tazelaar HD, Edwards WD, et al. Iatrogenic cardiac papillary fibroelastoma: a study of 12 cases (1990 to 2000). *Hum Pathol.* 2002;33:1165-1169.

28. Little WC, Freeman GL. Pericardial disease. *Circulation.* 2006;113:1622-1632.

29. Marcus RH, Sareli P, Pocock WA, et al. The spectrum of severe rheumatic mitral valve disease in a developing country. Correlations among clinical presentation, surgical pathologic findings, and hemodynamic sequelae. *Ann Intern Med.* 1994;120:177-183.

30. Maron BJ, Towbin JA, Thiene G, et al. Contemporary definitions and classification of the cardiomyopathies. *Circulation.* 2006;113:1807-1816.

31. McDonnell PJ, Moore GW, Miller NR, et al. Temporal arteritis. A clinicopathologic study. *Ophthalmology.* 1986;93:518-530.

32. Mitchell RN, Schoen FJ. Blood vessels. In: Kumar V, Abbas AK, Fausto N, Aster JC, eds. *Robbins and Cotran Pathologic Basis of Disease.* 8th ed. Philadelphia, PA: Saunders Elsevier; 2010:487-528.

33. Olson LJ, Subramanian R, Edwards WE. Surgical pathology of pure aortic insufficiency: a study of 225 cases. *Mayo Clin Proc.* 1984;59:8935-8941.

34. Passik CS, Ackermann DM, Pluth JR, et al. Temporal changes in the causes of aortic stenosis: a surgical pathologic study of 646 cases. *Mayo Clin Proc.* 1987;62:119-123.

35. Roberts WC, Honig HS. The spectrum of cardiovascular disease in the Marfan syndrome: a clinico-morphologic study of 18 necropsy patients and comparison to 151 previously reported necropsy patients. *Am Heart J.* 1982;104:115-135.

36. Sabet HY, Edwards WD, Tazelaar HD, et al. Congenitally bicuspid aortic valves: a surgical pathology study of 542 cases (1991 through 1996) and a literature review of 2,715 additional cases. *Mayo Clin Proc.* 1999;74:14-26.

37. Schoen FJ, Mitchell RN. The heart. In: Kumar V, Abbas AK, Fausto N, Aster JC, eds. *Robbins and Cotran Pathologic Basis of Disease.* 8th ed. Philadelphia, PA: Saunders Elsevier; 2010:529-587.

38. Shah KB, Inoue Y, Mehra MR. Amyloidosis and the heart. *Arch Intern Med.* 2006;166:1805-1813.

39. Shehata BM, Patterson K, Thomas JE, et al. Histiocytoid cardiomyopathy: three new cases and a review of the literature. *Pediatr Dev Pathol.* 1998;1:56-69.

40. Simula DV, Edwards WD, Tazelaar HD, et al. Surgical pathology of carcinoid heart disease: a study of 139 valves from 75 patients spanning 20 years. *Mayo Clin Proc.* 2002; 77: 139-147.

41. Szuba A, Cooke JP. Thromboangiitis obliterans. An update on Buerger's disease. *West J Med.* 1998;168:255-260.

42. Taubert KA, Shulman ST. Kawasaki disease. *Am Fam Physician.* 1999;59:3093-3102, 3107-3108.

43. Tazelaar HD, Locke TJ, McGregor CG. Pathology of surgically excised primary cardiac tumors. *Mayo Clin Proc.* 1992;67:957-965.

44. Uemura A, Morimoto S, Hiramitsu S, et al. Histologic diagnostic rate of cardiac sarcoidosis: evaluation of endomyocardial biopsies. *Am Heart J.* 1999;138:299-302.

45. Veinot JP. Diagnostic endomyocardial biopsy pathology—general biopsy considerations, and its use for myocarditis and cardiomyopathy. *Can J Cardiol.* 2002;18:55-65.

46. Veinot JP. Diagnostic endomyocardial biopsy pathology: secondary myocardial diseases and other clinical indications—a review. *Can J Cardiol.* 2002;18:287-296.

47. Virmani R, Kolodgie F, Farb A, et al. Pathologic evaluation of carotid endarterectomy. *Pathol Case Rev.* 2001;6:236-243.

48. Weitzenblum E. Chronic cor pulmonale. *Heart.* 2003;89: 225-230.

49. Yi ES, Colby TV. Wegener's granulomatosis. *Semin Diag Pathol.* 2001;18:34-46.

CHAPTER 8

CYTOLOGY: GYNECOLOGIC

1. The following changes are seen on a liquid-based Pap test from a 21-year-old woman (see Figure 8-1). The most appropriate interpretation would be

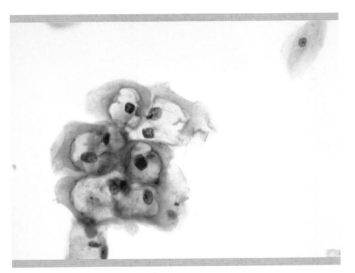

FIGURE 8-1

(A) Atrophy, negative for intraepithelial lesion or malignancy
(B) Low-grade squamous intraepithelial lesion (LSIL)
(C) High-grade squamous intraepithelial lesion (HSIL)
(D) Repair, negative for intraepithelial lesion or malignancy
(E) Squamous cell carcinoma (SCC)

2. Which of the following statements is true regarding the microorganism present in this Pap test (see Figure 8-2)?

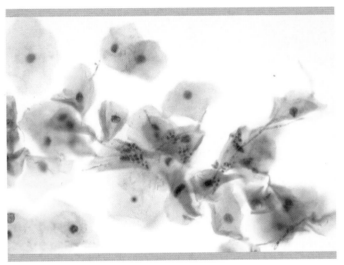

FIGURE 8-2

(A) *Candida glabrata* is the most common organism
(B) Classically shows both yeast and hyphae from cervical samples
(C) Considered a sexually transmitted disease
(D) Most common cause of abnormal vaginal discharge
(E) Presence on Pap test does not always correlate with symptomatic infection

3. A Pap test was performed on a 31-year-old woman and demonstrates the following cytologic findings (see Figure 8-3). What is the next best/acceptable step in the management of this woman?

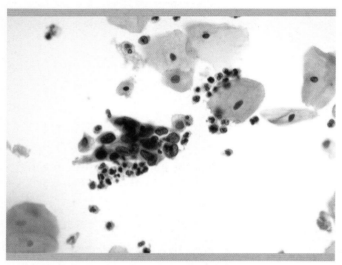

FIGURE 8-3

(A) Cervical colposcopy with endocervical sampling
(B) Colposcopy, endocervical sampling, and endometrial sampling
(C) Reflex human papilloma virus testing, and colposcopy if positive
(D) Repeat Pap in 6–12 months
(E) Routine screening in 3 years

4. A 42-year-old woman presents for annual exam. A representative field from her Pap test is shown (see Figure 8-4). What clinical history is important to correlate with this finding?

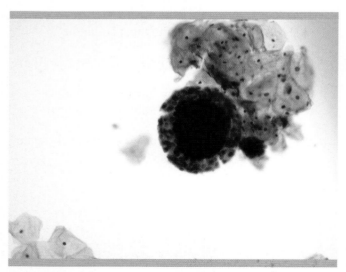

FIGURE 8-4

(A) Body mass index (BMI)
(B) Diethylstilbestrol (DES) exposure
(C) History of squamous dysplasia
(D) Last menstrual period
(E) Prior loop electrosurgical excision procedure (LEEP) conization

5. A 22-year-old woman presents for her annual Pap test (see Figure 8-5). The best interpretation of this is

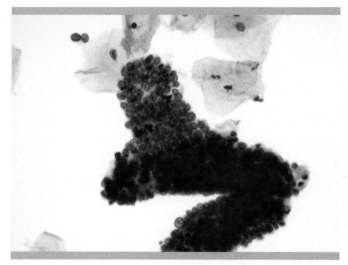

FIGURE 8-5

(A) Adenocarcinoma in situ
(B) Endocervical adenocarcinoma
(C) Exfoliated endometrial cells
(D) Normal endocervical cells
(E) Tubal metaplasia

6. A 23-year-old woman presents for routine follow-up. Her Pap test shows the following changes (see Figure 8-6). The best interpretation for this Pap test is

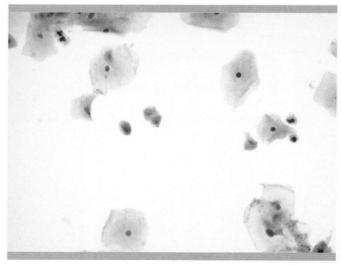

FIGURE 8-6

(A) Atypical squamous cells of undetermined significance (ASC-US)
(B) Low-grade squamous intraepithelial lesion (LSIL)
(C) Negative for intraepithelial lesion or malignancy; fungal organisms consistent with *Candida* species present
(D) Negative for intraepithelial lesion or malignancy; reactive cellular changes present
(E) Negative for intraepithelial lesion or malignancy; *Trichomonas vaginalis* present

7. A 29-year-old woman presents for follow-up and a Pap test is performed (see Figure 8-7). The most likely clinical history that would correlate with this cervical cytology would be

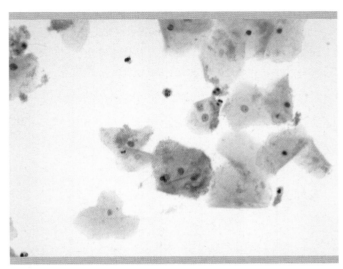

FIGURE 8-8

(A) Ammonia or "fishy" odor to vaginal discharge
(B) Blisters on the cervix or vulva
(C) Intrauterine device present
(D) Strawberry cervix (microhemorrhages)
(E) White, thick discharge

9. The most important criterion to determine if the cells present in this Pap test (see Figure 8-9) are atypical is

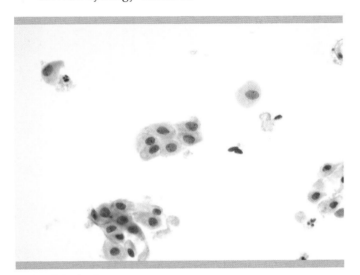

FIGURE 8-7

(A) Follow-up for polycystic ovarian disease
(B) Human papilloma virus positive at last Pap
(C) Postpartum follow-up
(D) Pregnancy week 30 exam
(E) Radiation therapy for Hodgkin disease

8. A 27-year-old woman presents for her annual physical and a Pap test is performed (see Figure 8-8). The most likely clinical finding at exam is

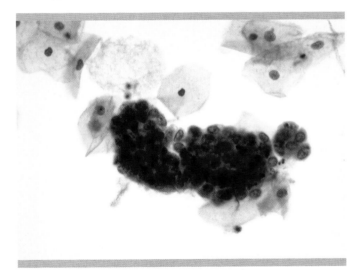

FIGURE 8-9

(A) Feathering
(B) High nuclear-to-cytoplasmic ratio
(C) Increase in nuclear size
(D) Presence of small nucleoli
(E) Three-dimensional arrangement

10. A Pap test was performed on a 37-year-old woman, and demonstrates the following cytologic findings (see Figure 8-10). The best interpretation for this is

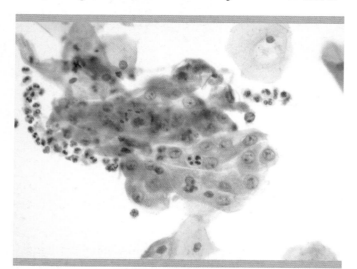

FIGURE 8-10

(A) Low-grade squamous intraepithelial lesion (LSIL)
(B) High-grade squamous intraepithelial lesion (HSIL)
(C) Negative for intraepithelial lesion or malignancy, atrophy
(D) Negative for intraepithelial lesion or malignancy, repair
(E) Squamous cell carcinoma (SCC)

11. The organism present in this Pap test (see Figure 8-11) is classically seen in association with what other infectious organism?

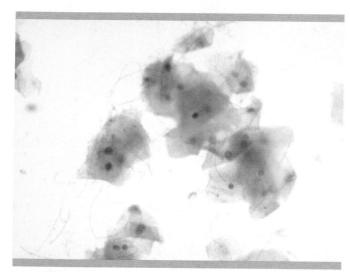

FIGURE 8-11

(A) *Candida*
(B) *Gardnerella*
(C) Herpes
(D) *Lactobacillus*
(E) *Trichomonas*

12. A 32-year-old woman with infertility problems has the following vaginal smear appearance (see Figure 8-12). This appearance is associated with which of the following states?

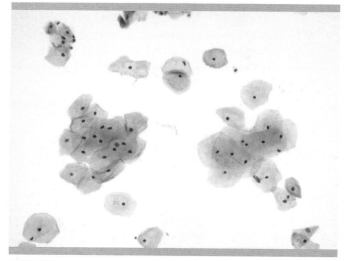

FIGURE 8-12

(A) Granulosa cell tumor of ovary
(B) Newborn girl
(C) Postmenopausal
(D) Pregnancy
(E) Second half of menstrual cycle

13. A 38-year-old woman has the following Pap test appearance (see Figure 8-13). What is the most likely clinical finding in this patient?

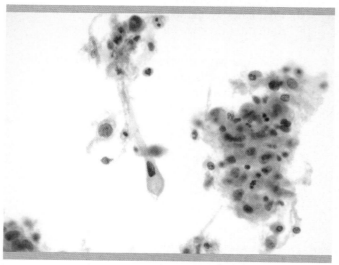

FIGURE 8-13

(A) Cervical mass
(B) Ovarian mass
(C) Pregnancy
(D) Uterine enlargement and bleeding
(E) Vaginal atrophy

14. A 22-year-old woman has a Pap test performed (see Figure 8-14). Features that favor a benign interpretation over an atypical interpretation of the central group of cells include all of the following except

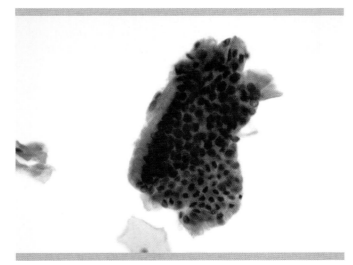

FIGURE 8-14

(A) Abundant tall columnar cytoplasm
(B) Flat strips and sheets
(C) High nuclear-to-cytoplasmic (N:C) ratio
(D) Honeycomb arrangement
(E) Nuclear enlargement up to 4 times normal cells

15. A 21-year-old woman with no prior history comes in for an annual examination. A Pap test is performed (see Figure 8-15). The changes in this figure most likely represent

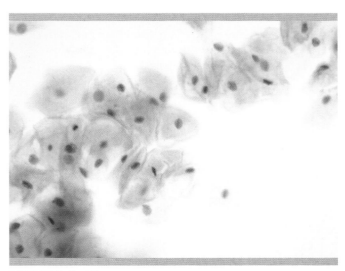

FIGURE 8-15

(A) Bacterial vaginosis
(B) Coverslipping artifact
(C) Glycogen deposition
(D) Keratohyaline granules
(E) Koilocytic change

16. A 52-year-old woman presents for annual screening. The changes on her Pap test (see Figure 8-16) are most likely secondary to

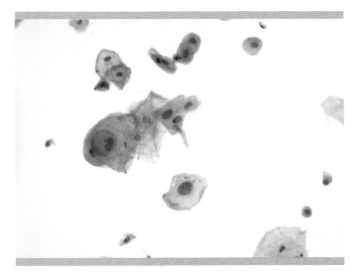

FIGURE 8-16

(A) Herpes simplex infection
(B) History of radiation therapy
(C) Human papilloma virus-related cervical dysplasia
(D) Intrauterine device (IUD)
(E) Invasive squamous cell carcinoma

17. A 31-year-old woman presents for her annual Pap test (see Figure 8-17). This finding is most commonly associated with which of the following processes in women under 50?

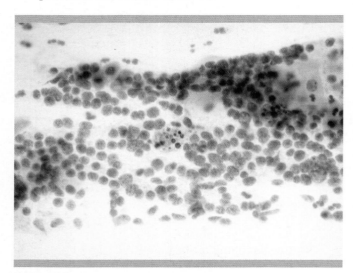

FIGURE 8-17

(A) *Candida*
(B) *Chlamydia*
(C) Lymphoma
(D) Small cell carcinoma
(E) *Trichomonas*

18. A 38-year-old woman presents for her annual Pap test, which shows the following findings (see Figure 8-18). Which of the following statements is true regarding this process?

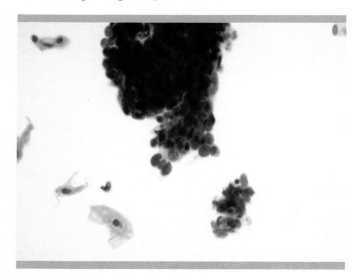

FIGURE 8-18

(A) Likely represents metastasis from an occult lung primary
(B) May be associated with a background of low-grade squamous intraepithelial lesion (LSIL)
(C) Most commonly associated with human papilloma virus type 16
(D) Rapid development can occur in the interval between screening Pap tests
(E) Treated similar to conventional squamous cell carcinoma

19. A 28-year-old woman who is 34 weeks pregnant has a Pap test (see Figure 8-19). Based on the findings present, which of the following changes in clinical management is indicated?

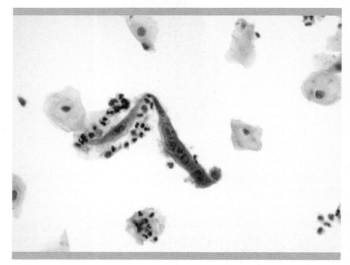

FIGURE 8-19

(A) Cesarean section instead of vaginal delivery
(B) Colposcopy immediately, with biopsy
(C) Deferred colposcopy until 6 weeks postpartum
(D) Therapy with antifungal cream
(E) Therapy with metronidazole (Flagyl)

20. A 25-year-old pregnant woman presents for her first prenatal visit, and has a Pap test performed. Rare cells are seen (see Figure 8-20), which most likely represent?

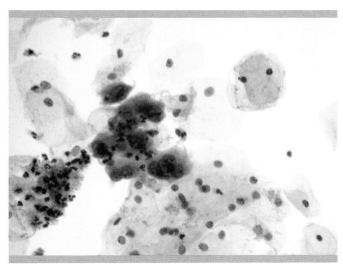

FIGURE 8-20

(A) Aria–Stella reaction
(B) Clear cell carcinoma
(C) Decidual cells
(D) Endometrial adenocarcinoma
(E) Intrauterine device (IUD) effect

21. A 29-year-old woman presents for her annual Pap test. The following changes are seen (see Figure 8-21). The most likely clinical finding at exam is

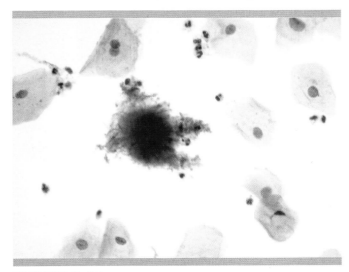

FIGURE 8-21

(A) Ammonia or "fishy" odor to vaginal discharge
(B) Blisters on the cervix or vulva
(C) Intrauterine device present
(D) Strawberry cervix (microhemorrhages)
(E) White, thick discharge

22. A 27-year-old woman has a Pap test performed (see Figure 8-22). Which of the following cytomorphologic changes is not a feature of this cell type?

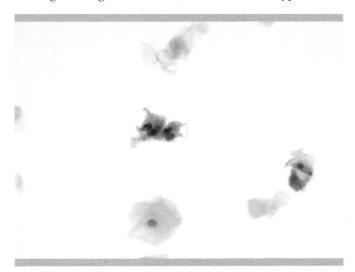

FIGURE 8-22

(A) Coarse chromatin
(B) Crowded clusters
(C) Increased nuclear-to-cytoplasmic ratio
(D) Pseudostratified nuclei
(E) Vacuolated cytoplasm

23. A 43-year-old woman undergoes a Pap test (see Figure 8-23). The best interpretation for this finding is

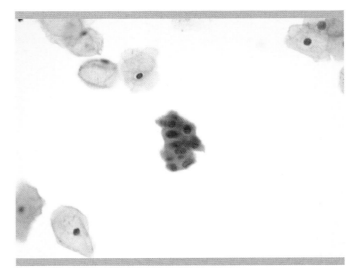

FIGURE 8-23

(A) Atypical squamous cells of undetermined significance (ASC-US)
(B) High-grade squamous intraepithelial lesion (HSIL)
(C) Negative for intraepithelial lesion or malignancy (NILM), hyperkeratosis present
(D) NILM, parakeratosis present
(E) NILM, reactive cellular changes present

24. A 22-year-old woman presents for her annual Pap test (see Figure 8-24). The structures present at the center of the figure are

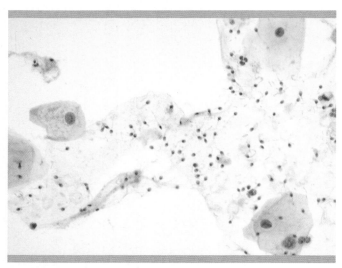

FIGURE 8-24

(A) *Candida albicans* hyphae
(B) *Leptothrix*
(C) Psammoma bodies
(D) Spermatozoa
(E) *Trichomonas vaginalis*

25. A 25-year-old woman presents for Pap test screening. The following changes are seen (see Figure 8-25). What is the most appropriate next clinical step?

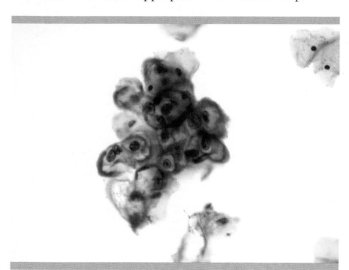

FIGURE 8-25

(A) Cervical colposcopy
(B) Endometrial sampling
(C) Reflex human papilloma virus testing, and colposcopy if positive

(D) Repeat Pap in 6–12 months
(E) Routine screening in 3 years

26. A 35-year-old woman undergoes Pap test screening. Her Pap test demonstrates an unusual finding (see Figure 8-26 photomicrograph). This finding is most commonly associated with which of the following conditions?

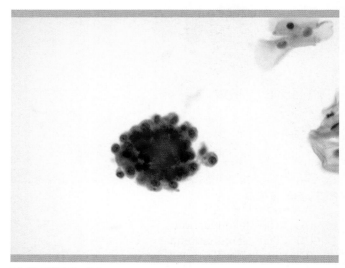

FIGURE 8-26

(A) Abnormal bleeding
(B) High-grade intraepithelial lesion (HSIL)
(C) Intrauterine device (IUD)
(D) Pregnancy
(E) *Trichomonas* infection

27. A 37-year-old woman presents for Pap test screening. The following cells are seen (see Figure 8-27). What type of contraception is she most likely using?

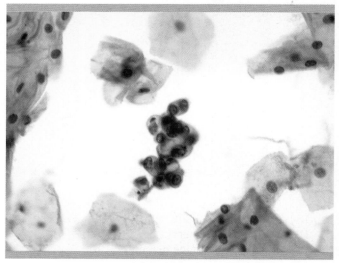

FIGURE 8-27

(A) Birth control pill (estrogen/progestin)
(B) Condoms
(C) Depo-Provera (progestin injections)
(D) Intrauterine device (IUD)
(E) None

28. A 49-year-old woman with a history of invasive ductal carcinoma of the breast presents for annual Pap test screening. Her cervix exam is normal, and her Pap test shows rare atypical cells (see Figure 8-28) in an otherwise normal-appearing background. The most likely source of the malignant cells is

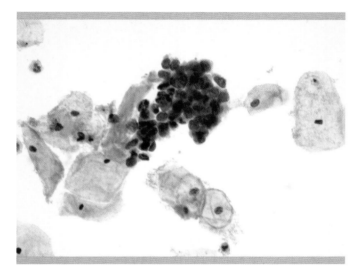

FIGURE 8-28

(A) Endocervical adenocarcinoma
(B) Endometrial adenocarcinoma
(C) Invasive squamous cell carcinoma
(D) Large cell lymphoma
(E) Metastatic breast carcinoma

29. A 31-year-old woman presents for a screening Pap test. The presence of abundant cells with the following features (see Figure 8-29) can be associated with all of the following conditions except

FIGURE 8-29

(A) Cervical condyloma
(B) Invasive well-differentiated squamous cell carcinoma
(C) Pregnancy
(D) Uterine prolapse
(E) Vulvar contamination

30. A 35-year-old woman with a history of a hysterectomy in the past due to fibroids has a Pap test performed, with the following finding (see Figure 8-30). Which of the following is the most likely reason for this finding in this patient?

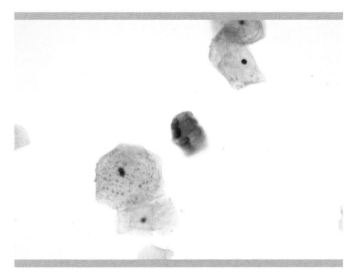

FIGURE 8-30

(A) Atrophy
(B) Diethylstilbestrol (DES) exposure as a child
(C) Endocervical adenocarcinoma
(D) Endometrial adenocarcinoma
(E) Fallopian tube prolapse

31. A 43-year-old woman presents for Pap test screening which shows the following changes (see Figure 8-31). This finding has been found in association with all of the following conditions except

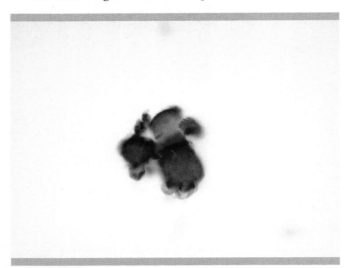

FIGURE 8-31

(A) Atrophy
(B) Cervical polyp
(C) Endometrial carcinoma
(D) Endometriosis
(E) Ovarian carcinoma

32. A 31-year-old woman presents for Pap test screening. This structure (see Figure 8-32) is most likely

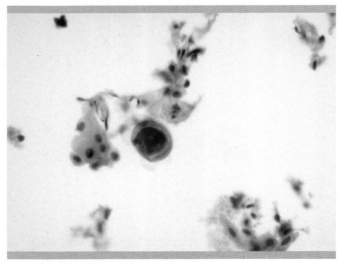

FIGURE 8-32

(A) *Actinomyces*
(B) Cocklebur
(C) Herpes simplex changes
(D) Pollen
(E) Psammoma body

33. A 27-year-old woman has a Pap test performed at her 22-week prenatal checkup. The following changes are seen (see Figure 8-33). What is the next best step in clinical management of this woman?

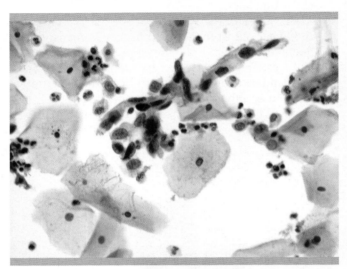

FIGURE 8-33

(A) Cervical colposcopy with endocervical sampling
(B) Cervical colposcopy without endocervical sampling
(C) Reflex human papilloma virus testing, and colposcopy if positive
(D) Repeat Pap at 6 weeks postpartum
(E) Routine screening in 3 years

34. A 32-year-old woman undergoes conventional Pap test screening, and the clinician notices significant ferning of the mucus on the slide. This most commonly corresponds with
(A) High levels of estrogen immediately before ovulation
(B) High levels of estrogen postovulation
(C) High levels of progesterone immediately before ovulation
(D) High levels of progesterone postovulation
(E) Pregnancy

35. In the past, vaginal smears have been used to evaluate women for infertility using the maturation index (MI). Which of the following hormonal states is correctly paired with the MI expected (parabasal: intermediate:superficial cells)?
(A) Newborn 0:90:10
(B) Premenstrual child 0:80:20
(C) Preovulatory 0:60:40
(D) Postmenopausal 20:80:0
(E) Postovulatory 0:40:60

36. A 34-year-old woman has a Pap test that contains clusters of hyperchromatic crowded groups. All of the following findings can cause hyperchromatic crowded groups except
    (A) Atrophy
    (B) Benign endometrial cells
    (C) Endocervical adenocarcinoma in situ
    (D) High-grade squamous intraepithelial lesion (HSIL)
    (E) Low-grade squamous intraepithelial lesion (LSIL)

37. The peak age range for women with a diagnosis of invasive squamous cell carcinoma is
    (A) 25–30 years old
    (B) 30–35 years old
    (C) 35–40 years old
    (D) 40–45 years old
    (E) 45–50 years old

38. What percentage of LSIL lesions will regress without further management within 2 years?
    (A) <5%
    (B) 20%
    (C) 50%
    (D) 80%
    (E) >95%

39. Which of the following human papilloma virus (HPV) subtypes is considered high risk?
    (A) 6
    (B) 11
    (C) 31
    (D) 40
    (E) 42

40. A woman has a vaginal smear with a maturation index (MI) of 0:80:20. Which of the following conditions could be associated with this MI?
    (A) Granulosa cell tumor of the ovary
    (B) Pregnancy
    (C) Preovulation
    (D) Polycystic ovarian disease
    (E) Postmenopause

41. During a human papilloma virus (HPV) infection of the cervical squamous epithelium, which of the following changes is associated with integration of the HPV genome into the host cell genome?
    (A) Disruption of the E1-E2 region of the virus genome
    (B) Irreversible infection by human immunodeficiency virus (HIV)

(C) Morphologic change from high-grade squamous intraepithelial lesion (HSIL) to invasive squamous cell carcinoma
(D) Overexpression of E6, which binds to retinoblastoma (Rb) protein
(E) Overexpression of E7, which binds to p53 protein

42. What is the single most important risk factor in the development of cervical squamous cell carcinoma?
    (A) Altered immune status (e.g., human immunodeficiency virus (HIV), leukemia)
    (B) HLA variation
    (C) Persistent human papilloma virus (HPV) infection
    (D) Microtrauma
    (E) Smoking

43. A 38-year-old woman has a Pap test, which is interpreted as high-grade squamous intraepithelial lesion (HSIL). A satisfactory colposcopy was performed, and the biopsy and endocervical curettage are negative for dysplasia. According to the 2012 ASCCP management guidelines, what is the next best step in the management of this woman?
    (A) Human papilloma virus testing alone at 6 months
    (B) Repeat colposcopy at 2 years
    (C) Repeat Pap test alone at 12 months
    (D) Repeat Pap test with human papilloma virus (HPV) cotesting at 12 months
    (E) Routine screening in 3 years

44. A 41-year-old woman presents for a screening Pap test, and benign-appearing exfoliated endometrial cells are present without other changes. Her last menstrual period is provided, and she is in day 9 of her cycle. The 2001 Bethesda System for Reporting Cervical Cytology recommends which of the following interpretations?
    (A) Atypical endometrial cells
    (B) Epithelial cell abnormality. Other: Endometrial cells present in a woman ≥40 years of age
    (C) Negative for intraepithelial lesion or malignancy (changes consistent with menstrual smear)
    (D) Negative for intraepithelial lesion or malignancy (no comment regarding endometrial cells)
    (E) Negative for intraepithelial lesion. Other: Endometrial cells present in a woman ≥40 years of age.

45. A 28-year-old woman presents for a screening Pap test, and an interpretation of "atypical squamous cells of undetermined significance (ASC-US)" is made. Assuming reflex human papilloma virus (HPV) testing is performed on this sample, what is the 2012 ASCCP recommended management of this woman?
    (A) If HPV negative: endocervical and endometrial sampling
    (B) If HPV negative: cervical colposcopy
    (C) If HPV negative: repeat Pap at 12 months
    (D) If HPV positive: cervical colposcopy
    (E) If HPV positive: repeat Pap at 12 months

46. A cell on a Pap test has a high nuclear to cytoplasmic ratio (close to 1:1). All of the other features listed below would be compatible with an interpretation of high-grade squamous intraepithelial lesion (HSIL) according to the 2001 Bethesda System for Reporting Cervical Cytology except
    (A) Densely keratinized cytoplasm
    (B) Irregular nuclear membrane
    (C) Nuclear hyperchromasia
    (D) Small cell size
    (E) Vesicular chromatin

47. A 36-year-old woman has a Pap test, which is interpreted as atypical glandular cells, not otherwise specified (AGC, NOS). According to the 2012 ASCCP management guidelines, what is the next best clinical management step?
    (A) Cervical colposcopy with endocervical sampling
    (B) Colposcopy, endocervical sampling, and endometrial sampling
    (C) Reflex human papilloma virus (HPV) testing, and colposcopy if positive
    (D) Repeat Pap in 6–12 months
    (E) Routine screening in 3 years

48. A 21-year-old woman presents for her initial Pap test. An interpretation of low-grade squamous intraepithelial lesion (LSIL) is made. According to the 2012 ASCCP management guidelines, what is the next best step in management of this process?
    (A) Cervical colposcopy with endocervical sampling
    (B) Colposcopy, endocervical sampling, and endometrial sampling
    (C) Reflex human papilloma virus testing, and colposcopy if positive
    (D) Repeat Pap in 12 months
    (E) Routine screening in 3 years

49. A 32-year-old woman has a negative Pap test, but human papilloma virus (HPV) testing is positive. According to the 2012 ASCCP management guidelines, what next step in the clinical management of this woman is most appropriate?
    (A) Diagnostic excisional procedure
    (B) HPV genotyping
    (C) Immediate colposcopy
    (D) Repeat HPV testing
    (E) Repeat Pap test and HPV testing in 24 months

50. A 57-year-old postmenopausal asymptomatic woman presents for a Pap test. An interpretation of "negative for squamous intraepithelial lesion, endometrial cells present in a woman over 40", is made. The endometrial cells are not atypical. According to the 2012 ASCCP management guidelines, what is the next best clinical management step for this woman?
    (A) Colposcopy with endocervical sampling and endometrial sampling
    (B) Endometrial sampling
    (C) Reflex human papilloma virus testing and colposcopy if positive
    (D) Repeat Pap test in 12 months
    (E) Routine screening in 3 years

51. Two vaccines have recently been developed against high-risk human papilloma virus subtypes 16 and 18. Both of these vaccines are manufactured using what process?
    (A) Killed virus particles
    (B) Live attenuated virus
    (C) Recombinant DNA vectors
    (D) Virus-like particles
    (E) Virus particles conjugated to a hapten

52. A 37-year-old woman has a Pap test performed, and an interpretation of "atypical squamous cells, cannot exclude a high-grade squamous intraepithelial lesion (ASC-H)", is made. According to the 2012 ASCCP management guidelines, what is the next best step in the clinical management of this woman?
    (A) Cervical colposcopy
    (B) Cervical colposcopy and endometrial sampling
    (C) Reflex human papilloma virus testing, and colposcopy only if positive
    (D) Repeat Pap in 12 months
    (E) Routine screening in 3 years

53. A 41-year-old woman has a Pap test performed, and it is interpreted as "atypical squamous cells, cannot exclude high-grade squamous intraepithelial lesion (ASC-H)". Why is aggressive management recommended for this result?

(A) The risk of cervical intraepithelial neoplasia 1 (CIN1) on biopsy is 40–50%
(B) The risk of CIN1 on biopsy is >80%
(C) The risk of CIN2 or worse on biopsy is 10–15%
(D) The risk of CIN2 or worse on biopsy is 40–50%
(E) The risk of CIN2 or worse on biopsy is >80%

54. During human papilloma virus (HPV)-related carcinogenesis, which of the following HPV-derived genes is responsible for an increase in p16 protein?
(A) E5
(B) E6
(C) E7
(D) L1
(E) L2

55. A 19-year-old woman presents to her primary care physician and requests the human papilloma virus vaccine Gardasil. She asks what percentage of cervical cancers this vaccine can prevent, and if she will also be protected from cervical warts. She also asks if she will need to continue to have Pap tests after finishing the vaccination series. What do you tell her?
(A) 70% of cervical cancers; it covers cervical warts; she does not need further screening
(B) 70% of cervical cancers; it covers cervical warts; she does need further screening
(C) 70% of cervical cancers; it does not cover cervical warts; she does need further screening
(D) 95% of cervical cancers; it covers cervical warts; she does not need further screening
(E) 95% of cervical cancers; it does not cover cervical warts; she does need further screening

56. Liquid-based Pap tests (e.g., ThinPrep and SurePath) were developed to overcome many limitations of conventional Pap tests, such as obscuring elements and poor fixation. What is another advantage of liquid-based Pap tests over conventional Pap tests?
(A) Ancillary testing on residual specimen
(B) Clustering of atypical cells for easier identification
(C) Easier evaluation of glandular clusters
(D) Less intense nuclear staining
(E) Reduced number of cells evaluated

57. Which of the following workloads can a cytopathologist perform and be within acceptable limits (without using automated screening)?
(A) Primary screening of 30 Pap tests and secondary review of 50 Pap tests in 3 hours of work
(B) Primary screening of 50 Pap tests and secondary review of 30 Pap tests in 3 hours of work
(C) Primary screening of 80 Pap tests in 6 hours of work
(D) Primary screening of 100 conventional Pap tests in 6 hours of work

(E) Primary screening of 200 liquid-based Pap tests in 8 hours of work

58. Which of the following quality control methods is required by a cytology laboratory that screens Pap tests, according to the Clinical Laboratory Improvement Amendments (CLIA) 1988 regulations?
(A) Correlation of all concurrently performed cervical biopsies with Pap test prior to final sign-out
(B) Correlation of all follow-up biopsies for all Pap tests after sign-out
(C) Rescreening of all negative high-risk Pap tests prior to final sign-out
(D) Rereview of all Pap tests in the last 5 years prior to the first interpretation of high-grade squamous intraepithelial lesion (HSIL)
(E) Random rescreening of at least 10% of negative Pap tests prior to final sign-out

59. Which of the following scenarios is an appropriate use of high-risk human papilloma virus (HPV) testing for the detection of cervical neoplasia?
(A) Follow-up of a 32-year-old woman with cervical intraepithelial neoplasia 1 (CIN1) 6 months ago and negative colposcopy
(B) Initial triage of a 19-year-old woman with atypical squamous cells of undetermined significance (ASC-US)
(C) Initial triage of a 31-year-old woman with atypical squamous cells, cannot exclude high-grade intraepithelial lesion (ASC-H)
(D) Initial triage of a postmenopausal woman with low-grade squamous intraepithelial lesion (LSIL)
(E) Primary HPV testing in a 29-year-old woman

60. The ThinPrep Imaging System (TIS) is the most widely used imaging system for cytology specimens, and is FDA approved for primary screening of cervical cytology. Which of the following statements is accurate regarding the TIS?
(A) Full manual review is required for all cases with an abnormality in at least one field of view
(B) There is no difference in sensitivity for the detection of atypical squamous cells of undetermined significance (ASC-US) or worse compared with manual review
(C) Slides can be filed without examination by a cytotechnologist if no abnormalities are identified by the imager
(D) The imager identifies 20 fields of view, which a cytotechnologist must review
(E) There is no difference in cytotechnologist productivity using this system, only increased detection of dysplasia

61. A 26-year-old woman has a Pap test interpretation of atypical squamous cells of undetermined significance (ASC-US), and reflex human papilloma virus testing is positive. At colposcopy, no lesions are identified, but the examination is considered unsatisfactory, as the transition zone cannot be visualized. Why is visualization of the transitional zone important for a satisfactory colposcopy?
    (A) Glandular epithelium is more susceptible to human papilloma virus infection
    (B) Most squamous lesions cannot be visualized in the ectocervix
    (C) Most squamous lesions involve the endocervix
    (D) Squamous metaplasia is more likely to involve the endocervix
    (E) The squamocolumnar junction is the site of most initial human papilloma virus infections

62. Pap test screening can be discontinued for which of the following women?
    (A) A 58-year-old woman who underwent hysterectomy for severe squamous dysplasia 10 years ago and has had 2 negative vaginal Pap tests
    (B) A 63-year-old woman with no prior abnormal paps and three consecutive negative Pap tests in the last 10 years
    (C) A 70-year-old woman with a history of diethylstilbestrol (DES) exposure and three consecutive negative Pap tests within the last 10 years
    (D) A 71-year-old woman with a history of atypical squamous cells of undetermined significance (ASC-US) at age 66 and three consecutive negative Pap tests since that time
    (E) A 79-year-old woman with a previous high-grade squamous intraepithelial lesion (HSIL) at age 34 and 3 consecutive negative Pap tests in the last 10 years

63. A 27-year-old woman is in the second half of her menstrual cycle, and a vaginal test performed has the following appearance (see Figure 8-34). Which of the following is true regarding the maturation index (MI) and appropriateness for her menstrual cycle?

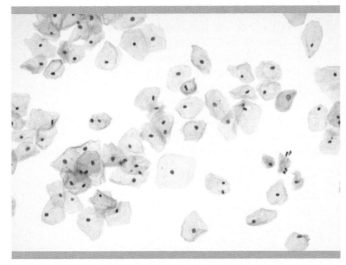

FIGURE 8-34

(A) Appropriate for phase, MI: 0/20/80
(B) Appropriate for phase, MI: 0/80/20
(C) Inappropriate for phase, MI: 0/20/80
(D) Inappropriate for phase, MI: 0/80/20
(E) Inappropriate for phase, MI: 60/40/0

64. A 25-year-old woman had a Pap test performed. The changes seen (see Figure 8-35) represent

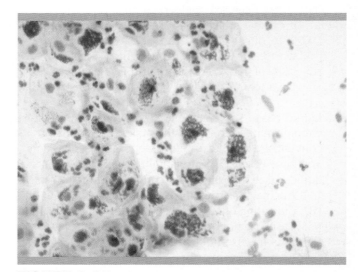

FIGURE 8-35

(A) Bacterial vaginosis
(B) Coverslipping artifact
(C) Glycogen deposition
(D) Keratohyaline granules
(E) Koilocytic change

65. A 32-year-old woman has the following changes present on her Pap test (see Figure 8-36). This change is most commonly associated with what clinical finding?

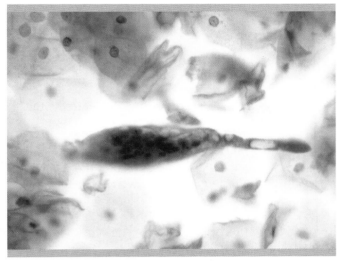

FIGURE 8-36

(A) Cervical tuberculosis
(B) *Chlamydia*
(C) Intrauterine device (IUD)
(D) Pregnancy
(E) Squamous cell carcinoma

66. A 27-year-old woman has the following Pap test (see Figure 8-37). The best interpretation for this finding is

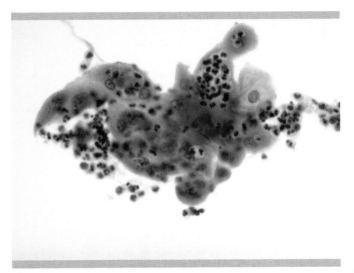

FIGURE 8-37

(A) Low-grade squamous intraepithelial lesion (LSIL)
(B) High-grade squamous intraepithelial lesion (HSIL)
(C) Negative for intraepithelial lesion or malignancy, atrophy
(D) Negative for intraepithelial lesion or malignancy, reactive changes
(E) Squamous cell carcinoma (SCC)

67. A 34-year-old woman presents for a Pap test, and a representative field is shown (see Figure 8-38). The best interpretation for this Pap test is

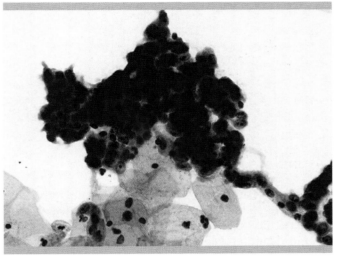

FIGURE 8-38

(A) Adenocarcinoma in situ
(B) Endocervical adenocarcinoma
(C) Exfoliated endometrial cells
(D) Normal endocervical cells
(E) Tubal metaplasia

68. A 51-year-old woman has a screening liquid-based Pap test performed, which has the following appearance (see Figure 8-39). Assuming that the figure is representative of the overall cellularity in each high-power field, in what setting would this Pap test not be adequate for an interpretation of negative for intraepithelial lesion or malignancy (NILM)?

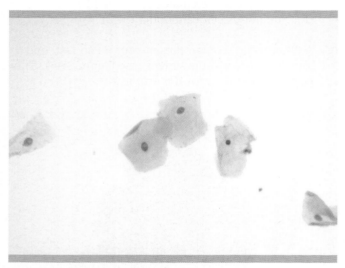

FIGURE 8-39

   (A) SurePath Pap test with atypical squamous cells
   (B) SurePath Pap test with no abnormalities
   (C) ThinPrep Pap test with atypical glandular cells
   (D) ThinPrep Pap test with atypical squamous cells
   (E) ThinPrep Pap test with no abnormalities

69. A 32-year-old woman has a Pap test with an interpretation of adenocarcinoma in situ (AIS). Colposcopy is performed, and biopsies are negative for neoplasia. According to the 2012 ASCCP management guidelines, what is the next best step in clinical management of this woman?
   (A) Diagnostic excision
   (B) Human papilloma virus testing
   (C) Repeat colposcopy in 1 year
   (D) Repeat Pap test at 6 months
   (E) Routine screening in 3 years

70. An atypical squamous cell is seen on a Pap test. What size should the nucleus be to qualify for an interpretation of low-grade squamous intraepithelial lesion (LSIL)?
   (A) 2.0–2.5 times the size of a normal intermediate cell nucleus
   (B) 2.5–3 times the size of a normal intermediate cell nucleus
   (C) 2.5–3 times the size of a normal superficial cell nucleus
   (D) >3 times the size of a normal intermediate cell nucleus

   (E) >3 times the size of a normal superficial cell nucleus

71. Which of the following statements regarding human papilloma virus (HPV) is not true?
   (A) HPV can contaminate objects as a potential source of transmission
   (B) Most HPV infections are transient
   (C) Most infections are asymptomatic
   (D) The peak age for HPV infection is 25–35 years old
   (E) The risk of infection is directly related to the number of sexual partners

72. A Pap test from a 34-year-old woman demonstrates atypical endocervical cells. Which of the following features, if present, would be worrisome for the presence of an invasive adenocarcinoma?
   (A) Coarse nuclear chromatin
   (B) Feathering
   (C) Granular, bloody background
   (D) Small nucleoli
   (E) Three-dimensional groups

73. In a Pap test, the arrangement of atypical glandular cells with palisading nuclei and nuclear and cytoplasmic tags protruding from the periphery is a feature of which of the following processes?
   (A) Endocervical adenocarcinoma in situ
   (B) Endometrial adenocarcinoma
   (C) Reactive glandular cells
   (D) Repair
   (E) Tubal metaplasia

74. A 34-year-old woman has a negative Pap test, which is limited due to absence of endocervical cells or a transition zone component. She has never had an abnormal Pap previously. Human papilloma virus testing was not performed. When should a repeat Pap test be performed?
   (A) 3 months
   (B) 6 months
   (C) 12 months
   (D) 3 years
   (E) 5 years

75. A 25-year-old woman has a Pap test performed, which is interpreted as atypical squamous cells of undetermined significance (ASC-US). Human papilloma virus (HPV) testing was performed and was positive. What percentage of women with these results will have a significant lesion (cervical intraepithelial neoplasia 2 or worse) on cervical biopsy?
   (A) <10%
   (B) 25–30%

(C) 45–50%
(D) 65–70%
(E) >80%

76. The Focal Point Primary Screening System (previously AutoPap) was approved by the FDA for primary screening of Pap tests in 1998. Which of the following statements accurately describes how this system works?
(A) Conventional smears, SurePath, and ThinPrep Pap tests can be screened on this instrument
(B) Slides are ranked according to the probability that an abnormality is present
(C) There is no difference in laboratory productivity using this system, only increased detection of dysplasia
(D) This system is approved for the screening of high-risk samples
(E) Up to 35% of slides can be filed without a cytotechnologist review

77. Which of the following statements is incorrect regarding human papilloma virus (HPV)?
(A) HPV is a double-stranded DNA virus
(B) Infection of basal cells is required
(C) Most infections are integrated into the host genome
(D) The HPV "early" genes (E6, E7) regulate transcription
(E) The HPV "late" genes (L1, L2) encode for capsid proteins

78. One of the most commonly used tests to detect human papilloma virus (HPV) in cervical samples is the hybrid capture test. Which of the following statements is true regarding this test methodology?
(A) All high-risk HPV subtypes can be identified using this modality in a cost-effective manner
(B) Antibodies against DNA–RNA hybrids are used
(C) Can detect a minimum of 1000 viral copies
(D) False-negative results are a common problem
(E) Hybrid capture is a DNA amplification-based test

79. The 2001 Bethesda System for Reporting Cervical Cytology includes the category "atypical squamous cells of undetermined significance (ASC-US)." Which of the following findings, if present in a Pap test, would qualify for an interpretation of ASC-US?
(A) Cell clusters with "feathering" and apoptotic bodies
(B) High nuclear to cytoplasmic ratio with coarse chromatin
(C) Nuclear enlargement 2.5–3 times larger than surrounding normal intermediate cells with minimal nuclear hyperchromasia

(D) Nuclear enlargement >3 times larger than surrounding normal intermediate cells with cytoplasmic perinuclear cavitation
(E) Nuclear enlargement 3.5–4 times larger than surrounding normal intermediate cells with irregular nuclear chromatin

80. The absence of a Barr body in almost all squamous epithelial cells during hormonal evaluation of an infertile woman on a vaginal smear is suggestive of which of the following clinical syndromes?
(A) Congenital atresia of the uterus
(B) Down syndrome
(C) Pituitary hypofunction
(D) Polycystic ovarian syndrome
(E) Turner syndrome

81. A Pap test from a 52-year-old woman demonstrates a high-grade squamous intraepithelial lesion (HSIL). Which of the following features, if present, would be worrisome for the presence of an invasive carcinoma?
(A) Coarse chromatin
(B) High nuclear-to-cytoplasmic ratio
(C) Irregular nuclear contours
(D) Macronucleoli
(E) Nuclear hyperchromasia

82. ThinPrep and SurePath are the two most commonly used liquid-based preparations for Pap tests in the United States. Each of these preparations uses a different mechanism to produce slides. Which of the following preparation mechanisms is appropriately paired with the correct system?
(A) SurePath: Centrifugation onto a filter
(B) SurePath: Liquid density gradient without centrifugation
(C) SurePath: Vacuum filtration
(D) ThinPrep: Liquid density gradient with centrifugation
(E) ThinPrep: Vacuum filtration

ANSWERS

1. **(B) Low-grade squamous intraepithelial lesion (LSIL).**
The squamous cells in this figure demonstrate the classic features diagnostic of LSIL: nuclear enlargement more than 3 times the size of nearby intermediate cells, nuclear hyperchromasia, coarse nuclear chromatin, and irregular nuclear contour. Binucleation is also a common finding. The cytoplasm demonstrates classic perinuclear cavitation (koilocytosis) that has a sharp delineation from the surrounding cytoplasm.

2. **(E) Presence on Pap test does not always correlate with symptomatic infection.**
   The photomicrograph demonstrates *Candida* species in a liquid-based Pap test. This is the most common vaginal and cervical fungal infection, and is most commonly *Candida albicans. Candida* grows predominantly as yeast buds, and forms pseudohyphae but not true hyphae. A classic appearance is the appearance of "shish kebab" or "spearing" of squamous cells. It is not considered a sexually transmitted disease, as it can occur in virgins and is part of the normal vaginal flora. Many asymptomatic women can demonstrate *Candida* organisms on Pap smears. Bacterial vaginosis is the most common cause of abnormal vaginal discharge.

3. **(A) Cervical colposcopy with endocervical sampling.**
   The findings present in the figure are classic for an interpretation of high-grade squamous intraepithelial lesion (HSIL). Single cells and small sheets of squamous cells with hyperchromatic, irregular nuclei are present that have significantly reduced amount of cytoplasm, leading to a high nuclear-to-cytoplasmic ratio. The significant nuclear contour irregularity and coarse chromatin differentiate HSIL from the parabasal cells of atrophy. The nuclei of HSIL may be larger than surrounding intermediate nuclei, but are not usually as enlarged as seen in low-grade squamous intraepithelial lesion (LSIL). The 2012 ASCCP guidelines for the management of women with abnormal cervical cytology recommend either an immediate diagnostic excisional procedure or immediate colposcopy with endocervical sampling in women with a Pap test interpretation of HSIL. Repeat Pap testing or triage with human papilloma virus testing is considered unacceptable. Endometrial biopsy is not required for women with an HSIL interpretation.

4. **(D) Last menstrual period.**
   The photomicrograph demonstrates a cluster of exfoliated small endometrial cells with no atypical features and the classic exodus "wreath" appearance of central dense stromal cells surrounded by glandular epithelium. The presence of normal-appearing exfoliated endometrial cells in a woman over the age of 40 should be reported in order to prevent missing endometrial pathology. However, in most women, particularly in those who are still menstruating, the risk of neoplasia is very low. In particular, in women over 40 with a provided last menstrual period that places the Pap test within the first half of her cycle, the laboratory can put an additional comment that the finding of endometrial cells correlates with the menstrual history provided. A prior loop electrosurgical excision procedure

(LEEP) procedure can result in a short endocervix and lead to direct sampling of the lower uterine segment. Diethylstilbestrol (DES) exposure is associated with the development of vaginal adenosis and clear cell carcinoma of the vagina. A high body-mass index (BMI) is often associated with endometrial adenocarcinoma in younger women, but, given the obesity epidemic in the United States, it is of less utility in most cases. A history of squamous dysplasia is common in women who develop endocervical neoplasia.

5. **(A) Adenocarcinoma in situ.**
   The photomicrograph demonstrates classic features of adenocarcinoma in situ: strips of endocervical cells with nuclear crowding and overlap, nuclear hyperchromasia and granular chromatin, mitotic figures, and apoptotic bodies. The classic feature of "feathering" is best seen on conventional Pap smears, and consists of nuclear and cytoplasmic tags protruding from the periphery of the group (like the feathers on an Indian headdress), seen focally in the lower portion of this figure. No tumor diathesis should be present, and nucleoli are generally inconspicuous; if these features are present, consider a diagnosis of adenocarcinoma. Tubal metaplasia is commonly mistaken for atypical endocervical cells, because of the nuclear crowding, overlap, and hyperchromasia, but other features of adenocarcinoma in situ (AIS) should not be present, and the presence of ciliary tufts on the surface is reassuring.

6. **(E) Negative for intraepithelial lesion or malignancy;** *Trichomonas vaginalis* **present.**
   The photomicrograph demonstrates squamous cells with reactive changes associated with *Trichomonas vaginalis* organisms in the background. These organisms are pear-shaped-to-oval, with a tiny pale nucleus that is eccentrically located. Eosinophilic granules in the cytoplasm are frequently seen, and although these organisms have a flagellum, it is not usually identified. *Trichomonas* can cause mild nuclear enlargement and perinuclear halos, but the changes are usually insufficient for an interpretation of atypical squamous cells of undetermined significance.

7. **(C) Postpartum follow-up.**
   The photomicrograph demonstrates a background of atrophy on her Pap test, characterized by a predominance of parabasal cells. Atrophy is most commonly seen in women who are postmenopausal or premenstrual. In a 29-year-old woman who is otherwise normal, this pattern would be unusual except in women who are postpartum, particularly women who are lactating. The withdrawal of pregnancy-related hormones can lead to this

pattern postpartum until the ovaries start to cycle normally again. Polycystic ovarian disease would result in a high estrogen state, with a corresponding superficial cell predominance. Pregnant women usually show intermediate predominance, unless a problem with the pregnancy has developed. Radiation therapy will typically show enlarged cells with bizarre nuclei, low nuclear-to-cytoplasmic ratios, and two-toned cytoplasm. The presence of human papilloma virus-positive testing on a previous Pap test can be present in any Pap test pattern, but most likely would show some nuclear changes indicative of dysplasia if infection was ongoing.

8. **(A) Ammonia or "fishy" odor to vaginal discharge.**
The photomicrograph demonstrates squamous epithelial cells, which are covered in coccobacilli, with loss of the normal lactobacilli of the cervical flora. This is highly suggestive of bacterial vaginosis, caused by *Gardnerella vaginalis*, which clings to squamous cells giving a "clue cell" appearance. Bacterial vaginosis most commonly causes a thin, gray, "fishy," or ammonia smelling discharge. Blisters can be a sign of herpes simplex infection, while a thick white discharge is more commonly associated with *Candida* infection. The classic finding of a "strawberry cervix," which is caused by many microhemorrhages on the cervix surface, is associated with *Trichomonas* infection. Intrauterine devices can be associated with *Actinomyces* infection.

9. **(C) Increase in nuclear size.**
The photomicrograph demonstrates a cluster of endometrial cells present in a liquid-based Pap test. The most important feature of atypical endometrial cells is nuclear enlargement, typically larger than the size of an intermediate cell nucleus. Both benign and atypical endometrial cells will have high nuclear-to-cytoplasmic ratios and a three-dimensional arrangement. Small nucleoli can be seen in both benign and neoplastic endometrial cells, particularly in liquid-based paps where better nuclear detail is visualized; however, large prominent nucleoli are a feature of atypical endometrial cells. Feathering is a feature of endocervical adenocarcinoma in situ.

10. **(D) Negative for intraepithelial lesion or malignancy, repair.**
The photomicrograph demonstrates features consistent with repair. Repair most commonly shows flat monolayer sheets of squamous cells with dense cytoplasm, distinct cytoplasmic borders, prominent nucleoli, and a streaming nuclear polarity (or "school of fish" appearance, where all of the oval nuclei are polarized and oriented in the same direction). It is not uncommon in repair to have

an inflammatory background, and mitotic figures can be seen. Although the nuclei are enlarged, this is usually less than that seen in dysplasia (around 2 times larger than intermediate nuclei), and the nuclear chromatin is open or finely granular. Other features of dysplasia, including marked nuclear enlargement, coarse chromatin, and variation in size or shape of nucleoli, should be absent; if present, an interpretation of atypical repair/atypical squamous cells of undetermined significance (ASC-US) should be rendered.

11. **(E) Trichomonas.**
The photomicrograph demonstrates long filamentous bacteria commonly known as *Leptothrix*, which is not generally considered clinically significant. *Leptothrix* is most commonly seen in association with *Trichomonas*; however, it is common for *Trichomonas* to be present without *Leptothrix* organisms. Whenever *Leptothrix* is seen on a Pap test, a close examination for *Trichomonas* is important to exclude this clinically important disease.

12. **(A) Granulosa cell tumor of ovary.**
In the past, the vaginal smears have been used to evaluate the hormonal cycling of women with infertility problems. The maturation index is counted as a ratio of parabasal-to-intermediate-to-superficial cells. In this case, the maturation index is 0/10/90, indicating a predominance of superficial cells. Superficial cells predominate in states with an excess of estrogen. This includes the first half of the menstrual cycle (preovulation), estrogen secreting tumors (such as granulosa cell tumor of the ovary), exogenous estrogen administration (hormone replacement therapy), or lack of estrogen metabolism (cirrhosis). Intermediate cells predominate in progesterone-rich states, such as pregnancy, the second half of the menstrual cycle (postovulation), and newborn girls (who get progesterone from their mother). Parabasal cells predominate in low hormonal states, such as postmenopausal atrophy and premenarche.

13. **(A) Cervical mass.**
The photomicrograph demonstrates features of a keratinizing squamous cell carcinoma: single cells with dense orangeophilic cytoplasm and spindled-to-tadpole shape in a background of tumor diathesis. Other cells with features of high-grade squamous intraepithelial lesion (HSIL) are present in the figure. Other features of squamous cell carcinoma on Pap test include macronucleoli and marked variation in nuclear size and shape. Squamous cell carcinoma on a Pap test is most likely associated with a cervical mass, although some women may have a normal exam. Uterine enlargement and bleeding

can be seen in association with endometrial carcinoma. Atrophy can be mistaken for a high-grade squamous intraepithelial lesion or carcinoma, due to the presence of granular debris and pseudo-parakeratotic cells, but will not show the nuclear pleomorphism or nuclear chromatin changes of neoplasia. Pregnancy most commonly results in a predominance of intermediate squamous cells, so-called "navicular cells." Ovarian carcinoma when present on a Pap test classically shows rare malignant cell clusters in an otherwise clean background of normal squamous cells.

14. **(C) High nuclear-to-cytoplasmic (N:C) ratio.**
Endocervical cells, such as those in the photomicrograph, can be difficult to evaluate for the presence of glandular neoplasia. Features that are reassuring for a benign or reactive process include arrangement in flat sheets or strips, honeycomb arrangement, and abundant cytoplasm. Significant nuclear enlargement can occur in reactive endocervical cells, and the nuclei may be four or more times larger than quiescent endocervical cell nuclei. One of the most useful features of endocervical glandular neoplasia is a high N:C ratio. Other features of neoplasia include three-dimensional groups, disorganized or crowded nuclei, feathered edges, coarse chromatin, and mitotic figures.

15. **(C) Glycogen deposition.**
The photomicrograph demonstrates intermediate squamous cells with a perinuclear deposition of golden-yellow material consistent with glycogen. When marked accumulation of glycogen occurs, the intermediate cells can have an elongated shape with distinct cell borders, called *navicular cells*, which is most commonly seen during pregnancy. This change is most commonly confused with koilocytic change due to human papilloma virus; however, the koilocytic halos of human papilloma virus are optically clear and associated with nuclear changes of dysplasia.

16. **(B) History of radiation therapy.**
The photomicrograph demonstrates bizarre squamous cells with large nuclei, abundant cytoplasm, and cytoplasmic vacuolization and polychromasia, but with a retained low nuclear-to-cytoplasmic (N:C) ratio. These changes are most consistent with prior ionizing radiation; this patient had a history of rectal carcinoma, which was treated with radiation therapy. A key morphologic feature helpful in discriminating between human papilloma virus-related dysplasia and radiation effect is the very low N:C ratio despite significant nuclear and cytoplasmic enlargement. Invasive squamous cell carcinoma may demonstrate increased cytoplasm with a

change in color, but this is generally related to keratin (orangeophilic appearance) and is associated with marked nuclear atypia, prominent nucleoli, and a background of tumor diathesis.

17. **(B) *Chlamydia*.**
The photomicrograph demonstrates a loose group of polymorphous lymphocytes associated with a tingible body macrophage, consistent with follicular cervicitis. Features that help to distinguish follicular cervicitis from small cell carcinoma and high-grade squamous intraepithelial lesion (HSIL) are the lack of nuclear molding, lack of clustering, and absence of epithelial groups. Features that help to distinguish follicular cervicitis from lymphoma are the range of lymphocyte size and appearance and the presence of tingible body macrophages. Follicular cervicitis in premenopausal women is associated with *Chlamydia* infection in over 50% of cases. However, follicular cervicitis is also common in postmenopausal women with atrophy, and is not associated with *Chlamydia* in this patient subset.

18. **(D) Rapid development can occur in the interval between screening Pap tests.**
The photomicrograph contains cells from a small cell undifferentiated (neuroendocrine) carcinoma of the cervix. This diagnosis can be difficult to make, due to the overlap of features with many other malignancies, including high-grade squamous intraepithelial lesion (HSIL), lymphoma, melanoma, and glandular neoplasia. Features that favor a diagnosis of small cell undifferentiated carcinoma of the cervix include small uniform cells with scant cytoplasm, hyperchromasia, stippled chromatin, and arrangement as single cells or in groups with nuclear molding or crush artifact. A background of tumor diathesis is common. This interpretation should be reserved for tumors that do not show evidence of glandular or squamous differentiation. These tumors are highly associated with human papilloma virus 18, and are often associated with a background or history of HSIL. Unfortunately, the rapid development of these tumors can result in progression from a previously normal Pap test to carcinoma in the interval between screening tests. Although these tumors are rare, it is unlikely to be a metastasis from an occult lung primary. Immunohistochemical staining for TTF-1 is not helpful; up to 33% of primary cervical small cell undifferentiated carcinomas can be positive for TTF-1. Treatment usually consists of aggressive chemotherapy, rather than initial surgical resection.

19. **(A) Cesarean section instead of vaginal delivery.**
The photomicrograph demonstrates squamous cells with multinucleation, nuclear molding, and

nuclear chromatin margination with viral inclusions, consistent with herpes simplex virus (HSV) infection. When changes of herpes simplex are found in a pregnant woman near term, cesarean section is recommended to prevent infection of the neonate with HSV during birth and risk of herpes neonatorum, which is rare but can be fatal. Antiviral agents, such as acyclovir, can be used to prevent active lesions during pregnancy in women with a history of HSV. A pregnant woman with the finding of low-grade squamous intraepithelial lesion (LSIL) or atypical squamous cells of undetermined significance (ASC-US) on Pap test typically results in colposcopy that is deferred until 6 weeks postpartum, while the finding of high-grade squamous intraepithelial lesion (HSIL) should prompt immediate colposcopy, despite pregnancy, but definitive excisions should be deferred until postpartum. Metronidazole is the most commonly used therapy for *Trichomonas*, and is safe during pregnancy. Antifungal creams are routinely used in the management of *Candida* infection during pregnancy.

20. **(A) Aria–Stella reaction.**
The photomicrograph demonstrates rare clusters of cells with abundant cytoplasm, atypical nuclei with hyperchromasia, and prominent nucleoli. Significant nuclear pleomorphism can also be seen in this process. However, it is important to note the clean background and lack of other dysplastic cells. These findings, in a pregnant woman, are most consistent with Aria–Stella reaction. These cells are commonly confused with adenocarcinoma, particularly clear cell type, but this is very rare in young women in the post-diethylstilbestrol (DES) era. Intrauterine devices (IUDs) can cause a similar effect on glandular cells, but an IUD would not be present in a pregnant woman. Decidual cells are rarely seen in pregnant women, and are the size of parabasal or intermediate cells with large nuclei and bland chromatin.

21. **(C) Intrauterine device present.**
The photomicrograph demonstrates balls of fluffy or "wooly" filamentous branching bacteria with a dark purple coloration, consistent with *Actinomyces*. This finding in a Pap test is most commonly associated with the presence of an intrauterine device (IUD). Bacterial vaginosis most commonly causes a thin, gray, "fishy," or ammonia smelling discharge. Blisters can be a sign of herpes simplex infection, while a thick white discharge is more commonly associated with *Candida* infection. The classic finding of a "strawberry cervix," which is caused by many microhemorrhages on the cervix surface, is associated with *Trichomonas* infection.

22. **(A) Coarse chromatin.**
The photomicrograph demonstrates tubal metaplasia on a Pap test, with the classic presence of terminal bars and cilia. When cilia are degenerated or lost, other features of tubal metaplasia can be worrisome for a glandular neoplasm, including crowded, three-dimensional clusters, increased nuclear-to-cytoplasmic ratio, and pseudostratified nuclei. One helpful feature that can be seen is the presence of vacuolated cytoplasm. Also, the chromatin of these cells, when not degenerated, is often fine and evenly distributed. The presence of coarse chromatin should prompt careful evaluation for other features of glandular neoplasia.

23. **(A) Atypical squamous cells of undetermined significance (ASC-US).**
The photomicrograph shows parakeratotic cells with dense orangeophilic cytoplasm and hyperchromatic nuclei. However, unlike normal parakeratosis, there is some nuclear enlargement and irregular nuclear contours. According to the 2006 Bethesda System for Reporting Cervical Cytology, atypical parakeratotic cells should be interpreted as ASC-US, atypical squamous cells of cannot exclude high-grade squamous intraepithelial lesion (ASC-H), or a squamous intraepithelial lesion, depending on the degree of abnormality. These cells show enough nuclear atypia to be interpreted as ASC-US; in contrast, normal parakeratotic cells would be classified under negative for intraepithelial lesion or malignancy (NILM), and it is optional to report them.

24. **(D) Spermatozoa.**
The photomicrograph demonstrates spermatozoa on a Pap test. Spermatozoa, or sperm, have small oval heads with a biphasic staining pattern, short necks, and long tails. They can be seen as long as 10 days after intercourse, but the numbers decrease rapidly after a day. The tail can be confused with infectious organisms, including *Candida* sp. and *Leptothrix*. The first sign of degeneration is loss of the tail, leaving only tiny sperm heads.

25. **(A) Cervical colposcopy.**
The photomicrograph demonstrates squamous cells with significant nuclear enlargement, nuclear hyperchromasia, coarse chromatin, and perinuclear koilocytic halos, consistent with low-grade squamous intraepithelial lesion (LSIL). According to the ASCCP 2012 consensus guidelines for the management of women with abnormal cervical cytology, the next best step in management is cervical colposcopy, with biopsy if a lesion is identified. According to the ALTS trial, women with a Pap test interpretation of LSIL have a 20–30% risk of cervical intraepithelial neoplasia 2 (CIN2) or worse at colposcopy within 2 years.

26. **(D) Pregnancy.**

The photomicrograph demonstrates a cocklebur (also known as a pseudoactinomycotic radiate granule). Cockleburs are radiating arrays of golden, refractile material that is not composed of hemosiderin or hematoidin. They are seen most commonly in pregnant women, and the presence of cockleburs does not have any association with maternal or fetal problems. They are believed to form from stagnating secretions containing degenerating cells, and are often surrounded by macrophages and inflammation. Cockleburs are rarely seen in women with intrauterine devices (IUDs), who more commonly have *Actinomyces* infection.

27. **(D) Intrauterine device (IUD).**

The photomicrograph demonstrates a cluster of atypical glandular cells with prominent nucleoli and vacuolization in a clean background. These types of cells are commonly seen in association with an IUD. These cells can be mistaken for adenocarcinoma; the clean background, open chromatin, and clinical history of an IUD should help to prevent misdiagnosis. Progestin injections result in an intermediate cell predominance or atrophy. Birth control pills containing estrogen and progesterone will show a mixture of superficial and intermediate cells. No specific changes are associated with condom use.

28. **(E) Metastatic breast carcinoma.**

The photomicrograph demonstrates rare markedly atypical cells arranged in a glandular cluster, but with a background of normal squamous cells and no tumor diathesis. This pattern is highly suggestive of metastasis (particularly fallopian tube or ovarian carcinomas). Invasive squamous cell carcinoma, endometrial adenocarcinoma, and endocervical adenocarcinoma almost always have an associated tumor diathesis, and the number of malignant cells is significantly higher. Involvement of the cervix by a large cell lymphoma would typically have more single cells and frequently will also show a necrotic background.

29. **(C) Pregnancy.**

The photomicrograph demonstrates abundant hyperkeratotic cells, which classically are anucleated and can have pink or orangeophilic cytoplasm. These cells may show keratohyaline granules. While a few hyperkeratotic cells are unremarkable, the presence of numerous hyperkeratotic anucleated squamous cells may be indicative of a hyperkeratotic squamous neoplasm, ranging from condyloma to a well-differentiated squamous cell carcinoma. Therefore, a comment in these cases on the presence of abundant hyperkeratotic cells is indicated to prompt clinical correlation; women with no clinical reason for hyperkeratosis (like prolapse) should be closely followed. A pregnant woman, in contrast, typically has a predominance of intermediate cells, and pregnancy alone should not cause hyperkeratosis.

30. **(E) Fallopian tube prolapse.**

The photomicrograph demonstrates a group of benign glandular cells in a background of superficial squamous cells. The finding of benign-appearing glandular cells in a post-hysterectomy woman can be related to several different possibilities: the history is wrong or she had a supracervical hysterectomy, vaginal adenosis, fallopian tube prolapse into the vaginal apex granulation tissue, or atrophic parabasal cells that have a "glandular" appearance. Careful attention to exclude a well-differentiated adenocarcinoma is required. In this patient, given the background of normal squamous maturation and lack of history of neoplasia, the most likely reason is fallopian tube prolapse. Vaginal adenosis caused by diethylstilbestrol (DES) requires in utero exposure.

31. **(A) Atrophy.**

The photomicrograph demonstrates a concentrically laminated calcified structure, consistent with a psammoma body. This is a very rare finding in Pap tests, and can be associated with a wide variety of conditions, both benign and malignant, including use of powders, pregnancy, intra-uterine device (IUD), ovarian cysts, endometriosis, endosalpingitis, cervical polyps, ovarian carcinomas (particularly serous carcinoma), endometrial carcinomas (particularly uterine serous carcinoma), and nongynecologic malignancies. Atrophy can show "blue blobs," which are mummified and degenerated parabasal cells and can mimic psammoma bodies, but psammoma bodies have not been specifically associated with an atrophic pattern.

32. **(D) Pollen.**

The photomicrograph demonstrates a strange particle with a waxy texture, irregular contour, and an internal structure reminiscent of plant matter. This most likely represents pollen, and is a contaminant from the air during processing. It is important to recognize this as not representing a psammoma body (which can have associations with malignant conditions), a cocklebur (which is associated with pregnancy), or infectious organisms. You never know what you will find in a Pap test!

33. **(B) Cervical colposcopy without endocervical sampling.**

The photomicrograph demonstrates cells with high nuclear-to-cytoplasmic ratio, hyperchromasia, coarse chromatin, and nuclear membrane irregularities, consistent with an interpretation of high-grade squamous intraepithelial lesion (HSIL). In a pregnant woman, the 2012 ASCCP guidelines for the management of women with abnormal cervical cytology recommends cervical colposcopy, with biopsy of any lesions worrisome for cervical intraepithelial neoplasia 2 (CIN2) or worse. Endocervical sampling is contraindicated in a pregnant woman. There is no role for reflex human papilloma virus testing due to the high probability of a significant lesion after a Pap test interpretation of HSIL. While a diagnostic excision may be postponed until after parturition, immediate colposcopy to exclude an invasive squamous cell carcinoma is recommended.

34. **(A) High levels of estrogen immediately before ovulation.**
    Although this finding is not reported on Pap test screening, the ferning pattern of endocervical mucus was first identified by Dr. Papanicolaou in 1946. It occurs at midcycle, at the point of peak estrogen production immediately preovulation, and is caused by the crystallization of cervical mucus as it dries. Estrogen treatment can also result in a ferning pattern. This phenomenon, along with spinnbarkeit (cervical mucus forming a thread when pulled apart), can be used to evaluate women for fertility, but this practice has gone out of favor with other modern testing modalities.

35. **(A) Newborn 0:90:10.**
    The maturation index (MI) has been used on vaginal smears to evaluate the hormonal cycle of women with infertility. The MI is listed as the percentage of each cell type: parabasal:intermediate:superficial (e.g., 0:40:60 in someone with no parabasal cells, 40% intermediate cells, and 60% superficial cells). Superficial cells predominate in high estrogen states, such as preovulation (e.g., 0:40:60), while intermediate cells predominate in high progesterone states, such as postovulation or pregnancy (e.g., 0:60:40). Parabasal cells predominate in premenstrual and postmenopausal women (e.g., 80:20:0) with the exception of newborns, who are exposed to maternal hormones and usually have an intermediate predominance (e.g., 0:90:10).

36. **(E) Low-grade squamous intraepithelial lesion (LSIL).**
    Hyperchromatic crowded groups on Pap tests are defined as three-dimensional aggregates of cells that show nuclear overlap and nuclear hyperchromasia. Most clusters of hyperchromatic crowded groups are benign, and can be caused by benign endometrial cells, atrophy, tubal metaplasia, or fragments of reactive endocervical glandular cells. However, some neoplasms can show a similar hyperchromatic crowded appearance, including endocervical adenocarcinoma, high-grade squamous intraepithelial lesion (particularly carcinoma in situ), and endometrial adenocarcinoma. LSIL cells generally have sufficient cytoplasm to prevent the crowding seen with these other processes. Careful attention to the nuclear features of hyperchromatic crowded groups is needed to discriminate benign from neoplastic processes: chaotic architecture, coarse chromatin, feathered edges, and background dysplasia favor a neoplastic process.

37. **(C) 35–40 years old.**
    Women of any age can develop invasive squamous cell carcinoma (although it is decidedly rare in teenagers), but the peak age at diagnosis is 39. More women with invasive squamous cell carcinoma are diagnosed in the 35–40 years old age group than any other. This reflects the natural history of squamous intraepithelial lesions, which typically take 10–15 years from human papilloma virus infection to development of invasive carcinoma.

38. **(C) 50%.**
    A significant number of cervical dysplasias will regress spontaneously, and dysplasia is more likely to regress if it is lower grade and in a younger woman. One study reported that approximately 50% of low-grade squamous intraepithelial lesions (LSIL) or cervical intraepithelial neoplasia 1 (CIN1) lesions would regress within 2 years, compared with around 33% of high-grade squamous intraepithelial lesion (HSIL), CIN2, or CIN3 lesions. In comparison, less than 20% of LSIL will progress to a higher-grade lesion, and 25% of HSIL will progress within 2 years.

39. **(C) 31.**
    A human papilloma virus (HPV) subtype is considered high risk if it has been found in cervical cancer. For all HPV subtypes, very few infections develop into cancer. The two high-risk HPV subtypes most strongly associated with cervical cancer are 16 and 18, and the other more common high-risk subtypes include 31 and 33. HPV subtypes 6, 11, 40, and 42 are all considered low risk.

40. **(B) Pregnancy.**
    A maturation index of 0:80:20 indicates a predominance of intermediate cells, which is usually associated with high progesterone states (postovulation, most oral contraceptives, etc.) or pregnancy. Preovulation, polycystic ovarian disease, and granulosa cell tumor of the ovary are all states with a high estrogen levels, while postmenopause is associated with very little hormone production and atrophy.

41. **(A) Disruption of the E1-E2 region of the virus genome.**
Integration of the human papilloma virus (HPV) genome into the host cell DNA is one of the most important steps in cervical carcinogenesis. Since the HPV genome is circular, integration results in disruption of part of the HPV genome, most commonly in the E1-E2 region, resulting in inactivation of the E2 gene. As E2 also acts as an inhibitor of E6/E7 transcription, integration results in overexpression of the E6 and E7 proteins. E6 binds to p53 protein, and E7 binds to RB protein, therefore preventing p53-mediated apoptosis and Rb-inhibition of cell cycle progression. This leads to rapid cell proliferation without cell death. Integration of the HPV genome is associated with transformation morphologically from a low-grade squamous intraepithelial lesion (LSIL) to a high-grade squamous intraepithelial lesion (HSIL) lesion (both HSIL and invasive squamous cell carcinoma are associated with integrated HPV).

42. **(C) Persistent human papilloma virus (HPV) infection.**
Persistent human papilloma virus (HPV) infection is the single most important risk factor for the development of cervical carcinoma. All of the other conditions listed above are additional risk factors for the development of cervical carcinoma, and most are thought to play a role in development of carcinoma because these conditions increase the probability of persistent HPV infection. Other risk factors, such as number of male vaginal sexual partners, high-risk sexual partners, and microtrauma, increase the risk of carcinoma by increasing the risk of exposure and infection by HPV.

43. **(D) Repeat Pap test with human papilloma virus (HPV) cotesting at 12 months.**
After a Pap test interpretation of high-grade squamous intraepithelial lesion (HSIL), the likelihood of a significant cervical lesion (cervical intraepithelial neoplasia 2 or worse) is >80%. Therefore, even if the initial colposcopic biopsy is negative for dysplasia, the 2012 ASCCP guidelines for management of women with abnormal cervical cytology recommend either a diagnostic excision, or repeat cytology and human papilloma virus testing every 12 months for the next 2 years. The option of observation with repeat Pap and HPV testing should only occur in women with an adequate initial colposcopy and negative endocervical curettage. If any repeat Pap test is abnormal or the HPV test is positive, repeat colposcopy should be performed. Repeat Pap test alone or HPV testing alone at 6 or 12 months are unacceptable. Repeat colposcopy at 2 years may delay diagnosis and is an unacceptable option alone.

44. **(E) Negative for intraepithelial lesion. Other: Endometrial cells present in a woman >40 years of age.**
According to the 2001 Bethesda System for Reporting Cervical Cytology, the presence of exfoliated endometrial cells on a Pap test from a woman 40 years of age or older should be reported, regardless of menstrual history. Benign endometrial cells in this situation are reported in the "Other" category, and a separate statement regarding the presence or absence of a squamous lesion should be included. If the menstrual history is provided and the woman is in phase (day 1–12), an additional comment can be added stating that the findings correlate with the menstrual history. Recent studies have shown that the risk of malignancy is very low in women who are asymptomatic and over 40 but premenopausal with benign endometrial cells on a Pap test; however, due to the problem of inaccurate reporting of clinical history and last menstrual period, laboratories are encouraged to still report endometrial cells in this population.

45. **(D) If HPV positive: cervical colposcopy.**
Reflex human papilloma virus (HPV) testing is recommended for Pap tests with an interpretation of "atypical squamous cells of undetermined significance," as it helps to better identify women who require colposcopy. The 2012 ASCCP guidelines for the management of women 25 or older with abnormal cervical cytology recommend colposcopy in women with ASC-US and a positive HPV result, and cotesting by cervical cytology and HPV testing at 3 years for women with a negative HPV result. If reflex HPV testing is not performed, physicians should repeat Pap testing at 1 year.

46. **(E) Vesicular chromatin.**
An interpretation of high-grade squamous intraepithelial lesion (HSIL) most commonly is made in the presence of cells that have coarse chromatin, nuclear hyperchromasia, irregular nuclear contours, and high nuclear to cytoplasmic ratios. These cells can be very small (close to basal cells) or larger, similar to the size of nuclei in a low-grade squamous intraepithelial lesion (LSIL) type cell. Most of the time the cytoplasm will be lacy and delicate or metaplastic, but occasionally the cytoplasm can be densely keratinized (keratinizing HSIL). The presence of vesicular chromatin, particularly with smooth nuclear contours, would favor benign parabasal cells, which can have a very high nuclear-to-cytoplasmic ratio.

47. **(B) Colposcopy, endocervical sampling, and endometrial sampling.**
An interpretation of atypical glandular cells, not otherwise specified (AGC, NOS) is associated

with a sufficient risk of neoplasia that immediate colposcopy with endocervical sampling is recommended in all women, according to the ASCCP 2012 guidelines for management of women with abnormal cervical cytology. In a woman over 35 or a woman under 35 with risk factors for endometrial neoplasia, endometrial sampling should also be performed, as in this case. At this time, there is no role for human papilloma virus testing prior to colposcopy.

48. **(D) Repeat Pap in 12 months.**

The 2012 ASCCP guidelines for the management of women with abnormal cervical cytology made an exception for younger women (ages 21 to 24). Unlike women over 24, the appropriate management of a younger woman with an interpretation of low-grade squamous intraepithelial lesion (LSIL) is to repeat her Pap test in 12 months, not to undergo colposcopy. This is due to the low probability of a significant cervical lesion in this population, and the increased risk of morbidity due to unnecessary procedures. If the subsequent Pap at 12 months shows atypical squamous cells, cannot exclude high-grade intraepithelial lesion (ASC-H), or high-grade squamous intraepithelial lesion (HSIL), then colposcopy is recommended. Also, if persistent abnormal but milder results (atypical squamous cells of undetermined significance (ASC-US) or LSIL) are present at both 12 and 24 months, then referral to colposcopy is recommended. Reflex human papilloma virus testing is not recommended in the management of younger women with LSIL.

49. **(B) HPV genotyping.**

Primary human papilloma virus (HPV) screening used in conjunction with Pap testing has been recommended for women over 30 as a more sensitive way to detect persistent HPV infections earlier. However, this has resulted in the problem of managing women who are negative by cytology, but positive for HPV testing. Several options are open to manage these women: repeat Pap testing and HPV cotesting in 12 months, or HPV genotyping. Due to the very low prevalence of significant disease in this patient subset, immediate colposcopy or a diagnostic excisional procedure is not recommended. If HPV genotyping is performed, immediate colposcopy is recommended if HPV subtypes 16 or 18 are identified, as these women are most likely to harbor a significant lesion. Otherwise, follow-up in 12 months using both tests is suggested.

50. **(B) Endometrial sampling.**

The finding of benign-appearing endometrial cells on a Pap test from a woman who is postmenopausal is concerning for possible endometrial pathology. Although it is uncommon for women with endometrial carcinoma to be asymptomatic, occasionally it can occur. Therefore, the 2012 ASCCP guidelines for the management of women with abnormal cervical cytology recommend endometrial sampling in these women. In this case, cervical colposcopy is not recommended due to the lack of evidence for a squamous lesion. Human papilloma virus has no association with endometrial pathology, and should not be used in this setting.

51. **(D) Virus-like particles.**

Both Gardasil and Cervarix vaccines are created using virus-like particles of human papilloma virus genotypes 16 and 18 (and 6 and 11 for Gardasil). Virus-like particles are empty protein shells created through recombinant technology to closely mimic the viral capsid L1 proteins found in human papilloma virus viruses. No live virus, killed virus, or viral DNA is present in the vaccine, so there is no risk of infection to the recipient. A hapten is not needed for this vaccine to mount a sufficient antibody response in the recipient.

52. **(A) Cervical colposcopy.**

An interpretation of atypical squamous cells, cannot exclude a high-grade squamous intraepithelial lesion (ASC-H) on Pap test is associated with a biopsy demonstrating cervical intraepithelial neoplasia 2 (CIN2) or worse in over 40% of women. Therefore, the 2012 ASCCP guidelines for the management of women with abnormal cervical cytology recommend immediate colposcopy. Endometrial sampling is not required in this setting. Reflex human papilloma virus testing is not recommended prior to colposcopy, due to the substantial risk of a significant lesion. However, if colposcopy with biopsy is negative, then human papilloma virus testing is recommended at the next cervical screening for further triage.

53. **(D) The risk of CIN2 or worse on biopsy is 40–50%.**

Most management decisions for women with abnormal Pap test results are based on the risk of a significant lesion (usually squamous, since that is more common) on subsequent biopsy. Most groups define a significant squamous lesion as CIN2 (moderate squamous dysplasia) or worse. Although the category "atypical squamous cells, cannot exclude high-grade squamous intraepithelial lesion (ASC-H)" has substantial inter-observer variability, multiple studies have demonstrated a significant risk (over 40%) of CIN 2 or worse on biopsy. This is considered sufficient risk that women with an ASC-H Pap test interpretation to go directly to colposcopy without reflex human papilloma virus testing. In contrast, an interpretation of high-grade squamous intraepithelial lesion (HSIL) is associated with CIN2 or worse on biopsy in over 80% of women.

54. **(C) E7.**

During human papilloma virus-related carcinogenesis, unrestricted production of the E7 protein (due to loss of the normal inhibitory feedback mechanisms after viral integration into the host genome) results in E7 binding to the retinoblastoma gene protein (Rb). Binding to Rb frees E2F, which then acts as a transcription factor to induce cell proliferation. E7 also induces cyclin A and cyclin E activity, which results in p16 (INK4A) overexpression. E6 binds to p53 to prevent cell-mediated apoptosis. L1 and L2 are viral capsid proteins that are essential for the production of normal viral proteins. There is very little known about the role of E5 in carcinogenesis at this time.

55. **(B) 70% of cervical cancers; it covers cervical warts; she does need further screening.**

Gardasil is the quadrivalent human papilloma virus (HPV) vaccine that covers HPV subtypes 16, 18, 6, and 11. Vaccination against HPV subtypes 6 and 11 should protect against the majority of cervical warts. The vaccination against HPV subtypes16 and 18 should protect against cervical cancers caused by those viruses, which account for 70% of cervical cancer. There may be some additional cross-protection from cervical cancer caused by other high-risk HPV subtypes, but how much is still uncertain. Since the HPV vaccine does not protect against all possible causes of cervical cancer, she will still need to undergo Pap test screening in the future.

56. **(A) Ancillary testing on residual specimen.**

Probably the largest advantage that liquid-based Pap tests have over conventional paps, besides reduction of obscuring elements and better fixation, is the availability of the residual vial for ancillary testing. High-risk human papilloma virus testing can be performed on the vial as a reflex for atypical squamous cells of undetermined significance (ASC-US) results, as well as other studies (such as immunohistochemical staining for p16(INK4A)) that are still in research development. Less intense nuclear staining and reduced number of cells evaluated are disadvantages of liquid-based Pap tests, although in theory the reduced sample may be more representative of the overall cervical sample than in conventional Pap test. Liquid-based Pap tests are notorious for disaggregating cell clusters, making identification of atypical cells more difficult. Finally, the evaluation of glandular cells in liquid-based Pap tests is generally regarded as more difficult than on conventional Pap tests, due to the tendency of

glandular cells to form thick, three-dimensional aggregates that are difficult to see through, and cells at the periphery of groups are harder to evaluate.

57. **(A) Primary screening of 30 Pap tests and secondary review of 50 Pap tests in 3 hours of work.**

Any person who performs primary screening of Pap tests (cytopathologists, cytotechnologists, etc.) cannot primary screen more than 100 Pap tests in an 8-hour period (excluding the use of automated screening). This must be pro-rated at 12.5 Pap tests screened per hour for persons who work part time. This is not a target for screening, and the actual limit of slides screened per hour should be determined by each laboratory for each individual screener, based on experience and other quality control measures. The number of secondary review of Pap tests is not regulated and does not count toward this total. Therefore, the only answer that complies with 12.5 Pap tests or less per hour is primary screening of 30 Pap tests in 3 hours of work (10 per hour). Recently, several automated systems to assist in the screening of Pap tests have been implemented (e.g., ThinPrep Imaging System, Focal Point Slide Imager), and the counting of imager-assisted screened slides is more complex; simply, an imager-assisted screened slide that does not require a full manual review counts as 0.5 slides toward the daily 100 slide limit. The counting of imager-assisted screened Pap test slides that are abnormal, and require a full manual review, is more controversial and beyond the scope of this question.

58. **(E) Random rescreening of at least 10% of negative Pap tests prior to final sign-out.**

The Clinical Laboratory Improvement Amendments (CLIA) were passed by Congress in 1988 to establish quality standards for all laboratory testing to ensure the accuracy, reliability, and timeliness of patient test results regardless of where the test was performed. The cytology laboratory is required to follow several quality control measures related to Pap test screening. These include a 10% random rescreen of all negative Pap tests (including some but not all high-risk patients), review of histologic biopsy correlation for all Pap test interpretations of high-grade squamous intraepithelial lesion (HSIL) or worse, and review of all prior negative Pap tests in the last 5 years prior to the first interpretation of HSIL or worse. The other options listed above may be used in many laboratories, but are not required by CLIA 88.

59. **(D) Initial triage of a postmenopausal woman with low-grade squamous intraepithelial lesion (LSIL).**

Recent guidelines regarding appropriate and inappropriate situations to use high-risk human papilloma virus (HPV) DNA testing have been published. The most common recommendations are for reflex testing with HPV in women 25 and older with a Pap test result of atypical squamous cells of undetermined significance (ASC-US). However, reflex HPV testing is not recommended for women who are younger than 25 due to the high prevalence of occult HPV infection in this population. Primary HPV testing is recommended for women over the age of 30. A Pap test result of LSIL, atypical squamous cells of undetermined significance cannot exclude high-grade squamous intraepithelial lesion (ASC-H), high-grade squamous intraepithelial lesion (HSIL), or worse should not have reflex HPV testing performed, but instead go directly to colposcopy. An exception to this rule is postmenopausal women with an LSIL result, in whom HPV triage can be useful in directing further management. In general, HPV testing should not occur more frequently than 12 months apart, except during follow-up of women with cervical intraepithelial neoplasia 2 (CIN2) or worse.

60. **(A) Full manual review is required for all cases with an abnormality in at least one field of view.**
The ThinPrep Imaging System works by staining the Pap test slide with a special quantitative stain, which will allow measurement of nuclear characteristics and DNA content. The computer system then screens the entire slide, and identifies 22 fields of view for a cytotechnologist to screen. If no abnormalities are seen within these fields of view, no further review is performed and the case is signed out as negative. However, if any cellular abnormalities are identified within the fields of view, the entire slide must be manually rescreened. The FDA clinical trials demonstrated that the TIS showed an increased sensitivity for the detection of atypical squamous cells of undetermined significance (ASC-US) or worse, and increased specificity in the detection of high-grade squamous intraepithelial lesion (HSIL) in comparison to manual review. In addition, the workload of cytotechnologists was increased to a possible 200 imaged-slides (each counted as 1/2 slide toward the 100 slides/day limit) within an 8-hour workday. In contrast to the Focal Point Imager, all slides must have a cytotechnologist review 22 fields, even if the computer does not detect an abnormality.

61. **(E) The squamocolumnar junction is the site of most initial human papilloma virus infections.**
Human papilloma virus (HPV) infection is the most important risk factor for the development of cervical neoplasia. HPV preferentially infects the dividing cells of squamous epithelium, specifically the basal cells. Access to these cells is most commonly

available at the squamocolumnar junction, where glandular epithelium undergoes squamous metaplasia in response to injury or trauma. Therefore, most initial HPV infections occur in the transition zone, and squamous lesions spread outward from that site into the rest of the ectocervix or endocervix. Failure to visualize the transition zone during colposcopy results in a risk of unrecognized neoplasia. While glandular epithelium can be infected by HPV, it is much less common. The majority of squamous lesions in the ectocervix can be visualized during colposcopy using acetowhite and other topical agents, as long as the area is satisfactorily visualized.

62. **(E) A 79-year-old woman with a previous high-grade squamous intraepithelial lesion (HSIL) at 34 and 3 consecutive negative Pap tests in the last 10 years.**
The 2012 American Cancer Society screening guidelines for the prevention and early detection of cervical cancer recommend two possible exits from cervical screening for women. The first is in women who are 65 years of age or older and have had 3 consecutive negative Pap tests in the last 10 years, with some exceptions. The other exit is for women who undergo hysterectomy for benign disease without a history of cervical neoplasia. If a woman has had a history of cervical intraepithelial neoplasia 2 (CIN2) or cervical intraepithelial neoplasia 3 (CIN3), she can exit screening if she has had at least 20 years of follow-up and meets one of the two above criteria. However, women with a history of cervical or endometrial cancer, or a history of diethylstilbestrol (DES) exposure, should continue to undergo screening until they develop a life-limiting chronic condition.

63. **(B) Appropriate for phase, MI: 0/80/20.**
In the past, the Pap test has been used to evaluate the hormonal cycling of women with infertility problems. The MI is counted as a ratio of parabasal cell to intermediate cells to superficial cells, written as percentages of each type of cell X/X/X. According to her history, she is in the second half of her menstrual phase (postovulatory) and therefore should have an abundance of progesterone, leading to a predominance of intermediate cells. The photomicrograph demonstrates a Pap test, which is predominantly intermediate cells with no parabasal cells and a few superficial cells (0/80/20), which is appropriate for her menstrual cycle.

64. **(B) Coverslipping artifact.**
The photomicrograph demonstrates squamous epithelial cells covered with tiny, refractile, golden-brown speckles, a coverslipping artifact known as

cornflaking. This artifact occurs when xylene evaporates before the coverslip is applied, leaving small air-bubbles trapped on top of the cells. It is commonly mistaken for keratohyaline granules, which are small, dark blue-black granules covering squamous cells derived from hyperkeratotic epithelium with a granular cell layer.

65. **(D) Pregnancy.**
The photomicrograph demonstrates a multinucleated giant cells with a cytoplasmic tail (or extension) and nuclei concentrated in the center of the cell. These findings are consistent with a syncytiotrophoblast, which is almost never seen except in association with pregnancy. It can mimic histiocytes or malignancy. Although some authors have suggested the finding of syncytiotrophoblasts is worrisome for premature delivery, there is limited evidence to support this claim due to the rarity of this finding.

66. **(D) Negative for intraepithelial lesion or malignancy, reactive changes.**
The squamous cells demonstrate mild nuclear enlargement (less than twofold larger than a normal intermediate cell nuclei) and small perinuclear halos, combined with small nucleoli. There is a background of acute inflammation. These features are consistent with reactive changes and should not be interpreted as evidence of squamous neoplasia.

67. **(B) Endocervical adenocarcinoma.**
The photomicrograph shows features classic for endocervical adenocarcinoma: two- or three-dimensional clusters of glandular cells with enlarged pleomorphic nuclei and irregular nuclear membranes. Prominent nucleoli and the presence of a tumor diathesis are helpful features. It can be difficult in some cases to distinguish endocervical adenocarcinoma from endometrial adenocarcinoma; in this case, endocervical adenocarcinoma would be favored due to her young age. Another feature of endocervical adenocarcinoma not present in this figure is the presence of background squamous dysplasia.

68. **(B) SurePath Pap test with no abnormalities.**
The photomicrograph demonstrates 4–5 benign-appearing squamous cells in one high-power field. The minimum squamous cellularity criteria for adequacy are 8,000–12,000 squamous cells for a conventional Pap test and 5000 squamous cells for a liquid-based Pap test. The ThinPrep Pap test has a much larger diameter for cell evaluation (20 mm), and therefore requires an average of 3–4 squamous cells per high-power field to have adequate cellularity. In contrast, the SurePath Pap test has a much smaller diameter for cell evaluation (13 mm), and

therefore 7–8 squamous cells per high-power field are required to have adequate cellularity. However, any Pap test with abnormal cells (glandular or squamous) is considered adequate regardless of cellularity.

69. **(A) Diagnostic excision.**
An interpretation of adenocarcinoma in situ (AIS) on Pap test is highly associated with the presence of high-grade squamous dysplasia or endocervical neoplasia on biopsy. Therefore, after a negative colposcopy, the 2012 ASCCP guidelines for the management of women with abnormal cervical cytology recommend a diagnostic excision, preferably cold knife cone excision, to exclude a lesion high within the endocervical canal. Human papilloma virus (HPV) testing is not useful in this setting; while HPV16 and 18 are highly associated with endocervical adenocarcinoma, a negative HPV result can be present in a significant number of women.

70. **(D) >3 times the size of a normal intermediate cell nucleus.**
An interpretation of low-grade squamous intraepithelial lesion (LSIL) on Pap test would include cells with nuclear enlargement >3 times the size of a normal intermediate cell nucleus on the same slide, along with nuclear hyperchromasia, and irregular chromatin. A cell that has a nucleus 2.5–3 times the size of a normal intermediate cell nucleus with minimal nuclear hyperchromasia would fall into the atypical squamous cells of undetermined significance (ASC-US) category. Cells with a nuclear size less than 2.5 times the size of an intermediate cell nucleus would be interpreted as negative unless a high nuclear-to-cytoplasmic ratio with hyperchromatic chromatin suggestive of high-grade squamous intraepithelial lesion (HSIL) was present. Comparison with superficial cell nuclei is not performed because of pyknosis and inconsistent size.

71. **(D) The peak age for HPV infection is 25–35 years old.**
Human papilloma virus (HPV) is the most common sexually transmitted disease. Risk of infection is directly related to the number of sexual partners. The peak age of HPV infection mirrors the peak age of sexual activity with new partners, and women from 15 to 25 are most likely to test positive for HPV. Most infections are transient and asymptomatic, and less than 30% of women will show cytologic abnormalities within 5 years. HPV is a relatively hardy virus, and has been found on contaminated objects, such as shared underwear, previously used speculums, surgical gloves and even toilet seats, although transmission in this fashion is rare.

72. **(C) Granular, bloody background.**
When atypical glandular cells are present on a Pap test, the following features are highly concerning for the presence of invasive adenocarcinoma: tumor diathesis (granular, bloody background), macronucleoli, and nuclear clearing with uneven distribution of the chromatin. However, in some well-differentiated adenocarcinomas, tumor diathesis and macronucleoli may not be seen. Clinical correlation with the clinical exam is recommended before making an interpretation of an invasive endocervical adenocarcinoma.

73. **(A) Endocervical adenocarcinoma in situ.**
The cellular arrangement of atypical glandular cells with palisading nuclei and nuclear and cytoplasmic tags protruding from the periphery of the group on a Pap test is referred to as "feathering." This is one of the most important features that helps distinguish endocervical adenocarcinoma in situ from an interpretation of atypical endocervical cells, along with the finding of mitotic figures and apoptotic bodies.

74. **(D) 3 years.**
According to the 2012 ASCCP guidelines for the management of women with abnormal cervical cytology, absence of an endocervical cell or transitional zone (EC/TZ) component alone in a Pap test no longer requires repeat Pap test at an earlier interval than routine screening. For women over 30 with a negative HPV test, a return to routine screening with cotesting (Pap and HPV) at 5 years is acceptable. If HPV testing was not performed, a repeat Pap test should be performed at 3 years. If her HPV test is positive, repeat cotesting at 12 months or HPV genotyping are acceptable options.

75. **(B) 25–30%.**
The ASC-US LSIL Triage Study (ALTS) was performed to evaluate the ability of human papilloma virus (HPV) testing to triage patients with an atypical squamous cells of undetermined significance (ASC-US) result on Pap test for colposcopy. This trial demonstrated that 25–30% of women (age 20–30) with an interpretation of ASC-US who were HPV positive had cervical intraepithelial neoplasia 2 (CIN2) or worse on biopsy within 2 years. This rate was identical to the rate of CIN2 or worse in women with an interpretation of low-grade squamous intraepithelial lesion (LSIL) on Pap test. In comparison, women with a negative HPV result and an ASC-US interpretation had a risk of CIN2 or worse that was very similar to that of women with a negative Pap test result. Based on these findings, the recommended management of ASC-US HPV-negative women is follow-up at 3 years with

cotesting; for ASC-US HPV positive women it is colposcopy.

76. **(B) Slides are ranked according to the probability that an abnormality is present.**
The Focal Point System (previously AutoPap) analyzes slides SurePath or conventional Pap test slides (not ThinPrep) using a high-speed video microscope and image interpretation software, which evaluates the slides without human intervention. It measures many cellular features and compares them to thousands of reference images; finally, it ranks all slides in the group into quintiles according to the probability of an abnormality (quintile 1 most likely to be abnormal, quintile 5 least likely to be abnormal). Up to 25% of slides that are least likely to be abnormal are designated as "no further review" and can be filed without further review by a cytotechnologist. The remaining 75% are manually screened by a cytotechnologist. The instrument also identifies at least 15% of the slides that are most likely to be abnormal for rescreening for quality control. This system can therefore improve the entire laboratory's productivity, as well as improve detection of dysplasia. However, this system is not approved for the screening of high-risk samples; high-risk cases require full manual review.

77. **(C) Most infections are integrated into the host genome.**
Human papilloma virus (HPV) is an encapsulated, double-stranded DNA virus that infects cells that are still capable of cell division. In the cervix, HPV infects the basal cells or reserve cells, usually gaining access through microtrauma during sexual activity. The late genes (L1, L2) encode proteins for the capsid, while early genes (E6, E7, etc.) are responsible for regulating transcription and replication. Most infections are episomal (not integrated), but most high-grade squamous intraepithelial lesions and squamous cell carcinomas have integration of the HPV genome into the host DNA. Integration in this manner appears to be a critical step in the development of high-grade squamous lesions.

78. **(B) Antibodies against DNA–RNA hybrids are used.**
The hybrid capture test is a signal amplification test. Rather than amplifying the amount of target DNA present in the sample by polymerase chain reaction, it captures human papilloma virus (HPV) DNA by hybridizing it to a complementary RNA sequence, and then amplifying the signal using chemiluminescent-tagged antibodies against DNA–RNA hybrids. This helps prevent false-positive results, but the cutoff for positive results is around 5000 viral copies. Only a limited number of high-

risk HPV subtypes are usually tested for in a single assay. While theoretically all high-risk HPV subtypes could be incorporated into the test, it is too expensive, and many of the less common high-risk HPV subtypes are too infrequent, for this to be cost-effective.

79. **(C) Nuclear enlargement 2.5–3 times larger than surrounding normal intermediate cells with minimal nuclear hyperchromasia.**
The 2001 Bethesda System for Reporting Cervical Cytology defines the category of *atypical squamous cells of undetermined significance (ASC-US)* as cytologic changes suggestive of a squamous intraepithelial lesion, which is qualitatively or quantitatively insufficient for definitive interpretation. For an interpretation of ASC-US, cells must show squamous differentiation, increased nuclear size, and minimal nuclear hyperchromasia, chromatin clumping, irregularity, smudging, or multinucleation. Comparison with normal-appearing intermediate cells in the same slide is recommended, and nuclear enlargement of 2.5–3 times larger than normal intermediate cell nucleoli is recommended. Nuclear enlargement >3 times larger than surrounding normal intermediate cells, along with cytoplasmic perinuclear cavitation, and irregular nuclear chromatin, would be appropriately interpreted as low-grade squamous intraepithelial lesion (LSIL), while cell clusters with "feathering" and apoptotic bodies are concerning for adenocarcinoma in situ of the endocervix. Cells with a high nuclear-to-cytoplasmic ratio and coarse chromatin would either be interpreted as atypical squamous cells—cannot exclude high-grade squamous intraepithelial lesion (ASC-H) or high-grade squamous intraepithelial lesion (HSIL).

80. **(E) Turner syndrome.**
Although evaluation for infertility by examination for Barr bodies is infrequently used in current practice, it continues to have historical significance as one of the first genetic tests. A Barr body is the randomly selected inactivated X chromosome that should be present in each nucleus derived from a normal woman's somatic tissues (such as squamous epithelium). Morphologically, it appears as a dense triangular area of chromatin that is darker than the rest of the nuclear chromatin and attached to the lateral edge of the nuclear envelope. Turner syndrome is a genetic disease characterized by loss of one X chromosome; therefore, a woman with Turner syndrome will not have any inactivated X chromosomes to form Barr bodies. All of the other disorders listed earlier are not usually associated with abnormalities of the X chromosome.

81. **(D) Macronucleoli.**
Many of the morphologic changes seen in a high-grade squamous intraepithelial lesion overlap with those seen in an invasive squamous cell carcinoma; these include nuclear hyperchromasia, coarse nuclear chromatin, irregular nuclear contours, and high nuclear-to-cytoplasmic ratio. When seen, the following features are worrisome for an invasive carcinoma: macronucleoli, background tumor diathesis, and marked variation in cell shape (spindle cell, caudate cells, teardrop, etc.) with dense orangeophilic cytoplasm. Correlation with clinical findings, including cervical exam, is recommended prior to rendering an interpretation of invasive squamous cell carcinoma on a Pap test.

82. **(E) ThinPrep: Vacuum filtration.**
The ThinPrep system uses a vacuum to draw cells from the vial onto a TransCyt filter, which epithelial cells and organisms adhere to but debris, mucus, and blood pass through. Then the filter is touched to a slide, leaving a "touch imprint" of the cells on the filter, but without the filter remaining on the slide, forming a 20-mm diameter disc. In contrast, the SurePath system mixes the vial material with a liquid density gradient solution, which is then centrifuged; the gradient concentrates epithelial cells in one level, while blood, debris and inflammation sediments at a different level. Then an aliquot of the appropriate level containing epithelial cells is placed onto a slide and allowed to sediment using gravity, forming a 13-mm diameter disc. In both of these systems, epithelial cells are concentrated and background debris, blood, and inflammation are removed, but this results in different artifacts for each system. In the ThinPrep system, cells are more disaggregated but form a very thin monolayer, while in the SurePath system, the cells remain more three-dimensional, but this requires significantly more depth of focus while evaluating the slides.

SUGGESTED READING

1. Clinical Laboratory Improvement Amendments of 1988. Final Rule. (2003). http://www.cms.gov/Regulations-and-Guidance/Legislation/CLIA
2. Cutts FT, Franceschi S, Goldie S, et al. Human papillomavirus and HPV vaccines: a review. *Bull World Health Organ.* 2007;85(9):719-726.
3. Davey DD, Cox JT, Austin RM, et al. Cervical cytology specimen adequacy: patient management guidelines and optimizing specimen collection. *J Low Genit Tract Dis.* 2008; 12(2):71-81.
4. DeMay RM. *The Pap Test.* Chicago, IL: ASCP Press; 2005.
5. The Atypical Squamous Cells of Undetermined Significance/Low-Grade Squamous Intraepithelial Lesions Triage

Study (ALTS) Group. Human papillomavirus testing for triage of women with cytologic evidence of low-grade squamous intraepithelial lesions: baseline data from a randomized trial. *J Natl Cancer Inst.* 2000;92(5):397-402.

6. Lowy DR, Schiller JT. Prophylactic human papillomavirus vaccines. *J Clin Invest.* 2006;116(5):1167-1173.

7. Massad LS, Einstein MH, Huh WK, et al. 2012 Updated Consensus Guidelines for the Management of Abnormal Cervical Cancer Screening Tests and Cancer Precursors. *Journal of Lower Genital Tract Disease*, Volume 17, Number 5, 2013, S1YS27.

8. Melnikow J, Nuovo J, Willan AR, Chan BK, Howell LP. Natural history of cervical squamous intraepithelial lesions: a meta-analysis. *Obstet Gynecol.* 1998;92(4 Pt 2):727-735.

9. ASCUS-LSIL Traige Study (ALTS) Group. Results of a randomized trial on the management of cytology interpretations of atypical squamous cells of undetermined significance. *Am J Obstet Gynecol.* 2003;188(6):1383-1392.

10. Saslow D, Solomon D, Lawson HW, et al. American Cancer Society, American Society for Colposcopy and Cervical Pathology, and American Society for Clinical Pathology screening guidelines for the prevention and early detection of cervical cancer. *Am J Clin Pathol.* 2012;137(4):516-542.

11. Schiffman M, Solomon D. Findings to date from the ASCUS-LSIL Triage Study (ALTS). *Arch Pathol Lab Med.* 2003;127(8):946-949.

12. Sherman ME, Schiffman M, Cox JT. Effects of age and human papilloma viral load on colposcopy triage: data from the randomized Atypical Squamous Cells of Undetermined Significance/Low-Grade Squamous Intraepithelial Lesion Triage Study (ALTS). *J Natl Cancer Inst.* 2002;94(2):102-107.

13. Solomon D, Davey D, Kurman R, et al. The 2001 Bethesda System: terminology for reporting results of cervical cytology. *JAMA.* 2002;287(16):2114-2119.

14. Solomon D, Nayar R, eds. *The Bethesda System for Reporting Cervical Cytology.* 2nd ed. New York, NY: Springer; 2004.

15. Solomon D, Papillo JL, Davey DD. Statement on HPV DNA test utilization. *Am J Clin Pathol.* 2009a;131(6):768-769; discussion 770-763.

16. Solomon D, Papillo JL, Davey DD. Statement on human papillomavirus DNA test utilization. *Cancer.* 2009b;117(3):154-156.

17. Stoler MH, Wright TC Jr, Sharma A, et al. High-risk human papillomavirus testing in women with ASC-US cytology: results from the ATHENA HPV study. *Am J Clin Pathol.* 2011;135(3):468-475.

18. Wojcik EM, Booth CN. Automation in cervical cytology. *Pathology Case Reviews.* 2005;10(3):138-143.

19. Wright TC Jr, Stoler MH, Sharma A, et al. Evaluation of HPV-16 and HPV-18 genotyping for the triage of women with high-risk HPV+ cytology-negative results. *Am J Clin Pathol.* 2011;136(4):578-586.

CHAPTER 9

CYTOLOGY: NON-GYNECOLOGIC

1. An 82-year-old woman undergoes transthoracic fine-needle aspiration biopsy of a lung mass. The first pass shows the following finding (see Figure 9-1). What is the most likely source of these cells?

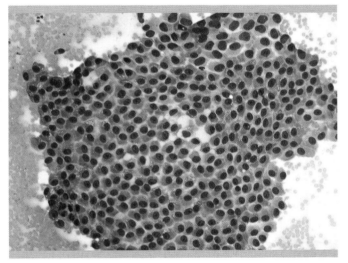

FIGURE 9-1

    (A) Alveolar macrophages
    (B) Benign bronchial cells
    (C) Non-small cell carcinoma
    (D) Pleural mesothelial cells
    (E) Small cell undifferentiated carcinoma

2. A 73-year-old man undergoes transthoracic fine-needle aspiration biopsy of a lung mass (see Figure 9-2). What is the best diagnosis?

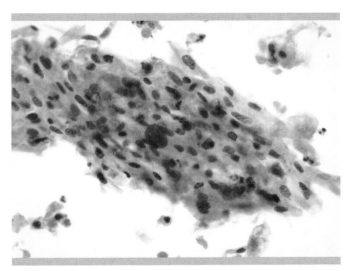

FIGURE 9-2

    (A) Adenocarcinoma
    (B) Reserve cell hyperplasia
    (C) Small cell undifferentiated carcinoma
    (D) Squamous cell carcinoma
    (E) Squamous metaplasia with reactive changes

3. A 43-year-old woman presents with an endobronchial mass and undergoes fine-needle aspiration biopsy (see Figure 9-3). What is the best diagnosis for this lesion?

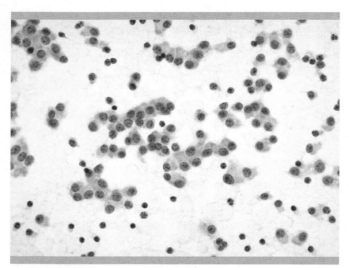

FIGURE 9-3

(A) Adenoid cystic carcinoma
(B) Pulmonary carcinoid tumor
(C) Plasmacytoma
(D) Small cell undifferentiated carcinoma
(E) Well-differentiated adenocarcinoma

4. A 75-year-old man with a 100-pack-year smoking history presents with a large hilar lung mass. Fine-needle aspiration biopsy is performed (see Figure 9-4). Which of the following immunohistochemical stains, if positive, would confirm the diagnosis?

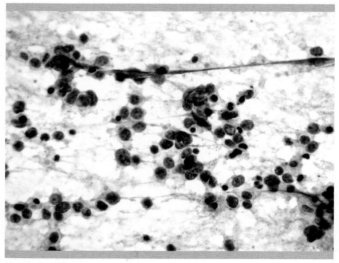

FIGURE 9-4

(A) CD20
(B) CD34

(C) Napsin A
(D) P63
(E) Synaptophysin

5. A 45-year-old man undergoes fine-needle aspiration biopsy of a renal mass. The following structure is seen in the aspirate sample (see Figure 9-5). From which of the following tissues does this structure likely originate?

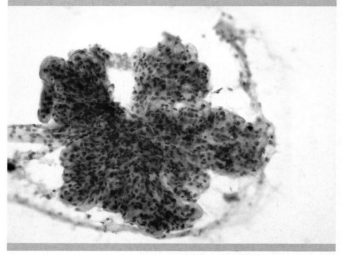

FIGURE 9-5

(A) Benign renal cortex
(B) Benign renal medulla
(C) Clear cell renal cell carcinoma
(D) Papillary renal cell carcinoma
(E) Renal medullary carcinoma

6. An 82-year-old man presents with a renal mass. Fine-needle aspiration biopsy is performed (see Figure 9-6). What cytogenetic abnormality is mostly likely present in this tumor?

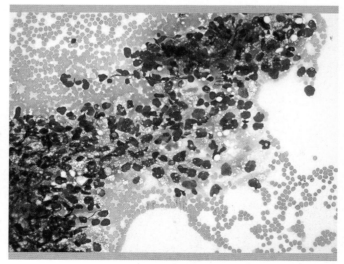

FIGURE 9-6

(A) Loss of chromosome 3 short arm (3p-)
(B) Loss of chromosome Y
(C) Trisomy 7
(D) *TSC1* gene inactivation
(E) Xp11.2 alterations

7. A 72-year-old man with a history of a "kidney tumor" presents with enlarged retroperitoneal lymph nodes. A fine-needle aspiration biopsy is performed (see Figure 9-7). Which of the following tumors is most likely to have this appearance?

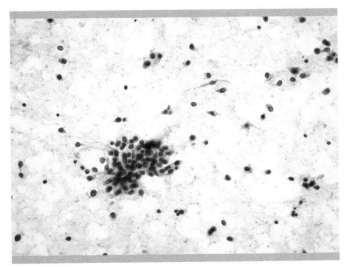

FIGURE 9-7

(A) Angiomyolipoma
(B) Clear cell renal cell carcinoma
(C) Oncocytoma
(D) Papillary renal cell carcinoma
(E) Urothelial carcinoma

8. A 44-year-old man with a history of cirrhosis is found to have a 3.0-cm liver mass. Fine-needle aspiration biopsy was performed (see Figure 9-8). What is the best diagnosis?

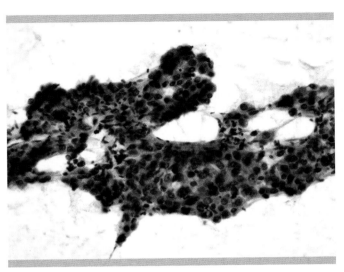

FIGURE 9-8

(A) Cholangiocarcinoma
(B) Focal nodular hyperplasia
(C) Metastatic colorectal carcinoma
(D) Regenerating cirrhotic nodule
(E) Well-differentiated hepatocellular carcinoma

9. A 37-year-old man presents with dry cough, fever, and bilateral pulmonary infiltrates. A bronchioloalveolar lavage is performed (see Figure 9-9, inset Gomori methenamine silver stain). What condition is this process associated with?

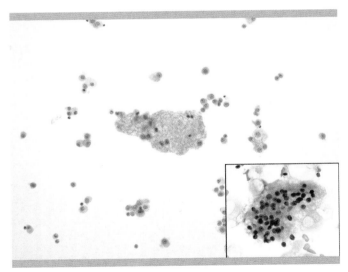

FIGURE 9-9

(A) Asbestos exposure
(B) Asthma
(C) Bird handling (e.g., pigeons)
(D) Heavy smoking history
(E) Suppressed immune function

Chapter 9 CYTOLOGY: NON-GYNECOLOGIC

10. A 62-year-old man presents with upper gastro-intestinal bleeding. At endoscopy, a polypoid submucosal mass is present in the body of the stomach, with relatively normal overlying mucosa. Endoscopic fine-needle aspiration biopsy is performed (see Figure 9-10). What immunohisto-chemical stain will confirm the diagnosis?

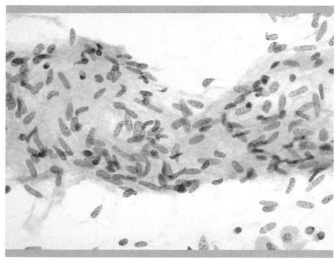

FIGURE 9-10

(A) C-kit (CD117)
(B) Cytokeratin
(C) Desmin
(D) HMB-45
(E) Myogenin

11. A 37-year-old man with poor dentition presents with enlarged right cervical neck lymph nodes. Fine-needle aspiration biopsy is performed (see Figure 9-11). Assuming this figure is representative of the entire aspirate sample, what is the best diagnosis?

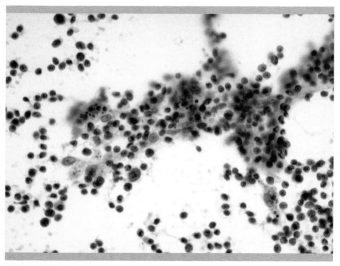

FIGURE 9-11

(A) Diffuse large B-cell lymphoma
(B) Mantle cell lymphoma
(C) Metastatic squamous cell carcinoma
(D) Reactive lymphoid hyperplasia
(E) Sarcoidosis

12. A 27-year-old man presents with bulky cervical lymphadenopathy, night sweats, and weight loss. Fine-needle aspiration biopsy of a neck lymph node is performed (see Figure 9-12). What is the next best step in the workup of this aspirate sample?

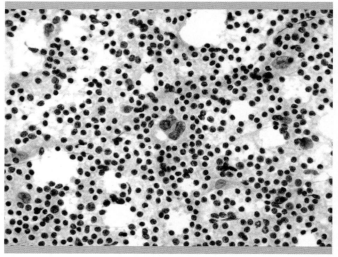

FIGURE 9-12

(A) Culture for acid-fast bacteria and fungi
(B) Flow cytometry
(C) Immunohistochemical staining for CD30, CD15, and CD20
(D) Immunohistochemical staining for cytokeratin and S-100
(E) Serologic studies for Epstein–Barr virus

13. A 45-year-old man presents with headache and neck stiffness. A cerebrospinal fluid sample is submitted for cytologic examination (see Figure 9-13). What special stain will highlight the capsule of this organism?

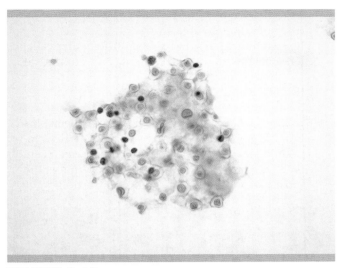

FIGURE 9-13

(A) Fontana–Masson
(B) Gomori methenamine silver (GMS)
(C) Mucicarmine
(D) Periodic acid Schiff (PAS)
(E) Ziehl–Neelson

14. A 44-year-old man undergoes fine-needle aspiration biopsy (FNA) of a solitary 2.5-cm solid thyroid nodule (see Figure 9-14). Assuming this figure is representative of the entire aspirate, what is the most appropriate next step in management of this lesion?

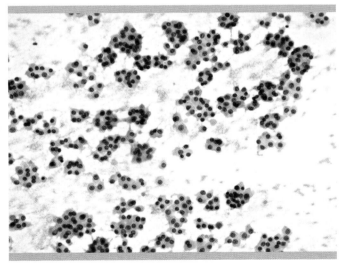

FIGURE 9-14

(A) Clinical follow-up only with ultrasound in 1 year
(B) Repeat FNA in 3 months
(C) Repeat FNA within a week
(D) Thyroid lobectomy
(E) Total thyroidectomy with central neck lymph node dissection

15. A 43-year-old man who recently emigrated from Egypt has a bladder mass, and a urine sample is submitted for cytologic examination (see Figure 9-15). This neoplasm is associated with what infectious organism?

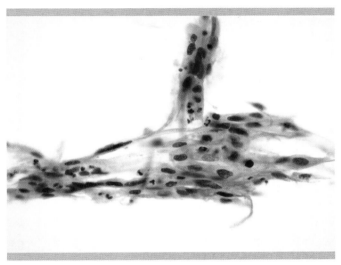

FIGURE 9-15

(A) *Clonorchis sinensis*
(B) Human papilloma virus
(C) Polyomavirus
(D) *Schistosoma hematobium*
(E) *Schistosoma mansoni*

16. A 71-year-old woman presents with hematuria. Cystoscopy of the bladder is negative for abnormalities, and a urine specimen at the time of cystoscopy is submitted for cytologic examination (see Figure 9-16). What is the most likely diagnosis?

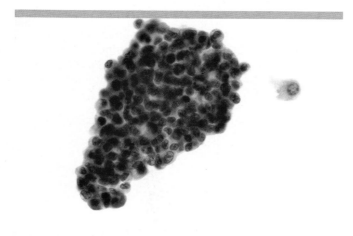

FIGURE 9-16

(A) Flat urothelial carcinoma in situ
(B) High-grade papillary urothelial carcinoma of the bladder
(C) Nephrolithiasis
(D) Polyoma virus infection
(E) Squamous cell carcinoma of the bladder

17. A 29-year-old woman undergoes fine-needle aspiration biopsy for a 1.8-cm thyroid nodule (see Figure 9-17). The most important cytologic feature for identification and diagnosis of this lesion is

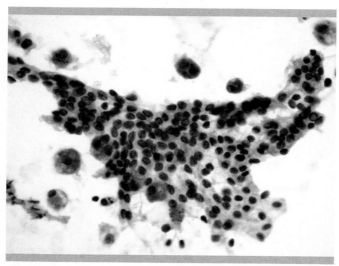

FIGURE 9-17

(A) Absence of colloid
(B) Abundant cytoplasm
(C) Architectural arrangement of follicular cells
(D) Background of cyst contents and multinucleated giant cells
(E) Nuclear atypia

18. A 33-year-old man undergoes fine-needle aspiration biopsy of a 1.0-cm right upper pole thyroid nodule (see Figure 9-18). His brother was recently diagnosed with the same neoplasm. What is the most likely mutation present in this lesion?

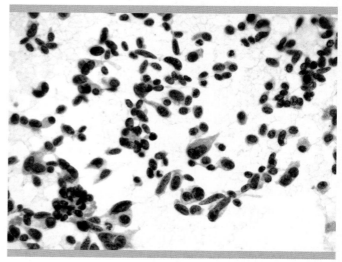

FIGURE 9-18

(A) *BRAF* point mutation
(B) *PAX8/PPARγ* translocation
(C) *RAS* point mutation
(D) *RET* point mutation
(E) *RET/PTC* translocation

19. An 89-year-old man presents with a rapidly growing thyroid mass causing respiratory stridor. The mass is very firm to palpation. A fine-needle aspiration biopsy is performed (see Figure 9-19). What is the most likely diagnosis?

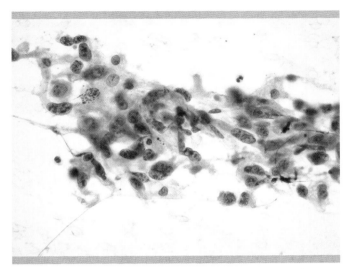

FIGURE 9-19

(A) Benign, reactive changes
(B) Metastatic squamous cell carcinoma
(C) Papillary thyroid carcinoma
(D) Pleomorphic sarcoma of the thyroid gland
(E) Undifferentiated (anaplastic) thyroid carcinoma

20. A 41-year-old woman undergoes thyroid fine-needle aspiration biopsy of a thyroid gland nodule (see Figure 9-20). What peripheral blood test is likely to be abnormal in this patient?

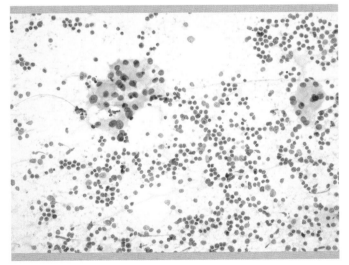

FIGURE 9-20

(A) Elevated serum calcitonin
(B) Elevated serum calcium
(C) Elevated serum thyroglobulin
(D) Elevated T3/T4 levels
(E) Positive antithyroglobulin antibodies

21. A 62-year-old man presents with a parotid mass. Fine-needle aspiration biopsy is performed (see Figure 9-21). What is the best diagnosis for this lesion?

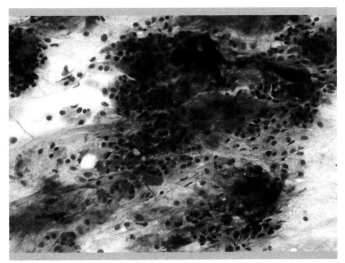

FIGURE 9-21

(A) Acinic cell carcinoma
(B) Adenoid cystic carcinoma
(C) Mucoepidermoid carcinoma
(D) Pleomorphic adenoma
(E) Warthin tumor

22. A 14-year-old boy presents with a parotid mass, and undergoes fine-needle aspiration biopsy (see Figure 9-22). All of the following statements are true regarding this lesion except

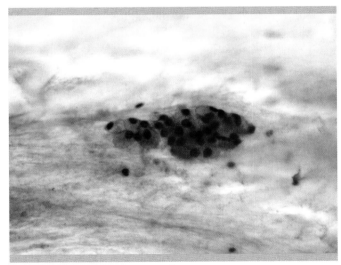

FIGURE 9-22

(A) Associated with a recurring translocation of chromosomes 11 and 19
(B) Can arise primarily within the mandibular bone
(C) Frequently a cause of false-negative aspirate results
(D) May appear oncocytic in fine-needle aspiration biopsy samples
(E) Second most common malignant salivary gland neoplasm in children

23. A 55-year-old woman presents with a submandibular mass, and undergoes fine-needle aspiration biopsy (see Figure 9-23). What is the most likely diagnosis?

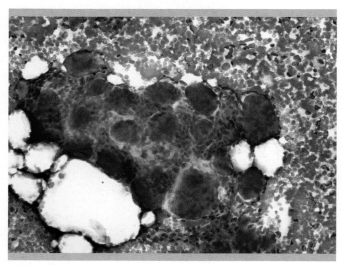

FIGURE 9-23

   (A) Acinic cell carcinoma
   (B) Adenoid cystic carcinoma
   (C) Mucoepidermoid carcinoma
   (D) Pleomorphic adenoma
   (E) Warthin tumor

24. A 58-year-old man has bilateral parotid lesions, and undergoes fine-needle aspiration biopsy (see Figure 9-24). This lesion is highly associated with what risk factor?

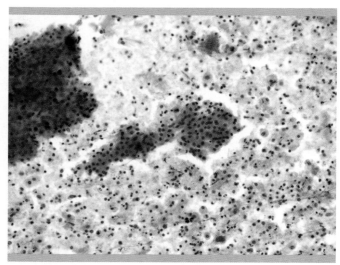

FIGURE 9-24

   (A) Alcohol
   (B) Human papilloma virus
   (C) Radiation exposure

   (D) Sjögren syndrome
   (E) Smoking

25. A 76-year-old man undergoes fine-needle aspiration biopsy of a parotid mass (see Figure 9-25). Immunohistochemical staining on the cell block demonstrates 3+ continuous membranous staining for HER2. What is the most likely diagnosis?

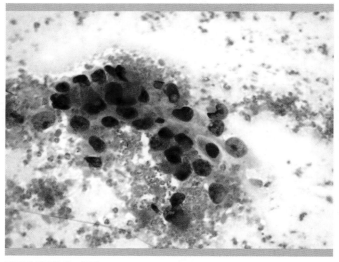

FIGURE 9-25

   (A) Adenocarcinoma, favor breast origin
   (B) Anaplastic large cell lymphoma
   (C) High-grade mucoepidermoid carcinoma
   (D) Malignant melanoma
   (E) Salivary duct carcinoma

26. A 52-year-old woman with an ovarian mass undergoes salpingo-oophorectomy. At the time of surgery, a pelvic washing is performed, which shows the following finding (see Figure 9-26). What is the best diagnosis for this washing?

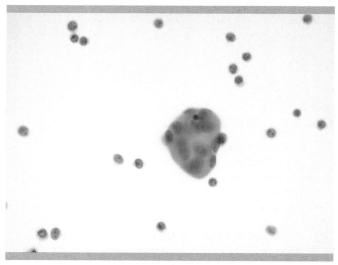

FIGURE 9-26

(A) Atypical cells, suspicious for a borderline serous tumor
(B) Atypical cells, suspicious for malignant mesothelioma
(C) Negative for malignancy
(D) Positive for malignancy, malignant mesothelioma
(E) Positive for malignancy, papillary serous carcinoma

27. A 65-year-old woman presents with a large right pleural effusion. Cytologic examination of the fluid demonstrates the following changes (see Figure 9-27). What is the most likely origin of these cells?

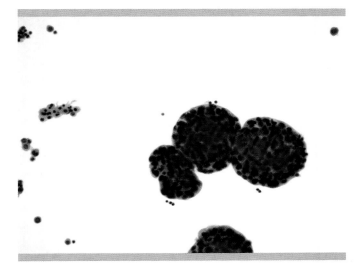

FIGURE 9-27

(A) Ductal carcinoma of the breast
(B) Gastric carcinoma
(C) Lobular carcinoma of the breast
(D) Lung carcinoma
(E) Reactive mesothelial cells

28. A 72-year-old woman presents with obstructive jaundice, and imaging shows a solid pancreatic head mass with irregular contours. Fine-needle aspiration biopsy is performed (see Figure 9-28). What is the best diagnosis for this aspirate?

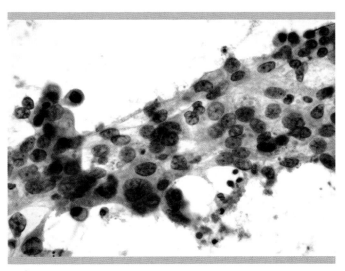

FIGURE 9-28

(A) Acinar cell carcinoma
(B) Chronic pancreatitis
(C) Ductal adenocarcinoma
(D) Intraductal papillary mucinous neoplasm
(E) Pancreatic endocrine neoplasm

29. A 61-year-old woman undergoes endoscopic ultrasound-guided fine-needle aspiration biopsy of a pancreatic tail mass (see Figure 9-29). What is the most likely diagnosis based on this cytomorphologic appearance?

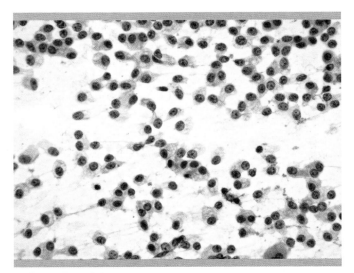

FIGURE 9-29

(A) Acinar cell carcinoma
(B) Chronic pancreatitis
(C) Ductal adenocarcinoma
(D) Intraductal papillary mucinous neoplasm
(E) Pancreatic endocrine neoplasm

30. A 68-year-old woman undergoes total hysterectomy and salpingo-oophorectomy for an ovarian mass. Pathologic examination demonstrates a high-grade papillary serous carcinoma confined to one ovary. A pelvic washing performed at the time of surgery shows the following change (see Figure 9-30). What effect does the pelvic washing finding have on the stage of her ovarian cancer?

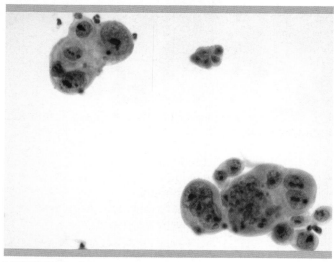

FIGURE 9-30

(A) No change to stage
(B) Upstage from T1a to T1c
(C) Upstage from T1 to T3
(D) Upstage from N0 to N1
(E) Upstage from M0 to M1

31. A 37-year-old woman undergoes fine-needle aspiration biopsy of a breast lesion (see Figure 9-31). Based on the cytologic features present, what is the most likely diagnosis?

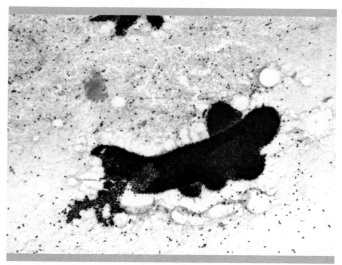

FIGURE 9-31

(A) Benign cyst
(B) Ductal carcinoma
(C) Fat necrosis
(D) Fibroadenoma
(E) Intraductal papilloma

32. A 42-year-old woman who is a smoker develops a tender lump underneath the nipple. Fine-needle aspiration biopsy is performed (see Figure 9-32). What is the most likely diagnosis?

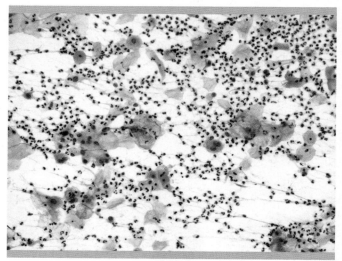

FIGURE 9-32

(A) Ductal carcinoma
(B) Fibroadenoma
(C) Intraductal papilloma
(D) Metastatic squamous cell carcinoma
(E) Subareolar abscess

33. A 72-year-old woman undergoes fine-needle aspiration biopsy of a breast mass (see Figure 9-33). The best diagnosis for this aspirate sample is

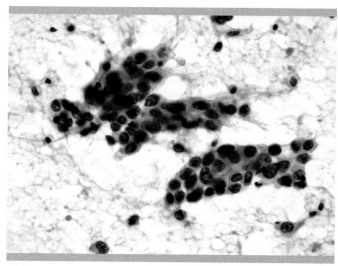

FIGURE 9-33

(A) Ductal carcinoma
(B) Fibroadenoma
(C) Intraductal papilloma
(D) Lobular carcinoma
(E) Subareolar abscess

34. A 59-year-old woman presents with a breast mass, and undergoes fine-needle aspiration biopsy (see Figure 9-34). What is the best diagnosis for this lesion?

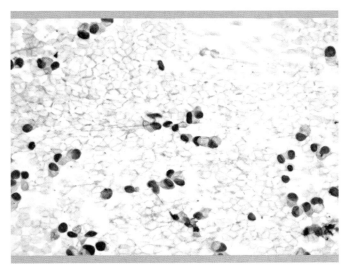

FIGURE 9-34

(A) Ductal carcinoma
(B) Fat necrosis
(C) Fibroadenoma
(D) Lobular carcinoma
(E) Metastatic signet ring carcinoma to the breast

35. A 23-year-old man presents with a rapidly growing mass in the lateral neck that measures 1.8 cm and is subcutaneous. Fine-needle aspiration biopsy is performed and is suggestive of nodular fasciitis (see Figure 9-35). All of the following are cytologic features of this lesion except

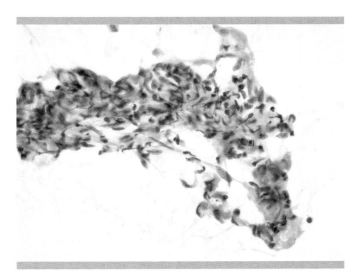

FIGURE 9-35

(A) Acute inflammation
(B) Frequent mitotic figures
(C) Marked nuclear hyperchromasia and atypia
(D) Myxoid background
(E) Spindled or stellate-shaped cells

36. Transbronchial fine-needle aspiration biopsy of a mediastinal lymph node demonstrates the following change (see Figure 9-36). What is the next best step in the evaluation of this lymph node?

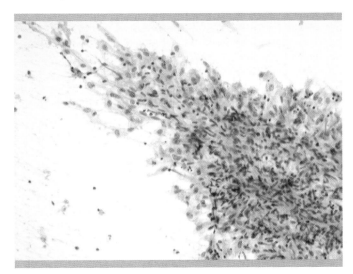

FIGURE 9-36

(A) Flow cytometry
(B) Gram stain on aspirate smears
(C) Immunohistochemistry on cell block material
(D) Microbiologic culture for fungi and acid-fast bacteria
(E) Serum angiotensin-converting enzyme (ACE) levels

37. A 7-year-old boy from Africa presents with a rapidly enlarging neck mass, and fine-needle aspiration biopsy demonstrates a monotonous population of atypical lymphocytes with dark blue cytoplasm and multiple cytoplasmic vacuoles. What gene is most likely altered in this neoplasm?
    (A) *BCL2*
    (B) *C-myc*
    (C) Immunoglobulin light chain
    (D) *N-myc*
    (E) T-cell receptor gamma chain

38. All of the following are cytologic features of mesothelial cells in effusion cytology except
    (A) Binucleation and multinucleation common
    (B) Clusters with cytoplasmic windows between cells
    (C) Clusters with smooth community borders
    (D) Dense inner cytoplasm with outer pale rim, so-called "lacy skirt"
    (E) Round-to-oval nucleus with small nucleolus

39. A 55-year-old woman has a history of invasive ductal carcinoma of the breast, and presents with a large pleural effusion. Atypical cells are present in her pleural effusion. Which of the following panels of immunohistochemical stains would be most useful in discriminating metastatic adenocarcinoma from reactive mesothelial cells in her effusion?
    (A) Calretinin, cytokeratins 5/6 (CK5/6), carcinoembryonic antigen (CEA), B72.3
    (B) Calretinin, CK5/6, WT-1, D2-40
    (C) CEA, B72.3, MOC-31, cytokeratin 7 (CK7)
    (D) CK7, AE1/3, CAM5.2
    (E) CK7, estrogen receptor, progesterone receptor

40. A 54-year-old man presents with bilateral pleural effusions, cavitary pulmonary lesions, and chronic cough. Examination of his pleural fluid demonstrates nearly 100% small mature lymphocytes and almost no mesothelial cells. What process is the most likely cause of this clinical picture?
    (A) *Aspergillus fumigatus*
    (B) Metastatic small cell undifferentiated carcinoma
    (C) *Mycobacterium tuberculosis*
    (D) Primary effusion lymphoma
    (E) Systemic lupus erythematosus

41. A 28-year-old man presents with a pleural effusion. Examination of the effusion demonstrates numerous eosinophils. Which of the following is a possible cause of this finding?

    (A) Empyema
    (B) Primary effusion lymphoma
    (C) Rheumatoid pleuritis
    (D) Spontaneous pneumothorax
    (E) Tuberculous pleuritis

42. When examining a pleural or peritoneal effusion cytology sample, all of the following findings are concerning for malignancy except
    (A) Large cell clusters (>50 cells)
    (B) Mitotic figures
    (C) Signet ring vacuoles
    (D) Smooth community borders to cell groups
    (E) Two distinct cell populations

43. In effusion cytology, some metastatic tumors will consist of predominantly single tumor cells rather than forming clusters. This pattern is called the "dispersed" or "mesothelial-type" pattern of metastasis. All of the following tumors commonly involve effusions with a dispersed pattern except
    (A) Lobular breast carcinoma
    (B) Malignant melanoma
    (C) Non-Hodgkin lymphoma
    (D) Ovarian serous carcinoma
    (E) Signet ring gastric carcinoma

44. A 32-year-old woman notices a well-circumscribed mass in her breast. Fine-needle aspiration biopsy is performed and shows a cellular aspirate composed of loosely cohesive epithelial cells with foamy cytoplasm and prominent nucleoli, in a background of proteinaceous material and stripped nuclei. These changes are most consistent with what diagnosis?
    (A) Ductal carcinoma
    (B) Fibroadenoma
    (C) Lactating adenoma
    (D) Lobular carcinoma
    (E) Mucinous carcinoma

45. All of the following are features of fat necrosis on fine-needle aspiration cytology except
    (A) Adipocytes
    (B) Amorphous granular background debris
    (C) Foamy histiocytes
    (D) Hypercellular epithelial fragments
    (E) Inflammation

46. Which of the following features favors a diagnosis of phyllodes tumor over fibroadenoma on fine-needle aspiration biopsy of the breast?
    (A) Branching fragments of ductal epithelium
    (B) Hypercellular stromal fragments

(C) Marked stromal atypia

(D) Overall high cellularity aspirate sample

(E) Spindle cells with short, oval nuclei

47. A woman undergoes fine-needle aspiration biopsy of a breast lesion, and the aspirate smears demonstrate abundant extracellular mucinous/myxoid material with admixed epithelial cells. All of the following lesions are in the differential diagnosis of this process except

(A) Colloid carcinoma

(B) Ductal carcinoma with mucinous features

(C) Fibroadenoma

(D) Mucocele-like lesion

(E) Tubular carcinoma

48. All of the following are cytologic features of pilomatricoma except

(A) Background of amorphous debris and calcification

(B) Background of naked nuclei

(C) Clusters of basaloid cells with high nuclear-to-cytoplasmic ratio

(D) Coarse hyperchromatic and irregular chromatin

(E) Ghost cells (anucleated squamous cells)

49. All of the following childhood tumors frequently have a small round blue cell appearance on fine-needle aspiration biopsy except

(A) Acute lymphoblastic lymphoma

(B) Ewing sarcoma/primitive neuroectodermal tumor

(C) Infantile fibrosarcoma

(D) Neuroblastoma

(E) Rhabdomyosarcoma

50. Which of the following features is seen in fine-needle aspiration samples of schwannoma?

(A) Epithelioid cells with plasmacytoid cytoplasm and binucleation

(B) Marked nuclear pleomorphism and tumor giant cells with prominent nucleoli

(C) Spindle cells with rounded, cigar-shaped nuclei

(D) Stellate, fibroblast-like spindle cells in an inflammatory background

(E) Wavy spindle cells with tapered nuclei

51. A 45-year-old woman undergoes fine-needle aspiration biopsy of a palpable breast mass. The aspirate smears demonstrate numerous naked nuclei in a granular background, and a few groups of intact polygonal cells have abundant granular

cytoplasm and small round nuclei with no significant pleomorphism. What immunohistochemical stain will be positive in this neoplasm?

(A) CD68

(B) Cytokeratin

(C) Desmin

(D) Myogenin

(E) S-100

52. A 49-year-old man presents with a deep thigh mass. A fine-needle aspiration biopsy is performed, and shows a prominent myxoid background with delicate branching vessels, cells with multiple cytoplasmic vacuoles, and round-to-spindled cells with scant cytoplasm. On the basis of this cytologic appearance, what cytogenetic translocation is most likely to be present in this lesion?

(A) t(X;17)(p11;q25)

(B) t(X;18)(p11;q11)

(C) t(2;13)(q35;q14)

(D) t(11;22)(q24;q12)

(E) t(12;16)(q13;p11)

53. Basaloid salivary gland neoplasms can show considerable overlap on fine-needle aspiration biopsy. Which of the following features, if present, would favor a diagnosis of basal cell adenoma?

(A) Fibrillary metachromatic matrix material

(B) High mitotic activity and necrosis

(C) Spheres of acellular, sharply demarcated metachromatic matrix material

(D) Squamous differentiation with nuclear atypia

(E) Thick ribbon of matrix material surrounding cell groups with peripheral palisading

54. Fine-needle aspiration biopsy of a parotid mass demonstrates polygonal cells with abundant cytoplasm and round central nucleoli. All of the following salivary gland lesions are in the differential diagnosis except

(A) Acinic cell carcinoma

(B) Adenoid cystic carcinoma

(C) Mucoepidermoid carcinoma

(D) Oncocytoma

(E) Warthin tumor

55. A parotid mass fine-needle aspiration biopsy contains extracellular metachromatic matrix material on Diff-Quik stain. Which of the following tumors can have this appearance on aspiration biopsy?

(A) Acinic cell carcinoma

(B) Epithelial myoepithelial carcinoma

(C) Mucoepidermoid carcinoma

(D) Myoepithelioma

(E) Salivary duct carcinoma

56. Which of the following salivary gland tumors is least likely to appear cystic on imaging?
    (A) Acinic cell carcinoma
    (B) Lymphoepithelial cyst
    (C) Polymorphous low-grade adenocarcinoma
    (D) Mucoepidermoid carcinoma
    (E) Warthin tumor

57. According to the 2007 Bethesda System for Reporting Thyroid Cytopathology, all of the following thyroid fine-needle aspirates would be considered adequate for interpretation except
    (A) Abundant colloid only
    (B) Abundant cyst contents only
    (C) Changes of chronic lymphocytic thyroiditis with 5 groups of 10 follicular cells
    (D) Only 3 groups of follicular cells with nuclear grooves, fine chromatin, and a nuclear pseudoinclusion
    (E) Scant colloid and 8 groups of 10 benign follicular cells

58. An interpretation of "suspicious for follicular neoplasm, Hürthle cell type" on a thyroid fine-needle aspiration biopsy requires all of the following cytologic findings except
    (A) Absence of lymphocytes
    (B) Absence of nuclear features of papillary thyroid carcinoma
    (C) At least 50% of the follicular cells have Hürthle cell change
    (D) Follicular cells with abundant cytoplasm, large nuclei, and prominent nucleoli
    (E) Minimal colloid

59. A 32-year-old woman undergoes fine-needle aspiration biopsy of a solitary thyroid nodule. The cytopathologist makes an interpretation of "atypia of undetermined significance." According to the 2007 Bethesda System for Reporting Thyroid Cytopathology recommendations, at excision what percentage of patients with this interpretation will have a malignant neoplasm?
    (A) <3%
    (B) 5–15%
    (C) 15–30%
    (D) 60–75%
    (E) 97–99%

60. In what clinical setting is a thyroid fine-needle aspiration biopsy considered clinically adequate with an interpretation of "nondiagnostic, cyst fluid only"?
    (A) Multilocular cyst 1.5 cm in size
    (B) Multilocular cyst 1.0 cm in size with microcalcifications
    (C) Solid nodule 2.0 cm in size
    (D) Unilocular cyst 2.5 cm in size
    (E) Unilocular cyst 4.5 cm in size

61. A 46-year-old woman undergoes fine-needle aspiration biopsy of a 1.5-cm unilocular cyst of the right thyroid. Approximately 5 mL of crystal clear fluid is aspirated, and the cyst collapses. Review of the aspirate smears demonstrates nearly acellular cyst fluid. What ancillary test can the pathologist perform to confirm the diagnosis?
    (A) Aspirate fluid calcitonin level
    (B) Aspirate fluid parathyroid hormone level
    (C) Aspirate fluid thyroglobulin level
    (D) Serum calcitonin level
    (E) Serum thyroglobulin level

62. A 46-year-old woman submits a urine specimen for cytologic examination. Several large papillary clusters of urothelial cells with a low nuclear-to-cytoplasmic ratio and minimal atypia are present. The differential diagnosis of this process includes all of the following except
    (A) Bladder papilloma
    (B) High-grade papillary urothelial carcinoma
    (C) Low-grade papillary urothelial carcinoma
    (D) Nephrolithiasis
    (E) Recent instrumentation of the bladder

63. Which of the following features, if present in a urine cytology sample, would favor a diagnosis of polyoma virus infection over a high-grade urothelial carcinoma?
    (A) Clusters of atypical cells
    (B) Extensive cellular degeneration
    (C) High nuclear-to-cytoplasmic ratio
    (D) Nuclear hyperchromasia
    (E) Round nuclei with smooth contours

64. A 55-year-old man with a history of high-grade urothelial carcinoma is seen for annual follow-up and a urine cytology specimen is submitted for a fluorescence in situ hybridization test (e.g., UroVysion™) to assess for recurrent disease. What type of genetic changes does this assay detect?

(A) Aneuploidy of multiple chromosomes (3, 7, 17)
(B) Break-apart probe for translocations involving chromosome 9p
(C) Fusion signal probe for translocations involving chromosome 17
(D) Homozygous deletion of chromosome 7
(E) Point mutation of chromosome 3

65. A 32-year-old woman presents with headaches, and a cerebrospinal fluid (CSF) sample is submitted for cytologic examination. The CSF sample demonstrates increased numbers of lymphocytes with occasional atypical lymphoid cells. All of the following processes can cause this appearance except
(A) Acute lymphoblastic leukemia with leptomeningeal involvement
(B) Borrelia burgdorferi (Lyme disease) infection
(C) *Neisseria meningitidis* infection
(D) Primary central nervous system lymphoma
(E) Viral meningitis

66. A premature baby girl with hydrocephalus and seizures has cerebrospinal fluid sample submitted for cytologic examination. Imaging does not demonstrate a mass lesion. The fluid demonstrates clusters of small dark cells with scant cytoplasm and nuclear molding. What is the most likely source of these cells?
(A) Germinal matrix cells
(B) Medulloblastoma
(C) Neuroblastoma
(D) Primary CNS lymphoma
(E) Small cell carcinoma

67. A sputum sample is submitted for cytologic examination in the workup of a patient with a lung mass. What cellular component is required to consider the sputum sample adequate?
(A) Alveolar macrophages
(B) Ciliated bronchial cells
(C) Goblet cells
(D) Mature squamous cells
(E) Metaplastic squamous cells

68. In a bile duct brushing, which of the following features would favor a diagnosis of adenocarcinoma over reactive changes?
(A) Abundant cytoplasm
(B) Cohesive clusters
(C) Large nuclei
(D) Marked nuclear size variation
(E) Prominent nucleoli

69. A woman presents with nipple discharge. Which of the following nipple discharge characteristics is most associated with an underlying malignancy?
(A) Bilateral discharge
(B) Bloody discharge
(C) Milky discharge
(D) Postpartum discharge
(E) Purulent discharge

70. A 45-year-old woman presents with unilateral bloody nipple discharge. A nipple discharge smear is made, and shows multiple cohesive three-dimensional clusters of small ductal cells with mild nuclear pleomorphism and scant cytoplasm. What is the best diagnosis for this cytology sample?
(A) Fibroadenoma
(B) Negative for malignancy, fibrocystic change
(C) Papillary lesion
(D) Positive for malignancy, ductal carcinoma
(E) Positive for malignancy, lobular neoplasia

71. Patients with Barrett's esophagus are at increased risk of developing invasive adenocarcinoma. What is the characteristic feature of Barrett's esophagus on esophageal brushing cytology?
(A) Atypical squamous cells
(B) Benign squamous cells
(C) Goblet cells
(D) Necrosis
(E) Sheets of columnar glandular epithelium

72. In a patient with known Barrett's esophagus, which of the following features would favor a diagnosis of high-grade dysplasia or adenocarcinoma over repair on an esophageal brushing cytology?
(A) Columnar glandular cells with interspersed goblet cells
(B) Honeycomb appearance
(C) Mitotic figures
(D) Numerous single atypical cells
(E) Vesicular chromatin with prominent nucleoli

73. Molecular testing for which of the following gene alterations can be performed on cytologic samples of metastatic colorectal carcinoma to determine tumor sensitivity to antiepidermal growth factor receptor (anti-EGFR) therapy?
(A) Epidermal growth factor receptor (EGFR) gene amplification
(B) *K-ras* point mutation
(C) *P53* gene amplification
(D) *RET* point mutation
(E) Vascular endothelial growth factor (VEGF) point mutation

74. An 18-year-old woman presents with malaise, pharyngitis, and bilateral cervical neck lymphadenopathy. Serologic studies demonstrate elevated IgM titers for Epstein–Barr virus. If fine-needle aspiration biopsy of a neck lymph node is performed, what is the most likely pattern seen?
    (A) Epithelioid histiocytes and well-formed granulomas
    (B) Extensive necrosis and marked acute inflammation
    (C) Monotonous large atypical lymphocytes with prominent nucleoli
    (D) Monotonous small mature lymphocytes lacking tingible body macrophages
    (E) Polymorphous lymphoid population containing abundant plasma cells and plasmacytoid lymphocytes

75. A man with a history of malignant melanoma undergoes fine-needle aspiration biopsy of an enlarged lymph node. All of the following are cytomorphologic features of malignant melanoma except
    (A) Binucleation with "mirror image" nuclei
    (B) Cohesive cell clusters
    (C) Large nuclei with prominent macronucleoli
    (D) Nuclear pseudoinclusions
    (E) Plasmacytoid appearance (eccentric nuclei)

76. All of the following are features of anaplastic large cell lymphoma on fine-needle aspiration biopsy except
    (A) Horseshoe-shaped nuclei with eccentric cytoplasm
    (B) Immunohistochemical staining for CD30
    (C) Large nuclei with prominent nucleoli
    (D) Marked nuclear pleomorphism
    (E) Background containing numerous lymphoglandular bodies

77. Merkel cell carcinoma is difficult to distinguish from small cell undifferentiated carcinoma of the lung on fine-needle aspiration biopsy. What immunohistochemical stain will be positive in Merkel cell carcinoma, but negative in small cell undifferentiated carcinoma of the lung?
    (A) CD56
    (B) Chromogranin
    (C) Cytokeratin 20
    (D) Synaptophysin
    (E) Thyroid transcription factor 1

78. Fine-needle aspiration biopsy of a liver mass demonstrates abundant normal-appearing hepatocytes arranged in small clusters and as single cells, without endothelial wrapping or transgressing vessels. No bile duct epithelium is seen. All of the following are possible correlates to this appearance except
    (A) Focal nodular hyperplasia
    (B) Hepatic adenoma
    (C) Hepatocellular carcinoma, fibrolamellar variant
    (D) Normal liver, the lesion was missed
    (E) Regenerating nodule of cirrhosis

79. Which of the following features, if seen on a liver fine-needle aspiration biopsy sample, would favor a diagnosis of well-differentiated hepatocellular carcinoma over a regenerating cirrhotic nodule?
    (A) Bile pigment
    (B) Marked variation in nuclear size
    (C) Nuclear pseudoinclusions
    (D) Prominent nucleoli
    (E) Thickened trabeculae

80. All of the following are cytomorphologic features of metastatic colorectal carcinoma to the liver on fine-needle aspiration biopsy except
    (A) Dirty necrosis
    (B) Hyperchromatic chromatin
    (C) Low cuboidal cells
    (D) Oval-to-cigar-shaped nuclei
    (E) Palisaded or picket-fence nuclear arrangement

81. A 45-year-old woman presents with a cystic pancreatic lesion. Which of the following features would favor a diagnosis of intraductal papillary mucinous neoplasm over a mucinous cystic neoplasm?
    (A) Atypical mucinous epithelium
    (B) Background of extracellular mucin
    (C) Connection with the main pancreatic duct
    (D) Elevated carcinoembryonic antigen (CEA) level in the cyst fluid
    (E) Location in the pancreas body

82. An endoscopic ultrasound-guided fine-needle aspiration biopsy of a pancreatic lesion is performed. Which of the following features would favor a diagnosis of well-differentiated pancreatic ductal adenocarcinoma over reactive changes in chronic pancreatitis?
    (A) Anisonucleocytosis
    (B) Cohesive epithelial sheets
    (C) Maintained nuclear polarity
    (D) Prominent nucleoli
    (E) Scattered mitotic figures

83. Which of the following techniques is the most sensitive, specific, and cost-effective for the evaluation and diagnosis of pancreatic lesions?
    (A) Computed tomography (CT)-guided fine-needle aspiration biopsy
    (B) Diagnostic surgical excision
    (C) Endoscopic ultrasound guided fine-needle aspiration biopsy (EUS-FNA)
    (D) Laparoscopic biopsy
    (E) Transabdominal ultrasound-guided fine-needle aspiration biopsy

84. Fine-needle aspiration biopsy of a 3.0-cm pancreatic cyst yields macrophages only. Ancillary testing with carcinoembryonic antigen (CEA) and amylase is performed on 2 mL of cyst fluid. Which of the following laboratory results would favor a diagnosis of pseudocyst?
    (A) CEA 5 ng/mL, amylase high
    (B) CEA 4 ng/mL, amylase low
    (C) CEA 220 ng/mL, amylase high
    (D) CEA 500 ng/mL, amylase low
    (E) CEA 1100 ng/mL, amylase high

85. All of the following are features of serous cystadenoma of the pancreas except
    (A) High risk of transformation to malignancy requires resection
    (B) Low carcinoembryonic antigen (CEA) level
    (C) Rare bland cuboidal cells with clear cytoplasm
    (D) Spongy appearance with central scar on ultrasound
    (E) Typically acellular cyst fluid without debris or inflammation

86. A 5-year-old presents with a large renal mass. Fine-needle aspiration biopsy demonstrates a small round cell tumor with occasional tubular structures and spindle cells. Immunohistochemical staining for cytokeratin and vimentin is positive in a subset of tumor cells. What other immunohistochemical stain is likely to be positive in this tumor?
    (A) CD34
    (B) CD99
    (C) Myogenin
    (D) Synaptophysin
    (E) WT1

87. Fine-needle aspiration biopsy of a renal mass in a 42-year old woman demonstrates spindled cells with stringy cytoplasm admixed with mature fibroadipose tissue. What immunohistochemical stain can confirm the diagnosis?
    (A) CD10
    (B) Cytokeratin 7
    (C) Epithelial membrane antigen
    (D) HMB-45
    (E) Inhibin

88. All of the following are cytologic features of seminoma except
    (A) Binucleation with nuclear pseudoinclusions
    (B) Cytoplasmic vacuolization
    (C) Dispersed single cell pattern
    (D) Large atypical cells with prominent macronucleoli
    (E) Tigroid background

89. Transthoracic fine-needle aspiration biopsy of a well-circumscribed peripheral lung nodule demonstrates fragments of fibroadipose tissue, immature cartilage, spindle cells, and bland glandular cells. What is the best diagnosis?
    (A) Carcinoid tumor
    (B) Nondiagnostic sample, thoracic wall sampling
    (C) Pulmonary hamartoma
    (D) Squamous cell carcinoma
    (E) Well-differentiated adenocarcinoma

90. An 81-year-old man presents with a large cavitary mass in the right upper lobe. Fine-needle aspiration biopsy demonstrates abundant necrosis and markedly atypical squamous cells. Besides a cavitary squamous cell carcinoma, what other disease process can have this appearance?
    (A) *Aspergillus fumigatus* fungal ball
    (B) Epithelioid hemangioendothelioma
    (C) *Pneumocystis* pneumonia
    (D) Sarcoidosis
    (E) Wegner's granulomatosis

91. Which of the following cytomorphologic features favors a diagnosis of lymphoma over small cell undifferentiated carcinoma of the lung?
    (A) High nuclear-to-cytoplasmic ratio
    (B) Lymphoglandular bodies
    (C) Nuclear molding
    (D) Paranuclear cytoplasmic blue bodies
    (E) Tightly cohesive cellular clusters

92. A 45-year-old man with a pancreatic mass undergoes fine-needle aspiration biopsy (see Figure 9-37). What is the most likely explanation for this appearance?

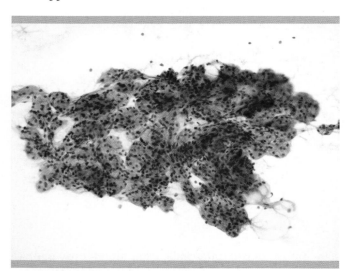

FIGURE 9-37

(A) Acinar cell carcinoma
(B) Chronic pancreatitis forming a mass-like lesion
(C) Ductal adenocarcinoma
(D) Metastatic renal cell carcinoma
(E) Normal pancreas; the lesion was missed

93. At endoscopy, esophageal brushings are performed, and show the following changes (see Figure 9-38). What clinical findings are most likely found in association with these changes?

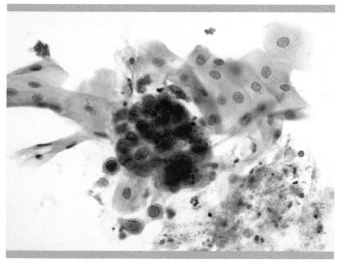

FIGURE 9-38

(A) Circumferential stenosis caused by a friable mass
(B) Multiple small shallow ulcers in the distal esophagus
(C) Salmon-colored patches near the gastroesophageal junction
(D) Submucosal mass in the upper third of the esophagus
(E) White pseudomembranes that scrape off the epithelium

94. A 48-year-old woman undergoes thyroid fine-needle aspiration biopsy; she has multiple nodules, and the largest is aspirated (see Figure 9-39). The most appropriate interpretation for this aspirate, presuming that the figure provided is representative of the entire aspirate sample, is

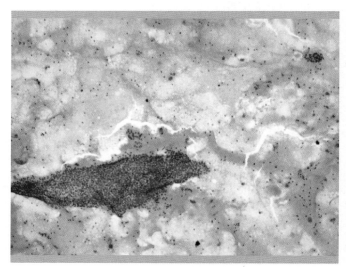

FIGURE 9-39

(A) Atypia of undetermined significance
(B) Benign
(C) Malignant
(D) Suspicious for follicular neoplasm
(E) Suspicious for malignancy

95. Transthoracic fine-needle aspiration biopsy of a peripherally located solitary, spiculated lung mass shows the following changes (see Figure 9-40). What is the most likely diagnosis?

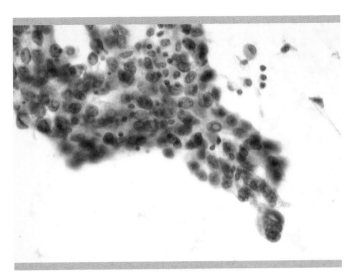

FIGURE 9-40

(A) Carcinoid tumor
(B) Metastatic papillary thyroid carcinoma
(C) Reactive bronchial cells
(D) Squamous cell carcinoma
(E) Well-differentiated lung adenocarcinoma

96. A 45-year-old man with hematuria submits a urine sample for cytologic examination. Rare cells with large, dark nuclei and cytoplasmic golden pigment are seen (see Figure 9-41). What is the most likely origin of these cells?

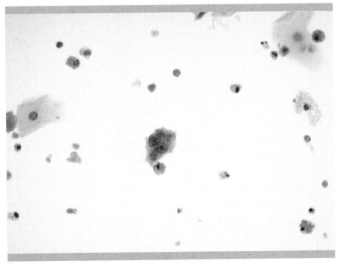

FIGURE 9-41

(A) Clear cell renal cell carcinoma
(B) High-grade urothelial carcinoma
(C) Seminal vesicle
(D) Squamous metaplasia of the trigone
(E) Urachal adenocarcinoma

97. A 75-year-old man who is a retired shipyard worker presents with dyspnea and a large left pleural effusion along with nodular thickening of the right pleural space. A portion of his right pleural effusion is submitted for cytologic examination, which shows large clusters of markedly atypical cells with scalloped borders and cytoplasmic windows. All of the following statements about this process are true except
(A) A distinctly different second population of benign mesothelial cells will be present in the effusion
(B) Electron microscopy will demonstrate long, thin microvilli (length-to-width ratio 15:1 or greater)
(C) Highly associated with asbestos exposure
(D) Immunohistochemical staining for calretinin will be positive in the neoplastic cells
(E) Low nuclear-to-cytoplasmic ratio is typical of this neoplasm

98. A 63-year-old woman undergoes fine-needle aspiration biopsy of a breast lesion associated with microcalcifications on mammography. The aspirate smears demonstrate atypical epithelial cells with marked pleomorphism and hyperchromasia arranged as disorganized clusters and single atypical cells in a background of necrosis. At subsequent excision, which of the following lesions is this woman likely to have?
(A) Fibroadenoma
(B) High-grade ductal carcinoma in situ
(C) Infiltrating lobular carcinoma
(D) Intraductal papilloma
(E) Low-grade ductal carcinoma in situ

99. Fine-needle aspiration biopsy of an enlarged lymph node demonstrates necrosis, epithelioid histiocytes, and numerous neutrophils. Which of the following processes commonly results in this appearance?
(A) Cat scratch disease
(B) Chronic lymphocytic leukemia/small cell lymphoma
(C) Rosai–Dorfman disease
(D) Sarcoidosis
(E) Tuberculous lymphadenitis

100. All of the following are features of solid pseudopapillary tumor of the pancreas on cytology samples except
(A) Absence of nuclear staining for β-catenin
(B) Branching papillary-like structures with a vascular core
(C) Lack of cellular cohesion
(D) Myxoid or hyaline stroma
(E) Small monotonous cuboidal cells

101. Distinction between oncocytoma and an eosino-philic variant of chromophobe renal cell carcinoma on kidney fine-needle aspiration biopsy can be very difficult. Which of the following cytologic features favors a diagnosis of oncocytoma?
    (A) Cytoplasmic clearing around the nucleus
    (B) Diffuse cytoplasmic staining for Hale's colloidal iron
    (C) Marked variation in nuclear size
    (D) Nuclear membrane irregularities
    (E) Round-nested architecture on cell block preparation

102. A 5-year-old girl has a rapidly growing orbital mass. Fine-needle aspiration biopsy demonstrates a small round blue cell tumor with interspersed larger cells with elongated, dense cytoplasm, and eccentric nuclei. An immunohistochemical stain for desmin is positive in the neoplastic cells. What is the best diagnosis?
    (A) Ewing sarcoma
    (B) Fibrosarcoma
    (C) Leiomyosarcoma
    (D) Rhabdomyosarcoma
    (E) Round cell liposarcoma

103. A parotid fine-needle aspiration biopsy demon-strates sheets of oncocyte-like cells in a back-ground of naked nuclei. Which of the following stains, if positive, would favor a diagnosis of acinic cell carcinoma?
    (A) Mucicarmine
    (B) P63
    (C) Periodic acid Schiff with diastase (PAS-D)
    (D) Phosphotungstic acid hematoxylin (PTAH)
    (E) S-100

104. A 52-year-old woman undergoes fine-needle aspi-ration biopsy of a thyroid nodule. The aspirate is interpreted as "suspicious for follicular neoplasm." According to the 2007 Bethesda System for Report-ing Thyroid Cytopathology, what is the risk of malignancy in this nodule?
    (A) <3%
    (B) 5–15%
    (C) 15–30%
    (D) 60–75%
    (E) 97–99%

105. Prominent ciliocytophthoria, or detached tufts of cytoplasm containing a terminal bar and cilia, in a lung washing is associated with what viral infec-tion?
    (A) Adenovirus
    (B) Cytomegalovirus
    (C) Herpes simplex virus
    (D) Measles virus
    (E) Respiratory syncytial virus

106. A nipple discharge sample from a 32-year-old woman shows abundant foamy histiocytes and a background of proteinaceous debris. Which of the following conditions is this form of nipple discharge most likely to be associated with?
    (A) Acute mastitis
    (B) Galactorrhea
    (C) Intraductal papilloma
    (D) Invasive ductal carcinoma
    (E) Tuberculous mastitis

107. Fine-needle aspiration biopsy of an enlarged lymph node demonstrates predominantly small mature lymphocytes, many of which are irregular or cleaved. Flow cytometry demonstrates a mono-typic population of lymphocytes that are κ light chain restricted and express CD10. What is the best diagnosis for this aspirate?
    (A) Burkitt lymphoma
    (B) Diffuse large B-cell lymphoma
    (C) Follicular lymphoma
    (D) Mantle cell lymphoma
    (E) Small lymphocytic lymphoma/chronic lymphocytic leukemia

108. Fine-needle aspiration biopsy of an acinar cell car-cinoma of the pancreas is characterized by all of the following cytologic features except
    (A) Cuboidal cells with granular cytoplasm
    (B) Cytoplasmic staining for periodic acid Schiff (PAS) stain that is diastase resistant
    (C) Granular background with naked nuclei
    (D) Marked nuclear pleomorphism and anisonucleocytosis
    (E) Sheets and acinar-like arrangement of cells

109. Fine-needle aspiration biopsy of a benign adrenal cortical nodule can show all of the following fea-tures except
    (A) Intact cells with abundant cytoplasm and indistinct cell borders
    (B) Frothy, granular background
    (C) Metachromatic fibrillary matrix material
    (D) Occasional spindle cells
    (E) Stripped naked nuclei

110. Molecular analysis for epidermal growth factor receptor (EGFR) mutation is performed on a fine-needle aspiration biopsy of metastatic lung carcinoma and is positive. What is the most likely cytomorphologic appearance of this tumor?
    (A) Adenocarcinoma with bronchioloalveolar features
    (B) Keratinizing squamous cell carcinoma
    (C) Mucinous adenocarcinoma
    (D) Nonkeratinizing squamous cell carcinoma
    (E) Small cell undifferentiated carcinoma

111. Fine-needle aspiration biopsy of a thymoma can show all of the following changes except
    (A) Admixed small mature lymphocytes
    (B) Immature lymphocytes that are positive for TdT
    (C) Loosely cohesive epithelioid cells
    (D) Nuclear pleomorphism
    (E) Short spindle cells arranged in fascicles and whorls

ANSWERS

1. **(D) Pleural mesothelial cells.**
The photomicrograph demonstrates a flat sheet of uniform cells with dense cytoplasm and cytoplasmic "windows," consistent with mesothelial cells obtained while transversing the pleural space. On fine-needle aspiration biopsy of the lung, it is important to recognize benign contaminants and not overinterpret these cells as sampling of a neoplasm. Mesothelial cells can be mistaken for a non-small cell carcinoma, particularly when reactive. Helpful features include characteristic mesothelial "windows" between cells, uniform appearance of the nuclei, and flat sheets without nuclear crowding or overlap. Transthoracic fine-needle aspiration biopsies may also contain fibrofatty tissue, skeletal muscle, and skin appendages. In contrast, trans-bronchial fine-needle aspiration biopsies may contain abundant benign bronchial cells, squamous cells (from squamous metaplasia of the bronchus), cartilage, and abundant mucin.

2. **(D) Squamous cell carcinoma.**
The photomicrograph demonstrates an aspirate of squamous cell carcinoma of the lung. Features that favor a diagnosis of squamous cell carcinoma include dense blue-to-orangeophilic cytoplasm with well-defined cell borders, bizarrely shaped cells with cytoplasmic extensions (tadpole or caudate shape), marked nuclear hyperchromasia, large irregular flat sheets of tumor cells, and keratin pearls. Squamous metaplasia with reactive atypia

can be seen in smokers and lining the cavity of a fungus ball, and on cytology specimens can show nuclear hyperchromasia, increased nuclear-to-cytoplasmic ratio, and prominent nucleoli. However, in contrast to squamous cell carcinoma, atypical squamous metaplasia will typically show uniform nuclei and orderly arrangement of the cells within small flat sheets.

3. **(B) Pulmonary carcinoid tumor.**
The photomicrograph demonstrates an aspirate of a pulmonary carcinoid tumor, characterized by a monotonous proliferation of plasmacytoid-to-spindled cells that lack cellular cohesion and have salt and pepper chromatin. Pulmonary carcinoid tumors most commonly present as obstructing proximal endobronchial tumors in nonsmokers. Typical and atypical carcinoid tumors show very similar cytomorphologic features; the possibility of an atypical carcinoid tumor should be suggested if mitotic figures are readily identified in the aspirate, but potential sampling error precludes definitive diagnosis of typical carcinoid tumors. Small cell undifferentiated carcinomas of the lung are also neuroendocrine tumors, but have significantly higher nuclear-to-cytoplasmic ratios, nuclear molding, increased mitotic activity, apoptotic bodies, and necrosis than carcinoid tumors. Adenoid cystic carcinomas also commonly present as endobronchial tumors in the trachea and large bronchi, but appear similar to their salivary gland counterparts on fine-needle aspiration biopsy. Plasmacytomas can be mistaken for carcinoid tumors because of the eccentrically located nuclei and lack of cellular cohesion, but perinuclear hoffs and cartwheel-like chromatin are seen in plasmacytomas. Well-differentiated adenocarcinomas will typically show more cellular cohesion than a carcinoid tumor, variable mucin vacuoles, and form honeycomb-like sheets, papillary structures, or gland-like structures.

4. **(E) Synaptophysin.**
The photomicrograph demonstrates an aspirate smear of small-cell undifferentiated carcinoma, which is characterized by abundant atypical cells with small nuclei, scant cytoplasm, uniform hyperchromatic chromatin, nuclear molding, and nuclear crush artifact. The background of small-cell undifferentiated carcinoma is usually necrotic with numerous apoptotic nuclei and mitotic figures. The cells generally lack cellular cohesion and are present as single cells or loose clusters. Small cell undifferentiated carcinomas are high-grade neuroendocrine tumors, and immunohistochemical staining will be positive for synaptophysin, chromogranin, and CD56, as well as cytokeratin

(usually dot-like perinuclear staining) and thyroid transcription factor 1. CD20 would be positive in a B-cell lymphoma. CD34 would be positive in vascular tumors, leukemias, and solitary fibrous tumor of the pleura. Napsin A shows cytoplasmic staining in pulmonary adenocarcinoma. P63 is positive in squamous cell carcinomas of the lung.

5. **(A) Benign renal cortex.**
The photomicrograph demonstrates a glomerulus on fine-needle aspiration biopsy, which appears as a dense, highly cellular aggregate of cells with a papillary appearance, which has numerous vascular structures and capillary loops. The presence of glomeruli on a kidney fine-needle aspiration sample is indicative of normal renal cortex sampling, and should not be mistaken for a papillary renal cell carcinoma. In contrast to papillary renal cell carcinoma, glomeruli lack atypia, are more cellular in the center of the structure, and contain distinctive capillary loops at the periphery of the structure. Aspirates of papillary renal cell carcinomas demonstrate papillary structures with fibrovascular cores and spherules of epithelium in a background of foamy macrophages. The papillae and spheres are lined by uniform cuboidal cells (in type 1 tumors) or by cells with large nuclei and prominent nucleoli (in type 2 tumors). Sampling of renal medulla is rare, and aspirates have limited cellularity, composed of small cuboidal cells with small nuclei. Aspirates of clear cell renal cell carcinoma are characterized by bloody smears containing cells with abundant, finely vacuolated cytoplasm arranged in sheets and loose clusters. Aspirates of medullary renal cell carcinoma are characterized by a high-grade malignant neoplasm with large nuclei and prominent nucleoli.

6. **(A) Loss of chromosome 3 short arm (3p-).**
The photomicrograph demonstrates an aspirate of clear cell renal cell carcinoma, characterized by cells with abundant foamy cytoplasm, which form sheets and loose aggregates. Other features of clear cell renal cell carcinoma on cytology include ill-defined wispy cell borders, large, round, eccentrically placed nuclei, and metachromatic (pink-purple) fibrillary material within the cell groups. Clear cell renal cell carcinomas are characterized by loss of the short arm of chromosome 3 (3p-) or alterations of the *VHL* gene. Loss of chromosome Y is seen in oncocytomas and some papillary renal cell carcinomas. Trisomy 7 is typically seen in papillary renal cell carcinomas. *TSC1* gene inactivation occurs in tuberous sclerosis, which results in angiomyolipomas of the kidney. Xp11.2 alterations occur in a unique subset of papillary renal cell

carcinomas that largely occur in children and young adults.

7. **(E) Urothelial carcinoma.**
The photomicrograph shows a fine-needle aspirate of urothelial carcinoma, characterized by loosely cohesive elongated cells with dense cytoplasm and hyperchromatic nuclei. The characteristic feature of urothelial carcinoma aspirates is the "cercariform" cell, or tadpole cell, which has long cytoplasmic extensions that are narrow in the middle and thicker at the ends. Angiomyolipomas are characterized by an admixture of spindle cells, mature fibroadipose tissue, and rarely thick vascular wall fragments on fine-needle aspiration samples. Aspirates of clear cell renal cell carcinoma are characterized by sheets and loose clusters of cells with abundant vacuolated cytoplasm. Aspirates of oncocytomas are characterized by cells with abundant, dense granular cytoplasm and central nuclei with small nucleoli. Aspirates of type 1 papillary renal cell carcinomas show papillae and epithelial spheres of small-to-medium-sized cuboidal cells in a background of foamy macrophages, and the cells frequently contain cytoplasmic hemosiderin.

8. **(E) Well-differentiated hepatocellular carcinoma.**
The photomicrograph demonstrates an aspirate of well-differentiated hepatocellular carcinoma, characterized by hepatocytes arranged in thickened trabeculae and cords with prominent endothelial wrapping, resulting in a very smooth sharp border to the groups. Also, transgressing vessels link the clusters of hepatocytes, imparting a papillary architecture to the sample. In contrast, aspirates of regenerating cirrhotic nodules and focal nodular hyperplasia are indistinguishable from normal liver, which will lack endothelial wrapping, thickened cords, and transgressing vessels. Aspirates of normal liver often show hepatocytes arranged as single cells and small clusters; larger clusters have a frayed, irregular border rather than a smooth contour. Cholangiocarcinoma will appear as a neoplastic proliferation of ductal epithelium, which are cohesive and form gland-like spaces. Metastatic colorectal carcinoma is commonly aspirated in the liver, and is characterized by the triad of dirty necrosis, abundant mucin, and tall columnar glandular epithelium with elongated, oval, hyperchromatic nuclei.

9. **(E) Suppressed immune function.**
The photomicrograph demonstrates acellular foamy casts containing debris with sharp borders (alveolar casts). The silver stain inset demonstrates cup-shaped organisms that lack budding, consistent

with *Pneumocystis* pneumonia. *Pneumocystis* organisms have an outer rounded cyst, which contains comma-shaped trophozoites. On Papanicolaou stains, the organisms are not visible except as negative images. On Romanowsky-type stains (e.g., Diff-Quik and Giemsa), the cysts are again seen only as a negative image, but the trophozoites appear as blue-purple dots. Silver stains, such as Gomori methenamine silver (GMS), are best at demonstrating the cup-shaped cysts and internal comma-shaped trophozoites of *Pneumocystis*. The differential diagnosis of alveolar casts includes pulmonary alveolar proteinosis. Pulmonary alveolar proteinosis will stain positive for periodic acid Schiff, and will be negative for organisms by GMS stain. *Pneumocystis* pneumonia occurs in patients with reduced or suppressed immune function, including patients with acquired immunodeficiency syndrome, bone marrow transplant, or solid organ transplant. Asbestos exposure is associated with ferruginous bodies and malignant mesothelioma. Asthma is associated with Charcot–Leiden crystals and Curschmann spirals. Bird handling, particularly pigeons, is associated with *Cryptococcus* infection, and less frequently *Histoplasma* infection. A heavy smoking history is associated with pigmented macrophages and development of malignancy.

10. **(A) C-kit (CD117).**
The photomicrograph demonstrates cohesive fragments of spindle cells with mild nuclear pleomorphism. This finding, when present in a patient with a submucosal stomach mass, is highly suggestive of a gastrointestinal stromal tumor (GIST). However, the differential diagnosis includes smooth muscle neoplasms, such as leiomyoma and leiomyosarcoma. Leiomyomas are very rare in the stomach, and are most commonly found in upper one-third of the esophagus. Leiomyosarcomas of the stomach are also very rare, and would show marked nuclear pleomorphism and mitotic figures. Immunohistochemical staining is required to confirm the diagnosis of GIST. GISTs are positive for CD34 and c-kit (CD117), while smooth muscle tumors will be positive for desmin and smooth muscle actin. Myogenin is a marker of skeletal muscle differentiation, and HMB-45 is positive in melanocytic tumors and perivascular epithelioid tumor (PEComa).

11. **(D) Reactive lymphoid hyperplasia.**
The photomicrograph shows a fine-needle aspirate example of reactive lymphoid hyperplasia. Poor dentition, leading to gingivitis and abscess formation, is a common cause of reactive lymphadenopathy in the neck. Reactive lymphoid hyperplasia on fine-needle aspiration biopsy is characterized by a polymorphous population of predominantly small mature lymphocytes, admixed with tingible body macrophages (histiocytes containing engulfed cellular debris) and germinal center fragments. The main differential diagnosis of reactive lymphoid hyperplasia is a low-grade lymphoma, such as small-cell lymphocytic lymphoma, mantle-cell lymphoma, or follicular lymphoma. The most important characteristics in differentiating reactive lymphoid tissue from a low-grade lymphoma are cellular pleomorphism and the presence of tingible body macrophages, which indicate the presence of normal germinal centers. In difficult cases lacking tingible body macrophages, ancillary testing (such as flow cytometry) may be required for definitive diagnosis. Higher-grade lymphomas, such as diffuse large B-cell lymphoma, may contain tingible body macrophages, but are characterized by large atypical lymphocytes, which are monotonous. Aspirates of sarcoidosis typically show nonnecrotizing granulomatous inflammation, including well-developed multinucleated giant cells. Aspirates of metastatic squamous cell carcinoma would show cohesive clusters of cells with more abundant cytoplasm and marked nuclear atypia.

12. **(C) Immunohistochemical staining for CD30, CD15, and CD20.**
The photomicrograph demonstrates large, atypical, binucleated cells with prominent nucleoli, in a background of small mature lymphocytes and rare eosinophils. This appearance is typical for Reed–Sternberg (RS) cells derived from classical Hodgkin lymphoma. Flow cytometry is of little help in the diagnosis of Hodgkin lymphoma, as the majority of lymphocytes in aspirates of Hodgkin lymphoma will be non-neoplastic. Immunohistochemical staining is helpful in identifying RS cells, as they are positive for CD30 and CD15, and usually negative for CD45 and CD20. This immunophenotype differs from most other reactive disorders that mimic Hodgkin lymphoma. Culture would be useful if suppurative or granulomatous lymphadenitis were present. Serologic studies for Epstein–Barr virus can be helpful in the diagnosis of infectious mononucleosis. While the atypical immunoblasts of infectious mononucleosis can mimic mononuclear RS cells, infectious mononucleosis will usually lack a background of neutrophils and eosinophils. Immunohistochemical staining for cytokeratin and S-100 is useful when metastatic carcinoma or malignant melanoma is in the differential diagnosis.

13. **(C) Mucicarmine.**

The photomicrograph demonstrates a cerebrospinal fluid (CSF) involved by *Cryptococcus neoformans*, which is characterized by small yeast forms with narrow-based budding. *Cryptococcus neoformans* is the most common fungal infection to involve the CSF, and is most commonly seen in immunocompromised patients (e.g., human immunodeficiency virus infection). *Cryptococcus* is distinguished from other infectious yeasts by the presence of a thick mucopolysaccharide capsule. This capsule is not seen on Papanicolaou stains, except as a negative image around the yeast. Special stains can be used to highlight the capsule to confirm the diagnosis of *Cryptococcus*; the capsule is positive for mucicarmine and Alcian blue stains. In contrast, Gomori methenamine silver (GMS) and periodic acid Schiff (PAS) will stain the fungal cell wall, and are not specific to *Cryptococcus*. Fontana–Masson silver stain will also stain the fungal cell wall of *Cryptococcus*, but this staining is unique among the budding yeasts that infect humans. Ziehl–Neelson stains acid-fast bacteria, and will not stain cryptococcal organisms.

14. **(D) Thyroid lobectomy.**

The photomicrograph demonstrates a thyroid fine-needle aspirate that is highly cellular, lacks colloid, and has follicular cells arranged in a repetitive microfollicular pattern. No nuclear features of papillary thyroid carcinoma are present. Thyroid aspirates with this appearance are best interpreted as "follicular neoplasm" or "suspicious for follicular neoplasm." This interpretation implies a 15–30% risk of malignancy; therefore, the recommended next step in clinical management is thyroid lobectomy, unless otherwise indicated clinically. The possible histologic processes that can result in a fine-needle aspiration biopsy interpretation of "follicular neoplasm" include cellular hyperplastic nodule, follicular adenoma, follicular carcinoma, and follicular variant of papillary thyroid carcinoma.

15. **(D) *Schistosoma hematobium*.**

The photomicrograph depicts a squamous cell carcinoma of the bladder, characterized by markedly atypical keratinizing and nonkeratinizing squamous epithelium. Squamous cell carcinoma of the bladder is highly associated with *Schistosoma hematobium* infection of the bladder. Schistosomiasis is endemic in areas of Africa, Asia, and South America, and is a trematode (or fluke) that commonly infects freshwater snails. *Schistosoma hematobium* is the primary cause of urinary schistosomiasis, while *Schistosoma mansoni* and

Schistosoma japonicum primarily cause intestinal schistosomiasis. Chronic bladder infection with *Schistosoma* organisms causes reactive changes, including squamous metaplasia, which over time can develop into squamous cell carcinoma of the bladder. *Clonorchis sinensis* is a liver fluke that causes biliary injury, obstruction, and cholangitis, and is associated with the development of cholangiocarcinoma. Polyomavirus, or BK virus, can infect urothelial cells producing a distinctive nuclear inclusion, but is not associated with the development of a urinary neoplasm. Human papilloma virus can infect squamous epithelium of the penis and cause condylomas and squamous cell carcinoma, but is not associated with the development of squamous cell carcinoma of the bladder.

16. **(A) Flat urothelial carcinoma in situ.**

The photomicrograph demonstrates urothelial cells with large hyperchromatic nuclei, coarse chromatin, and irregular nuclear contours with scant cytoplasm, consistent with a high-grade urothelial carcinoma. When cystoscopic examination of the bladder is negative for a lesion in this setting, the neoplastic cells are likely derived from an upper-tract high-grade urothelial carcinoma or flat urothelial carcinoma in situ of the bladder. Blind biopsies of the bladder are recommended for definitive diagnosis, along with cystoscopic examination of the upper urothelial tracts. In most cases, a papillary lesion of the bladder will be readily identified at the time of cystoscopy. While polyoma virus infection shows some overlap with high-grade urothelial carcinoma, the coarse chromatin and irregular nuclear contours in this case are diagnostic of malignancy. Kidney stones can result in urothelial atypia, but this is typically associated with exfoliation of clusters of urothelial cells, which are often vacuolated and have prominent nucleoli. Squamous cell carcinoma of the bladder is similar in appearance to squamous cell carcinoma at other sites, showing cells with abundant, dense, or keratinized cytoplasm and hyperchromatic nuclei with coarse chromatin.

17. **(E) Nuclear atypia.**

The photomicrograph demonstrates a thyroid aspirate of papillary thyroid carcinoma. The diagnosis of papillary thyroid carcinoma on both cytology and histology requires identification of characteristic nuclear changes. These nuclear changes include nuclear grooves, intranuclear cytoplasmic pseudoinclusions, fine chromatin, nuclear crowding, oval shape, irregular contour, peripherally located small nucleoli, and nuclear enlargement. Other changes, which are helpful but variably present and not required for diagnosis, include architectural changes (papillary fragments, flat sheets, or microfollicles), background changes (cyst contents, multinucleated giant cells, and psammoma bodies), ropy hard colloid (so-called "bubble-gum" colloid), and dense "squamoid" cytoplasm.

18. **(D) *RET* point mutation.**
The photomicrograph demonstrates a thyroid aspirate sample of medullary thyroid carcinoma, characterized by discohesive cells with a plasmacytoid appearance and granular "salt and pepper" chromatin. Medullary thyroid carcinoma is highly associated with *RET* gene point mutations that cause constitutive activation of the *RET* gene. These mutations are found in almost all hereditary forms of medullary thyroid carcinoma (including MEN 2 and familial medullary thyroid carcinoma syndrome) as well as many sporadic cases of medullary thyroid carcinoma. *BRAF* point mutations and *RET/PTC* translocations are most commonly found in papillary thyroid carcinomas. *RAS* point mutations and *PAX8/PPARγ* translocations are most commonly found in follicular neoplasms (adenomas and carcinomas).

19. **(E) Undifferentiated (anaplastic) thyroid carcinoma.**
The photomicrograph demonstrates a thyroid aspirate sample composed of markedly atypical spindled to epithelioid cells with bizarre pleomorphic nuclei in a background of necrosis. These changes, along with the clinical history provided, are most consistent with undifferentiated (anaplastic) thyroid carcinoma. While the cytologic changes are similar to those seen in a pleomorphic sarcoma, primary sarcomas of the thyroid gland are exceedingly rare. Metastasis to the thyroid gland can occur, most commonly renal cell carcinoma, but rarely cause airway obstruction and usually show cytologic features typically of the tumor of origin. The degree of atypia present in this aspirate is beyond that seen in well-differentiated thyroid carcinomas such as papillary thyroid carcinoma. When undifferentiated thyroid carcinomas are extensively necrotic, the aspirate sample may be paucicellular and any atypical cells may be interpreted as regressive or reactive change. However, the degree of atypia in undifferentiated thyroid carcinomas is beyond that seen in reactive/reparative change, and close attention to the clinical history is helpful in making the diagnosis.

20. **(E) Positive antithyroglobulin antibodies.**
The photomicrograph demonstrates a thyroid aspirate composed of Hürthle cells with abundant granular cytoplasm, a mixed lymphocytic infiltrate,

and tingible body macrophages. These changes are highly suggestive of chronic lymphocytic thyroiditis, which is most commonly associated with positive antithyroglobulin antibodies (or antimicrosomal antibodies). Patients with lymphocytic thyroiditis are usually hypothyroid rather than hyperthyroid (choice D), and thyroglobulin levels are minimally elevated to normal. Elevated serum calcitonin is seen in patients with medullary thyroid carcinoma. An elevated serum calcium may be seen in a patient with hyperparathyroidism, which can mimic a thyroid nodule.

21. **(D) Pleomorphic adenoma.**
The photomicrograph shows an aspirate smear containing abundant metachromatic fibrillary matrix, which is intimately admixed with plasmacytoid and spindled myoepithelial cells and ductal cells, consistent with a pleomorphic adenoma. In contrast, fine-needle aspiration biopsy of an adenoid cystic carcinoma would contain abundant small basaloid cells with scant cytoplasm, which surround but are not admixed with strips and balls of metachromatic stroma, which have sharp contours. Fine-needle aspiration biopsy of mucoepidermoid carcinomas varies greatly in appearance, but low-grade mucoepidermoid carcinomas typically contain abundant blue background mucin with groups of goblet cells, muciphages, and epidermoid cells. Fine-needle aspiration biopsy of acinic cell carcinomas typically shows large polygonal cells with vacuolated cytoplasm forming sheets and clusters in a background of naked nuclei. Fine-needle aspiration biopsies of Warthin tumors typically show a background of granular debris, sheets of oncocytic epithelium, and lymphocytes.

22. **(E) Second most common malignant salivary gland neoplasm in children.**
The photomicrograph demonstrates an example of a low-grade mucoepidermoid carcinoma on fine-needle aspiration biopsy, characterized by abundant extracellular mucin and rare goblet cells. Mucoepidermoid carcinomas are the most common malignant salivary gland tumor in both adults and children, and involve both major and minor salivary gland locations. Rarely, primary intraosseous mucoepidermoid carcinoma (central mucoepidermoid carcinoma) can occur within the mandibular bone. Low-grade mucoepidermoid carcinomas are the most frequent cause of false-negative results on fine-needle aspiration biopsy, as the aspirate may contain only extracellular mucin and histiocytes. The oncocytic variant of mucoepidermoid carcinoma is notorious for mimicking other oncocytic tumors of the salivary gland, notably Warthin

tumors and oncocytomas. Recently, a recurring translocation involving chromosomes 11 and 19 has been described in low-grade mucoepidermoid carcinomas t(11;19), which fuse the *MECT1* and *MAML2* genes.

23. **(B) Adenoid cystic carcinoma.**
The photomicrograph shows an aspirate smear containing small basaloid cells with scant cytoplasm, which surround acellular balls of metachromatic stroma that have sharp borders, consistent with adenoid cystic carcinoma. In contrast, fine-needle aspiration biopsies of pleomorphic adenomas contain metachromatic fibrillary matrix, which is intimately admixed with plasmacytoid and spindled myoepithelial cells and gland-forming ductal cells. Fine-needle aspiration biopsy of mucoepidermoid carcinomas varies greatly in appearance, but low-grade mucoepidermoid carcinomas typically contain abundant blue background mucin with groups of goblet cells, muciphages, and epidermoid cells. Fine-needle aspiration biopsies of acinic cell carcinomas typically show large polygonal cells with vacuolated cytoplasm forming sheets and clusters in a background of naked nuclei. Fine-needle aspiration biopsies of Warthin tumors typically show a background of granular debris, sheets of oncocytic epithelium, and lymphocytes.

24. **(E) Smoking.**
The photomicrograph demonstrates sheets of oncocytic cells in a background of granular debris and lymphocytes, consistent with a Warthin tumor. Very few salivary gland tumors have defined epidemiological associations. However, Warthin tumors are highly associated with smoking, and are eightfold more common in cigarette smokers.

25. **(E) Salivary duct carcinoma.**
The photomicrograph demonstrates high-grade malignant cells with large nuclei and prominent nucleoli in a background of necrosis. This appearance, in combination with the clinical history (elderly man with parotid mass) and immunohistochemical staining for HER2, is diagnostic of salivary duct carcinoma. Salivary duct carcinoma can arise de novo, or can be the malignant component of a carcinoma (e.g., pleomorphic adenoma). These tumors preferentially occur in older men, and histologically can resemble a high-grade ductal carcinoma of the breast. Immunohistochemical staining of salivary duct carcinomas will show positive staining for androgen receptor, HER2, and gross cystic disease fluid protein 15 (GCDFP-15), along with other ductal markers (cytokeratin 7, CEA, etc.). The other listed choices include tumors that can have high-grade malignant cells on a

parotid or periparotid fine-needle aspirate. Metastasis from an occult breast carcinoma to the parotid of an elderly man is exceptionally unlikely in this case, but immunohistochemical staining for androgen receptor can be used to discriminate these tumors if necessary.

26. **(C) Negative for malignancy.**
The photomicrograph demonstrates a collagen ball, which is characterized by spherical-to-oval balls of collagen surrounded by flat, bland mesothelial cells. The collagen has a blue color on Papanicolaou stains. Collagen balls are seen in up to 50% of pelvic washings, are benign, and have no known clinical significance. Their presence is not typically commented on in the final diagnosis. They should not be mistaken for evidence of a low-grade neoplasm, particularly when numerous. In comparison, a pelvic washing involved by a borderline serous tumor of the ovary would show clusters of mildly atypical cells that often have a papillary architecture and may be associated with psammoma bodies. Occasionally, true fibrovascular cores will be present, but the amorphous collagen stroma of a collagen ball is not seen. A high-grade papillary serous carcinoma in a pelvic washing will contain clusters of markedly atypical cells with nuclear pleomorphism, hyperchromasia, prominent nucleoli, and mitotic figures. Malignant mesothelioma is rarely sampled on pelvic washings, as this procedure is usually performed as part of a staging surgery for a gynecologic tumor. It should be noted that a diagnosis of "atypical" or "suspicious" on a washing cytology should be discouraged, as this procedure is used for staging purposes, and only "positive" or "negative" results are included in the staging protocols.

27. **(A) Ductal carcinoma of the breast.**
The photomicrograph demonstrates very large clusters of neoplastic cells with smooth community borders. These large spherical clusters are often called "cannonballs" or "proliferation spheres," and are seen almost exclusively in metastatic adenocarcinoma involving an effusion. This pattern is most commonly seen in metastatic ductal carcinoma of the breast, less commonly in metastatic ovarian carcinoma, and rarely in lung adenocarcinoma. In addition, breast carcinoma is the most common tumor to present with pleural effusion prior to recognition of the primary tumor site. In contrast, lobular carcinoma of the breast and signet ring cell carcinoma of the stomach are more likely to involve effusions as single cells or small clusters. Reactive mesothelial cells almost never form large spherical clusters, and will have a scalloped or "knobby" border.

28. **(C) Ductal adenocarcinoma.**

The photomicrograph demonstrates malignant ductal epithelium with marked variation in nuclear size, loss of the normal honeycomb glandular arrangement, and nuclear pleomorphism, consistent with ductal adenocarcinoma of the pancreas. Aspirates of ductal adenocarcinoma are typically highly cellular, may have a background of necrotic debris, and contain cohesive groups of ductal epithelium with nuclear atypia, including nuclear membrane irregularities, marked (usually at least fourfold) variation in nuclear size, loss of nuclear polarity (so-called "drunken honeycomb" appearance), and irregular chromatin. Other features of ductal adenocarcinoma include isolated single atypical cells, high nuclear-to-cytoplasmic ratio, and atypical mitotic figures. While intraductal papillary mucinous neoplasms can show significant nuclear atypia, which is indistinguishable from ductal adenocarcinoma, the clinical history (particularly lack of cystic appearance and connection with the main pancreatic duct) is more typical of a ductal adenocarcinoma.

29. **(E) Pancreatic endocrine neoplasm.**

The photomicrograph demonstrates an aspirate smear of a pancreatic endocrine neoplasm, characterized by a monotonous population of plasmacytoid cells with salt and pepper chromatin. Aspirates of pancreatic endocrine neoplasms are usually moderately to highly cellular, and the cells are largely single or form loose clusters. Immunohistochemical staining will confirm the diagnosis, as the cells will be positive for synaptophysin and chromogranin. In contrast, aspirates of acinar cell carcinomas are moderately cellular and are composed of cuboidal cells with abundant granular cytoplasm forming sheets and acinar-like structures, which have uniform nuclei with prominent nucleoli. Aspirates of chronic pancreatitis can be highly variable, but most often have minimal reactive ductal epithelium, chronic inflammation, and debris. Aspirates of ductal adenocarcinoma are characterized by highly cellular smears containing malignant appearing glandular cells with nuclear pleomorphism and a background of necrosis. Aspirates of intraductal papillary mucinous neoplasms typically contain abundant, thick mucin admixed with glandular epithelium. This epithelium can range from benign-appearing ductal cells to cells indistinguishable from invasive ductal adenocarcinoma.

30. **(B) Upstage from T1a to T1c.**

Pelvic and peritoneal washings are routinely performed as part of an oncologic surgery for patients with gynecologic malignancies. The presence of neoplastic cells in a pelvic or peritoneal wash is highly associated with reduced disease-free survival and overall survival, particularly for patients with an ovarian serous papillary carcinoma. Over 80% of patients with a stage I tumor (confined to one or both ovaries) with malignant cells in a washing will die of their disease, compared with only 35% of patients with the same stage and a negative washing cytology. This is reflected in the staging of ovarian carcinomas; a positive washing result will change the stage of a tumor confined to one ovary from T1a to T1c, and the overall stage will change from IA to IC. Peritoneal spread is not considered N1 or M1 disease. Stage T3 requires histologically confirmed evidence of involvement of the peritoneum beyond the pelvis by tumor.

31. **(D) Fibroadenoma.**

The photomicrograph demonstrates an aspirate sample composed of benign, three-dimensional sheets of ductal cells with a branching or "staghorn" appearance, along with a background of naked bipolar nuclei and rare stromal fragments, consistent with a fibroadenoma. The naked bipolar nuclei represent myoepithelial cells stripped from the benign epithelium when the aspirate slides are smeared. Other reassuring features are epithelium with uniform, well-spaced nuclei (or "honeycomb" appearance) and residual myoepithelial cells present on the epithelial strips, which have darker nuclei slightly out of the plane of focus of the epithelium (so-called "poppy seed" appearance). A breast cyst would be composed of predominantly histiocytes, with or without apocrine metaplasia. Ductal carcinoma is characterized by epithelial cells with reduced cohesion, marked pleomorphism and atypia, lack of myoepithelial cells, and coarse chromatin. Fine-needle aspiration biopsy of an intraductal papilloma would contain papillary structures with fibrovascular cores that are tightly cohesive and have a variable myoepithelial component. Fat necrosis is characterized by hypocellular smears containing vacuolated histiocytes and inflammation.

32. **(E) Subareolar abscess.**

The photomicrograph demonstrates an aspirate composed of abundant anucleated squamous cells, histiocytes, and acute inflammation. This, combined with the clinical setting of a tender mass under the nipple, is most consistent with a subareolar abscess. Subareolar abscesses tend to occur in women who smoke, and are caused by squamous metaplasia of the lactiferous ducts immediately under the nipple, which become clogged with keratin debris and rupture, resulting in an inflammatory response. Complete excision is required to prevent recurrence of this process. Metastatic squamous cell carcinoma to the breast is exceedingly rare, and would demonstrate atypical squamous epithelium.

33. **(A) Ductal carcinoma.**

The photomicrograph demonstrates a breast aspirate composed of markedly atypical epithelial cells, some of which are present as single cells, consistent with a diagnosis of ductal carcinoma. The major features of ductal carcinoma of the breast on fine-needle aspiration biopsy include high smear cellularity, atypical ductal epithelium with nuclear pleomorphism, groups arranged in syncytial or three-dimensional clusters, single atypical cells, absence of myoepithelial cells (or naked bipolar nuclei), and variable tumor diathesis. Fine-needle aspiration biopsy cannot reliably distinguish invasive ductal carcinoma from high-grade ductal carcinoma in situ, and therefore, the best diagnosis is ductal carcinoma, which encompasses both entities. Lobular carcinoma will typically have low cellularity aspirates with mildly atypical cells arranged as single cells or linear aggregates with intracytoplasmic lumens. A subareolar abscess would be located underneath the nipple, and aspirates contain anucleated squamous cells and marked acute inflammation. Intraductal papilloma aspirates demonstrate sheets and three-dimensional clusters of tightly cohesive ductal cells with associated myoepithelial cells and fibrovascular cores. Aspirates of fibroadenomas demonstrate a triad of branching benign ductal epithelium, stromal fragments, and a background of naked bipolar nuclei.

34. **(D) Lobular carcinoma.**

The photomicrograph demonstrates an aspirate sample composed of small epithelial cells arranged as single cells and small linear clusters, which have mild nuclear atypia and cytoplasmic vacuoles that contain mucin (so-called intracytoplasmic lumens). This appearance is diagnostic of lobular carcinoma of the breast. Other features of lobular carcinoma of the breast include low cellularity (due to the frequent stromal sclerosis seen in these tumors), high nuclear-to-cytoplasmic ratio, vesicular nuclei with inconspicuous or absent nucleoli, and linear arrangement of the cells. While signet ring cells are not specific to lobular carcinoma, when present in ductal carcinoma, they are associated with significantly more pleomorphism, higher smear cellularity, larger cell clusters, and larger nuclei. Metastasis of other carcinomas to the breast is very infrequent, and typically seen only in advanced disease. Aspirates of fat necrosis are characterized

by foamy histiocytes, amorphous debris, fibro-adipose tissue, and inflammation. Fibroadenoma cytology is characterized by the triad of staghorn fragments of benign epithelium, stromal fragments, and naked bipolar nuclei.

35. **(C) Marked nuclear hyperchromasia and atypia.**

The photomicrograph demonstrates an aspirate of spindle cells with a "tissue culture"-like appearance, which are loosely cohesive, and have vesicular chromatin and minimal atypia. This appearance, combined with the clinical history of a rapidly growing small (<2 cm) mass in the head and neck region of a young person, is highly suggestive of a diagnosis of nodular fasciitis. Other features of nodular fasciitis on fine-needle aspiration biopsy include stellate (myofibroblastic) cells, ganglion-like cells with eccentric nuclei and prominent nucleoli, background inflammation, and binucleated cells. Numerous mitotic figures can be seen, and do not indicate malignancy. However, significant hyperchromasia or nuclear atypia should prompt further evaluation for malignancy.

36. **(D) Microbiologic culture for fungi and acid-fast bacteria.**

The photomicrograph demonstrates non-necrotizing granulomatous inflammation, characterized by aggregates of epithelioid histiocytes with indented-, spindled-, or "boomerang-shaped" nuclei and lymphocytes. A background of necrosis (caseation) may be seen, particularly in infectious conditions. When granulomatous inflammation is recognized, microbiologic culture for fungi and acid-fast bacteria should be recommended to exclude an infectious process. Flow cytometry would be useful in cases of suspected lymphoma. Gram stain is useful when a typical bacterial infection is suspected, such as aspiration biopsy of an abscess cavity. Immunohistochemistry is useful in cases of malignancy to determine cell differentiation and origin (lung versus metastasis). Serum angiotensin converting enzyme (ACE) levels are often elevated in patients with sarcoidosis but this finding is not specific, and exclusion of an infectious process is required in all cases of suspected sarcoidosis.

37. **(B) *C-myc*.**

The cytologic description, in a child from Africa, is highly suggestive of endemic-type Burkitt lymphoma. Burkitt lymphomas are characterized by recurring translocations involving *c-myc*, most commonly t(8;14) involving *c-myc* and immunoglobulin G (IgG) heavy chain. Burkitt lymphomas are B-cell neoplasms, so T-cell receptor genes are not involved in neoplasia. *BCL2* is commonly involved in translocations in follicular lymphoma.

N-myc is amplified or mutated in a variety of neoplasms, including neuroblastomas. Immunoglobulin light chain is occasionally involved in a variety of lymphoid neoplasms, but is less common than immunoglobulin heavy chain rearrangement.

38. **(C) Clusters with smooth community borders.**
In effusion specimens, mesothelial cells are characterized by single cells or small groups that have moderate cytoplasm, which is dense near the nucleus and is pale at the periphery of the cell, giving rise to the term "lacy skirt." This lacy skirt is the result of numerous long, thin microvilli, which also result in clear spaces, or "windows" between mesothelial cells within a cluster. Binucleation and multinucleation are commonly seen in mesothelial cells, and the nucleus is usually round-to-oval with fine chromatin and contains a small nucleolus. When mesothelial cells are present in a cluster, the border of the group usually has a scalloped or "bumpy" appearance. In contrast, epithelial neoplasms in effusion specimens will characteristically have a smooth community border due to junctions, which hold epithelial cells together.

39. **(A) Calretinin, cytokeratins 5/6 (CK 5/6), carcinoembryonic antigen (CEA), B72.3.**
In effusion cytology, distinction of mesothelial cells (reactive or neoplastic) from metastatic adenocarcinoma can be difficult on cytologic features alone. Therefore, application of an appropriate immunohistochemical panel is recommended in many cases for definitive diagnosis. Immunohistochemical markers that are positive in mesothelial cells and typically negative in adenocarcinomas include calretinin, high-molecular-weight keratin (e.g., cytokeratins 5/6), WT-1, and D2-40 (also known as *podoplanin*). Immunohistochemical markers that are positive in adenocarcinomas and typically negative in mesothelial cells include CEA, B72.3, MOC-31, CD15 (LeuM1), and EP-4. Both adenocarcinomas and mesothelial cells will be positive for low-molecular-weight keratins, which include cytokeratin 7, AE1/3, and CAM5.2. According to recommendations of the Association of Directors of Anatomic and Surgical Pathology published in 2007, at least two mesothelial-specific markers and two markers typically negative in mesothelial cells should be used as a panel for the distinction of mesothelial proliferations from metastatic adenocarcinoma. The only choice in the question that includes two of each category is choice A. Choice B contains only mesothelial-specific markers. Choice C contains only nonmesothelial markers. Choice D contains stains that would be positive in both

mesothelial cells and adenocarcinoma. Specific markers such as estrogen receptor and progesterone are not helpful unless the prior breast carcinoma was positive for ER and PR. In addition, ER can occasionally be positive in mesothelial cells, limiting the utility of this marker.

40. **(C) *Mycobacterium tuberculosis.***
A pleural effusion composed of nearly 100% small mature lymphocytes with very few-to-absent mesothelial cells is the classic appearance of tuberculous pleuritis. The relative absence of mesothelial cells is believed to be secondary to trapping of mesothelial cells by fibrin deposition. While this appearance is not specific to tuberculosis (e.g., pleural involvement by low-grade lymphomas), the other possibilities listed in the question would not result in this effusion appearance. *Aspergillus fumigatus* infection rarely will involve the pleural space and has been associated with increased neutrophils and eosinophils. While pleural involvement by small-cell undifferentiated carcinoma can be overlooked as a chronic inflammatory infiltrate, on closer examination, the cells have coarse chromatin, nuclear molding, clumping of cell groups, and a background of apoptotic debris. Primary effusion lymphoma is a large-cell lymphoma that has prominent nucleoli. Systemic lupus erythematosus pleuritis is characterized by increased neutrophils, necrosis, and lupus erythematosus (LE) cells, which are neutrophils or macrophages engulfing nuclear fragments.

41. **(D) Spontaneous pneumothorax.**
An *eosinophilic pleural effusion* is defined as an effusion where eosinophils represent 10% or more of the total cellular composition of the effusion. The most common cause of eosinophilic pleural effusion is introduction of air into the pleural space. This can occur spontaneously, due to a spontaneous pneumothorax or lung-pleural fistula, or iatrogenically, due to repeated thoracocentesis or lung fine-needle aspiration biopsy. Other causes of eosinophilic pleural effusions include allergic processes, pulmonary infarct, pneumonia, fungal infection, parasitic infection, and involvement of the pleural space by a neoplasm. Tuberculous pleuritis is characterized by a marked lymphocytosis with very few mesothelial cells. Rheumatoid pleuritis is characterized by abundant multinucleated histiocytes, granular debris, and cholesterol crystals. Empyema is characterized by numerous neutrophils in a necrotic background. Primary effusion lymphoma is characterized by numerous large atypical lymphocytes with prominent nucleoli.

42. **(B) Mitotic figures.**

Identification of malignancy in a pleural or peritoneal effusion by cytology does not depend on any one feature. However, certain findings are highly associated with malignancy and should prompt careful review of the sample, along with clinical correlation and possible immunohistochemical stains. One of the most helpful features in the identification of metastatic carcinoma to mesothelial-lined spaces is the presence of two cell populations: normal mesothelial cells and an atypical cell population. Another useful feature is the presence of very large cell clusters; normal and reactive mesothelial cells will almost never form groups of more than 20 cells, and when present, can be a sign of malignant mesothelioma or metastatic carcinoma. When involving effusions, carcinomas are likely to have smooth community borders at the edge of cell groups, unlike reactive mesothelial cells that have scalloped or knobby borders. Vacuoles can be seen in normal and reactive mesothelial cells, but large vacuoles that displace and indent the nucleus are uncommon, and a worrisome sign for neoplasia. On the other hand, mitotic figures can be seen in many benign and reactive conditions. The presence of atypical mitotic figures should raise concern for malignancy.

43. **(D) Ovarian serous carcinoma.**

Ovarian serous carcinoma typically forms large groups, often with papillary architecture, in effusion cytology. Other features of ovarian serous carcinoma in effusion cytology include psammoma bodies, marked nuclear enlargement and pleomorphism, and cytoplasmic vacuolization. In contrast, all of the other options listed in the question present as effusions with a predominance of single cells. Lobular carcinoma of the breast is particularly subtle when involving effusion fluid, and many authors recommend performing immunohistochemistry on any effusion sample from a patient with a prior history of lobular breast carcinoma.

44. **(C) Lactating adenoma.**

The cytologic description provided is highly suggestive of lactational change, which can be seen in postpartum women, or may persist as a discrete nodule in nonlactating women where it is called a *lactating adenoma*. Lactational change is characterized by highly cellular aspirates of loosely cohesive or discohesive epithelial cells that have delicate foamy cytoplasm. This cytoplasm is often stripped, leading to a background of foamy, proteinaceous debris, and naked nuclei. The epithelial cells will show nuclear enlargement and prominent nucleoli features that should not be mistaken for malignancy. Features

that favor lactational change over ductal carcinoma include foamy background, relative monotony of the nuclei (despite enlargement and prominent nucleoli), absence of necrosis, presence of rare intact acinar structures, and young age of the patient.

45. **(D) Hypercellular epithelial fragments.**

Fat necrosis can mimic breast carcinoma both clinically and radiologically by presenting as a spiculated dense mass. Fat necrosis is often associated with prior trauma (breast injury, prior surgical procedure), although no history may be present at the time of evaluation. Fine-needle aspiration biopsy of fat necrosis is characterized by abundant histiocytes that are usually foamy and frequently form multinucleated giant cells. A background of amorphous, granular debris is commonly present, and dystrophic calcifications may be seen. Interspersed normal fat fragments are typically also present. The degree of inflammation is variable, but a chronic inflammatory infiltrate is typically seen except in the acute setting, where neutrophils are more common. The presence of high epithelial cellularity should raise concern for another process; an infiltrating ductal carcinoma may be present in association with fat necrosis if a prior biopsy was performed in the area.

46. **(C) Marked stromal atypia.**

The differentiation of fibroadenoma from phyllodes tumor on fine-needle aspiration biopsy is difficult, as both lesions are biphasic neoplasms composed of both epithelial and stromal cells. Overall cellularity is not helpful; fibroadenomas can be very cellular. The epithelial component of both lesions can be indistinguishable; branching fragments of ductal epithelium are frequently seen in both lesions. In addition, the stromal fragments in both lesions can be very hypercellular, and this feature does not reliably distinguish these tumors. Features that are most suggestive of phyllodes tumor include marked stromal atypia, numerous mitotic figures within the stromal component, spindle cells with elongated, thin nuclei, and marked epithelial atypia (which can be mistaken for ductal carcinoma). Fibroadenomas will typically have spindle cells with short, oval nuclei.

47. **(E) Tubular carcinoma.**

Extracellular myxoid or mucinous material on a breast fine-needle aspiration biopsy can be seen in a variety of benign and malignant neoplasms, including mucocele-like lesion, myxoid fibroadenomas, colloid carcinomas, and ductal carcinomas with mucinous features. Mucocele-like lesions are believed to arise from rupture of mucinous material in a duct into the surrounding breast parenchyma. On fine-needle aspiration biopsy, mucocele-like lesions show predominantly extra-cellular mucinous material with very few epithelial cells that are present in small groups and lack atypia. Fibroadenomas can have abundant myx-oid change in the stromal component, which can mimic a mucinous neoplasm on fine-needle aspi-ration biopsy, but will show the other features of fibroadenoma, including branching epithelial frag-ments and naked bipolar nuclei in the background. Colloid carcinoma on fine-needle aspiration biopsy of the breast typically demonstrates abundant extracellular mucinous material admixed with three-dimensional clusters of mildly atypical ductal cells. This appearance can significantly overlap with the findings in mucocele-like lesions; there-fore, any mucinous breast aspirate should be fol-lowed up with core or excisional biopsy for further evaluation. Focal mucinous differentiation can be seen in ductal carcinomas as well, which typically show more atypia and pleomorphism than colloid carcinomas on fine-needle aspiration biopsy, but excision is required for definitive classification. In contrast, tubular carcinomas are low-grade ductal neoplasms that on fine-needle aspiration biopsy have low cellularity and contain epithelial groups with minimal atypia that form angulated or rigid tubules, have comma-shaped projections, and do not contain mucinous material.

48. **(D) Coarse hyperchromatic and irregular chromatin.**
Pilomatricoma typically occurs in children and young adults, and presents as a firm subcutane-ous or deep dermal nodule. Fine-needle aspirate samples of pilomatricoma are characterized by the admixture of basaloid cells, ghost cells, and background of amorphous debris. The basaloid cells appear as cohesive clusters of small cells with scant cytoplasm and a high nuclear-to-cytoplasmic ratio. These basaloid cells have round-to-oval uniform nuclei with open fine chromatin and prominent nucleoli. The ghost cells are anucle-ated squamous cells that often appear refractile and commonly fragment on aspirate smears. A background of naked nuclei is common, as well as abundant amorphous debris that frequently will be calcified. In adults, pilomatricomas can be mistaken for squamous cell carcinomas. In this population, the presence of marked atypia, nuclear hyperchromasia, and coarse irregular chromatin is worrisome for malignancy.

49. **(C) Infantile fibrosarcoma.**
A pattern-based approach to the fine-needle aspira-tion biopsy of many soft tissue tumors is helpful in the evaluation of difficult cases. Patterns of soft tis-sue tumors include small round blue cell, spindled, myxoid, pleomorphic, epithelioid, and fat-containing tumors. Many tumors of childhood fall into the small round blue cell category, which is character-ized by small cells with scant cytoplasm and round contours that frequently lack cellular cohesion. Childhood soft tissue tumors with this pattern include Ewing sarcoma/primitive neuroectodermal tumor, neuroblastoma, and rhabdomyosarcoma. Acute lymphoblastic leukemia is the most common malignancy of childhood and can present as a soft tissue mass. Recognition of this differential diagno-sis is important in the triage of tissue for ancillary testing to confirm the diagnosis. In contrast, infan-tile fibrosarcoma is a highly cellular spindle cell proliferation with a herringbone pattern and, on fine-needle aspiration biopsy, retains a spindle cell appearance.

50. **(E) Wavy spindle cells with tapered nuclei.**
Aspirates of schwannomas typically show large cohesive fragments of spindle cells with wavy tapered nuclei. Nuclear palisading suggestive of Verocay bodies can be seen. In addition, rare, large hyperchromatic smudgy nuclei with intranuclear inclusions can be seen in schwannomas with "ancient change." Epithelioid cells with plasma-cytoid cytoplasm and binucleation are frequently seen in malignant melanomas and some carcino-mas. Marked nuclear pleomorphism, tumor giant cells, and prominent nucleoli are more typical of an undifferentiated pleomorphic sarcoma. Spindle cells with rounded, cigar-shaped nuclei are typical of smooth muscle neoplasms, such as leiomyomas. Stellate, fibroblast-like spindle cells in a myxoid or inflammatory background are seen in aspirates of nodular fasciitis.

51. **(E) S-100.**
The cytologic description is classic for a granular cell tumor of the breast. Granular cell tumors occur most frequently in the head and neck, particularly the oral cavity and larynx, but are infrequently aspirated in these sites. The second most com-mon location for granular cell tumor is the breast, which is the most common source of fine-needle aspirates of this lesion. Immunohistochemical staining for S-100 will be positive in granular cell tumor cells. CD68 would be positive in fat necro-sis, which would be expected to show histiocytes with grooved or kidney bean-shaped nuclei, foamy cytoplasm, and multinucleated giant cells. Desmin and myogenin would be positive in a rhabdo-myoma, a benign neoplasm that is exceedingly rare in the breast, which cytologically would show

multinucleated cells and dense fibrillary cytoplasm. Cytokeratin would be positive in epithelial lesions such as lactational change, which would demonstrate intact cells with abundant foamy cytoplasm, prominent nucleoli, and proteinaceous debris in the background.

52. **(E) t(12;16)(q13;p11).**
The cytologic description of a myxoid spindle cell lesion of the deep thigh with a delicate capillary network and round cells is highly suggestive of a myxoid liposarcoma. The characteristic translocation of myxoid liposarcoma is t(12;16)(q13;p11), and fluorescence in situ hybridization is frequently used to demonstrate this abnormality on cytologic preparations to confirm the diagnosis. Alveolar soft part sarcoma is characterized by a t(X;17)(p11;q25) translocation and, on fine-needle aspiration biopsy, shows large cells with abundant cytoplasm and prominent nucleoli that often form pseudoacinar structures. Synovial sarcoma characteristically has a t(X;18)(p11;q11) translocation and, on fine-needle aspiration biopsy, shows highly cellular aspirates containing alternating dispersed spindle cells and cohesive clusters. The t(2;13)(q35;q14) is one of the two translocations seen in alveolar rhabdomyosarcoma, which, on fine-needle aspiration biopsy, will appear as a small round blue cell tumor with occasional rhabdomyoblasts. Finally, Ewing sarcoma is characterized by a t(12;16)(q13;p11) translocation and, also, has a small round blue cell appearance with alternating light and dark cells on fine-needle aspiration biopsy.

53. **(E) Thick ribbon of matrix material surrounding cell groups with peripheral palisading.**
Basaloid neoplasms involving the salivary gland can show considerable overlap on fine-needle aspiration biopsy. This is problematic, as benign tumors (such as basal cell adenoma, cellular pleomorphic adenoma, and chronic sialadenitis) can be indistinguishable from malignant neoplasms (such as basal cell adenocarcinoma, adenoid cystic carcinoma, and basaloid squamous cell carcinoma). In many cases, only a descriptive report with a differential diagnosis can be provided. However, some features, when present, can be helpful in narrowing the differential diagnosis. The membranous subtype of basal cell adenoma is cytologically distinctive. This subtype of basal cell adenoma shows rimming of cellular groups by a thick rim of acellular matrix material that often surrounds the groups (as opposed to the cells surrounding spheres of acellular matrix material in an adenoid cystic carcinoma). At the interface, the basaloid cells frequently show peripheral palisading.

Fibrillary metachromatic matrix material is characteristic of pleomorphic adenomas. High mitotic activity and necrosis is more typical of high-grade carcinomas, such as basaloid squamous cell carcinoma and the solid type of adenoid cystic carcinoma. Spheres of acellular, sharply demarcated metachromatic matrix material is typical of adenoid cystic carcinoma. While squamous differentiation can be seen in basal cell adenomas, atypical squamous epithelium should not be seen, and is suggestive of a basaloid squamous cell carcinoma.

54. **(B) Adenoid cystic carcinoma.**
Cells with abundant cytoplasm, polygonal shape, and central nuclei are considered oncocytic or oncocyte-like on fine-needle aspiration biopsy. The presence of oncocyte-like cells in a salivary gland aspirate suggests a limited differential diagnosis that includes oncocytoma, Warthin tumor, oncocytic carcinoma, acinic cell carcinoma, mucoepidermoid carcinoma, and metastasis (particularly renal cell carcinoma). The ability of mucoepidermoid carcinoma to appear oncocyte-like is frequently forgotten; a key clue to this diagnosis is the admixture of mucus-containing goblet cells. In contrast, adenoid cystic carcinoma is characterized by cells that have small, dark, and angulated nuclei with minimal cytoplasm.

55. **(B) Epithelial myoepithelial carcinoma.**
Metachromatic (purple-pink) extracellular matrix material on Diff-Quik stained aspirates can be seen in a variety of benign and malignant salivary gland tumors. This list includes pleomorphic adenoma, carcinoma ex pleomorphic adenoma, adenoid cystic carcinoma, basal cell adenoma, basal cell adenocarcinoma, and epithelial myoepithelial carcinoma. Metachromatic matrix material that is fibrillary and admixed with myoepithelial cells is characteristic of pleomorphic adenomas, and can be seen in carcinoma ex pleomorphic adenoma. In most other tumors, the stroma is acellular, has sharp contours, and is not diagnostic for any one specific entity. Therefore, in most cases, a descriptive diagnosis with a comment listing the differential diagnostic possibilities is required. In contrast, all of the other tumors listed do not contain matrix material. In fact, the absence of chondromyxoid stroma is what distinguishes myoepithelioma from pleomorphic adenoma both on histology and cytology preparations.

56. **(C) Polymorphous low-grade adenocarcinoma.**
A variety of salivary gland lesions can be cystic, including benign and malignant tumors. Cystic salivary gland lesions can be divided into mucinous and nonmucinous types. Mucinous cystic lesions

include mucocele, retention cyst, Warthin tumor with mucinous metaplasia, and mucoepidermoid carcinoma. Nonmucinous cystic lesions include Warthin tumor, cystic pleomorphic adenoma, ductal papilloma, lymphoepithelial cyst, cystadenoma, acinic cell carcinoma, cystic squamous cell carcinoma, and cystadenocarcinoma. In particular, the papillary cystic variant of acinic cell carcinoma can be extensively cystic, and, in some cases, aspirates will contain only acellular cyst fluid and histiocytes. Low-grade mucoepidermoid carcinomas are almost always at least partially cystic, and Warthin tumors are by definition cystic with papillary oncocytic epithelium and lymphoid stroma. In contrast, polymorphous low-grade adenocarcinomas almost always present as slow-growing firm masses, most commonly in the palate.

57. **(B) Abundant cyst contents only.**
According to the 2007 Bethesda System for Reporting Thyroid Cytopathology, thyroid fine-needle aspirates must have at least 6 groups of 10 follicular cells that are well preserved and visualized to be adequate for interpretation, with three exceptions. The exceptions include abundant colloid, a thyroiditis pattern, or the presence of sufficient atypia to warrant another diagnostic category. In the choices listed in the question, choice E meets standard adequacy criteria, choice A meets the abundant colloid exception, and choice C meets the thyroiditis exception. Choice D shows atypia, sufficient for an interpretation of at least "atypia of undetermined significance" and some might consider an interpretation of "suspicious for malignancy," so it is also adequate. The presence of cyst contents, in the absence of at least 6 groups of 10 follicular cells, would not be considered adequate for interpretation and should have an interpretation of either "nondiagnostic" or "unsatisfactory" with a description of the aspirate contents. An interpretation of nondiagnostic should prompt repeat aspiration biopsy after an appropriate clinical interval (generally 3 months to prevent repair atypia on subsequent sample).

58. **(C) At least 50% of the follicular cells have Hürthle cell change.**
The criteria for a thyroid fine-needle aspiration biopsy interpretation of "suspicious for follicular neoplasm, Hürthle cell type" includes follicular epithelium with Hürthle cell change (abundant granular cytoplasm, large nuclei, and prominent nucleoli) along with an abnormal architectural pattern, which most often is characterized by little to no colloid and either microfollicles, single cells, or syncytial groups. The follicular epithelium in these aspirates should be composed exclusively or nearly exclusively of Hürthle cells. Aspirates that show an admixture of Hürthle cells and non-Hürthle cells, particularly in the presence of moderate-to-abundant colloid, are usually benign. Therefore, in an aspirate with high cellularity and abnormal architecture, at least 75% of the cells must show Hürthle cell change for an interpretation of "suspicious for follicular neoplasm, Hürthle cell type," and, if below this, an interpretation of "suspicious for follicular neoplasm" is more appropriate. Aspirate samples showing nuclear features of papillary thyroid carcinoma should not be placed into this category, and belong in the "suspicious for papillary thyroid carcinoma" or "positive for malignancy, papillary thyroid carcinoma" categories. As Hürthle cell metaplasia is prominent in cases of chronic lymphocytic thyroiditis, a significant lymphoid component in a thyroid aspirate with Hürthle cells is reassuring and, in most cases, is best interpreted as "benign, chronic lymphocytic thyroiditis" or at most "atypia of undetermined significance" with a comment regarding the possibility of Hürthle cell hyperplasia in the setting of chronic lymphocytic thyroiditis.

59. **(B) 5–15%.**
In the 2007 Bethesda System for Reporting Thyroid Cytopathology, the recommended estimated risk of malignancy for various interpretation categories has been published to further standardize reporting and management guidelines. Individual laboratories may use internal cytologic–histologic correlations to track and report their own risk of malignancy if they choose. The 2007 Bethesda System suggests a risk of malignancy around 5–15% for aspirates with an interpretation of "atypia of undetermined significance" or "follicular lesion of undetermined significance." A benign aspirate has a risk of less than 3%, an aspirate interpreted as "follicular neoplasm" or "suspicious for a follicular neoplasm" has a risk of 15–30%, an aspirate interpreted as "suspicious for malignancy" has a risk of 60–75%, and an aspirate interpreted as "malignant" has a risk of 97–99%.

60. **(D) Unilocular cyst 2.5 cm in size.**
The decision to categorize thyroid aspirates that contain cyst fluid only as "nondiagnostic" in the 2007 Bethesda System for Reporting Thyroid Cytopathology was somewhat controversial. Most thyroid aspirates that contain abundant cyst fluid will be derived from benign processes. However, because of the risk of a low-cellularity cystic papillary thyroid carcinoma, many stakeholders did not want to risk interpreting these aspirates as

"benign." Clinical evidence suggests that patients with a thyroid ultrasound demonstrating a unilocular cyst that is less than 3.0 cm in size are almost always benign in the absence of atypia on fine-needle aspiration biopsy. Since pathologists are not always privy to this information, the current recommendation is to report thyroid aspirates with cyst contents only as "nondiagnostic, cyst contents only," and the clinician should correlate ultrasound and clinical information. An interpretation of "nondiagnostic, cyst contents only" is considered clinically adequate in patients with a unilocular simple cyst that is less than 3.0 cm in size; repeat fine-needle aspiration biopsy is not required.

61. **(B) Aspirate fluid parathyroid hormone level.**
The clinical appearance of crystal clear cyst fluid from a lesion in the neck, usually near the thyroid gland, is highly suggestive of a parathyroid cyst. Most thyroid cysts will contain turbulent fluid that is often brown in color due to the presence of hemosiderin-laden macrophages. The astute pathologist can confirm the diagnosis by sending a portion of the cyst fluid for a parathyroid hormone level. The parathyroid hormone level in a parathyroid cyst will usually be markedly elevated, typically in thousands per milliliter. Most patients with a parathyroid cyst do not have hyperparathyroidism. Parathyroid adenomas can undergo central degeneration with cystic change, but these cysts often grossly appear more similar to thyroid cysts.

62. **(B) High-grade papillary urothelial carcinoma.**
Clusters of bland urothelial cells in a voided urine cytology specimen can be caused by a variety of processes, including kidney stones (nephrolithiasis), infection, urothelial papillomas, and low-grade urothelial carcinoma. Instrumented urines frequently will show similar changes, due to iatrogenic disruption of the urothelium off the basement membrane in fragments. In many cases, it is impossible to cytologically distinguish urothelial clusters of low-grade urothelial carcinoma from reactive conditions. In contrast, high-grade urothelial carcinoma may shed into the urine as papillary fragments, but the cells will show nuclear atypia, hyperchromasia, and increased nuclear-to-cytoplasmic ratio.

63. **(E) Round nuclei with smooth contours.**
Urothelial cells infected by polyoma virus are called *decoy cells* because they can mimic high-grade urothelial carcinoma. This is largely due to the fact that polyoma virus infection results in urothelial cells with hyperchromatic nuclei and scant cytoplasm (high nuclear-to-cytoplasmic ratio),

features that are shared with high-grade urothelial carcinoma. Features that favor the presence of urothelial carcinoma include clusters of atypical cells (polyoma cells are almost always exclusively single cells), coarse chromatin (rather than the glassy or opaque nuclear inclusion in polyoma infection), and irregular nuclear contours. Intact polyoma-infected urothelial cells will have very round nuclei with smooth nuclear contours. However, extensive cellular degeneration can occur in both polyoma virus infection and urothelial carcinoma, making distinction difficult in some cases.

64. **(A) Aneuploidy of multiple chromosomes (3, 7, 17, and 9p).**
UroVysion™ fluorescence in situ hybridization is FDA approved for the detection of recurrent urothelial carcinoma in urine cytology specimens in patients with a history of urothelial carcinoma and for the primary detection of urothelial carcinoma in patients with hematuria. This assay is based on the identification of common chromosomal alterations in high-grade urothelial carcinomas, specifically aneuploidy (gain in number) of multiple chromosomes. The UroVysion assay uses centromeric probes for chromosomes 3, 7, and 17 and a probe for the short arm of chromosome 9 (9p), and the number of signals for each chromosome is counted in the abnormal urothelial cells. *Positive for aneuploidy* is defined as a gain in 2 or more chromosomes (usually 3, 7, or 17) in 5 or more urothelial cells. Rarely, homozygous loss of chromosome 9p is seen in more than 50% of cells (or more than 12 cells), and is also a marker of urothelial carcinoma but is seen in lower-grade neoplasms. This assay does not examine for specific translocations or point mutations.

65. **(C) *Neisseria meningitidis* infection.**
The cytologic description of increased lymphocytes and occasional atypical lymphocytes in a cerebrospinal fluid (CSF) sample is commonly seen in a variety of reactive and neoplastic conditions. The most common infectious cause of CSF lymphocytosis is viral meningitis, followed by Lyme disease, syphilis, and some fungal infections (*Cryptococcus*, *Histoplasma*). However, lymphocytosis can also be caused by a neoplastic lymphoproliferative disorder, including both primary central nervous system lymphomas and secondary involvement by a systemic lymphoma (e.g., acute lymphoblastic lymphoma). Flow cytometry is often critical in distinguishing a reactive pleocytosis from a malignant lymphoma involving CSF. In contrast, *Neisseria meningitidis* is a gram-positive bacillus that causes acute, fulminant meningitis, which is characterized by

marked neutrophilic infiltrate that often contains bacterial organisms. Recognition of this pattern is critical as *Neisseria meningitidis* can be rapidly fatal.

66. **(A) Germinal matrix cells.**

In the pediatric population, the presence of small, dark, atypical cells with scant cytoplasm and nuclear molding in a cerebrospinal fluid (CSF) sample is highly concerning for an undifferentiated malignancy, such as medulloblastoma, neuroblastoma, or pineoblastoma. However, premature babies, particularly those with hydrocephalus and intraventricular hemorrhage, will frequently shed germinal matrix cells into the CSF. The germinal matrix is a highly cellular region of immature cells surrounding the ventricular spaces (subependymal) from which neurons and glial precursors are derived during fetal development. Germinal matrix can be seen in fetuses and premature neonates with a gestational age of less than 35 weeks. These cells are very similar in appearance to other childhood undifferentiated or anaplastic neuronal-derived tumors, and can mimic malignancy. Close clinical correlation is recommended to prevent overdiagnosis. While primary central nervous system lymphomas and small cell carcinomas can have a similar appearance, these tumors almost never occur in neonates.

67. **(A) Alveolar macrophages.**

Sputum is one of the easiest samples to obtain of the respiratory tract. While a single sputum sample has a low sensitivity in the detection of malignancy (less than 50%), multiple samples over time can significantly increase the detection of neoplasia (sensitivity up to 90%). Early morning deep cough samples are preferred. One problem with sputum samples is failure to acquire material from the lower respiratory tract. It is common to get samples that contain material only from the oral cavity and upper respiratory tract. Therefore, for a sputum sample to be considered adequate, abundant alveolar macrophages are required to ensure sampling of the lower respiratory tract. Mature squamous cells, metaplastic squamous cells, ciliated bronchial cells, and goblet cells can all be present in samples of the oral cavity and upper respiratory tract, and are not indicative of lower tract sampling.

68. **(D) Marked nuclear size variation.**

Bile duct epithelium can show significant reactive atypia that can be difficult to distinguish from adenocarcinoma. Both reactive and neoplastic epithelium can show nuclear enlargement, prominent nucleoli, and cohesive sheets and clusters of cells. Reactive epithelium will retain abundant cytoplasm, with a low nuclear-to-cytoplasmic ratio. However, well-differentiated adenocarcinomas commonly will also have abundant cytoplasm. It is the more poorly differentiated adenocarcinomas that have a high nuclear-to-cytoplasmic ratio, a feature that is helpful when present in the diagnosis of malignancy. Other features that favor a diagnosis of malignancy include numerous atypical cells, disorganized architecture (so-called "drunken honeycomb"), marked variation in nuclear size (often greater than three- to fourfold), irregular nuclear contour, and coarse chromatin.

69. **(B) Bloody discharge.**

When not associated with pregnancy or lactation, spontaneous nipple discharge is abnormal. The vast majority of spontaneous nipple discharges are associated with non-neoplastic processes such as prolactin secreting pituitary adenomas, hormonal abnormalities, mastitis, intraductal papillomas, and duct ectasia. In addition, only a small percentage of women with breast cancer will present with nipple discharge. Therefore, some authors advocate cytologic evaluation of nipple discharge only when unilateral and bloody. Up to 4% of unilateral bloody nipple discharges will be related to an underlying malignancy. Bilateral nipple discharges are almost always benign, and frequently hormonal in origin. Milky and purulent discharges are also common due to underlying benign disease, with less than 1% of patients having an underlying neoplasm.

70. **(C) Papillary lesion.**

The presence of three-dimensional cohesive clusters of mildly atypical ductal cells in a bloody nipple discharge is suggestive of a papillary lesion. The differential diagnosis includes intraductal papilloma and papillary carcinoma, which can be indistinguishable on cytology alone. In addition, intraductal carcinomas can be involved by ductal carcinoma in situ, which is difficult to determine by nipple discharge cytology. Therefore, when papillary fragments are present in a nipple discharge or aspirate sample, it is better to provide an interpretation of "papillary lesion" and favor benign or malignant, rather than providing an interpretation of "negative" or "positive" for malignancy. Further clinical workup, including excisional biopsy, is required for definitive diagnosis. Features that favor a benign papillary lesion include cohesive groups, myoepithelial cells, distinct fibrovascular cores, and moderate nuclear pleomorphism. Neoplastic papillary lesions will commonly show single atypical cells, an absence of myoepithelial cells, tall columnar cytoplasm, and cellular monotony.

Fibroadenomas almost never shed into nipple discharge specimens, and, on fine-needle aspiration biopsy, contain stromal fragments and naked bipolar nuclei, but the ductal component can be very similar in appearance to intraductal papillomas.

71. **(C) Goblet cells.**

Barrett's esophagus occurs when the normal squamous epithelium of the esophagus is replaced by intestinal-type glandular epithelium. Clinically, this change appears as salmon-colored patches, usually near the gastroesophageal junction. Intestinal metaplasia of the esophagus is associated with significantly increased risk of developing adenocarcinoma. Other glandular metaplasias of the esophagus can occur (gastric cardia or fundic types), but these are not associated with an increased risk of malignancy, and therefore are not included in the diagnosis of Barrett's esophagus. Therefore, the characteristic finding of Barrett's esophagus on brushing cytology is the presence of glandular epithelium containing goblet cells (cells containing a large mucin-filled vacuole that displaces or indents the nucleus, and appear as "holes" in sheets of glandular epithelium). Sheets of columnar glandular epithelium lacking goblet cells can result from inadvertent sampling of the gastric cardia or non-Barrett's type metaplasia. Benign squamous cells are a normal component of esophageal brushings. Atypical squamous cells can be seen in patients with squamous cell carcinoma of the esophagus. Necrosis is a feature of malignancy, including both adenocarcinoma and squamous cell carcinoma; in contrast, Barrett's esophagus typically has a clean background.

72. **(D) Numerous single atypical cells.**

Barrett's esophagus is a risk factor for the development of adenocarcinoma of the esophagus. Therefore, patients with this diagnosis must undergo regular surveillance to screen for progression. This surveillance can be performed by biopsy or brushing cytology; neither methodology is 100% sensitive, and these techniques can be complementary. Biopsy is better at diagnosing invasive adenocarcinoma. In contrast, brushing cytology will sample a larger surface area than a biopsy with fewer complications. One problem in cytology samples is that repair in glandular epithelium can result in substantial atypia that can mimic neoplasia. On brushing cytology, distinguishing high-grade dysplasia from invasive adenocarcinoma is not usually possible due to overlapping cytomorphologic features. Both repair and glandular neoplasia can have mitotic figures, large nuclei, and prominent nucleoli. Epithelium with reparative changes will

typically remain cohesive, while high-grade dysplasia and adenocarcinomas will typically show increasing numbers of atypical single cells. Other features that suggest neoplasia include coarse chromatin, irregular nuclear contours, marked nuclear variation in size and shape, loss of the normal honeycomb appearance, atypical mitotic figures, and necrosis. Brushing samples containing columnar glandular cells with interspersed goblet cells are diagnostic of Barrett's esophagus, but these findings are not indicative of malignancy.

73. **(B) *K-ras* point mutation.**

Fine-needle aspiration biopsies and other cytologic specimens are increasingly used to evaluate the utility of targeted systemic therapies for metastatic tumors. Perhaps the most commonly used targeted therapy is anti-epidermal growth factor receptor (anti-EGFR) therapy, which can be a tyrosine kinase inhibitor (such as gefitinib and erlotinib) or a monoclonal antibody specific to EGFR (such as cetuximab and panitumumab). In colorectal carcinoma, nearly 80% of tumors will show overexpression of the EGFR protein, and a subset will respond to anti-EGFR therapy. However, immunohistochemical expression of EGFR or gene amplification of EGFR is a poor predictor of response to anti-EGFR therapy in these patients. *K-ras* gene point mutation, when present in a colorectal carcinoma, is a strong predictor of failure to respond to anti-EGFR therapy. Therefore, all patients with colorectal carcinoma who are being considered for anti-EGFR therapy are recommended to undergo *K-ras* mutational analysis prior to the initiation of therapy. *BRAF* gene mutation is also a strong predictor of failure to respond to anti-EGFR therapy. *K-ras* gene mutational analysis has been validated on cytologic aspirate smears and liquid-based preparations.

74. **(E) Polymorphous lymphoid population containing abundant plasma cells and plasmacytoid lymphocytes.**

The clinical history of malaise, pharyngitis, and cervical lymphadenopathy in a young adult is typical for infectious mononucleosis. The presence of elevated IgM titers for Epstein–Barr virus confirms the diagnosis. Fine-needle aspiration biopsy of infectious mononucleosis is characterized by a polymorphous population of lymphocytes with an increased percentage of plasma cells and plasmacytoid lymphocytes, as well as increased numbers of immunoblasts and centroblasts. Germinal center fragments and tingible body macrophages are usually infrequent. The presence of epithelioid histiocytes and well-formed granulomas is suggestive of sarcoidosis. Extensive necrosis and marked acute inflammation in a lymph node aspirate is suggestive of a suppurative lymphadenitis, cat scratch disease being the prototype. Monotonous large atypical lymphocytes with prominent nucleoli are suggestive of a diffuse large B-cell lymphoma or anaplastic large cell lymphoma. A monotonous population of small mature lymphocytes lacking tingible body macrophages or germinal center fragments would be concerning for a low-grade lymphoma, such as follicular lymphoma.

75. **(B) Cohesive cell clusters.**
Malignant melanoma is frequently seen on fine-needle aspiration biopsy of lymph nodes. While malignant melanomas can vary widely in appearance, the classic features of malignant melanoma on cytologic preparations include epithelioid-to-spindled cells with large nuclei, prominent macronucleoli, and frequent binucleation and multinucleation. The binucleated cells often have two nuclei that appear identical, which are sometimes called "mirror image" nuclei. Frequently epithelioid cells have a plasmacytoid appearance with eccentric nuclei. Nuclear pseudoinclusions can be identified, which are helpful in discriminating malignant melanoma from other large-cell malignancies, such as diffuse large B-cell lymphoma. Melanin pigment, when present, is also very helpful. Another characteristic feature of malignant melanoma is a lack of cellular cohesion, usually resulting in aspirate smears containing single cells or loose clusters of only a few cells. The presence of cohesive clusters would be more typical of a metastatic carcinoma.

76. **(E) Background containing numerous lymphoglandular bodies.**
Fine-needle aspiration biopsies of anaplastic large cell lymphoma are characterized by intermediate-to-large cells with large nuclei, frequent binucleation and multinucleation, irregular nuclei, and marked nuclear pleomorphism. Most cells have abundant cytoplasm and are epithelioid in shape. The classic "hallmark" cell has a horseshoe-shaped nucleus. Reed–Sternberg-like cells are commonly seen, with two large mirror-image nuclei and prominent macronucleoli. Anaplastic large cell lymphomas will stain positive for CD30, are frequently positive for ALK protein and epithelial membrane antigen, and will typically be negative for CD45 (leukocyte common antigen) and CD20. In contrast to most other lymphoid neoplasms, lymphoglandular bodies are not typically seen in aspirates of anaplastic large cell lymphoma. This feature, along with the tendency of anaplastic large cell lymphoma cells to cluster and immunoreactivity for epithelial membrane antigen, can lead to misdiagnosis as an epithelial malignancy.

77. **(C) Cytokeratin 20.**
Aspirates of Merkel cell carcinoma are characterized by small cell undifferentiated carcinoma features (small cells, high nuclear-to-cytoplasmic ratio, stippled chromatin, nuclear molding, marked mitotic activity and apoptosis, absence of lymphoglandular bodies, and lack of cellular cohesion) and immunohistochemical staining in a dot-like pattern for cytokeratin 20 (CK20). Merkel cell carcinomas, also called *neuroendocrine carcinoma of the skin*, occur on the skin of elderly patients, usually in the head and neck. Immunohistochemical staining of Merkel cell carcinomas shows strong staining for synaptophysin, chromogranin, and CD56, dot-like perinuclear staining for CK20, and no staining for thyroid transcription factor 1, CD45, and CK7. The differential diagnosis includes high-grade lymphomas and metastasis from pulmonary small cell undifferentiated carcinoma. The absence of thyroid transcription factor 1 staining and presence of dot-like CK20 staining, along with the history of a skin lesion, distinguishes Merkel cell carcinoma from small cell undifferentiated carcinoma of the lung.

78. **(C) Hepatocellular carcinoma, fibrolamellar variant.**
The cytologic appearance of normal liver is morphologically indistinguishable from that of focal nodular hyperplasia, hepatic adenoma, and a regenerating nodule in the setting of cirrhosis. All of these aspirates will show normal or near-normal appearing hepatocytes that lack endothelial wrapping or transgressing vessels. They are also characterized by an absence of nuclear atypia, except regenerating cirrhotic nodules, which may show increased nuclear size and hyperchromasia. While hepatic adenomas are characterized by the absence of portal tracts and bile ducts on histology, this feature is unreliable on fine-needle aspiration biopsy. It is common for aspirates of normal liver and other reactive conditions to lack bile ducts. In contrast, the fibrolamellar variant of hepatocellular carcinoma is characterized by pleomorphic extremely large hepatocytes with large nuclei, abundant cytoplasm (a retained low nuclear-to-cytoplasmic ratio), and prominent nucleoli. Intracytoplasmic hyaline globules are common. These aspirates also frequently lack endothelial wrapping and transgressing vessels, but often contain fragments of dense fibrosis.

79. **(E) Thickened trabeculae.**

In a patient with a history of cirrhosis and a liver mass, the differential diagnosis includes hepatocellular carcinoma and a regenerating cirrhotic nodule. Regenerating cirrhotic nodules share some features with normal liver, including fragments of tissue with a frayed edge, background of single hepatocytes, and absence of endothelial wrapping and transgressing vessels. However, regenerating cirrhotic nodules also can show significant atypia, including large nuclei, prominent nucleoli, marked variation in nuclear size, and nuclear hyperchromasia. In contrast, hepatocellular carcinoma is characterized by thickened, irregular trabeculae of hepatocytes that will often show peripheral endothelial wrapping and transgressing vessels, increased nuclear-to-cytoplasmic ratio, prominent macronucleoli, and background of singe naked atypical nuclei. The thickened trabeculae can be highlighted by reticulin stain on cell block samples. Most well-differentiated hepatocellular carcinomas have a monotonous appearance that is distinctive compared with the marked pleomorphism seen in regenerative nodules. Both regenerative cirrhotic nodules and hepatocellular carcinomas can contain bile pigment, prominent nucleoli, and nuclear pseudoinclusions. It is important to note that rare endothelial cells at the periphery of hepatocyte clusters can be seen in benign liver lesions. Cases with abundant endothelial wrapping, along with other features such as thickened trabeculae and atypia, can be diagnosed as malignant with greater confidence.

80. **(C) Low cuboidal cells.**

The liver is the second most common site of metastasis in the abdomen, after lymph nodes. Therefore, fine-needle aspiration biopsy of metastatic lesions is more common than aspiration biopsy of primary liver tumors. While most metastatic adenocarcinomas cannot be reliably distinguished on cytomorphologic features alone, metastatic colorectal adenocarcinoma can often be identified due to its distinctive appearance. Fine-needle aspirate samples of metastatic colorectal carcinoma are characterized by tall columnar glandular cells with oval-to-cigar-shaped nuclei that typically show pseudostratification and palisading (all nuclei oriented perpendicular to the base of the gland), which are commonly referred to as a "picket-fence" arrangement. In addition, colorectal adenocarcinomas are characterized by a background of dirty necrosis and may contain abundant extracellular mucin. Low cuboidal cells are frequently seen in other adenocarcinomas, including

cholangiocarcinoma and metastatic pancreaticobiliary adenocarcinoma.

81. **(C) Connection with the main pancreatic duct.**

Distinction of an intraductal papillary mucinous neoplasm (IPMN) from a mucinous cystic neoplasm (MCN) requires careful clinical and radiologic correlation in addition to cytologic examination of cyst fluid. This is because aspirates of IPMN and MCN can be nearly indistinguishable by cytomorphologic features alone. Both can show abundant extracellular mucin, cyst contents, and mucinous epithelium that can range from normal appearing to overtly malignant. IPMNs will usually have more viscous, thick mucin than MCNs, but that distinction can be difficult to make on aspirate smears. In addition, both IPMN and MCN can have highly elevated carcinoembryonic antigen (CEA) levels in the cyst fluid. Elevated CEA levels are almost always present in IPMNs, but there is more variation in MCNs. The most common location of IPMNs is the head of the pancreas. The most common location of MCNs is the tail of the pancreas. Therefore, a pancreatic body tumor does not favor either tumor type. The most specific clinical and radiologic finding, which is required for the diagnosis of IPMN, is connection of the lesion with the main pancreatic duct. During endoscopic ultrasound-guided evaluation, this connection (or lack thereof) can usually be demonstrated.

82. **(A) Anisonucleocytosis.**

Well-differentiated pancreatic ductal adenocarcinomas can be difficult to distinguish from reactive ductal atypia. Both reactive and neoplastic epithelium will appear cohesive, and can have mitotic figures. Reactive epithelium will also retain nuclear polarity and a low nuclear-to-cytoplasmic ratio, but in well-differentiated adenocarcinomas, particularly mucinous adenocarcinomas, the nuclear-to-cytoplasmic ratio can remain low and only minimal loss of polarity may be seen. Prominent nucleoli are more typical of reactive changes than adenocarcinoma, which usually has vesicular nuclei, irregular nuclear contours, and variably sized nucleoli. The features that are most specific for malignancy in a pancreatic aspirate sample include irregular nuclear membranes, single atypical cells, and anisonucleocytosis (variation in nuclear size), particularly fourfold or more variation in nuclear size within a group.

83. **(C) Endoscopic ultrasound-guided fine-needle aspiration biopsy (EUS-FNA).**

EUS-FNA has rapidly become the diagnostic modality of choice in the evaluation of pancreatic lesions. The sensitivity and specificity of EUS-FNA in the detection of pancreatic carcinoma has been reported as up to 93% and 100%, respectively. EUS-FNA allows for highly sensitive and detailed ultrasound evaluation of pancreatic lesions, which is more accurate in the staging of pancreatic cancer than computed tomography (CT), magnetic resonance imaging (MRI), or transabdominal ultrasound. In addition, during EUS evaluation of a pancreatic mass, FNA can be performed with minimal risk of complications and allows definitive diagnosis for further treatment. EUS-FNA can be performed under light sedation rather than full anesthesia. The addition of rapid on-site evaluation by cytopathologists at the time of EUS-FNA has made this modality even more sensitive and specific, and also can further reduce the risk of complications by reducing the number of passes needed for a diagnosis.

84. **(A) CEA 5 ng/mL, amylase high.**
Ancillary testing with carcinoembryonic antigen (CEA), amylase, mucin stains, and CA 19-9 has been used to improve the diagnosis of cystic pancreatic lesions on fine-needle aspiration biopsy. This is because almost all mucinous cystic lesions are neoplastic, while the majority of nonmucinous cystic lesions are benign. However, there can be significant cytomorphologic overlap between benign and neoplastic cystic lesions on fine-needle aspiration biopsy. An elevated CEA level (over 192 ng/mL) is nearly always diagnostic of a mucinous neoplasm, such as mucinous cystic neoplasm or intraductal papillary mucinous neoplasm (answers C, D, and E). The aspirate smears of mucinous neoplasms also typically contain thick visible mucin, which can be confirmed on mucin stains, and will have elevated CA 19-9 levels. Amylase in these tumors can be high or low. In contrast, pancreatic pseudocysts will have very low CEA levels, and the destruction of pancreatic tissue results in extremely high levels of amylase (answer A). Other tests, including mucin staining and CA 19-9, are usually negative. Serous cystadenomas of the pancreas will have very low CEA, amylase, and CA 19-9 levels and a negative mucin stain (answer B).

85. **(A) High risk of transformation to malignancy requires resection.**
The diagnosis of serous cystadenoma of the pancreas requires correlation of cytologic, clinical, and radiologic features. Aspirate smears of serous cystadenomas usually contain histiocytes and no or very little epithelium, which, when present, appears as bland cuboidal cells with clear cytoplasm. Background debris and inflammation are not seen, unlike aspirates of chronic pancreatitis.

Mucin should be absent, and carcinoembryonic antigen (CEA) testing of the cyst fluid will usually be extremely low, as will enzyme levels (such as amylase). The radiologic appearance is characteristic, with a spongy appearance and a central scar or fibrous area. Thankfully, nearly all serous cystadenomas of the pancreas are benign. Therefore, as the cytologic features of serous cystadenoma are so nonspecific, the primary role of cytology in the evaluation of these tumors is to exclude a more significant neoplasm, particularly a mucinous cystic neoplasm.

86. **(E) WT1.**
Small round blue cell tumors of childhood include Wilms tumor, neuroblastoma, rhabdomyosarcoma, lymphoma/leukemia, and Ewing sarcoma/ primitive neuroectodermal tumor (PNET). All of these tumors are characterized by small cells with scant cytoplasm and hyperchromatic nuclei on fine-needle aspiration biopsy. Wilms tumors occur within or near the kidney of young children. Aspirates of Wilms tumors are notable for three components: blastemal cells (classic small round blue cells), a primitive epithelial component (often arranged in tubules and pseudoglomeruli), and a stromal component (small loosely arranged spindle cells). Wilms tumors are positive for WT1, and will have cytokeratin staining in the epithelial component and vimentin staining in the spindle cell component. CD34 will be positive in acute leukemias; CD99 will be positive in Ewing sarcoma/PNET; myogenin will be positive in rhabdomyosarcoma; and synaptophysin will be positive in neuroblastoma.

87. **(D) HMB-45.**
Fine-needle aspiration biopsy samples of angiomyolipomas of the kidney are characterized by variable amounts of spindle cells with stringy cytoplasm, mature fibroadipose tissue, and thick-walled blood vessels. The spindle cells are usually small, with delicate-to-stringy cytoplasm, and can be predominant in the sample, mimicking a sarcoma or sarcomatoid carcinoma. Significant atypia may be seen in the spindle cell component, but is usually interspersed with more benign-appearing spindle cells. The presence of mature fibroadipose tissue is helpful when admixed with spindle cells, and may show areas of fat necrosis. Immunohistochemical staining for HMB-45 and MelanA (MART1) will be positive in the spindle cells, confirming the diagnosis. Angiomyolipomas may also be positive for smooth muscle actin, but will be negative for epithelial markers, CD10, and inhibin.

88. **(A) Binucleation with nuclear pseudoinclusions.**
Seminomas are the most common germ cell tumor in men, and aspirates are characterized by large atypical cells with large vesicular nuclei, prominent macronucleoli, and fragile cytoplasm that often appears vacuolated or has cytoplasmic blebs. The background can appear "tigroid," which refers to alternating linear areas of light and dark debris in the background, due to stripped glycogenated cytoplasm. This feature is not always present, however. Immunohistochemical staining with placental alkaline phosphatase (PLAP) is positive, a useful finding in the differential diagnosis with large cell lymphoma. Binucleation and nuclear pseudoinclusions are features of malignant melanoma and are not seen in seminoma.

89. **(C) Pulmonary hamartoma.**
Pulmonary hamartomas classically appear as well-circumscribed round lesions in the peripheral lung. On fine-needle aspiration biopsy, they appear as an admixture of various cellular components, including adipose tissue, spindle cells, fibromyxoid stroma, cartilage, and benign epithelial cells (usually glandular cells). Usually, the fibromyxoid and cartilaginous elements predominate and allow recognition of this lesion. When the glandular component predominates, differentiation from a well-differentiated adenocarcinoma can be difficult. Pulmonary hamartoma should be considered in the differential diagnosis of any peripheral well-circumscribed nodule that contains epithelial cells. The presence of immature cartilage and glandular cells would not be typical of thoracic wall sampling and, with the clinical history provided, a nondiagnostic interpretation would not be the best choice.

90. **(A) *Aspergillus fumigatus* fungal ball.**
Intracavitary fungus balls in the lung can result in significant reactive squamous atypia, which can mimic a squamous cell carcinoma on fine-needle aspiration biopsy. This change is most notable in *Aspergillus* sp. infections, but can be seen with other fungal infections as well. Usually, fungal hyphae can be demonstrated, either on Papanicolaou stained smears or with special stains (e.g., silver stain). However, it is possible to have fungal colonization of a necrotic and cavitary squamous cell carcinoma as well. Therefore, careful correlation with clinical and radiologic features is recommended. In some cases, surgical excision may be required to exclude malignancy. However, cytologic features that favor a reactive squamous atypia include smudgy chromatin, absence of well-preserved malignant squamous cells, and low squamous cellularity.

91. **(B) Lymphoglandular bodies.**
On fine-needle aspiration biopsy, it can be very difficult to distinguish small cell undifferentiated carcinoma from lymphoid proliferations, particularly high-grade lymphomas. Both small cell undifferentiated carcinoma and a high-grade lymphoma will have small-to-intermediate-sized cells with a high nuclear-to-cytoplasmic ratio, a predominantly dispersed, single cell pattern, and increased mitotic activity. Nuclear molding and nuclear crush artifact are classically considered features of small cell undifferentiated carcinoma, but aspirates of high-grade lymphomas can also demonstrate these changes. Cytoplasmic paranuclear blue bodies are a feature of small cell undifferentiated carcinoma that most lymphomas lack. Lymphoglandular bodies are fragments of cytoplasm from disrupted lymphocytes that form very small light-blue bodies in the background of both benign and neoplastic lymphoid proliferations. Numerous lymphoglandular bodies should raise concern for a possible lymphoid neoplasm, although aspirates of other tumors with a prominent lymphoid component (e.g., lymphoepithelial carcinoma) will also contain lymphoglandular bodies. Tightly cohesive clusters are suggestive of an epithelial neoplasm, such as basaloid squamous cell carcinoma, and are less commonly seen in small cell undifferentiated carcinoma.

92. **(E) Normal pancreas; the lesion was missed.**
The photomicrograph demonstrates normal pancreatic tissue; the aspirate is composed predominantly of well-formed acinar structures containing cells with abundant granular cytoplasm. The cohesive and regularly arranged nature of these acinar cells and absence of single cells or a granular background favors normal pancreas over an acinar cell carcinoma. Chronic pancreatitis usually leads to significant acinar cell atrophy, such that aspirate smears are predominantly composed of fibrosis, debris, inflammation, and reactive ductal epithelium. Aspirate smears of ductal adenocarcinoma contain very little acinar tissue and have abundant atypical glandular cells with marked nuclear pleomorphism and atypia. Metastatic renal cell carcinoma to the pancreas is very rare, but when present, the cells are largely discohesive or form sheets rather than well-formed acini and have a prominent capillary network.

93. **(B) Multiple small shallow ulcers in the distal esophagus.**
The photomicrograph demonstrates multinucleated cells with viral inclusions and molding, consistent with herpes esophagitis. Herpes esophagitis

usually appears as multiple shallow small ulcers in the distal esophagus. In contrast, *Candida* esophagitis appears as white pseudomembranes on the esophageal squamous epithelium, which sometimes will scrape off. Barrett's esophagus will appear clinically as salmon-colored patches in the distal esophagus and, on brushing cytology, is characterized by goblet cells in the sample. Leiomyomas typically occur in the upper one-third of the esophagus and result in a submucosal mass; therefore, brushing cytology will be normal in appearance, as the leiomyoma is not sampled.

94. **(B) Benign.**
The photomicrograph demonstrates a thyroid aspirate composed of abundant colloid and groups of follicular cells forming flat sheets without atypia. These changes are consistent with a colloid nodule, and therefore should be interpreted as "benign." Thyroid aspirate samples can be considered benign when sufficient follicular epithelium is present to meet adequacy requirements (6 groups of 10 follicular cells at minimum), and no cytologic or architectural atypia is present. Cytologic atypia includes nuclear features of papillary thyroid carcinoma. Architectural atypia includes high cellularity in the absence of colloid and repetitive microfollicular groups. Flat sheets of follicular cells, which lack nuclear changes of papillary thyroid carcinoma, are a reassuring finding, particularly when found in association with abundant colloid.

95. **(E) Well-differentiated lung adenocarcinoma.**
The photomicrograph demonstrates a proliferation of glandular epithelium forming sheets and acinar-like structures that have fine, open chromatin, prominent nucleoli, nuclear grooves, and nuclear pseudoinclusions, consistent with a well-differentiated lung adenocarcinoma. Nuclear grooves and nuclear pseudoinclusions are more prominent in the bronchioloalveolar subtype of lung adenocarcinomas. While the nuclear features can overlap with a papillary thyroid carcinoma, the clinical history of a solitary, spiculated lung lesion is typical of a lung adenocarcinoma. In contrast, most patients with metastatic papillary thyroid carcinoma will have multiple lung lesions. Other features of a well-differentiated lung adenocarcinoma include foamy cytoplasm, mucin vacuoles, and psammoma bodies. Well-differentiated adenocarcinomas can also be difficult to distinguish from benign bronchial cells. Features that favor a well-differentiated adenocarcinoma include absence of cilia, disorganized "drunken honeycomb" structure, irregular nuclear contours, nuclear pseudoinclusions, and variation in nuclear size. Aspirates of

carcinoid tumors are characterized by monotonous plasmacytoid cells arranged singly or in loosely cohesive clusters. Aspirates of squamous cell carcinoma are characterized by cells with dense blue to orangeophilic cytoplasm with well-defined cell borders, bizarrely shaped cells with cytoplasmic extensions (tadpole or caudate shape), marked nuclear hyperchromasia, large irregular flat sheets of tumor cells, and keratin pearls.

96. **(C) Seminal vesicle.**
The photomicrograph demonstrates a seminal vesicle cell, which is characterized by the presence of a large nucleus with hyperchromasia and golden-brown lipofuscin pigment in the cytoplasm. This pigment is particularly helpful in separating benign seminal vesicle cells from neoplasms of the bladder and kidney. In the urine, squamous cells are commonly seen due to metaplasia of the trigone and/or contamination during collection, and these cells have abundant polygonal cytoplasm with small round nuclei. High-grade urothelial carcinomas are characterized by clusters and single cells with large, hyperchromatic, and irregular nuclei with scant cytoplasm. Urachal adenocarcinomas are very rarely identified in urine cytology, and, when present, typically appear as high-grade adenocarcinomas with vacuolated cytoplasm and large nuclei with prominent nucleoli. Clear cell renal cell carcinoma is also very rarely found in urine cytology samples, and, when present, appears as large cells with abundant granular or vacuolated cytoplasm in clusters.

97. **(A) A distinctly different second population of benign mesothelial cells will be present in the effusion.**
The clinical presentation and description of the effusion sample are highly suggestive of diffuse malignant mesothelioma of the pleura. This disease is highly associated with prior asbestos exposure, which commonly occurred in shipyard workers prior to the 1980s. Malignant mesothelioma in effusion cytology is characterized by cells showing characteristic features of mesothelial origin (low nuclear-to-cytoplasmic ratio, large round-to-oval nuclei, lacy skirt, clusters with scalloped edges, windows between cells), which are atypical. It can be very difficult to distinguish malignant mesothelioma on effusion cytology from reactive mesothelial cells. Helpful features include high cellularity, very large (>50 cell) clusters or "mulberry clusters," papillary architecture, and marked nuclear enlargement. Unlike most metastatic adenocarcinomas, malignant mesotheliomas usually lack the helpful feature of

two distinct cell populations on cytologic examination. Instead, there often is a continual spectrum of cells ranging from more bland-appearing mesothelial cells to clearly neoplastic cells in the same sample. Although rarely used in current diagnostic algorithms, electron microscopy of malignant mesotheliomas will demonstrate long, thin microvilli along the cell surface, which usually have a length-to-width ratio of 15:1 or higher. Both benign and malignant mesothelial cells will be positive for calretinin immunohistochemistry. Unfortunately, there are no highly sensitive or specific immunohistochemical markers of neoplasia for mesothelial cells in effusion cytology.

98. **(B) High-grade ductal carcinoma in situ.**
The cytologic description is diagnostic of ductal carcinoma, characterized by markedly atypical epithelial cells that show loss of cohesion and a background of necrosis. Fine-needle aspiration biopsy cytology cannot reliably distinguish invasive ductal carcinoma from a high-grade (usually comedo-type) ductal carcinoma in situ. Therefore, core or excisional biopsy is recommended for definitive classification. In contrast, low-grade ductal carcinoma in situ is difficult to distinguish from benign proliferative breast disease. Low-grade ductal carcinoma in situ on fine-needle aspiration biopsy typically shows cohesive groups of monotonous cells lacking myoepithelial cells and mild nuclear atypia; necrosis is typically absent. Infiltrating lobular carcinoma on fine-needle aspiration biopsy most commonly demonstrates single, small epithelial cells with intracytoplasmic vacuoles containing secretions and mild nuclear atypia. Both fibroadenoma and intraductal papilloma will show fragments of benign epithelial cells with associated myoepithelial cells on fine-needle aspiration biopsy unlike the aspirate sample described in the question.

99. **(A) Cat scratch disease.**
Fine-needle aspirates of suppurative lymphadenitis are characterized by necrosis, numerous neutrophils, and poorly formed granulomas composed of epithelioid histiocytes. Suppurative lymphadenitis is classically caused by cat scratch disease, which is the result of infection with *Bartonella henselae*, a gram-negative bacteria that is best demonstrated on Warthin–Starry special stains. Other causes of suppurative lymphadenitis include other bacterial infections, actinomycosis, and *Coccidioides immitis*. Rarely, *Mycobacterium tuberculosis* infection can cause a suppurative lymphadenitis, but more commonly shows necrotizing granulomatous inflammation without significant neutrophils. Sarcoidosis is characterized by well-formed, non-

necrotizing granulomatous inflammation and multinucleated giant cells. Rosai–Dorfman disease or sinus histiocytosis with massive lymphadenopathy is characterized by numerous histiocytes engulfing lymphocytes and red blood cells (emperipolesis) and small mature lymphocytes. Chronic lymphocytic leukemia/small cell lymphoma is characterized by a monotonous population of small mature lymphocytes with clumped chromatin.

100. **(A) Absence of nuclear staining for β-catenin.**
Solid pseudopapillary tumor of the pancreas most commonly occurs in tail of the pancreas in young women, and appears at least partially cystic on imaging. On aspirate smears, solid pseudopapillary tumors are typically highly cellular and contain a monotonous population of cuboidal cells with small round nuclei and inconspicuous nucleoli. Nuclear grooves are common. The characteristic finding is branching papillary-like structures composed of a central vessel, myxoid or hyaline stroma, and a single or several layers of neoplastic cells. In other areas, the cuboidal cells will fall apart due to a lack of cellular cohesion, and appear as single cells or loose clusters. Immunohistochemical staining for β-catenin is diagnostic; solid pseudopapillary tumors will have strong nuclear staining, while other pancreatic tumors will lack nuclear staining for this marker.

101. **(E) Round nested architecture on cell block preparation.**
Fine-needle aspiration biopsy of oncocytic renal lesions can be extremely challenging. Oncocytoma and the eosinophilic variant of chromophobe renal cell carcinoma share many cytologic features, including polygonal cells with abundant granular cytoplasm, well-defined cell borders, central or slightly eccentric nucleoli, and occasional binucleation. Since the difference in management and prognosis of these tumors is significant in many cases, it is prudent to render an interpretation of "oncocytic neoplasm (oncocytoma versus chromophobe)" and recommend surgical excision. Some cytomorphologic features that favor a diagnosis of chromophobe renal cell carcinoma include nuclear hyperchromasia, irregular nuclear contours, perinuclear cytoplasmic halos, and marked variation in nuclear size (anisonucleocytosis). Hale's colloidal iron stain will be diffusely positive in chromophobe renal cell carcinomas but can show focal apical cytoplasmic staining in oncocytomas as well. Perhaps the most useful feature in the distinction of oncocytoma from chromophobe renal cell carcinoma is the cell architecture on cell block. The presence of rounded nests of tumor cells

favors oncocytoma, while a trabecular growth pattern favors a chromophobe renal cell carcinoma.

102. **(D) Rhabdomyosarcoma.**
The cytologic description provided is highly suggestive of an embryonal rhabdomyosarcoma, which is supported by the clinical history (child with an orbital soft tissue mass) and immunohistochemical staining (positive for desmin). Embryonal rhabdomyosarcomas characteristically appear on fine-needle aspiration biopsy as small round blue cell neoplasms with variable admixed strap cells, which have more abundant cytoplasm, eccentric nuclei and may occasionally show cytoplasmic cross striations. Other small round blue cell tumors of childhood include Ewing sarcoma/PNET, neuroblastoma, and acute lymphoblastic leukemia. However, Ewing sarcoma/PNET will be positive for CD99, and neuroblastoma will be positive for synaptophysin and chromogranin. Fibrosarcomas and leiomyosarcomas will typically show a predominance of spindle cells with variable pleomorphism. Round cell liposarcomas are uncommon in children, occur more commonly in the extremities, particularly the thigh and, on fine-needle aspiration biopsy, show large atypical round cells with marked pleomorphism.

103. **(C) Periodic acid Schiff with diastase (PAS-D).**
The presence of oncocytic or oncocyte-like cells on a fine-needle aspiration biopsy has a limited differential diagnosis, which includes oncocytoma, Warthin tumor, oncocytic carcinoma, acinic cell carcinoma, mucoepidermoid carcinoma, and metastasis (particularly renal cell carcinoma). Special stains (histochemical and immunohistochemical) can help to differentiate these tumors when adequate tissue is present. Acinic cell carcinomas characteristically show cytoplasmic staining in a granular pattern with PAS-D. PAS-D highlights the zymogen granules of acinar differentiation. In contrast, oncocytomas will stain positive with phospho-tungstic acid hematoxylin (PTAH), which highlights the abundant mitochondria in the cytoplasm. S-100 is positive in granular cell tumors. Mucicarmine and p63 are positive in mucoepidermoid carcinomas, which can show oncocytic change.

104. **(C) 15–30%.**
In the 2007 Bethesda System for Reporting Thyroid Cytopathology, the recommended estimated risk of malignancy for various interpretation categories has been published to further standardize reporting and management guidelines. Individual laboratories may use internal cytologic–histologic correlations to track and report their own risk of malignancy if they choose. The 2007 Bethesda System suggests a risk of malignancy around 15–30% for aspirates with an interpretation of "suspicious for follicular neoplasm" or "suspicious for follicular neoplasm, Hürthle cell type." A benign aspirate has a risk of less than 3%, an aspirate interpreted as "atypia of undetermined significance" or "follicular lesion of undetermined significance" has a risk of 5–15%, an aspirate interpreted as "suspicious for malignancy" has a risk of 60–75%, and an aspirate interpreted as "malignant" has a risk of 97–99%.

105. **(A) Adenovirus.**
Ciliocytophthoria occurs when fragmentation of bronchial cells results in detached tufts of bronchial cytoplasm containing the terminal bar and cilia. This change can be seen in sputum samples and bronchioloalveolar lavage samples. When prominent, ciliocytophthoria is highly associated with adenovirus infection. Adenovirus also can cause prominent nuclear inclusions that can be basophilic or eosinophilic within pneumocytes. In contrast, respiratory syncytial virus and measles virus cause multinucleated giant cells with inclusions, cytomegalovirus results in prominent intranuclear and cytoplasmic inclusions, and herpes simplex virus results in multinucleated cells with nuclear inclusions and molding.

106. **(B) Galactorrhea.**
Spontaneous nipple discharges that are physiologic in nature usually are composed of abundant proteinaceous debris and foamy histiocytes. Physiologic nipple discharge with this appearance includes normal lactation and hormonal imbalances such as galactorrhea due to a prolactin producing pituitary adenoma. Acute mastitis will typically result in a bloody nipple discharge with marked acute inflammation and necroinflammatory debris. Tuberculous mastitis will typically result in a nipple discharge containing epithelioid histiocytes and multinucleated giant cells; an acid-fast stain will confirm the presence of acid-fast bacteria. Intraductal papillomas typically cause a bloody nipple discharge containing papillary epithelial clusters. Invasive ductal carcinomas will rarely cause nipple discharge, which is invariably bloody and may contain single atypical ductal cells.

107. **(C) Follicular lymphoma.**
The cytomorphologic description and flow cytometry results are most consistent with a follicular lymphoma. Follicular lymphomas typically appear on aspirate smears as a monotonous population of predominantly small mature lymphocytes, which have irregular contours, causing the nuclei looking "cleaved." Occasional larger centroblasts can be seen. Grading of follicular lymphoma is difficult on

aspirate smears, as grading is based on the number of larger lymphocytes per high power field on histologic sections. By flow cytometry, follicular lymphomas are positive for CD10 and negative for CD5. Other lymphomas can be positive for CD10, including diffuse large B-cell lymphoma and Burkitt lymphoma. However, diffuse large B-cell lymphomas typically appear as large atypical cells rather than small-cleaved lymphocytes. Burkitt lymphoma appears as a monotonous population of intermediate size lymphocytes that have scant, vacuolated cytoplasm and multiple small nucleoli. Mantle cell lymphoma and small lymphocytic lymphoma/chronic lymphocytic leukemia are both positive for CD5 and negative for CD10.

108. **(D) Marked nuclear pleomorphism and anisonucleocytosis.**
Aspirates of acinar cell carcinoma of the pancreas are typically moderately to highly cellular and composed of sheets, acinar-like aggregates, and individual cuboidal cells with delicate granular cytoplasm and uniform nuclei. Commonly, the background contains abundant granular material and naked nuclei, secondary to cytoplasmic rupture during the smearing process. Periodic acid Schiff staining will be positive in the cytoplasm, which will be resistant to diastase digestion. The nuclei of acinar cell carcinoma are typically round-to-oval, uniform, and have prominent nucleoli. Minimal atypia is usually present. In contrast, marked nuclear pleomorphism and anisonucleocytosis are features of ductal adenocarcinoma of the pancreas. The greatest challenge in the diagnosis of acinar cell carcinoma is distinguishing it from normal pancreatic acinar epithelium. Normal acinar cells have similar delicate granular cytoplasm and round nuclei, but form tightly cohesive packets of cells forming acini, rather than the loosely cohesive-to-discohesive appearance of acinar cell carcinomas.

109. **(C) Metachromatic fibrillary matrix material.**
Fine-needle aspiration biopsy of benign adrenal cortical nodules (cortical hyperplasia and cortical adenomas) is characterized by numerous stripped nuclei, a background of foamy or frothy granular material, and occasional intact cells with abundant vacuolated cytoplasm with indistinct cell borders. Occasional spindled cells may be seen, which likely represents sampling of the adrenal stroma. In some cases, cellular fragments with entrapped endothelial cells are identified. The presence of necrosis, mitotic figures, and marked nuclear pleomorphism is worrisome for an adrenal cortical carcinoma. Metachromatic stromal material is seen in aspirates of clear cell renal cell carcinomas.

110. **(A) Adenocarcinoma with bronchioloalveolar features.**
A subset of lung carcinomas contains point mutations in the epidermal growth factor receptor (EGFR) gene, and these tumors have a favorable response to anti-EGFR therapy. Anti-EGFR responsive tumors most commonly occur in Asian nonsmoking women, and these tumors are nearly always adenocarcinomas. The most common appearance of EGFR mutated adenocarcinomas is a nonmucinous adenocarcinoma with bronchioloalveolar features. Adenocarcinomas with bronchioloalveolar features traditionally show flat monolayers of glandular epithelium with nuclear grooves and nuclear inclusions and lack prominent nucleoli. Mucinous adenocarcinomas (with abundant extracellular mucin), squamous cell carcinomas, and small cell undifferentiated tumors nearly always lack this mutation, and molecular testing is not necessary on these tumors. In contrast to colorectal carcinomas, in which EGFR mutation is not correlated with anti-EGFR therapy response, lung adenocarcinomas with EGFR mutation are significantly more responsive to anti-EGFR therapy than non-EGFR–mutated tumors.

111. **(D) Nuclear pleomorphism.**
Fine-needle aspiration biopsy of thymomas varies depending on the histologic subtype. For thymomas with a predominant medullary component (type A thymomas), aspirates are composed predominantly of bland short spindle cells that are often arranged in fascicles and whorls, and admixed with small mature lymphocytes. For thymomas with a predominantly cortical component (type B thymomas), aspirates are composed predominantly of immature lymphoid cells and inconspicuous, loosely cohesive epithelioid or polygonal cells with minimal atypia. The immature lymphoid cells are positive for TdT and CD1a by immunocytochemistry or flow cytometry. In contrast, the presence of significant nuclear pleomorphism, including nuclear hyperchromasia, prominent nucleoli, irregular nuclear contours, variation in nuclear size and shape, and increased mitotic activity, is highly concerning for a thymic carcinoma or other epithelial malignancy and should not be seen in a thymoma.

SUGGESTED READING

1. Absher KJ, Truong LD, Khurana KK, Ramzy I. Parathyroid cytology: avoiding diagnostic pitfalls. *Head Neck.* 2002; 24(2):157-164.

2. Baloch ZW, LiVolsi VA, Asa SL, et al. Diagnostic terminology and morphologic criteria for cytologic diagnosis of thyroid lesions: a synopsis of the National Cancer Institute Thyroid Fine-Needle Aspiration State of the Science Conference. *Diagn Cytopathol*. 2008;36(6):425-437.

3. Bardales RH, Stelow EB, Mallery S, Lai R, Stanley MW. Review of endoscopic ultrasound-guided fine-needle aspiration cytology. *Diagn Cytopathol*. 2006;34(2):140-175.

4. Bayon MN, Drut R. Cytologic diagnosis of adenovirus bronchopneumonia. *Acta Cytol*. 1991;35(2):181-182.

5. Brachtel EF, Iafrate AJ, Mark EJ, Deshpande V. Cytomorphological correlates of epidermal growth factor receptor mutations in lung carcinoma. *Diagn Cytopathol*. 2007;35(5):257-262.

6. Brimo F, Michel RP, Khetani K, Auger M. Primary effusion lymphoma: a series of 4 cases and review of the literature with emphasis on cytomorphologic and immunocytochemical differential diagnosis. *Cancer*. 2007;111(4):224-233.

7. Butnor KJ, Sporn TA, Ordonez NG. Recommendations for the reporting of pleural mesothelioma. *Hum Pathol*. 2007;38(11):1587-1589.

8. Chhieng DC, Cangiarella JF, Symmans WF, Cohen JM. Fine-needle aspiration cytology of Hodgkin disease: a study of 89 cases with emphasis on false-negative cases. *Cancer*. 2001;93(1):52-59.

9. Choi KU, Kim JY, Park DY, et al. Recommendations for the management of cystic thyroid nodules. *ANZ J Surg*. 2005;75(7):537-541.

10. Ciatto S, Bravetti P, Cariaggi P. Significance of nipple discharge clinical patterns in the selection of cases for cytologic examination. *Acta Cytol*. 1986;30(1):17-20.

11. Cibas ES, Ali SZ. The Bethesda system for reporting thyroid cytopathology. *Am J Clin Pathol*. 2009;132(5:658-665.

12. Collins BT, Elmberger PG, Tani EM, Bjornhagen V, Ramos RR. Fine-needle of Merkel cell carcinoma of the skin with cytomorphology and immunocytochemical correlation. *Diagn Cytopathol*. 1998;18(4):251-257.

13. Crapanzano JP. Fine-needle aspiration of renal angiomyolipoma: cytological findings and diagnostic pitfalls in a series of five cases. *Diagn Cytopathol*. 2005;32(1):53-57.

14. Edge SB, BD, Carducci MA, Compton CC (eds.). *AJCC Cancer Staging Manual*. 7th ed. New York, NY: Springer; 2009.

15. Erozan YS, Frost JK. Cytopathologic diagnosis of cancer in pulmonary material: a critical histopathologic correlation. *Acta Cytol*. 1970;14(9):560-565.

16. Glant MD. Cytopathology of lymph nodes in nonspecific reactive hyperplasia. Prognostication and differential diagnoses. *Am J Clin Pathol*. 1997;108(4 Suppl 1):S31-S55.

17. Hughes JH, Cohen MB. Is the cytologic diagnosis of esophageal glandular dysplasia feasible? *Diagn Cytopathol*. 1998;18(4):312-316.

18. Jaffey PB, Varma SK, DeMay RM, McLucas EJ, Campbell GA. Blast-like cells in the cerebrospinal fluid of young infants: further characterization of clinical setting, morphology and origin. *Am J Clin Pathol*. 1996;105(5):544-547.

19. Jayaram G, Elsayed EM, Yaccob RB. Papillary breast lesions diagnosed on cytology. Profile of 65 cases. *Acta Cytol*. 2007;51(1):3-8.

20. Jorgensen JL. State of the Art Symposium: flow cytometry in the diagnosis of lymphoproliferative disorders by fine-needle aspiration. *Cancer*. 2005;105(6):443-451.

21. Kawahara A, Harada H, Akiba J, Yokoyama T, Kage M. Fine-needle aspiration cytology of basal cell adenoma of the parotid gland: characteristic cytological features and diagnostic pitfalls. *Diagn Cytopathol*. 2007;35(2):85-90.

22. Krishnamurthy S, Ashfaq R, Shin HJ, Sneige N. Distinction of phyllodes tumor from fibroadenoma: a reappraisal of an old problem. *Cancer*. 2000;90(6):342-349.

23. Lopez-Ferrer P, Jimenez-Heffernan JA, Vicandi B, Ortega L, Viguer JM. Fine needle aspiration cytology of breast fibroadenoma. A cytohistologic correlation study of 405 cases. *Acta Cytol*. 1999;43(4):579-586.

24. Nemanqani D, Mourad WA. Cytomorphologic features of fine-needle aspiration of liposarcoma. *Diagn Cytopathol*. 1999;20(2):67-69.

25. Nikiforov YE. Molecular diagnostics of thyroid tumors. *Arch Pathol Lab Med*. 2011;135(5):569-577.

26. Pacini F, Castagna MG, Cipri C, Schlumberger M. Medullary thyroid carcinoma. *Clin Oncol (R Coll Radiol)*. 2010;22(6):475-485.

27. Pereira TC, Saad RS, Liu Y, Silverman JF. The diagnosis of malignancy in effusion cytology: a pattern recognition approach. *Adv Anat Pathol*. 2006;13(4):174-184.

28. Perez-Guillermo M, Masgrau NA, Garcia-Solano J, Sola-Perez J, de Agustin y de Agustin P. Cytologic aspect of fibrolamellar hepatocellular carcinoma in fine-needle aspirates. *Diagn Cytopathol*. 1999;21(3):180-187.

29. Plaza JA, Mayerson J, Wakely PE Jr. Nodular fasciitis of the hand: a potential diagnostic pitfall in fine-needle aspiration cytopathology. *Am J Clin Pathol*. 2005;123(3):388-393.

30. Policarpio-Nicolas ML, Wick MR. False-positive interpretations in respiratory cytopathology: exemplary cases and literature review. *Diagn Cytopathol*. 2008;36(1):13-19.

31. Schindler S, Nayar R, Dutra J, Bedrossian CW. Diagnostic challenges in aspiration cytology of the salivary glands. *Semin Diagn Pathol*. 2001;18(2):124-146.

32. Seethala RR, Dacic S, Cieply K, Kelly LM, Nikiforova MN. A reappraisal of the MECT1/MAML2 translocation in salivary mucoepidermoid carcinomas. *Am J Surg Pathol*. 2010;34(8):1106-1121.

33. Selvaggi SM. Diagnostic pitfalls of peritoneal washing cytology and the role of cell blocks in their diagnosis. *Diagn Cytopathol*. 2003;28(6):335-341.

34. Sgrignoli A, Abati A. Cytologic diagnosis of anaplastic large cell lymphoma. *Acta Cytol*. 1997;41(4):1048-1052.

35. Sherman ME, Mark EJ. Effusion cytology in the diagnosis of malignant epithelioid and biphasic pleural mesothelioma. *Arch Pathol Lab Med*. 1990;114(8):845-851.

36. Silverman JF, Masood S, Ducatman BS, Wang HH, Sneige N. Can FNA biopsy separate atypical hyperplasia, carcinoma in situ, and invasive carcinoma of the breast? Cytomorphologic criteria and limitations in diagnosis. *Diagn Cytopathol*. 1993;9(6):713-728.

37. Singh HK, VK, Elsheikh TM, Silverman JF. The diagnostic utility of fine-needle aspiration biopsy of soft-tissue sarcomas in the core needle biopsy era. *Pathology Case Reviews*. 2007;12((January/February):36-43.

38. Sohn JH, Kim LS, Chae SW, Shin HS. Fine needle aspiration cytologic findings of breast mucinous neoplasms: differential diagnosis between mucocelelike tumor and mucinous carcinoma. *Acta Cytol*. 2001;45(5):723-729.

39. Sokolova IA, Halling KC, Jenkins RB, et al. The development of a multitarget, multicolor fluorescence in situ hybridization assay for the detection of urothelial carcinoma in urine. *J Mol Diagn*. 2000;2(3):116-123.

40. Stanley MW, Steeper TA, Horwitz CA, Burton LG, Strickler JG, Borken S. Fine-needle aspiration of lymph nodes in patients with acute infectious mononucleosis. *Diagn Cytopathol*. 1990;6(5):323-329.

41. Stastny JF, Wakely PE Jr., Frable WJ. Cytologic features of necrotizing granulomatous inflammation consistent with cat-scratch disease. *Diagn Cytopathol*. 1996; 15(2):108-115.

42. Troncone G, Malapelle U, Cozzolino I, Palombini L. KRAS mutation analysis on cytological specimens of metastatic colorectal cancer. *Diagn Cytopathol*. 2010;38(12):869-873.

43. Troxell ML, Bangs CD, Cherry AM, Natkunam Y, Kong CS. Cytologic diagnosis of Burkitt lymphoma. *Cancer*. 2005; 105(5):310-318.

44. Us-Krasovec M, Golouh R, Auersperg M, Besic N, Ruparcic-Oblak L. Anaplastic thyroid carcinoma in fine needle aspirates. *Acta Cytol*. 1996;40(5):953-958.

45. Wang HH, Sovie S, Zeroogian JM, Spechler SJ, Goyal RK, Antonioli DA. Value of cytology in detecting intestinal metaplasia and associated dysplasia at the gastroesophageal junction. *Hum Pathol*. 1997;28(4):465-471.

46. Wang J, Cobb CJ, Martin SE, Venegas R, Wu N, Greaves TS. Pilomatrixoma: clinicopathologic study of 51 cases with emphasis on cytologic features. *Diagn Cytopathol*. 2002; 27(3):167-172.

47. Wiatrowska BA, Zakowski MF. Fine-needle aspiration biopsy of chromophobe renal cell carcinoma and oncocytoma: comparison of cytomorphologic features. *Cancer*. 1999; 87(3):161-167.

48. Zuna RE, Behrens A. Peritoneal washing cytology in gynecologic cancers: long-term follow-up of 355 patients. *J Natl Cancer Inst*. 1996;88(14):980-987.

CHAPTER 10

DERMATOPATHOLOGY

1. All of the following are true regarding Langerhans cells in the skin except
   (A) CD138 positive
   (B) Prominently seen in allergic contact dermatitis
   (C) S-100 positive
   (D) They are dendritic cells
   (E) They are involved with antigen presentation

2. Specialized apocrine glands, Moll glands, are located where in the body?
   (A) External ear canal
   (B) Eyelid
   (C) Nail bed
   (D) Near the oral cavity
   (E) Scalp

3. Eccrine glands can express all of the following immunoreactivities except
   (A) Calponin
   (B) CEA
   (C) Cytokeratin 7
   (D) HMB-45
   (E) p63

4. All of the following disorders represent a form of spongiotic dermatitis except
   (A) Atopic dermatitis
   (B) Erythema multiforme
   (C) Irritant contact dermatitis
   (D) Pityriasis rosea
   (E) Seborrheic dermatitis

5. Erythrocyte extravasation is most commonly encountered in which of the following?
   (A) Atopic dermatitis
   (B) Dyshydrosis
   (C) Irritant contact dermatitis
   (D) Nummular dermatitis
   (E) Pityriasis rosea

6. Which of the following is the least likely cause of allergic contact dermatitis?
   (A) Dermatophytosis
   (B) Latex
   (C) Nickel
   (D) Perfume
   (E) Poison ivy

7. A 4-year-old girl with a history of asthma presents with ill-defined plaques composed of pruritic, crusted papules in the antecubital fossae. A biopsy shows focal spongiosis with superficial perivascular lymphocytes, epidermal hyperplasia and parakeratosis. The most likely diagnosis is which of the following?
   (A) Atopic dermatitis
   (B) Dyshidrotic dermatitis
   (C) Pityriasis alba
   (D) Psoriasis
   (E) Seborrheic dermatitis

8. A 12-year-old male presents with multiple-round or oval erythematous patches and plaques distributed in a "Christmas tree"-like pattern on the trunk. All of the following are features commonly seen on a biopsy of this entity except
   (A) Epidermal necrosis
   (B) Exocytosis of lymphocytes
   (C) Parakeratosis
   (D) Red cell extravasation
   (E) Spongiosis

9. A 26-year-old male presents with an acute onset of coin-sized plaques on the scalp, elbows and knees. He is diagnosed with guttate psoriasis. Which of the following conditions are likely to be associated with his presentation?
   (A) Allergic rhinitis
   (B) Exposure to erythromycin
   (C) Lymphoma
   (D) Streptococcal pharyngitis
   (E) Syphilis genital infection

10. Which of the following would be least effective in treating psoriasis?
    (A) Antibiotics
    (B) Corticosteroids
    (C) Phototherapy
    (D) Retinoids
    (E) Vitamin D3 analogs

11. A 49-year-old male is diagnosed with necrolytic migratory erythema on a skin biopsy from the groin. The clinician should be advised to look for evidence of which of the following in this patient?
    (A) Glucagonoma
    (B) Lung carcinoma
    (C) Non-Hodgkin lymphoma
    (D) Pheochromocytoma
    (E) Vitamin B12 deficiency

12. Which of the following is least likely to be seen in Stevens–Johnson syndrome?
    (A) Involvement of mucosal sites
    (B) May be triggered by *Mycoplasma pneumoniae* infection
    (C) Prominent hemorrhagic crusting
    (D) Recent drug exposure
    (E) Widespread sloughing of the epidermal surface (>10% of total body surface area)

13. All of the following are morphologic features more suggestive of a fixed drug reaction versus erythema multiforme except
    (A) Greater spongiosis
    (B) Involvement of deep perivascular plexus
    (C) Keratinocyte necrosis
    (D) Prominent melanophages
    (E) Psoriasiform epidermal hyperplasia

14. A 45-year-old male presents with flat-topped violaceous papules and plaques involving the wrist, forearm and oral mucosa. Some of the lesions show small white lines on the surface. A biopsy is taken and shown in Figure 10-1. The best diagnosis for this lesion is which of the following?

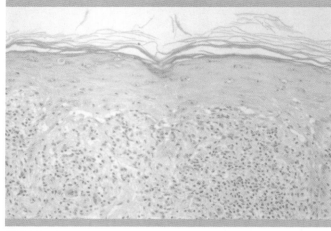

FIGURE 10-1

    (A) Erythema multiforme
    (B) Lichen planus
    (C) Lichen sclerosis
    (D) Lupus erythematosus
    (E) Mycosis fungoides

15. All of the following histologic features may be seen in the setting of lupus erythematosus involving the skin except
    (A) Civatte bodies
    (B) Epidermal atrophy
    (C) Hyperkeratosis and follicular plugging
    (D) Interface dermatitis
    (E) Perivascular chronic inflammation

16. All of the following are features typical of dermatomyositis except
    (A) Associated with malignancy
    (B) Gottron papules
    (C) Max-Joseph spaces
    (D) Perifascicular muscle atrophy
    (E) Violaceous poikiloderma

17. A 26-year-old bone marrow transplant patient presents with erythematous macules on the face and hands about 6 weeks after transplantation. A diagnosis of acute graft versus host disease is being entertained. A biopsy shows vacuolar epidermal alterations with necrotic keratinocytes and subepidermal microvesicles. The lesion is best characterized as which grade?
    (A) Grade 0
    (B) Grade 1
    (C) Grade 2
    (D) Grade 3
    (E) Grade 4

18. Which of the following least likely presents with granulomatous dermatitis?
    (A) Granuloma annulare
    (B) Leprosy
    (C) Necrobiosis lipoidica
    (D) Pityriasis lichenoides
    (E) Sarcoid

19. A 9-year-old presents with multiple small papules and plaques. On biopsy, palisaded granulomas with increased Alcian blue positive interstitial mucin and eosinophils are seen. The best diagnosis for this entity is which of the following?
    (A) Dermatofibroma
    (B) Granuloma annulare
    (C) Necrobiosis lipoidica
    (D) Rheumatoid nodule
    (E) Sarcoid

20. Kaposi sarcoma is associated with infection by which of the following human herpes viruses (HHV)?
    (A) HHV-1
    (B) HHV-2
    (C) HHV-6
    (D) HHV-8
    (E) HHV-12

21. A 46-year-old woman with a history of rheumatoid arthritis presents with tender, nonpruritic erythematous plaques on the head and neck. Biopsy of one of the neck lesions shows a dense neutrophilic infiltrate in the dermis with edema and minimal vascular damage. The most likely diagnosis is which of the following?
    (A) Cellulitis
    (B) Dermatitis herpetiformis
    (C) Polymorphous light eruption
    (D) Sweet syndrome
    (E) Vasculitis

22. Urticaria can be a manifestation of all of the following exposures except
    (A) Basal cell carcinoma
    (B) Parasitic infection
    (C) Radiocontrast media
    (D) Shellfish consumption
    (E) Sun exposure

23. Erythema migrans is associated with which of the following conditions?
    (A) Lyme disease
    (B) Lymphoma
    (C) Poxvirus exposure
    (D) Rheumatoid arthritis
    (E) Syphilis infection

24. All of the following are findings associated with plasmacytosis mucosae except
    (A) A monoclonal kappa or lambda population is present
    (B) Cells stain with CD138 antibody
    (C) Includes Zoon balanitis
    (D) There is minimal cytologic atypia
    (E) Usually presents as a solitary lesion

25. Morphea on the scalp and trunk are associated with which of the following entities?
    (A) Chronic graft versus host disease
    (B) Dermatomyositis
    (C) Lupus erythematosus
    (D) Rheumatoid arthritis
    (E) Scleroderma

26. Nephrogenic systemic fibrosis is typically associated with which of the following conditions
    (A) Oncocytomas of the kidney
    (B) Polycystic kidney disease
    (C) Renal cell carcinoma
    (D) Renal transplantation
    (E) von Hippel-Lindau syndrome

27. Comedones are associated with which of the following organisms?
    (A) No organism is associated with comedones
    (B) *Propionibacterium acnes*
    (C) *Pseudomonas aeruginosa*
    (D) *Staphylococcus aureus*
    (E) *Staphylococcus epidermidis*

28. Eosinophilic folliculitis is associated with which of the following viral infections?
    (A) CMV
    (B) Hepatitis A
    (C) Hepatitis B
    (D) HIV
    (E) HTLV I

29. Rosacea is marked by central facial erythema that can be exacerbated by all of the following except
    (A) Exercise
    (B) Hot drinks
    (C) Peanuts
    (D) Spicy foods
    (E) Sunlight

30. All of the following are associated with a neutrophilic lobular panniculitis except
    (A) Alpha-1-antitrypsin
    (B) Arthropod bite reaction
    (C) Infection
    (D) Pancreatic fat necrosis
    (E) Ruptured folliculitis

31. The most common form of panniculitis is represented by which of the following?
    (A) Erythema nodosa
    (B) Lipodystrophy
    (C) Lupus profundus
    (D) Sarcoidosis
    (E) Scleroderma

32. All of the following are true regarding lupus profundus except
    (A) Alcian blue stain highlights stromal mucin
    (B) It is a form of lymphocytic lobular panniculitis
    (C) May contain lymphoid follicles
    (D) Most cases have a clonal T cell population
    (E) Presents as an erythematous tender nodule or plaque

33. Erythema induratum represents a form of lobular panniculitis associated with which of the following?
    (A) Leukemia
    (B) Polyarteritis nodosa
    (C) Rosai–Dorfman disease
    (D) Sarcoidosis
    (E) Tuberculosis

34. The findings in this biopsy shown in Figure 10-2 are best described as which of the following?

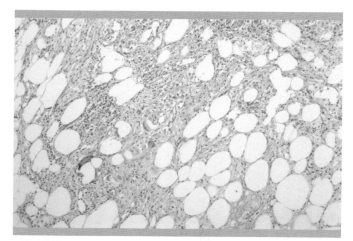

FIGURE 10-2

(A) Interface dermatitis
(B) Nodular fasciitis
(C) Panniculitis
(D) Spongiotic dermatitis
(E) Vasculitis

35. Bowenoid papulosis is most commonly associated with which HPV type?
    (A) Type 1
    (B) Type 2
    (C) Type 4
    (D) Type 10
    (E) Type 16

36. An 8-year-old presents with a centrally umbilicated, pearly papule. The biopsy shown in Figure 10-3 is most consistent with an infection by which of the following organisms?

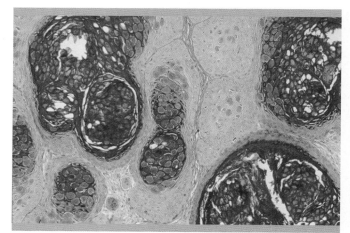

FIGURE 10-3

(A) Cytomegalovirus
(B) Herpes simplex virus type II
(C) Polyoma virus
(D) Poxvirus
(E) Varicella zoster

37. Intracytoplasmic eosinophilic inclusions, known as Guarnieri bodies, are associated with which of the following?
    (A) Epstein–Barr versus infection
    (B) Milker nodules
    (C) Molluscum contagiosum
    (D) Polyoma virus infection
    (E) Varicella zoster infection

38. A 19-year-old male presents with fever, stomatitis, and oval vesicles with an erythematous rim on the hands and feet. A diagnosis of hand-foot-and-mouth disease is made. The most likely etiology is which of the following organisms?
    (A) BK virus
    (B) Cowpox
    (C) Coxsackie virus
    (D) Enterovirus 17
    (E) Monkeypox

39. An immunocompromised a 62-year-old male presents with multiple ulcerated lesions. One of the lesions is biopsied and shown in Figure 10-4. The best diagnosis for this lesion is an ulcer due to which of the following?

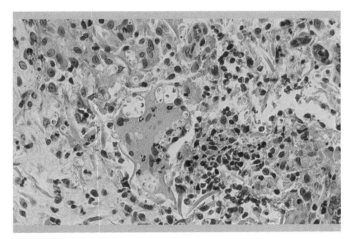

FIGURE 10-4

    (A) Blastomycosis
    (B) *Candida*
    (C) Chromomycosis
    (D) *Cryptococcus*
    (E) *Fusarium*

40. Ecthyma is caused most commonly by which of the following organisms?
    (A) Group A *Streptococcus*
    (B) Group B *Streptococcus*
    (C) *Staphylococcus aureus*
    (D) *Staphylococcus epidermidis*
    (E) *Streptococcus pneumoniae*

41. A 62-year-old male presents with pruritic reddish-brown patches in the axillae. A diagnosis of erythrasma is being entertained clinically. Which of the following organisms is most likely

responsible for the clinical lesions, if this is the correct diagnosis?
    (A) *Candida albicans*
    (B) *Corynebacterium minutissimum*
    (C) Group B *Streptococcus*
    (D) *Staphylococcus aureus*
    (E) *Streptococcus pyogenes*

42. Rickettsialpox skin infection caused by *Rickettsia akari* is transmitted by the bite of which vector?
    (A) Flea
    (B) Louse
    (C) Mite
    (D) Mosquito
    (E) Tick

43. All of the following are true regarding lymphogranuloma venereum except
    (A) Can be treated with antibiotics
    (B) Caused by *Calymmatobacterium granulomatis*
    (C) Initially presents with a painless vesicle, papule or ulcer
    (D) May histologically show areas of necrosis
    (E) Patients may develop fistulae and strictures

44. The lesion shown in Figure 10-5 was excised from a 42-year-old male who presented with a partially ulcerated nodule on the right arm. A Fite stain shows occasional positive staining organisms. The most likely etiology is which of the following?

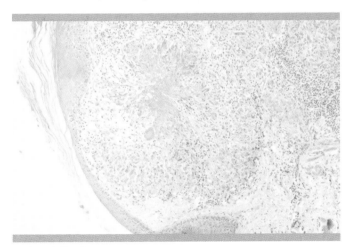

FIGURE 10-5

    (A) Actinomyces
    (B) Klebsiella
    (C) Mycobacteria
    (D) Mycoplasma
    (E) Nocardia

45. New cases of this disease (in Question 44) are most likely to be encountered where in the United States?
    (A) Alaska
    (B) California
    (C) Florida
    (D) Maine
    (E) Texas

46. All of the following are features of lepromatous leprosy except
    (A) Can involve peripheral nerves
    (B) Cutaneous lesions are often symmetric and poorly demarcated
    (C) Frequently involves the trunk or extremities
    (D) Associated with an increased incidence of vitiligo
    (E) Occurs in patients with a poor immune response

47. Fish tank granuloma is associated with infection by which of the following organisms?
    (A) *Mycobacterium bovis (M. bovis)*
    (B) *M. haemophilum*
    (C) *M. leprae*
    (D) *M. marinum*
    (E) *M. ulcerans*

48. A 62-year-old diabetic woman with poor oral hygiene recently had two teeth pulled. She subsequently develops ulcerated and draining nodules on the face and neck. The most likely diagnosis is which of the following?
    (A) Actinomycosis
    (B) Botryomycosis
    (C) Cat scratch disease
    (D) Cryptococcosis
    (E) Nocardiosis

49. The lesion shown in Figure 10-6 arises in a 69-year-old male with a history of leukemia and recent bone marrow transplant. *M. leprae* is cultured and responds to treatment. The pathology best fits with which of the following?

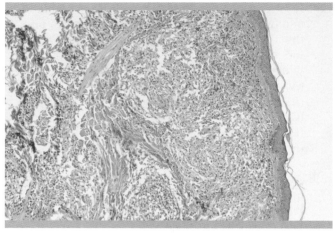

FIGURE 10-6

    (A) Erythema nodosum leprosum
    (B) Histoid leprosy
    (C) Lepromatous leprosy
    (D) Lucio phenomenon
    (E) Tuberculoid leprosy

50. The presence of necrotizing granulomatous inflammation on a skin biopsy in the setting of an infection by *Treponema pallidum* is characteristic of which of the following?
    (A) Condyloma lata
    (B) Initial infection with syphilis
    (C) Primary syphilis
    (D) Secondary syphilis
    (E) Tertiary syphilis

51. All of the following dermatophytosis-associated organisms are typically transmitted from human to human (anthropophilic) except
    (A) *Epidermophyton floccosum*
    (B) *Microsporum gypseum*
    (C) *Trichophyton concentricum*
    (D) *Trichophyton mentagrophytes interdigitale*
    (E) *Trichophyton rubrum*

52. The clinical differential diagnosis of tinea pedis includes all of the following lesions except
    (A) Allergic contact dermatitis
    (B) Candidiasis
    (C) Erythema nodosum
    (D) Impetigo
    (E) Interdigital erythrasma

53. All of the following are true regarding tinea versicolor except
    (A) Caused by *Malassezia furfur*
    (B) Cultured on blood agar plate
    (C) Epidermis may show hyperkeratosis and acanthosis
    (D) Mostly involves upper trunk or arms
    (E) Well-demarcated macules and patches

54. All of the following are dematiaceous fungi that may be responsible for causing phaeohyphomycosis infection except
    (A) *Alternaria*
    (B) *Bipolaris*
    (C) *Cladosporium*
    (D) *Pityrosporum*
    (E) Wangiella

55. The lesion illustrated in Figure 10-7 is most likely caused by which of the following organisms?

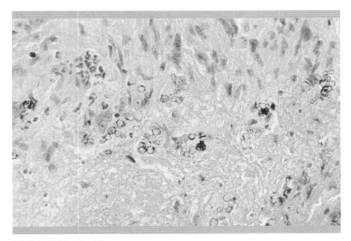

FIGURE 10-7

    (A) *Alternaria*
    (B) *Curvularia*
    (C) *Fonsecaea*
    (D) *Sporothrix*
    (E) *Leishmania*

56. A "Mariner's wheel" type of budding is characteristic of infection by which of the following yeast?
    (A) *Alterneria*
    (B) *Blastomyces*
    (C) *Coccidioides*
    (D) *Cryptococcus*
    (E) *Paracoccidioides*

57. Which of the following clinical conditions are associated with the lesion illustrated in Figure 10-8?

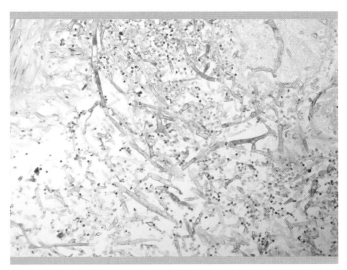

FIGURE 10-8

    (A) Crohn disease
    (B) Diabetes
    (C) Emphysema
    (D) Hemochromatosis
    (E) Renal failure

58. All of the following are true regarding the lesion illustrated in Figure 10-9 except

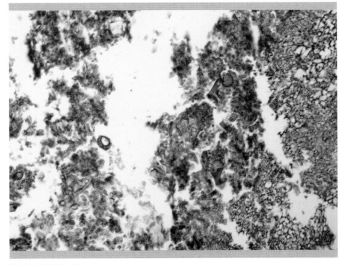

FIGURE 10-9

    (A) Acute angle branching hyphae
    (B) Fruiting bodies are commonly seen in skin lesions
    (C) Granulomatous inflammation
    (D) Increased risk in burn victims
    (E) Vascular invasion common

59. The sandfly serves as a vector for the transmission of which of the following infections?
    (A) Amebiasis
    (B) Leishmaniasis
    (C) Lobomycosis
    (D) Rhinosporidiosis
    (E) Schistosomiasis

60. A 27-year-old woman presents with a rosacea-like eruption. Follicular dilation with inflammation is seen on a biopsy. Organisms consistent with Demodex are seen. The organism represents which of the following?
    (A) Fly larvae (myiasis)
    (B) Fungus
    (C) Louse
    (D) Mite
    (E) Parasite

61. All of the following are true regarding scabies infestation of the skin except
    (A) Eosinophil infiltrates
    (B) Highly infectious
    (C) Necrotizing granulomatous inflammation
    (D) Preferentially involves interdigital and flexural areas
    (E) Pruritic lesions

62. A 64-year-old male presents with a verrucous, crusted nodule. A biopsy is taken and shown in Figure 10-10. The best diagnosis is which of the following?

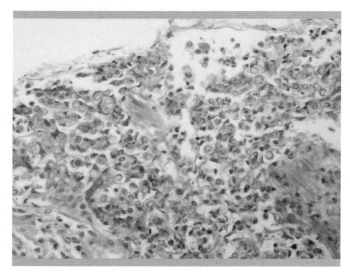

FIGURE 10-10

(A) Blastomycosis
(B) Coccidioidomycosis
(C) Cryptococcosis
(D) Histoplasmosis
(E) Paracoccidioidomycosis

63. A 19-year-old sustains head trauma during a camping trip. She develops an ulcerated lesion on her right lower leg. The lesion is biopsied and shown in Figure 10-11. The best diagnosis is which of the following?

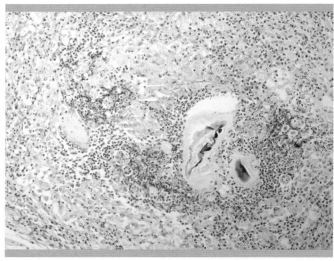

FIGURE 10-11

(A) Cimicosis
(B) Myiasis
(C) Pediculosis
(D) Scabies
(E) Tick bite

64. A 59-year-old female who recently travelled to India presents with white papules and nodules with a central black dot and erythematous halo on the feet. She liked to take long walks on the beaches. The most likely diagnosis is which of the following?
    (A) Cimicosis
    (B) Pediculosis
    (C) Spider bites
    (D) Tick bites
    (E) Tungiasis

65. A 6-year-old from Central America presents with subcutaneous nodules and a history of black fly bites. The nodules are most likely due to which of the following?
    (A) Cysticercosis
    (B) *Dirofilaria*
    (C) Onchocerciasis
    (D) Protothecosis
    (E) Schistosomiasis

66. In entertaining a diagnosis of cutaneous vasculitis, the optimal time for a skin biopsy is how many hours after the appearance of the lesion?
    (A) 12 hours
    (B) 36 hours
    (C) 60 hours
    (D) 1 week
    (E) None. It cannot be diagnosed on a biopsy

67. All of the following represent small vessel, neutrophilic, immune complex-mediated vasculitides of the skin except
    (A) Cutaneous leukocytoclastic vasculitis
    (B) Erythema elevatum diutinum
    (C) Henoch–Schönlein purpura
    (D) Rickettsial infection
    (E) Urticarial vasculitis

68. All of the following are likely clinical manifestations of a small vessel vasculitis except
    (A) Limb claudication
    (B) Purpura
    (C) Splinter hemorrhage
    (D) Urticaria
    (E) Vesiculobullous lesions

69. All of the following are chronic signs of healed lesions associated with cutaneous vasculitis except
    (A) Endarteritis obliterans
    (B) Intimal proliferation
    (C) Intraluminal fibrin thrombi
    (D) Neovascularization of vessel adventitia
    (E) Onion-skinning or lamination of vessel walls

70. All of the following represent type IV delayed hypersensitivity-mediated vasculitides except
    (A) Chronic graft versus host disease
    (B) Cryoglobulinemic vasculitis
    (C) Dego disease
    (D) Giant cell arteritis
    (E) Sneddon syndrome

71. The most common immunoreactant found in blood vessels by direct immunofluorescent (DIF) studies in the setting of cutaneous vasculitis is which of the following?
    (A) C3
    (B) C5
    (C) IgA
    (D) IgG
    (E) IgM

72. Predominant IgM vascular deposits on a skin biopsy are most suggestive of which of the following?
    (A) Churg–Strauss syndrome
    (B) Cryoglobulinemic vasculitis
    (C) Henoch–Schönlein purpura
    (D) Lupus erythematosus vasculitis
    (E) Wegener granulomatosis (granulomatosis with polyangiitis)

73. A patient with cutaneous vasculitis accompanied by ocular disease most likely has which of the following?
    (A) Henoch–Schönlein purpura
    (B) Microscopic polyangiitis
    (C) Polyarteritis nodosa
    (D) Urticarial vasculitis
    (E) Wegener granulomatosis (granulomatosis with polyangiitis)

74. A 62-year-old woman with a diagnosis of cutaneous vasculitis has a positive pANCA test. Which of the following diagnoses is least likely?
    (A) Churg–Strauss syndrome
    (B) Microscopic polyangiitis
    (C) Polyarteritis nodosa
    (D) Rheumatoid vasculitis
    (E) Wegener granulomatosis (granulomatosis with polyangiitis)

75. The most common group of malignancies associated with paraneoplastic vasculitis includes which of the following?
    (A) Breast carcinomas
    (B) Leukemias
    (C) Lung carcinomas
    (D) Lymphoproliferative disorders
    (E) Melanomas

76. In which of the following conditions is acantholysis due to loss of cell-to- cell contact between keratinocytes the mechanism of blister formation?
    (A) Acute allergic contact dermatitis
    (B) Bullous pemphigoid
    (C) Heat
    (D) Pemphigus
    (E) Polymorphous light eruption

77. All of the following conditions are associated with corneal or subcorneal blister formation in the skin except
    (A) Bullous impetigo
    (B) Pemphigus foliaceus
    (C) Pemphigus vulgaris
    (D) Pustular psoriasis
    (E) Staphylococcal scalded skin syndrome

78. Miliaria in neonates is due to which of the following?
    (A) Blockage of apocrine ducts
    (B) Blockage of eccrine ducts
    (C) Hair follicle plugging
    (D) Infection
    (E) Overproduction of sebaceous glands

79. Bullous impetigo is associated with a superficial infection by which of the following organisms?
    (A) Staphylococcus aureus (S. aureus)
    (B) S. epidermidis
    (C) S. saprophyticus
    (D) S. hemolyticus
    (E) S. hominis

80. In which of the following conditions is IgG antibody directed against desmoglein I and not desmoglein 3?
    (A) Acropustulosis of infancy
    (B) Darier disease
    (C) Pemphigus foliaceus
    (D) Pemphigus vulgaris
    (E) Polymorphous light eruption

81. All of the following are true regarding Darier disease except
    (A) Biopsy shows acantholysis and dyskeratosis
    (B) Can appear as greasy, brown crusted, keratotic papules
    (C) Corps ronds may be seen
    (D) May involve the oral mucosa
    (E) X-linked disorder

82. The biopsy shown in Figure 10-12 is from the axilla of a 49-year-old male with flaccid blisters. DIF studies are negative. Several family members have the same disease. The best diagnosis for this condition is which of the following?

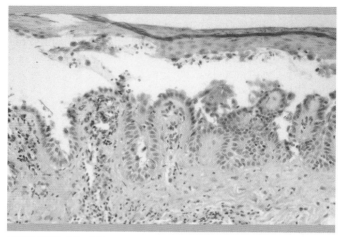

FIGURE 10-12

    (A) Grover disease
    (B) Hailey–Hailey disease
    (C) Herpetic dermatitis
    (D) IgA pemphigus
    (E) Pemphigus foliaceus

83. Cicatricial pemphigoid can be distinguished from epidermolysis bullosa acquisita by which of the following?
    (A) Clinical presentation
    (B) Direct immunofluorescence
    (C) Indirect immunofluorescence
    (D) Location of the bullae
    (E) Salt split skin test

84. Linear IgA bullous dermatosis may be drug induced. The most common drug that has been associated with this disorder is which of the following?
    (A) Corticosteroids
    (B) Penicillin
    (C) Proprandol
    (D) Sulfapyridine
    (E) Vancomycin

85. The biopsy shown here in Figure 10-13 is from a 26-year-old male who presented with pruritic grouped papules and vesicles on the elbows, knees, and neck. By DIF, granular IgA deposits are seen in the dermal papillae. Which of the following disorders are associated with this condition?

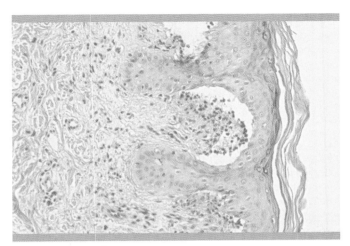

FIGURE 10-13

(A) Crohn disease
(B) Gluten-sensitive enteropathy
(C) Hepatitis C infection
(D) HIV infection
(E) Oral ulcers

86. Epidermolysis bullosa acquisita is an immune-mediated bullous disorder associated with autoimmune antibodies to which of the following?
(A) Type I collagen
(B) Type II collagen
(C) Type V collagen
(D) Type VI collagen
(E) Type VII collagen

87. A 28-year-old woman presents with blisters that develop on exposure to sunlight. A biopsy of one of the hand lesions is shown in Figure 10-14. All of the following are true regarding the disorder except

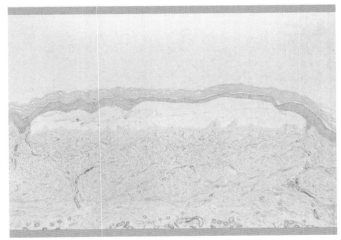

FIGURE 10-14

(A) Associated with marked eosinophilic dermal infiltrates
(B) Causes subepidermal blistering
(C) Hyaline deposits around papillary dermal vessels
(D) May see IgG deposits at the dermoepidermal junction
(E) Rigid papillae at the blister base may be seen

88. Localized or pretibial myxedema is associated with which of the following conditions?
(A) Acromegaly
(B) Hypercortisolism
(C) Hyperthyroidism
(D) Hypercortisolism
(E) Hypothyroidism

89. The lesion illustrated in Figure 10-15 from the finger of a 58-year-old male is best diagnosed as which of the following?

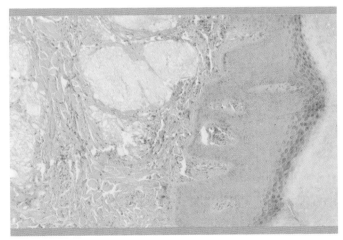

FIGURE 10-15

(A) Gout
(B) Ochronosis
(C) Pilomatricoma
(D) Pseudogout
(E) Rheumatoid nodule

90. All of the following are risk factors for the development of the condition in Question 89 except
(A) Alcohol
(B) Family history
(C) Gender
(D) Smoking
(E) Thiazide diuretic use

91. All of the following are true regarding the
    condition illustrated in Figure 10-16 except

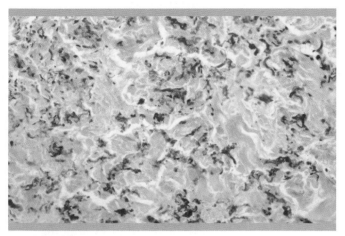

FIGURE 10-16

    (A) Affects elastic fibers in the eye and cardiovas-
         cular systems
    (B) Autosomal-recessive condition
    (C) Findings present at birth
    (D) Mutations of the ABCC6 gene
    (E) Presents as yellowish papules

92. The presence of numerous café-au-lait macules is
    associated with which of the following conditions?
    (A) Carney complex
    (B) Neurofibromatosis type I
    (C) Neurofibromatosis type II
    (D) Tuberous sclerosis
    (E) von Hippel-Lindau syndrome

93. Which of the following drugs is least likely to
    result in hyperpigmentation of the skin?
    (A) Amiodarone
    (B) Clofazimine
    (C) Corticosteroids
    (D) Imipramine
    (E) Minocycline

94. All of the following are true regarding vitiligo
    except
    (A) Associated with Graves disease
    (B) Decreased melanin pigment
    (C) Decreased number of intraepidermal
         melanocytes
    (D) No gender predilection
    (E) Present at birth

95. Hypopigmented macules known as ash-leaf
    spots are associated with which of the following
    conditions?
    (A) Carney complex
    (B) Neurofibromatosis type I
    (C) Neurofibromatosis type II
    (D) Tuberous sclerosis
    (E) von Hippel-Lindau syndrome

96. All of the following conditions are nonscarring
    forms of alopecia except
    (A) Alopecia areata
    (B) Androgenetic alopecia
    (C) Lupus erythematosus
    (D) Senescent baldness
    (E) Trichotillomania

97. Approximately what percent of hair are in the
    telogen or resting phase?
    (A) 10%
    (B) 25%
    (C) 50%
    (D) 75%
    (E) 90%

98. A 46-year-old male presents with a balding patch
    marked by follicular hyperkeratosis. A biopsy
    is taken and shown in Figure 10-17. The best
    diagnosis is which of the following?

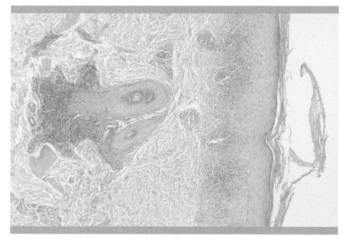

FIGURE 10-17

    (A) Lichen planopilaris
    (B) Loose anagen hair syndrome
    (C) Pressure-induced alopecia
    (D) Traction alopecia
    (E) Trichotillomania

99. Which of the following cysts is the most common of all cutaneous cysts?
    (A) Dermoid cyst
    (B) Follicular cyst of infundibular type
    (C) Sebaceous duct cyst
    (D) Trichilemmal cyst
    (E) Verrucous cyst

100. Which of the following cysts is associated with Gardner syndrome and Gorlin syndrome?
    (A) Epidermoid cyst
    (B) Infundibular cyst
    (C) Milium
    (D) Pilar cyst
    (E) Steatocystoma

101. All of the following are true regarding the cutaneous cyst shown here in Figure 10-18 except

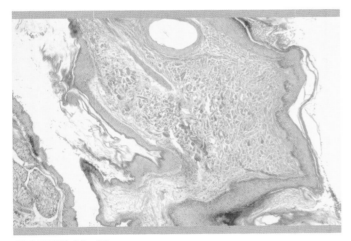

FIGURE 10-18

    (A) Cysts have a granular layer
    (B) Located in the dermis
    (C) May have a autosomal-dominant inheritance pattern
    (D) Most commonly affects the trunk
    (E) Often presents as multiple cysts

102. The most common location for dermoid cysts of the skin is which of the following?
    (A) Chest
    (B) Lower back
    (C) Nose
    (D) Periorbital region
    (E) Scalp

103. The lesion illustrated here in Figure 10-19 arose on the back of a 64-year-old male. It is best diagnosed as which of the following?

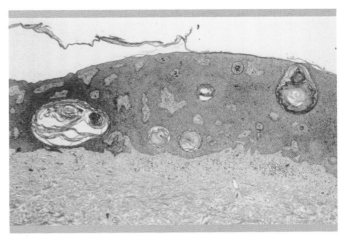

FIGURE 10-19

    (A) Actinic keratosis
    (B) Epidermal nevus
    (C) Seborrheic keratosis
    (D) Squamous cell carcinoma
    (E) Verruca vulgaris

104. All of the following may arise in the background of a seborrheic keratosis except
    (A) Basal cell carcinoma
    (B) Bowen disease
    (C) Melanoma
    (D) Nevus
    (E) Pilomatricoma

105. The lesion illustrated here in Figure 10-20 in this 69-year-old male is best classified as which of the following?

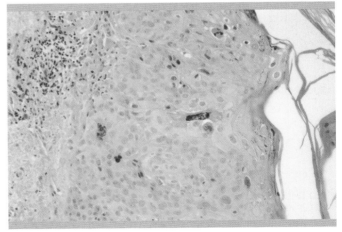

FIGURE 10-20

    (A) Actinic keratosis
    (B) Benign keratosis
    (C) Lentigo maligna
    (D) Seborrheic keratosis
    (E) Squamous cell carcinoma in situ

106. Which of the following is not a risk factor for the development of invasive squamous cell carcinoma of the skin?
     (A) Arsenic
     (B) Impetigo
     (C) Organ transplantation
     (D) Ultraviolet radiation
     (E) Xeroderma pigmentosum

107. All of the following are unfavorable pathologic parameters in cutaneous squamous cell carcinoma except
     (A) Degree of stromal inflammatory response
     (B) Depth >4 mm invasion
     (C) Lymphovascular invasion
     (D) Poor differentiation
     (E) Width >2 cm

108. Which of the following immunomarkers is least likely to be positive in squamous cell carcinoma?
     (A) 34βE12
     (B) CAM 5.2
     (C) Cytokeratins 5/6
     (D) EMA
     (E) p63

109. A 76-year-old male presents with a rapidly growing nodule with rolled borders and a central keratin plug on the right arm. The lesion is excised and shown here in Figure 10-21. The best diagnosis for the lesion is which of the following?

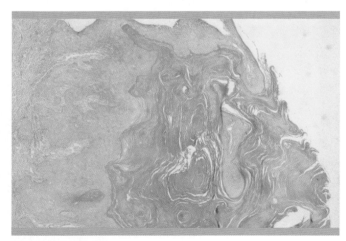

FIGURE 10-21

     (A) Bowen disease
     (B) Keratoacanthoma
     (C) Seborrheic keratosis
     (D) Squamous cell carcinoma
     (E) Verruca vulgaris

110. The lesion in Question 109 is associated with which of the following conditions?
     (A) Cowden disease
     (B) Epidermal nevus syndrome
     (C) Gorlin syndrome
     (D) Muir–Torre syndrome
     (E) Tuberous sclerosis

111. All of the following features are consistent with a desmoplastic trichoepithelioma (Figure 10-22) versus a sclerosing basal cell carcinoma except

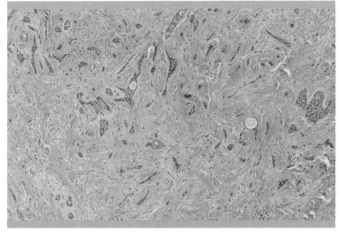

FIGURE 10-22

     (A) Keratin cyst formation
     (B) Minimal cytologic atypia
     (C) Minimal mitotic activity
     (D) More apoptotic bodies
     (E) Papillary mesenchymal bodies present

112. Which of the following skin lesions is associated with Cowden syndrome?
     (A) Basal cell carcinoma
     (B) Pilomatricoma
     (C) Syringoma
     (D) Trichoblastoma
     (E) Trichilemmoma

113. All of the following are true regarding the lesion shown in Figure 10-23 except

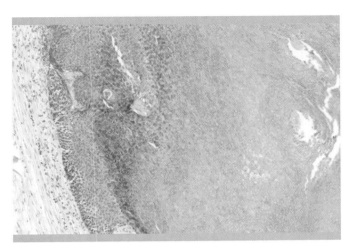

FIGURE 10-23

(A) Calcifications are commonly found
(B) Familial occurrence associated with myasthenia gravis
(C) Majority arise in the first 2 decades of life
(D) Stains positively with beta-catenin
(E) Usually presents as multifocal lesions

114. Which of the following markers will generally stain basal cell carcinoma and not adenoid cystic carcinoma?
(A) Ber-EP4
(B) CAM 5.2
(C) Cytokeratin 7
(D) EMA
(E) S-100 protein

115. The lesion shown in Figure 10-24 is most likely to be located where on the body?

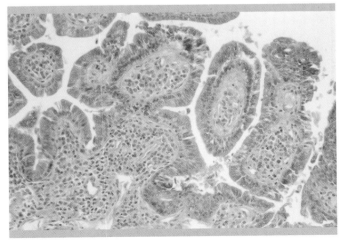

FIGURE 10-24

(A) Arms
(B) Face
(C) Inguinal region
(D) Toes
(E) Trunk

116. The lesion illustrated in Figure 10-25 was excised from the neck of a 62-year-old male. The best diagnosis is which of the following?

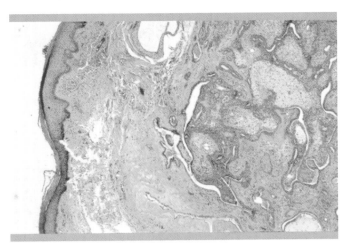

FIGURE 10-25

(A) Benign mixed tumor
(B) Cylindroma
(C) Microcystic adnexal carcinoma
(D) Poroma
(E) Spiradenoma

117. The lesion shown in Figure 10-26 presented in a 76-year-old male in the scrotal area. The lesion demonstrates positive staining with CAM 5.2 and is negative for S-100 protein. The best diagnosis for this lesion is which of the following?

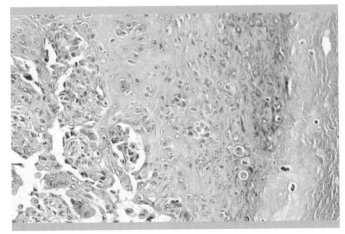

FIGURE 10-26

(A) Extramammary Paget disease
(B) Hidradenocarcinoma
(C) Intraepidermal sebaceous carcinoma
(D) Melanoma
(E) Squamous cell carcinoma in situ

118. All of the following syndromes are associated with lentiginous lesions except
    (A) Carney complex
    (B) Gorlin syndrome
    (C) Laugier–Hunziker syndrome
    (D) Leopard syndrome
    (E) Peutz–Jeghers syndrome

119. All of the following are histologic features characteristic of a dysplastic melanocytic nevus except
    (A) Architectural disorder
    (B) Bridging of nests
    (C) Circumscribed and symmetric lesion
    (D) Single cell proliferation of melanocytes in between rete ridges
    (E) Variation in the size and shape of nests

120. A 12-year-old presents with a red papule on the right cheek. The lesion is marked by a proliferation of large epithelioid and spindled cells with a wedge-shaped and symmetric growth pattern and sharp peripheral borders. Pink globules are noted at the dermal-epidermal junction. The findings are most suggestive of which of the following?
    (A) Dysplastic melanocytic nevus
    (B) Lentigo simplex
    (C) Ordinary compound nevus
    (D) Solar lentigo
    (E) Spitz nevus

121. All of the following are findings associated with a cellular blue nevus except
    (A) Childhood development
    (B) Localization to the reticular dermis
    (C) May lack a nested growth pattern
    (D) Nodular expanded growth pattern
    (E) Prominent mitoses

122. All of the following are clinical features concerning for melanoma except
    (A) Asymmetrical lesion
    (B) Change in appearance
    (C) Irregular border
    (D) Large size (>1 cm)
    (E) Uniform coloration

123. All of the following are risk factors for the development of melanoma except
    (A) Age >50 years
    (B) Multiple seborrheic keratoses
    (C) Pale skin
    (D) Ultraviolet light exposure
    (E) Xeroderma pigmentosum

124. A melanoma that fills and expands the papillary dermis but does not extend to involve the reticular dermis is best designated by which Clark level?
    (A) Clark level I
    (B) Clark level II
    (C) Clark level III
    (D) Clark level IV
    (E) Clark level V

125. Which of the following parameters is the most powerful predictor of prognosis in melanoma?
    (A) Clark level
    (B) Lymphovascular invasion
    (C) Mitotic rate
    (D) Perineural invasion
    (E) Tumor thickness

126. Of the antibodies listed, which has the least specificity for detecting metastatic melanoma in lymph nodes?
    (A) HMB-45
    (B) Melan A (A103/M2-7C10)
    (C) MITF (C5/D5)
    (D) S-100 protein
    (E) TRP-1 (TA-99)

127. All of the following features support a diagnosis of melanoma versus Spitz nevus except
    (A) Confluence of nests along the dermal-epidermal junction
    (B) Lack of maturation
    (C) Mitotic figures
    (D) Rhabdoid features
    (E) Well-demarcated peripheral margin

128. All of the following features support a diagnosis of dermatofibrosarcoma protuberans versus dermatofibroma except
    (A) CD34 positivity
    (B) Foamy histiocytes
    (C) Infiltrative growth
    (D) No collagen trapping
    (E) No epidermal hyperplasia

129. Angiofibromas are associated with which of the following conditions?
    (A) Basal cell nevus syndrome
    (B) Cowden syndrome
    (C) Neurofibromatosis type I
    (D) Sturge–Weber syndrome
    (E) Tuberous sclerosis

130. A 26-year-old male with a left forearm nodule is diagnosed with nodular fasciitis. Of the stains listed, which is the most likely to be positive in this lesion?

(A) Cytokeratins AE1/3
(B) Desmin
(C) HMB-45
(D) Smooth muscle actin
(E) S-100 protein

131. Which of the following lesions is associated with Carney complex?
(A) Basal cell carcinoma
(B) Cutaneous myxoma
(C) Cylindroma
(D) Myofibroma
(E) Neurofibroma

132. Angiomatoid fibrous histiocytoma is associated with all of the following except
(A) Anemia
(B) CD34 positivity
(C) Commonly arises in the extremities
(D) Dense fibrous capsule
(E) Polyclonal gammopathy

133. A 36-year-old female presents with a painless mass arising in the right upper arm. Histologically, the lesion is marked by fibrosis and myxoid stroma composed of spindled to stellate cells. The tumor demonstrates a t(7;16)(q34; p11) translocation. The best diagnosis for this mass is which of the following?
(A) Dermatofibroma
(B) Epithelioid sarcoma
(C) Low-grade fibromyxoid sarcoma
(D) Malignant fibrous histiocytoma
(E) Spindle cell lipoma

134. The lesion shown in Figure 10-27 arises in a 49-year-old male on the leg. The lesion demonstrates positive staining with HHV-8 antibody. The best diagnosis for the lesion is which of the following?

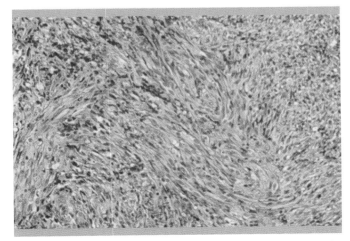

FIGURE 10-27

(A) Angiolymphoid hyperplasia with eosinophilia
(B) Angiosarcoma
(C) Dabska tumor
(D) Epithelioid hemangioendothelioma
(E) Kaposi sarcoma

135. The presence of small intraepidermal aggregates of lymphoid cells called Pautrier microabscesses is characteristic of which of the following?
(A) Chronic eczema
(B) Mycosis fungoides
(C) Psoriasis
(D) Tinea infection
(E) Vitiligo

136. Sézary syndrome associated with cutaneous T cell lymphoma is characterized by all of the following except
(A) Atypical hyperconvoluted cells in the peripheral blood
(B) CD4 positivity in circulating atypical cells
(C) Erythroderma
(D) Lymphadenopathy
(E) T cell clonality by polymerase chain reaction

137. The large atypical mononuclear cells of lymphomatoid papulosis characteristically stain with which of the following?
(A) CD3
(B) CD5
(C) CD7
(D) CD8
(E) CD30

138. Which of the following leukemias accounts for the greatest number of new cases of cutaneous involvement per year?
(A) Acute lymphoblastic leukemia
(B) Acute myeloid leukemia
(C) Chronic lymphocytic leukemia
(D) Chronic myeloid leukemia
(E) Hairy cell leukemia

139. Which of the following markers is most useful in confirming that this lesion is a mastocytoma? (See Figure 10-28.)

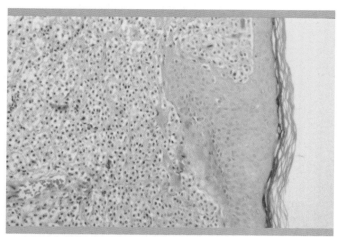

FIGURE 10-28

(A) CD1
(B) CD19
(C) CD30
(D) CD117
(E) CD136

140. All of the following are true regarding Hand–Schüller–Christian disease except
(A) About 80% of patients have cutaneous disease
(B) Birbeck granules are seen in the Langerhans cells
(C) Langerhans cells stain with CD1a
(D) Lytic skull lesions often seen
(E) May develop diabetes insipidus

141. An 8-year-old male presents with a solitary, rubbery, brown-yellow 3 mm papule on the face that is biopsied and shown in Figure 10-29. The lesion demonstrates positive staining with CD68 antibody and does not stain with CD1a and Melan-A antibodies. The best diagnosis is which of the following?

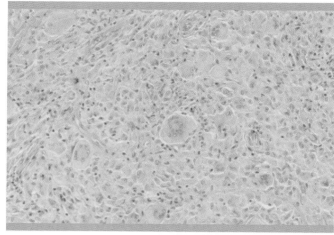

FIGURE 10-29

(A) Balloon cell nevus
(B) Granular cell tumor
(C) Juvenile xanthogranuloma
(D) Langerhans cell histiocytosis
(E) Mastocytoma

142. The lesion shown in Figure 10-30 presented as a yellow papule on the elbow in a patent with hypertension, diabetes, and hypertriglyceridemia/hypercholesterolemia. The best diagnosis is which of the following?

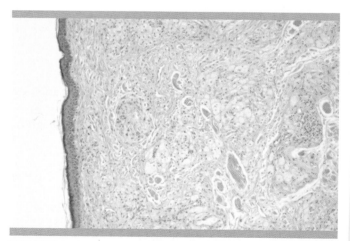

FIGURE 10-30

(A) Histocytosis X
(B) Leishmaniasis
(C) Leprosy
(D) Necrobiotic xanthogranuloma
(E) Xanthoma

143. The lesion shown in Figure 10-31 stains with cyto-keratin CAM 5.2 and is associated with which of the following conditions?

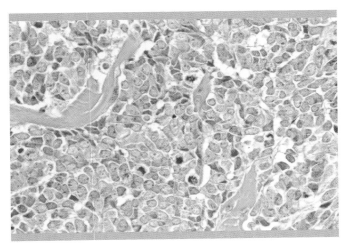

FIGURE 10-31

   (A) Emphysema
   (B) Leukemia
   (C) Organ transplantation
   (D) Pancreatic cancer
   (E) Tuberous sclerosis

144. All of the following are true regarding the lesion seen in Question 143 except
   (A) Chromogranin positive
   (B) Electron dense granules on electron microscopy
   (C) Paranuclear CK20 positivity
   (D) Positive for Merkel cell virus by polymerase chain reaction
   (E) Positive for TTF-1 antibody

145. Which of the following tumors is least likely to metastasize to the skin?
   (A) Breast carcinoma
   (B) Colorectal carcinoma
   (C) Lung carcinoma
   (D) Melanoma
   (E) Pancreatic carcinoma

146. Metastasis to the umbilicus (Sister Mary Joseph nodules) most likely represents spread from cancer in what organ?
   (A) Breast
   (B) Colon
   (C) Pancreas
   (D) Stomach
   (E) Uterus

147. Which of the following immunomarkers would be most useful in distinguishing a cutaneous metastasis from a lung adenocarcinoma versus a breast carcinoma?
   (A) CA125
   (B) CEA
   (C) CK7
   (D) CK8
   (E) TTF-1

148. A metastatic clear cell carcinoma in the skin most likely originates from which of the following primaries?
   (A) Endometrial carcinoma
   (B) Lung carcinoma
   (C) Ovarian carcinoma
   (D) Pancreatic carcinoma
   (E) Renal cell carcinoma

149. Which of the following immunomarkers is least useful in distinguishing a Merkel cell carcinoma from a metastatic pulmonary neuroendocrine carcinoma?
   (A) CK7
   (B) CK20
   (C) MCV (Merkel cell virus)
   (D) Synaptophysin
   (E) TTF-1

150. In differentiating a metastatic small cell neuroendocrine carcinoma from a metastatic neuroblastoma, which of the following immunomarkers would be most useful?
   (A) CD99
   (B) Chromogranin
   (C) Neurofilament protein
   (D) Synaptophysin
   (E) TdT

ANSWERS

1. **(A) CD138 positive.**
   Langerhans cells represent dendritic cells that function in antigen presentation and travel between the skin and adjoining lymph nodes. These cells stain positively with antibodies to S-100 protein and CD1a. Ultrastructurally, they demonstrate evidence of Birbeck granules. They are particularly prominent in allergic contact dermatitis. CD138 is a plasma cell marker and does not stain Langerhans cells.

2. **(B) Eyelid.**
   Specialized apocrine glands are found in the external ear canal ceruminous glands and eyelids (Moll glands).

3. **(D) HMB-45.**
Eccrine glands demonstrate positive staining with antibodies to CAM 5.2, cytokeratin 7, CEA, and EMA. The myoepithelial cell component of the glands can be highlighted with antibodies to S-100 protein, p63, calponin, and smooth muscle actin. Neither component of eccrine glands will stain positively with antibody to HMB-45, which typically targets melanocytic cells.

4. **(B) Erythema multiforme.**
Spongiotic dermatoses represent a variety of lesions including atopic dermatitis, Nummular dermatitis, seborrheic dermatitis, dyshidrosis, allergic contact dermatitis, irritant contact dermatitis, papular dermatitis, and pityriasis rosea. Erythema multiforme does not present typically as a spongiotic dermatitis but belongs to a group of disorders designated as interface dermatitis.

5. **(E) Pityriasis rosea.**
Of the entities listed, a prominent erythrocyte extravasation is most commonly encountered in the setting of pityriasis rosea.

6. **(A) Dermatophytosis.**
Acute allergic contact dermatitis usually manifests as papules, vesicles, or plaques arranged in a linear fashion at the point of contact with the offending agent. Offending agents may include poison ivy, latex, perfumes, certain plants, preservatives, antibiotics, or certain metals such as nickel. Dermatophyte infections are not typically associated with allergic contact dermatitis.

7. **(A) Atopic dermatitis.**
Atopic dermatitis often presents with a history of asthma, allergic rhinitis, or allergic conjunctivitis. It most typically presents in infancy or childhood. The skin is often pruritic before an actual lesion can be visualized. Biopsies are marked by superficial perivascular lymphocytic inflammation, which may be accompanied by follicular spongiosis, dermal eosinophils, and lymphocyte exocytosis. The lesions may show evidence of epidermal hyperplasia and parakeratosis with chronicity. These histologic findings described in this 4-year-old girl are most consistent with that of atopic dermatitis. Pityriasis alba is characterized by hypopigmented scaly patches on the face of dark-complected children. Dyshidrotic dermatitis is characterized by small vesicles, often on fingers and toes, which are typically pruritic. Seborrheic dermatitis is common in adulthood and is marked by soft greasy scale and erythema with preferential involvement of the scalp, eyebrows, nasolabial, and retroauricular skin folds and upper trunk. Psoriasis is marked by hyperplasia with hyperkeratosis, often accompanied by collections of neutrophils.

8. **(A) Epidermal necrosis.**
The lesion described in this 12-year-old male is most consistent with that of pityriasis rosea. Of the histologic features described, epidermal necrosis is not a typical feature of this entity.

9. **(D) Streptococcal pharyngitis.**
The gross features described in this 26-year-old male are consistent with that of a guttate psoriasis. This form of psoriasis is classically associated with streptococcal pharyngitis or other forms of infection.

10. **(A) Antibiotics.**
A variety of treatments can be employed in managing psoriasis. These treatments include vitamin D3 analogs, corticosteroids, retinoids, phototherapy, and a variety of biologic therapies including inhibitors of tumor necrosis factor-alpha, CD2, or CD11a. Antibiotics are generally not employed for the primary management of psoriasis.

11. **(A) Glucagonoma.**
Necrolytic migratory erythema is marked by pronounced pallor of the upper epidermis associated with necrolysis and eventually necrosis. This lesion is usually associated with an islet cell glucagon secreting malignancy or a glucagonoma.

12. **(E) Widespread sloughing of the epidermal surface (>10% of total body surface area).**
Stevens–Johnson syndrome is a generalized severe acute reaction, which is marked by involvement of multiple mucosal sites by lesions with hemorrhagic crusts. The syndrome is usually triggered by recent drug exposure or infection from organisms such as *Mycoplasma pneumoniae*. Widespread sloughing of the epidermal surface involving >10% of the total body surface area is characteristic of toxic epidermal necrolysis, which is the most severe form of the spectrum of erythema multiforme disorders.

13. **(C) Keratinocyte necrosis.**
Fixed drug reactions are histologically marked by vacuolar alterations with single or clustered keratinocyte necrosis. Features that favor fixed drug reaction versus erythema multiforme include psoriasiform epidermal hyperplasia, more prominent spongiosis, and more common involvement of the deep perivascular plexus by an eosinophilic and or neutrophilic infiltrate. Prominent numbers of melanophages may also be evident in a fixed drug reaction.

14. **(B) Lichen planus.**
The histologic findings illustrated in the figure in association with the clinical presentation are most consistent with lichen planus. The lesion typically presents in middle-aged individuals; mucosal involvement is quite common (in up to 75% of

affected individuals). The small fine white lines on the surface of lesions are referred to as Wickham striae. Histologically, the pathology is marked by a band-like lymphocytic infiltrate with associated epidermal hyperplasia, hypergranulosis, sawtoothing of the epidermis, and Civatte bodies (remnants of apoptotic keratinocytes).

15. **(A) Civatte bodies.**

Civatte bodies, which represent remnants of apoptotic keratinocytes, are classically observed in lichen planus. The features listed here are commonly encountered in cutaneous lupus erythematosus. Hyperkeratosis with follicular plugging, basement membrane thickening, and periadnexal lymphocytic infiltrates are more typical of discoid lupus.

16. **(C) Max-Joseph spaces.**

Dermatomyositis may present in either childhood or adulthood. The adult form is associated with an increased incidence of malignancy. Skin lesions are most frequently marked by violaceous poikiloderma. Additionally, a heliotropic rash around the eyes, Gottron papules over the knuckles, ragged cuticles, and calcinosis cutis are all common features of dermatomyositis. A muscle biopsy may demonstrate evidence of perifascicular atrophy accompanied by perivascular chronic inflammation. Max-Joseph spaces represent focal subepidermal clefts formed by confluent vacuoles, typically encountered in the setting of lichen planus.

17. **(D) Grade 3.**

The grading approach that is sometimes used in evaluating acute graft versus host disease involves the presence of vacuolar alterations (grade 1), necrotic keratinocytes (grade 2), subepidermal microvesicles (grade 3), and epidermal separation (grade 4). The absence of epidermal separation with the presence of the other three listed features on biopsy is consistent with a grade 3 acute graft versus host disease.

18. **(D) Pityriasis lichenoides.**

A variety of skin lesions are associated with granulomatous inflammation including sarcoid, granuloma annulare, rheumatoid nodules, necrobiosis lipoidica, foreign body giant cell reaction, infection, or necrobiotic xanthogranuloma. Pityriasis lichenoides is not associated with granulomatous dermatitis.

19. **(B) Granuloma annulare.**

Granuloma annulare typical affects extremities (particularly hands and arms) in children and young adults. The lesions are marked by small papules and plaques and on biopsy demonstrate evidence of palisaded granulomas with interstitial mucin material. Eosinophils are also commonly seen.

20. **(D) HHV-8.**

Kaposi sarcoma is often observed in the setting of immunocompromised individuals in association with HHV-8 infection.

21. **(D) Sweet syndrome.**

Sweet syndrome, also known as acute febrile neutrophilic dermatosis, typically presents in middle-aged adults and may be associated with infection, chronic disease, malignancy, or certain drug exposures. The syndrome typically presents as erythematous plaques, which may be tender but are usually not pruritic. These lesions most commonly involve the head and neck and upper extremity regions, but may be found anywhere. Histologically, these lesions are marked by a dense infiltrate of neutrophils with dermal edema and minimal vascular damage.

22. **(A) Basal cell carcinoma.**

Urticaria is marked by pruritic and erythematous papules or plaques that occur transiently on any part of the body. Urticaria may be associated with a wide variety of exposures including drugs such as aspirin, opiates, or radiocontrast media; infections, particularly parasitic; and foods such as shellfish, nuts, and chocolate. Cold, heat, pressure, or sun exposure induced urticaria is well known to exist. Emotional stress or exercise may induce urticaria and urticaria may be associated with systemic malignancy. Of the conditions listed as optional answers for this question, basal cell carcinoma is least likely to be associated with urticaria.

23. **(A) Lyme disease.**

Erythema migrans or erythema chronicum migrans is the most common cutaneous manifestation of Lyme disease due to an infection by Borrelia burgdorferi. The lesion is characterized by an annular border marked by superficial or deep perivascular chronic inflammation with variable numbers of eosinophils and neutrophils. The overlying epidermis usually looks fairly normal.

24. **(A) A monoclonal kappa or lambda population is present.**

Plasmacytosis mucosae forms a group of noninfectious disorders affecting mucosal surfaces and marked by prominent numbers of plasma cells. Among the lesions that fall under this generally heading include Zoon balanitis and Zoon vulvitis. It usually presents as a solitary lesion with prominent numbers of plasma cells, which would stain with antibody to CD138. Minimal cytologic atypia is evident. The numbers of kappa and lambda staining plasma cells are within normal limits and monoclonal populations are generally not present.

25. **(E) Scleroderma.**
Morphea represents a localized form of scleroderma. Morphea typically presents in adults, although it may occur in children, and usually involves the scalp, trunk, or extremities. The lesion presents as an indurated plaque, which may be erythematous and show pigmentary alterations. Prominent dermal fibrosis extending into the subcutaneous tissue with inflammation at the dermal–subcutaneous junction is typical.

26. **(D) Renal transplantation.**
Nephrogenic systemic fibrosis has classically been associated with acute or chronic renal failure and renal transplantation. The lesions are marked by a proliferation within the dermis of epithelioid and spindled cells with increased collagen fibers and occasional multinucleated giant cells. Over time, the lesions may evolve to resemble a scar.

27. **(B) *Propionibacterium acnes.***
Comedones represent the lesions of acnes vulgaris. They may present as open comedones (black heads) or closed comedones (white heads). *Propionibacterium acnes* is the bacteria usually associated with this lesion.

28. **(D) HIV.**
Eosinophilic folliculitis presents as a prominent eosinophilic infiltrate involving the follicles. One form of this disorder is noted to be associated with HIV infection.

29. **(C) Peanuts.**
Rosacea is usually not the target of a biopsy, since it is clinically easily recognizable. The condition may be worsened by exposure to heat, spicy foods, exercise, hot drinks, and sunlight. Peanuts are generally not typically associated with an exacerbation of this disorder.

30. **(B) Arthropod bite reaction.**
There are a variety of conditions well known to be associated with a lobular pattern of panniculitis. When this is seen and accompanied by prominent number of neutrophils, the differential diagnosis includes infection, ruptured folliculitis or cyst, pancreatic fat necrosis, and alpha-1 antitrypsin deficiency. An arthropod bite reaction typically does not present with a neutrophilic lobular panniculitis.

31. **(A) Erythema nodosa.**
Erythema nodosum represents the most common form of panniculitis. It typically presents in adolescents and young adults, more commonly in women than men, and often involving the lower extremities in a bilateral fashion. The lesion presents as erythematous nodules that are often tender but typically do not ulcerate. Histologically, the pathology is that of a septal panniculitis with variable numbers of granulomas.

32. **(D) Most cases have a clonal T cell population.**
Lupus profundus occurs in approximately 1–3% of patients with discoid and systemic lupus erythematosus. It more commonly affects women who are young and middle-aged. It most commonly involves the trunk and proximal extremities and other sites exposed to trauma. Histologically, the disorder is marked by a lymphocytic lobular panniculitis with prominent numbers of plasma cells and lymphoid follicles. An Alcian blue stain may highlight the presence of stromal mucin. There is usually no detectable clonal T cell population in these cases. The lesion presents as an erythematous tender subcutaneous nodule or plaque.

33. **(E) Tuberculosis.**
Erythema induratum represents a form of lobular panniculitis. This disorder is most commonly associated with tuberculosis, but may be seen with other forms of *Mycobacterium* infection. This disorder classically affects the lower legs and tends to show symmetric involvement. Granulomatous inflammation is a prominent feature of this disorder.

34. **(C) Panniculitis.**
Findings in this biopsy show evidence of a panniculitis. The lesion is marked by prominent numbers of histocytic cells with variable numbers of acute and other chronic inflammatory cells. This particular patient was eventually diagnosed with Weber–Christian disease, which can manifest as a lobular panniculitis. Weber–Christian disease represents an uncommon form of idiopathic panniculitis. Most commonly seen in women, it often is marked by bilateral involvement of the thighs and lower legs.

35. **(E) Type 16.**
Bowenoid papulosis has been associated with HPV 16 and less frequently with other HPV types such as 18, 35, and 39. The lesions typically present as multiple brown-red, small verrucous papules on the genitalia in young adults.

36. **(D) Poxvirus.**
The lesion shown in the figure is marked by acanthotic squamous epithelium with prominent numbers of eosinophilic inclusion bodies known as Henderson–Patterson bodies. These histologic findings are quite consistent with a diagnosis of molluscum contagiosum. This disorder is caused by poxvirus infection. Patients are most commonly children who present with small, centrally umbilicated, pearly papules involving the face and trunk.

37. **(B) Milker nodules.**
Guarnieri bodies are intracytoplasmic eosinophilic inclusion that may be seen in association with parapoxvirus infections such as one may see Milker nodule or orf.

38. **(C) Coxsackie virus.**
    The presentation described in this patient is suggestive of hand-foot-and-mouth disease. This represents a viral exanthem, which can be caused by a variety of enteroviruses but most commonly by Coxsackie virus type A16.

39. **(D) *Cryptococcus*.**
    Small budding fungal organisms arranged in the background of acute and chronic inflammation with readily identifiable histiocytes and occasional giant cells are most consistent with *Cryptococcus*. Cryptococcal organisms typically measure 5–15 microns in diameter (about the size of 1 to 2 red blood cells).

40. **(A) Group A *Streptococcus*.**
    Ecthyma represents a contagious superficial pyogenic infection of the skin. Ecthyma represents ulceration in the setting of impetigo, caused by group A *Streptococcus*.

41. **(B) *Corynebacterium minutissimum*.**
    Erythrasma is a chronic infectious condition involving the intertriginous areas of the skin. It is caused by *Corynebacterium minutissimum*, a gram-positive lipophilic bacteria.

42. **(C) Mite.**
    Rickettsialpox is caused by the organism *Rickettsia akari*, which is transmitted by a mite. Histologically, prominent lymphocytic vasculitis with fibrin thrombi, endothelial cell swelling and extravasation of red blood cells is noted. Marked subepidermal edema with lymphocytic exocytosis is a frequent feature of rickettsialpox.

43. **(B) Caused by *Calymmatobacterium granulomatis*.**
    Lymphogranuloma venereum is a sexually transmitted disease caused by *Chlamydia trachomatis*. *Calymmatobacterium granulomatis* is responsible for causing granuloma inguinale or Donovanosis. The initial presentation of lymphogranuloma venereum is a painless papule, vesicle, or ulcer that resolves in a few days. Several weeks later, a painful regional lymphadenopathy develops with constitutional symptoms. Eventually in the tertiary stage of the disease, ulcers, fistulae, strictures, or lymphedema may develop. A biopsy, if ulceration is present, shows areas of necrosis. Oral antibiotic treatment is effective in managing this infection.

44. **(C) Mycobacteria.**
    The abnormality seen in this biopsy along with the clinical history is consistent with tuberculoid leprosy, which is caused by the organism *Mycobacterium leprae*. The organism is an intracellular obligate, gram-positive, acid-fast organism. Fite and Ziehl–Neelsen stains can be helpful in identifying the organism. Polymerase chain reaction testing is a more sensitive test for the diagnosis. Histologically, tuberculoid leprosy is marked by nonnecrotizing granulomatous inflammation with the presence of well-formed epithelioid granulomas, often surrounded by a rim of benign appearing lymphocytes.

45. **(E) Texas.**
    Leprosy is still predominantly a disease of developing counties, especially in tropical areas. In the United States, it still is encountered in Texas and Louisiana.

46. **(C) Frequently involves the trunk or extremities.**
    Lepromatous leprosy occurs in patients who are immunocompromised or have an absent host immune response. The lesions are typically symmetrical, poorly demarcated, erythematous or hypopigmented macules, patches, and nodules. Earlobes and nasal mucosa are frequently involved because of the lower temperature of these body parts. Peripheral nerves are frequently involved. Because of an association with autoantibody development, there is an increased instance of vitiligo in these patients. Involvement of the trunk or extremities is more commonly encountered in tuberculoid leprosy.

47. **(A) *M. marinum*.**
    So-called fish tank granulomas are classically associated with infection by *M. marinum*. This is the most common nontuberculous *Mycobacterium* to cause skin infections. At the site of trauma and exposure to a water environment, a nodule may form.

48. **(A) Actinomycosis.**
    Cutaneous actinomycosis most commonly presents with cervicofacial involvement, usually associated with poor oral hygiene or a dental extraction, as is the case in this patient. The lesions may become ulcerated and draining abscesses with sulfur granules. The granules are composed of thin filamentous branching bacteria that have a beaded appearance. Deposits may peripherally be associated with eosinophilic material that is referred to as the Hoeppli–Splendore reaction.

49. **(C) Lepromatous leprosy.**
    The biopsy shown in the figure represents an example of lepromatous leprosy, which is typically characterized by a diffuse sheet of histocytic cells. Many of these patients have a history of being immunocompromised. Tuberculoid leprosy is marked more by nonnecrotizing granulomatous inflammation. Histoid leprosy is a rare nodular variant of the lepromatous leprosy that usually develops in long-standing cases and may be related to drug resistance; the clinical history does not appear to fit with this scenario. Erythema nodosum

leprosum is an immune complex-mediated reaction associated with multidrug therapy. The Lucio phenomenon represents a diffuse non-nodular form of lepromatous leprosy, usually observed in Mexican patients and associated with vasculitic changes.

50. **(E) Tertiary syphilis.**
Tertiary syphilis is characterized by the presence of necrotizing granulomatous inflammation. Primary syphilis is marked by ulceration with a prominent lymphoplasmacytic neutrophilic infiltrate. Secondary syphilis is characterized by mixed lichenoid and psoriasiform patterns with prominent numbers of lymphocytes, plasma cells, and neutrophils; granulomas may occasionally be present.

51. **(B) *Microsporum gypseum.***
There are a variety of fungal organisms that are responsible for causing dermatophytosis that can be transmitted from human to human. All of the organisms listed here fall into that category with the exception of *Microsporum gypseum*, which is acquired from contaminated soil exposure (geophilic).

52. **(C) Erythema nodosum.**
Tinea pedis represents a dermatophytosis that typically involves the feet. Differential diagnostic considerations include interdigital erythrasma, *Candida* infection, impetigo, psoriasis, and eczematous dermatitis caused by allergic contact dermatitis, atopic dermatitis, or dyshidrotic dermatitis. Erythema nodosum represents a deeper-seated panniculitis.

53. **(B) Cultured on blood agar plate.**
Tinea versicolor is caused by an infection from *Malassezia furfur*. *Malassezia furfur* represents a lipophilic fungus. Culture conditions in the microbiology laboratory required overlaying oil on the culture plate; simple culturing on a blood agar plate will not grow the organisms. The disorder involves mostly the upper trunk and arms of young adults and presents as well-demarcated macules and patches with variable color. The organism can be seen on hematoxylin and eosin stained sections as a budding yeast and short pseudohyphae. The epidermis typically shows hyperkeratosis and acanthosis with mild perivascular dermal chronic inflammation.

54. **(D) *Pityrosporum.***
All of the organisms listed may be responsible for causing phaeohyphomycosis that represents cutaneous or subcutaneous infection by dematiaceous fungi with pigmented hyphae, except *Pityrosporum. Pityrosporum ovale* is another name for *Malassezia furfur*, which is associated with tinea versicolor.

55. **(C) Fonsecaea.**
The figure shows an inflammatory background marked by the presence of round brown fungal forms, so-called copper pennies. This finding is characteristic of chromomycosis, which is most commonly caused by the organism *Fonsecaea pedrosoi*.

56. **(E) *Paracoccidioides.***
Paracoccidioides is caused by a dimorphic fungus that is endemic in South America (*Paracoccidioides brasiliensis*). Histologically, the organism appears as a Mariner wheel, characterized by a central large yeast form with smaller daughter yeast forms attached by narrow neck buds around the perimeter.

57. **(B) Diabetes.**
The fungal organisms illustrated in the figure are hyphae with broad, ribbon-like, irregular contours. They lack septations and branch at right angles. This morphology is consistent with organisms that cause Zygomycosis. Patients with diabetes are at increased risk of developing infection by this organism, particularly in the periorbital or sinus regions of the head.

58. **(B) Fruiting bodies are commonly seen in skin lesions.**
The figure shows fruiting bodies associated with hyphal forms consistent with *Aspergillus* infection. Although fruiting heads are shown in this figure, they are very unusual in the setting of a skin biopsy. The organism may present as an abscess or with granulomatous inflammation. The hyphae are septated with acute angle branching. Increased risk of infection in patients with burns, wounds, or intravenous catheters is not uncommon. The organism is angioinvasive.

59. **(B) Leishmaniasis.**
Leishmaniasis is an infection caused by a hemoflagellate parasite that is transmitted by a sandfly vector. Typically, organisms are histologically identified within macrophages.

60. **(D) Mite.**
The patient described here is presenting with Demodicosis caused by Demodex, a mite. On biopsy the mite can actually be visualized, often within follicular ostia.

61. **(C) Necrotizing granulomatous inflammation.**
Histologically, scabies typically results in perivascular superficial and deep inflammatory infiltrates with prominent number of eosinophils. The mites that cause scabies (*Sarcoptes scabiei*) or their eggs, larvae, or excreta may be visualized in the stratum corneum. Prominent numbers of eosinophils may be seen. Necrotizing granulomatous inflammation is not

a feature of scabies. The infection is highly conta-
gious, preferentially involves interdigital and flexural
areas, and presents as intensely pruritic papules.

62. **(A) Blastomycosis.**
The biopsy shown in the figure is marked by
large budding yeast forms, many of which
contain a central protoplasmic body. The yeast
measures 15–20 microns in diameter. Infection
by *Blastomyces dermatitidis* is endemic along the
Mississippi and Ohio Rivers, Great Lakes, and
southeast United States. Yeast forms are usually
seen in the background of an abscess.

63. **(B) Myiasis.**
Myiasis represents an infestation of living tissues
by fly larvae or maggots. Larvae may be seen in
the dermis or subcutaneous tissue and are usually
surrounded by a heavy inflammatory infiltrate
marked by prominent numbers of eosinophils and
fibrosis. A larvae is actually shown in this biopsy.
Cimicosis represents an infestation by bedbugs
(*Cimex lectularius*). Bedbugs may be found in
cracks and crevices in walls, furniture, mattresses,
or under carpeting. The bedbugs are usually
active during the night. Pediculosis is due to lice
infestation.

64. **(E) Tungiasis.**
Tungiasis is the result of skin infestation by the
sand flea (*Tunga penetrans*), which is found in Central and South America, India, tropical Africa, and
Pakistan. The flea usually burrows into the skin on
the foot after exposure to contaminated sand.

65. **(C) Onchocerciasis.**
Onchocerciasis is caused by larvae of the
Onchocerca volvulus, which is transmitted via
blackflies in Africa and Central and South America.
The organism is a thread-like worm measuring
0.25–0.45 mm in diameter and 20–50 cm in length.
Microfilariae can be identified in lymphatic vessels
or dermis on biopsy.

66. **(B) 36 hours.**
An optimal time for taking the skin biopsy is
24–48 hours after the appearance of a vasculitic
lesion. Remember, a negative biopsy does not
necessarily rule out a diagnosis of vasculitis, since
the process is often only focally present.

67. **(D) Rickettsial infection.**
Rickettsial and many viral infections are usually
responsible for causing a small vessel lymphocytic
vasculitis. Neutrophilic immune complex mediated
DIF positive vasculitis includes all of the other
entities listed.

68. **(A) Limb claudication.**
Limb claudication, along with asymmetric blood
pressures, absence of pulses, aortic dilatation, and

bruits, is usually associated clinically with large
vessel involvement by vasculitis. All of the other
lesions listed here may be seen in the setting of
small vessel cutaneous vasculitis.

69. **(C) Intraluminal fibrin thrombi.**
The signs of chronic vasculitis or healed lesions of
vasculitis include lamination or onion-skinning of
blood vessel walls, luminal obliteration or endarteritis obliterans, intramural or medial proliferation
of cellular elements resulting in luminal occlusion, segmental or complete loss of elastic lamina
with scar tissue, reactive angioendotheliomatosis,
and neovascularization of vessel adventitia. The
presence of intramural and/or intraluminal fibrin
deposition and/or fibrinoid necrosis are features of
acute vasculitis.

70. **(B) Cryoglobulinemic vasculitis.**
Cryoglobulinemic vasculitis is an example of a type
III immune complex-mediated process. All the other
conditions listed here represent examples of type IV
delayed hypersensitivity vasculitis. Other examples
of type III immune complex-mediated vasculitis
included Henoch–Schönlein purpura, cutaneous
leukocytoclastic angiitis, and polyarteritis nodosa.

71. **(A) C3.**
The most common immunoreactant found in blood
vessels by DIF is C3. Less commonly, IgM, IgA,
IgG, and fibrinogen are noted.

72. **(B) Cryoglobulinemic vasculitis.**
The presence of a prominently IgM vascular
deposits by direct immunofluorescence is most
commonly observed with cryoglobulinemic vasculitis and sometimes with rheumatoid vasculitis.
Henoch–Schönlein purpura may be associated with
IgA vascular deposits.

73. **(E) Wegener granulomatosis (granulomatosis
with polyangiitis).**
Of the diseases listed here, Wegener granulomatosis
most commonly demonstrates evidence of ocular
disease in up to 50–60% of cases.

74. **(D) Rheumatoid vasculitis.**
Evidence of pANCA can be noted in a variety of
vasculitic conditions including microscopic polyangiitis, Churg–Strauss syndrome, polyarteritis
nodosa, and Wegener granulomatosis. In <2% of
cases of rheumatoid vasculitis, pANCA observed.

75. **(D) Lymphoproliferative disorders.**
Paraneoplastic vasculitis is most commonly
observed in the setting of a lymphoproliferative
disorder but may be seen with other types of
malignancy. Paraneoplastic vasculitis should be
considered in patients with evidence of recurrent
purpura and hematologic abnormalities including
cytopenia and monoclonal gammopathy.

76. **(D) Pemphigus.**
    Pemphigus is marked by acantholysis and results in blister formation due to loss of cell-to-cell contact between keratinocytes. In acute allergic contact dermatitis, spongiosis results from intercellular edema, leading to cell separation. Heat and friction can cause physical trauma, resulting in cell-to-cell disruption or death. Bullous pemphigoid is a defect, resulting in basement membrane zone destruction. Polymorphous light eruption results in disruption of the subbasement membrane zone, resulting in dermolysis.

77. **(C) Pemphigus vulgaris.**
    All of the conditions listed here are associated with corneal or subcorneal blistering with the exception of pemphigus vulgaris, which results in suprabasilar blistering. Suprabasilar blistering may also be seen in paraneoplastic pemphigus and Darier disease.

78. **(B) Blockage of eccrine ducts.**
    Miliaria is the result of the blockage of eccrine ducts. This condition usually presents in children, particularly in neonates.

79. **(A) *Staphylococcus aureus*.**
    Bullous impetigo typically effects school-age children and presents as vesicles containing cloudy fluid. The blister often breaks, resulting in erosions and a honey-colored crust. The lesions are contagious and are caused by infection by *Staphylococcus aureus* phage group 2, type 71.

80. **(C) Pemphigus foliaceus.**
    Pemphigus foliaceus is associated with a pathogenic IgG antibody directed against desmoglein 1, a desmosomal cadherin. In pemphigus vulgaris, antibodies are directed against desmoglein 3 but may also be seen targeting desmoglein 1.

81. **(E) X-linked disorder.**
    Darier disease is an autosomal-dominant, not X-linked, disorder associated with mutations in the ATP2A2 gene. The lesions may involve the oral mucosa or seborrheic areas and occasionally the palmoplantar surfaces and nails. They can appear as greasy, crusted, brown keratotic papules. Biopsies are marked by acantholysis and dyskeratosis. Corps ronds represent large acantholytic keratinocytes in the spinous layer. Additionally, corps grains, which are small oval cells in the upper granular cell or corneal layer marked by nuclear pyknosis and shrunken eosinophilic cytoplasm, are also a feature of this disorder.

82. **(B) Hailey–Hailey disease.**
    Hailey–Hailey disease is a benign familial pemphigus condition that has an autosomal-dominant pattern of inheritance and is associated with mutations in ATP2C1. DIF studies are generally negative. The disease typically presents in adulthood and involves intertriginous sites with the development of flaccid blisters. Grover disease is an acquired or nonhereditary condition; therefore, one would not expect to see several family members with the similar disorder.

83. **(E) Salt split skin test.**
    Bullous pemphigoid can be distinguished from epidermolysis bullosa acquisita by utilizing the salt split skin test. In bullous pemphigoid, IgG is deposited on the blister roof or the epidermal side of the split skin. In epidermolysis bullosa acquisita, the immune deposits are located on the floor of the blister.

84. **(E) Vancomycin.**
    Linear IgA bullous dermatosis may be idiopathic or related to drug use. Almost half of drug-induced cases are related to vancomycin use. The disease manifests with clear or hemorrhagic blisters, which may be discrete or arranged in a pattern referred to as the "cluster of jewels sign." Linear IgA deposits are noted at the basement membrane zone.

85. **(B) Gluten-sensitive enteropathy.**
    The findings described in this patient are typical of dermatitis herpetiformis. This disorder is associated with an increased risk of gluten-sensitive enteropathy.

86. **(E) Type VII collagen.**
    Epidermolysis bullosa acquisita is an immunologically mediated bullous disorder resulting from antibodies to type VII collagen. Type VII collagen is a major component of the anchoring fibrils located at the dermal-epidermal junction.

87. **(A) Associated with marked eosinophilic dermal infiltrates.**
    The pathology shown in the figure, along with the clinical history, is suggestive of porphyria cutanea tarda. This disorder results in subepidermal blistering. The dorsum of the hands is the most frequently involved site. Cases may be familial or sporadic, often associated with hepatic injury. Exposure to the sun often elicits a reaction. Histologically, there is minimal or no inflammation. Prominent numbers of eosinophils are not seen. Hyaline deposits around papillary dermal vessels and festooning, which is marked by ridged papillae at the blister base, are noted. IgG deposits may be present at the dermoepidermal junction and the papillary dermis.

88. **(C) Hyperthyroidism.**
    Localized or pretibial myxedema is often associated with hyperthyroidism and may be seen in Graves disease. Histologically, mucin deposition is observed in the mid and lower dermis. The

epidermis may show evidence of hyperkeratosis and follicular plugging.

89. **(A) Gout.**
The lesion illustrated in the figure shows amorphous material corresponding to gout crystals, associated with an adjacent granulomatous reaction. The urate crystals are best visualized after alcohol fixation; formalin fixation will dissolve the needle-like crystals. In pseudogout, the crystals are rhomboid in shape and represent calcium pyrophosphate.

90. **(D) Smoking.**
Of the conditions listed, smoking is not generally associated with the development of gout. Additionally, increased age, obesity, and a history of hypertension or diabetes are also associated with the development of gout.

91. **(C) Findings present at birth.**
The condition illustrated in the figure is marked by the presence of fragmented elastic fibers consistent with pseudoxanthoma elasticum. The finding is usually not present at birth but can develop in childhood or adolescence. The condition is inherited as an autosomal-recessive disorder and is associated with mutations of the ABCC6 gene. Elastic fibers within the eyes and cardiovascular system are also affected by the disease. Skin lesions appear as yellowish papules, especially on the neck and flexural regions. The papules may coalesce to form cobblestone-like plaques.

92. **(B) Neurofibromatosis type I.**
Café-au-lait macules are associated with neurofibromatosis type I and Albright syndrome. Isolated lesions are quite common and may be observed in up to 10–20% of the adult population. The lesions are histologically marked by increased melanin and pigment deposition within basilar keratinocytes.

93. **(C) Corticosteroids.**
A variety of substances are known to be associated with drug-induced hyperpigmentation of the skin. Of the medicines listed as an option, corticosteroids are not known to be associated with hyperpigmentation. Additionally, certain drugs used to treat cancers, antimalarial agents, heavy metals, and hormones may also produce the cutaneous hyperpigmentation.

94. **(E) Present at birth.**
Vitiligo is present in up to 2% of the population and typically presents in late adolescence or young adulthood. There is no gender predilection. The disorder is associated with other autoimmune diseases, particularly of the thyroid gland (Graves disease or Hashimoto thyroiditis) or uveitis. Lesions are marked by decreased melanin pigment and a decreased number of intraepidermal melanocytes. Often, there is a lymphocytic infiltrate at the dermal-epidermal junction.

95. **(D) Tuberous sclerosis.**
The ash-leaf spot of macule is classically associated with tuberous sclerosis. It is often one of the earliest skin findings in tuberous sclerosis and may be present at birth. Histologically, there is a normal distribution of melanocytes in these lesions but a decreased amount of epidermal melanin.

96. **(C) Lupus erythematosus.**
Of the conditions listed here, lupus erythematosus is associated with scarring and is an example of a scarring alopecia. Other examples of scarring alopecia include lichen planopilaris, alopecia mucinosa, classic pseudopelade, and central centrifugal cicatricial alopecia.

97. **(A) 10%.**
Approximately 10–15% of hair is in the telogen or resting phase, which lasts approximately 100 days. Approximately 80–90% of hair is in the anagen or active phase, which lasts from 2 to 7 years. The catagen or involutional phase accounts for approximately 1% of hair and lasts approximately 2–3 weeks.

98. **(A) Lichen planopilaris.**
Lichen planopilaris represents a scarring form of alopecia. The pathology is characterized by hyperkeratotic follicular papules and spines surrounded by mild erythema and accompanied by perifollicular chronic inflammation, which is shown in this illustration. The inflammation is mostly present at the lower portion of the dilatated infundibulum. The disorder is often accompanied by destruction of sebaceous glands.

99. **(B) Follicular cyst of infundibular type.**
Follicular infundibular cysts or epidermoid cysts account for approximately 80% of all cutaneous cysts. These may occur anywhere but are most frequently seen on the face or neck. They present as dermal nodules. The cysts are lined by infundibular type squamous epithelium with a granular cell layer and basket weave stratum corneum. Ruptured cysts may elicit a granulomatous inflammatory reaction.

100. **(A) Epidermoid cyst.**
Epidermoid cysts are known to be associated with both Gardener and basal cell nevus (Gorlin) syndrome.

101. **(A) Cysts have a granular layer.**
The lesion illustrated in the figure is consistent with a steatocystoma multiplex. This cyst

is derived from the sebaceous duct. It typically presents in the second to fourth decades of life, often with onset around puberty. It may have an autosomal-dominant pattern of inheritance in some cases. The solitary cyst form (steatocystoma simplex) usually presents in adulthood. Trunk areas are most commonly involved and patients usually present with flesh colored to yellow papules or nodules. Lesions arise in the dermis. Histologically, the cyst is lined by squamous epithelium that is devoid of a granular cell layer.

102. **(D) Periorbital region.**
Dermoid cysts are usually located in midline areas, particularly in the head and neck region. They usually are present at birth or detected in early childhood. Of the locations listed here, the periorbital region is the most common site of origin.

103. **(C) Seborrheic keratosis.**
The lesion illustrated in the figure represents an example of a seborrheic keratosis. Histologically, it is marked by hyperkeratosis with epidermal thickening and the presence of epidermal keratin cysts. Seborrheic keratosis typically arises in older individuals and can be found almost anywhere on the body except on the palms and soles.

104. **(E) Pilomatricoma.**
Occasionally, other lesions may rise in the background of a seborrheic keratosis. These lesions may include squamous cell carcinoma (usually Bowen disease), basal cell carcinoma, nevi, and melanoma. Pilomatricoma has not been known to generally arise in the background of a seborrheic keratosis.

105. **(E) Squamous cell carcinoma in situ.**
The lesion shown in the figure shows full thickness atypia in the squamous epithelium with disorganized architecture consistent with squamous cell carcinoma in situ.

106. **(B) Impetigo.**
There are a variety of risk factors that have been defined for squamous cell carcinoma in situ. Among these risk factors include UV radiation, immunosuppression via organ transplantation or HIV infection, ionizing radiation, infection with human papilloma virus, exposure to certain chemical carcinogens such as arsenic, chronic inflammatory conditions such as a burn, genetic disorders of DNA repair such as xeroderma pigmentosum, and light skin. Impetigo is generally not thought of as being a significant risk factor for the development of squamous cell carcinoma.

107. **(A) Degree of stromal inflammatory response.**
A variety of risk factors have been identified that predict prognosis in squamous cell carcinoma. Among these predictive parameters include a width of >2 cm, a depth of invasion of >4 mm, lymphovascular or perineural invasion, and poor differentiation. The degree of stromal inflammatory response is generally not been predictive of outcome in these tumors.

108. **(B) CAM 5.2.**
Squamous cell carcinomas may stain with a variety of immunohistochemical markers including cytokeratins AE1/3, EMA, p63, cytokeratins 5/6, MNF-116, and 34βE12. Squamous cell carcinomas typically do not stain with antibodies to cytokeratin CAM 5.2, SMA, S-100 protein, and Ber-EP4.

109. **(B) Keratoacanthoma.**
The lesion shown in the figure represents an example of a keratoacanthoma. The lesion has a cup-shaped architecture with a central keratin plug. The edges extend upward to form the lips of the cup around the perimeter of the keratin plug. This lesion is commonly encountered in elderly individuals. There is an increased risk of developing keratoacanthoma in the setting of UV exposure, exposure to certain chemical carcinogens, in immunosuppressed patients, in patients with a history of trauma, and with HPV infection.

110. **(D) Muir–Torre syndrome.**
Keratoacanthomas have been described arising in association with a number of syndromes including Muir–Torre. Muir–Torre syndrome is also associated with the development of sebaceous tumors and other malignancies. Keratoacanthomas may also be seen arising in the setting of Grzybowski syndrome and Ferguson–Smith syndrome.

111. **(D) More apoptotic bodies.**
The lesion shown in the figure represents a desmoplastic trichoepithelioma. In contrast to sclerosing basal cell carcinomas, desmoplastic trichoepitheliomas are marked by papillary mesenchymal bodies, keratin cysts, absent or mild atypia, and absent or rare mitotic activity. Apoptotic bodies are more likely to be encountered with basal cell carcinoma rather than trichoepithelioma.

112. **(E) Trichilemmoma.**
Tricholemmomas typically arise as solitary lesions on the face of young individuals. A subset of these tumors may be encountered in the setting of Cowden syndrome. The lesion histologically is marked by a dermal nodule composed of small cuboidal keratinocytes with a lobular growth pattern, often associated with a follicle. Clear cell change may be focally present in the lesion.

113. **(E) Usually presents as multifocal lesions.**
The lesion illustrated in the figure represents a pilomatricoma. This lesion typically presents as

a well-circumscribed nodule in the dermis or superficial subcutis. This lesion is composed of basaloid cells with mitotic figures and ghost cells with absent nuclei. An associated foreign body giant cell reaction and calcifications are often noted in these tumors. They usually present as a solitary nodule and are not multifocal. The majority of patients are in their first 2 decades of life. There is an association of pilomatricoma with myasthenia gravis and Gardner syndrome. They show nuclear and cytoplasmic staining with beta-catenin antibody.

114. **(A) Ber-EP4.**
Ber-EP4 stains basal cell carcinomas but generally does not stain adenoid cystic carcinomas. Cyto-keratin 7, CAM 5.2, and EMA do not stain basal cell carcinomas and often stain adenoid cystic carcinomas. S-100 protein is not useful in differential diagnosis.

115. **(B) Face.**
The image shown in the figure represents a syringocystadenoma papilliferum. This lesion is marked by papillary fronds that project into a cystic lumen lined by apocrine-type epithelial cells. It most commonly arises on the scalp or face.

116. **(A) Benign mixed tumor.**
The lesion illustrated in the figure represents a benign mixed tumor of skin or chondroid syringoma. This lesion most often arises on the head and neck in middle-aged or elderly individuals. This tumor consists of a combination of both epithelial duct components with epithelial and myoepithelial cells, as well as a mesenchymal component.

117. **(A) Extramammary Paget disease.**
The lesion illustrated in the figure shows atypical cells located in the surface squamous epithelium consistent with extramammary Paget disease. These cells stain positively with cytokeratin antibodies but are negative for melanoma markers including S-100 protein and melan A. These often arise in elderly individuals in the genital and perianal region, as well as the axilla and eyelids.

118. **(B) Gorlin syndrome.**
There are a variety of conditions associated with lentiginous lesions. Among these conditions are Laugier–Hunziker syndrome, which is marked by mucosal and cutaneous lentigines and melano-nychia; Peutz–Jeghers syndrome, which is associated with hamartomatous gastrointestinal polyps; Carney complex, which is associated with atrial myxomas, mucocutaneous myxomas, and blue nevi; and Leopard syndrome, which is marked by

ECG abnormalities, ocular hypertelorism, pulmonic stenosis, abnormalities of the genitalia, retarded growth, skeletal abnormalities, and deafness. Gorlin syndrome is not associated with lentiginous lesions.

119. **(C) Circumscribed and symmetric lesion.**
Dysplastic melanocytic nevi are associated with architectural disorder, a slight asymmetry, and a slightly irregular border. Focal single cell prolifera-tion of melanocytes along and in between the rete ridges may be present. Nests of cells may vary in size and shape, and bridging fusion of nests may be evident.

120. **(E) Spitz nevus.**
The typical Spitz nevus presents in children and young adults as a pink papule on the face or extremity. These lesions are symmetric and often wedge-shaped with a sharp peripheral border. They are composed microscopically of large spindled and epithelioid cells that show evidence of matura-tion. Pink globules, known as Kamino bodies, may be present in some but not all cases.

121. **(E) Prominent mitoses.**
The cellular blue nevus is a lesion that typically arises on the sacral area, foot, and scalp, usually in childhood. These are well-circumscribed, gray-blue nodules, which are localized to the reticular dermis. They grow in a nodular expansile growth pattern. They generally lack a nested growth pattern and mitotic activity is sparse.

122. **(E) Uniform coloration.**
Clinical features that raise the possibility of a melanoma include asymmetry in the lesion, irregular borders, color variegation, a diameter of >6 mm, and a change in the pigmentation of the lesion.

123. **(B) Multiple seborrheic keratoses.**
Well-established risk factors for the development of malignant melanoma include a family history of melanoma, the presence of numerous melanocytic nevi, light skin, ultraviolet light exposure, age >50 years, and the presence of underlying genetic conditions such as xeroderma pigmentosum. Seborrheic keratoses are not usually thought of as significant risk factor for the development of melanoma.

124. **(C) Clark level III.**
Clark levels are one of the histologic parameters associated with prognosis in melanoma. A Clark level I lesion represents intraepidermal or in situ melanoma. A Clark level II lesion shows partial invasion of the papillary dermis. A Clark level III lesion refers to melanomas that fill and/or expand the papillary dermis. A Clark level IV lesion involves

the reticular dermis. A Clark Level V lesion refers to melanomas that involve the subcutaneous fat or deeper tissues, such as skeletal muscle or bone.

125. **(E) Tumor thickness.**
Tumor thickness, measured with an ocular micrometer, represents the most powerful predictor of prognosis in melanoma. The other features listed as options also represent prognostic features in melanoma.

126. **(D) S-100 protein.**
Of the antibodies listed, S-100 protein has the lowest specificity for the diagnosis of metastatic melanoma to lymph nodes. Of the markers listed, S-100 protein has the highest sensitivity in this setting.

127. **(E) Well-demarcated peripheral margin.**
All of the features listed are features suggestive of melanoma versus Spitz nevus except a well-demarcated peripheral margin. Additionally, melanomas have an asymmetric growth pattern with intraepidermal melanocytic proliferation and ill-defined peripheral demarcation. There is a relative lack of maturation of cells, as the tumor expands. Necrosis of melanocytes and marked nuclear atypia are also features more commonly encountered in melanoma. Melanomas also usually lack the pink globules that are frequently seen in Spitz nevus.

128. **(B) Foamy histiocytes.**
The presence of foamy histiocytes is more commonly encountered in dermatofibroma versus dermatofibrosarcoma protuberans. The other features listed are more typical of dermatofibrosarcoma protuberans.

129. **(E) Tuberous sclerosis.**
Angiofibromas represent lesions that appear as flesh-colored papules, usually in childhood, involving the central face and nasolabial folds. These lesions are characterized by ectatic blood vessels embedded in a collagenous stroma. They are associated with tuberous sclerosis and are referred to as adenoma sebaceum in this setting.

130. **(D) Smooth muscle actin.**
Of the stains listed here, nodular fasciitis is most likely to demonstrate some positive staining with antibody to smooth muscle actin. Nodular fasciitis also shows vimentin immunoreactivity. Nodular fasciitis does not characteristically stain with antibodies to desmin, cytokeratins, and S-100 protein.

131. **(B) Cutaneous myxoma.**
Cutaneous myxomas may arise as sporadic lesions or in association with Carney complex. Carney complex represents an autosomal-dominant condition associated with abnormalities on chromosomes 2p and 17q. Patients with Carney complex

also develop cardiac myxomas, spotty pigmentation, endocrine overactivity, and psammomatous melanotic schwannomas.

132. **(B) CD34 positivity.**
Angiomatoid fibrous histiocytoma usually arises on the extremities in young patients. They frequently are accompanied by systemic symptoms including fever and weight loss. These lesions are marked by a dense fibrous capsule with lymphoid aggregates at the periphery and by a proliferation of histocytic to spindled cells with blood-filled pseudovascular spaces. They usually demonstrate positive staining with antibodies to EMA, desmin, and CD68. They may be associated with polyclonal gammopathy and anemia.

133. **(C) Low-grade fibromyxoid sarcoma.**
The lesions described in this case are suggestive of a low-grade fibromyxoid sarcoma. These commonly arise as painless intramuscular masses on the extremities or trunk in young- to middle-aged adults. They may on occasion arise in the superficial subcutis or dermis. They are characterized by alternating fibrous to myxoid stroma, and marked by bland spindled to stellate cells. These lesions commonly demonstrate t(7;16)(q34;p11).

134. **(E) Kaposi sarcoma.**
The lesion shown in the figure is marked by a proliferation of spindled cells with slit-like vascular lumens. Extravasated red blood cells are commonly noted, and lymphocytes and plasma cells may be seen at the periphery. Positive staining with antibody to HHV-8 is characteristic of this lesion.

135. **(B) Mycosis fungoides.**
Mycosis fungoides represents the most common form of cutaneous T cell lymphoma. The lesion is marked by band-like lymphocytic infiltrate with a proliferation of atypical lymphocytic cells. The cells generally are CD4 positive and may show loss of CD7. Small aggregates of intraepidermal lymphocytes, referred to as Pautrier microabscesses, are commonly encountered in this lesion.

136. **(B) CD4 positivity in circulating atypical cells.**
Sézary syndrome represents a leukemic form of cutaneous T cell lymphoma. Patients usually present with erythroderma, lymphadenopathy, and neoplastic cells in the skin, blood, and lymph nodes. Many of the circulating cells demonstrate loss of T cell antigens including loss of markers CD2, CD3, CD4, and CD5. T cell clonality can be demonstrated by polymerase chain reaction. Atypical hyperconvoluted cells may be evident in the peripheral circulation.

137. **(E) CD30.**
Lymphomatoid papulosis may occur at any age, but has a peak incidence in middle-aged adults.

Patients present with small papules, which appear in crops. The lesions are marked by wedge-shaped infiltrate associated with epidermal hyperplasia and ulceration. In many forms of this disease, large cells, which may be positive for CD30, are observed in the lesion. The inflammatory infiltrate often consists of small lymphocytes, neutrophils, and variable numbers of eosinophils.

138. **(C) Chronic lymphocytic leukemia.**
Chronic lymphocytic leukemia represents the leukemia type that has the greatest number of new cases of cutaneous involvement diagnosed each year. This is closely followed by acute myeloid leukemia.

139. **(D) CD117.**
The lesion shown in the figure represents a mastocytoma, which is a mass composed of mast cells. Cells sometimes have a granular cytoplasm with a fried egg appearance. Mast cells will stain with antibodies to CD117 and tryptase and may also be highlighted with stains such as sulfated alcian blue, Giemsa, and toluidine blue.

140. **(A) About 80% of patients have cutaneous disease.**
Hand–Schüller–Christian disease is typically a disorder of older children characterized by osteolytic skull lesions, hypopituitarism, diabetes insipidus, and exophthalmos. Skin lesions are only evident in about a third of cases, not 80%. These lesions are marked by the presence of Langerhans cells, which may stain positively with antibodies to CD1a and S-100 protein. Ultrastructurally, Birbeck granules may be evident in the Langerhans cells.

141. **(C) Juvenile xanthogranuloma.**
The biopsy shown in the figure is consistent with juvenile xanthogranuloma. The biopsy shows a dermal infiltrate of mononuclear cells with abundant eosinophilic or foamy cytoplasm. Occasional Touton giant cells are present. These lesions usually present in childhood and involve skin from the upper part of the body. The lesions stain with antibodies to histocytic markers such as CD68 or HAM56 and do not stain with Langerhans cell marker CD1a or melanoma marker melan A.

142. **(E) Xanthoma.**
The lesion shown in the figure histologically is marked by an increased number of bland foamy histiocytes in the dermis. This lesion is often associated with hypercholesterolemia, dyslipoproteinemia, and hypertriglyceridemia.

143. **(C) Organ transplantation.**
The lesion shown in the figure histologically is consistent with a Merkel cell carcinoma. This is typically present in older adults, who are often immunosuppressed via infection or organ transplantation. Merkel cell carcinomas often involve the head and neck or extremity region and prognosis depends on their stage and histologic parameters such as evidence of lymphatic spread.

144. **(E) Positive for TTF-1 antibody.**
The lesion shown in Question 143 represents a Merkel cell carcinoma. This lesion ultrastructurally demonstrates electron dense granules. It demonstrates dot-like immunoreactivity with antibodies to certain cytokeratin markers such as cytokeratin 20 and CAM 5.2. It will stain with neuroendocrine markers such as synaptophysin and chromogranin. It does not stain with TTF-1 antibody, which is more commonly encountered with neuroendocrine lung carcinomas. Positivity for Merkel cell virus by polymerase chain reaction can be demonstrated in up to 80% of these tumors.

145. **(E) Pancreatic carcinoma.**
Of the tumors listed here, the one that is least likely to metastasize to the skin is pancreatic carcinoma.

146. **(D) Stomach.**
Metastases to the umbilicus have been termed Sister Mary Joseph nodules. The underlining primary tumor is most commonly a gastric adenocarcinoma, but occasionally carcinomas from other primary sites, including many of those listed as other options in this question, may result in this manifestation of cutaneous metastasis.

147. **(E) TTF-1.**
In differentiating between cutaneous metastases from a lung adenocarcinoma and breast carcinoma, TTF-1 would be most useful, in that many lung adenocarcinomas will demonstrate positive staining with TTF-1 and most breast carcinomas will not stain with TTF-1. Both lung and breast may stain with antibodies to cytokeratin 8, cytokeratin 7, variably with CEA and occasionally with CA125.

148. **(E) Renal cell carcinoma.**
A metastatic clear cell carcinoma to the skin, although it may come from a variety of sites of origin, most commonly represents a metastatic clear cell renal cell carcinoma.

149. **(D) Synaptophysin.**
Of the antibodies listed, synaptophysin may demonstrate positive staining in both Merkel cell carcinoma and metastatic pulmonary neuroendocrine carcinoma. Cytokeratin 7 is generally positive in lung cancer and not Merkel cell carcinoma, and cytokeratin 20 is more commonly positive in Merkel cell carcinoma and not lung cancer. TTF-1 immunoreactivity is seen in lung cancer, and MCV or Merkel cell virus antibody staining is a feature of most Merkel cell tumors.

150. **(B) Chromogranin.**

In differentiating a metastatic small cell neuroendocrine carcinoma from a metastatic neuroblastoma, the most useful marker of those listed would be chromogranin; small cell neuroendocrine carcinomas generally stain positively and neuroblastomas do not stain. Both tumors may stain with a neurofilament protein antibody and synaptophysin. Both tumors generally do not stain with antibodies to CD99 and TdT.

SUGGESTED READING

1. Ahmed AR. Diagnosis of bullous disease and studies in the pathogenesis of blister formation using immunopathological techniques. *J Cutan Pathol*. 1984;11:237-248.
2. Ahmed I, Piepkon MW, Rabkin MS, et al. Histopathologic characteristics of dysplastic nevi. Limited association of conventional histologic criteria with melanoma risk group. *J Am Acad Dermatol*. 1990;22:727-733.
3. Anhalt GJ. Paraneoplastic pemphigus. *Adv Dermatol*. 1996;12:77-96.
4. Antman K, Chang Y. Kaposi's sarcoma. *N Engl J Med*. 2000;342:1027-1038.
5. Bataille V. Genetics of familial and sporadic melanoma. *Clin Exp Dermatol*. 2000;25:464-470.
6. Betti R, Inselvini E, Carducci M, et al. Age and site prevalence of histologic subtypes of basal cell carcinomas. *Int J Dermatol*. 1995;34:174-176.
7. Binder SW, Asnong C, Paul E, et al. The histology and differential diagnosis of Spitz nevus. *Semin Diagn Pathol*. 1993;10:36-46.
8. Boyd AS, Nelder KH. Lichen planus. *J Am Acad Dermatol*. 1991;25:593-619.
9. Breathnach SM. Amyloid and amyloidosis. *J Am Acad Dermatol*. 1988;18:1-16.
10. Brownstein MH, Shapiro L. Desmoplastic trichoepithelioma. *Cancer*. 1977;40:2979-2986.
11. Busam KJ (ed.). *Dermatopathology*. Philadelphia, PA: Saunders Elsevier; 2010.
12. Cancrini C, Angelini F, Colavita M, et al. Erythema nodosum: a presenting sign of early onset sarcoidosis. *Clin Exp Rheumatol*. 1998;16:337-339.
13. Chan JK, Suster S, Wenig BM, et al. Cytokeratin 20 immunoreactivity distinguishes Merkel cell (primary cutaneous neuroendocrine) carcinomas and salivary gland small cell carcinomas from small cell carcinomas of various sites. *Am J Surg Pathol*. 1997;21:226-234.
14. Churg J, Churg A. Idiopathic and secondary vasculitis: a review. *Mod Pathol*. 1989;2:144-160.
15. Clemente C, Cochran AJ, Elder DE, et al. Histopathologic diagnosis of dysplastic nevi: concordance among pathologists convened by the World Heath Organization Melanoma Programme. *Hun Pathol*. 1991;22:313-319.
16. Cohen PR, Kurzock R. Sweet's syndrome and cancer. *Clinics Dermatol*. 1993;11:149-157.
17. Cooper PH. Angiosarcomas of the skin. *Semin Diagn Pathol*. 1987;4:2-17.
18. Cribier B, Caille A, Heid E, et al. Erythema nodosum and associated diseases. A study of 129 cases. *Int J Dermatol*. 1998;37:667-672.
19. Dabski K, Winkelmann RK. Generalized granuloma annulare: clinical and laboratory findings in 100 patients. *J Am Acad Dermatol*. 1989;20:39-47.
20. Darmstadt GL, Lane AT. Impetigo: an overview. *Pediatr Dermatol*. 1994;11:293-303.
21. del Carmen Farina M, Gezundez I, Pique E, et al. Cutaneous tuberculosis: a clinical, histopathologic, and bacteriologic study. *J Am Acad Dermatol*. 1995;33:433-440.
22. Dineen AM, Dicken CH. Scleromyxedema. *J Am Acad Dermatol*. 1995;33:37-43.
23. Epstein JH. Polymorphous light eruption. *Dermatol Clin*. 1986;4:243-251.
24. Epstein JH, Tuffanelli DL, Epstein WL. Cutaneous changes in the porphyrias. A microscopic study. *Arch Dermatol*. 1973;107:689-698.
25. Ferrara JLM, Deeg HJ. Graft-versus-host disease. *N Engl J Med*. 1991;324:667-674.
26. Gemmell CG. Staphylococcal scalded skin syndrome. *J Med Microbiol*. 1995;43:318-327.
27. Hall RP. Dermatitis herpetiformis. *J Investig Dermatol*. 1992;99:873-881.
28. Hassab-el Naby HM, Tam S, White WL Jr, et al. Mixed tumors of the skin. A histological and immunohistochemical study. *Am J Dermatopathol*. 1989;11:413-428.
29. Headington JT. Tumors of the hair follicle. A review. *Am J Pathol*. 1976;85:479-514.
30. Helwig EB. Eccrine acrospiroma. *J Cutan Pathol*. 1984;11:415-420.
31. Johnson TM, Rowe DE, Nelson BR, et al. Squamous cell carcinoma of the skin (excluding lip and oral mucosa). *J Am Acad Dermatol*. 1992;26:467-484.
32. Kamino H, Jacobson M. Dermatofibroma extending into the subcutaneous tissue. Differential diagnosis from dermatofibrosarcoma protuberans. *Am J Surg Pathol*. 1990;14:1156-1164.
33. Koulu L, Stanley JR. Clinical, histologic, and immunopathologic comparison of pemphigus vulgaris and pemphigus foliaceus. *Semin Dermatol*. 1988;7:82-90.
34. Kovacs SO, Kovacs SC. Dermatomyositis. *J Am Acad Dermatol*. 1998;39:899-920.
35. Lloyd J, Flanagan AM. Mammary and extramammary Paget's disease. *J Clin Pathol*. 2000;53:742-749.
36. Love JR, Dubin HV. Xanthomas and lipoproteins. *Cutis*. 1978;21:801-805.
37. Mambo NC. Eccrine spiradenoma: clinical and pathologic study of 49 tumors. *J Cutan Pathol*. 1983;10:312-320.
38. Mahood JM. Erythema annulare centrifugum: a review of 24 cases with special reference to its association with underlying disease. *Clin Exp Dermatol*. 1983;8:383-387.
39. Marrogi AJ, Dehner LP, Coffin CM, et al. Benign cutaneous histiocytic tumors in childhood and adolescence, excluding Langerhans' cell proliferations. A clinicopathologic and immunohistochemical analysis. *Am J Dermatopathol*. 1992;14:8-18.

40. Mehregan DA, Van Hale HM, Muller SA. Lichen planopilaris: clinical and pathologic study of forty-five patients. *J Am Acad Dermatol.* 1992;27:935-942.
41. Mihm MC, Clark WH, Reed RJ, et al. Mast cell infiltrates of the skin and the mastocytosis syndrome. *Hum Pathol.* 1973;4:231-239.
42. Munn S, Chu AC. Langerhans cell histiocytosis of the skin. *Hematol Oncol Clin North Am.* 1998;12:269-286.
43. Powell FC, Su WPD, Perry HO. Pyoderma gangrenosum: classification and management. *J Am Acad Dermatol.* 1996;34:395-409.
44. Radentz WH, Vogel P. Congenital common blue nevus. *Arch Dermatol.* 1990;126:124-125.
45. Ralfkiaer E. Immunohistological markers for the diagnosis of cutaneous lymphomas. *Semin Diagn Pathol.* 1991;8:62-72.
46. Requena L, Sangüeza OP. Cutaneous vascular proliferation. Part II. Hyperplasias and benign neoplasms. *J Am Acad Dermatol.* 1997;37:887-919.
47. Requena L, Sangüeza OP. Cutaneous vascular proliferations. Part III. Malignant neoplasms, other cutaneous neoplasms with significant vascular component, and disorders erroneously considered as vascular neoplasms. *J Am Acad Dermatol.* 1998;38:143-175.
48. Rigel DS, Rivers JK, Kopf AW, et al. Dysplastic nevi. Markers for increased risk for melanoma. *Cancer.* 1989;63:386-389.
49. Sangüeza OP, Salmon JK, White CR Jr, et al. Juvenile xanthogranuloma: a clinical, histopathologic and immunohistochemical study. *J Cutan Pathol.* 1995;22:327-335.
50. Santa Cruz DJ. Sweat gland carcinomas: a comprehensive review. *Semin Diagn Pathol.* 1987;4:38-74.
51. Sehgel VN. Leprosy. *Dermatologic Clinics.* 1994;12:629-644.
52. Shapiro PE, Pinto FJ. The histologic spectrum of mycosis fungoides/Sezary syndrome (cutaneous T-cell lymphoma). A review of 222 biopsies, including newly described patterns and the earliest pathologic changes. *Am J Surg Pathol.* 1994;18:645-667.
53. Skelton HG, Smith KJ, Laskin WB, et al. Desmoplastic malignant melanoma. *J Am Acad Dermatol.* 1995;32:717-725.
54. Taylor RM. Histopathology of contact dermatitis. *Clin Dermatol.* 1986;4:18-22.
55. Tellechea O, Reis JP, Baptista AP. Desmoplastic trichilemmoma. *Am J Dermatopathol.* 1992;14:107-104.
56. Thivolet J, Barthelemy H. Bullous pemphigoid. *Semin Dermatol.* 1988;7:91-103.
57. Tonneson M, Soter NA. Erythema multiforme. *J Am Acad Dermatol.* 1979;1:357-364.
58. Vanatta PR, Bangert JL, Freeman RG. Syringocystadenoma papilliferum. A plasmacytotropic tumor. *Am J Surg Pathol.* 1985;9:678-683.
59. Wade TR, Ackerman AB. The many faces of seborrheic keratoses. *J Dermatol Surg Oncol.* 1979;5:378-382.
60. Webster G. Seborrheic dermatitis. *Int J Dermatol.* 1991;30:843-844.
61. Weedon D, Little JH. Spindle and epithelioid cell nevi in children and adults. A review of 211 cases of the Spitz nevus. *Cancer.* 1977;40:217-225.
62. Weyers W, Euler M, Diaz-Cascajo C, et al. Classification of cutaneous malignant melanoma: a reassessment of histopathologic criteria for the distinction on different types. *Cancer.* 1999;86:288-299.
63. Wick MR, Goeliner JR, Wolfe JT 3rd, et al. Adnexal carcinomas of the skin. I. Eccrine carcinomas. *Cancer.* 1985;56:1147-1162.
64. Wick MR, Mills SE. Intravascular lymphomatosis: clinicopathologic features and differential diagnosis. *Semin Diagn Pathol.* 1991;8:91-101.
65. Willemze R. Lymphomatoid papulosis. *Dermatol Clin.* 1985;3:735-747.
66. Yammamoto T, Ohkubo H, Nishioka K. Skin manifestations associated with rheumatoid arthritis. *J Dermatol.* 1995;22:324-329.
67. Zackheim HS, McCalmont TH. Mycosis fungoides: the great imitator. *J Am Acad Dermatol.* 2002;47:914-918.
68. Zelickson BD, Muller SA. Generalized pustular psoriasis. A review of 63 cases. *Arch Dermatol.* 1991;12:1339-1345.
69. Zitelli JA, Grant MG, Abell E, et al. Histologic patterns of congenital nevocytic nevi and implications for treatment. *J Am Acad Dermatol.* 1984;11:402-409.

CHAPTER 11

ENDOCRINE PATHOLOGY

1. A 45-year-old woman has a pancreatic body mass that is excised. Amorphous pink material is present, entrapping the neoplastic cells (see Figure 11-1). Congo red staining is positive within this material. What is the most likely hormone secreted by this tumor?

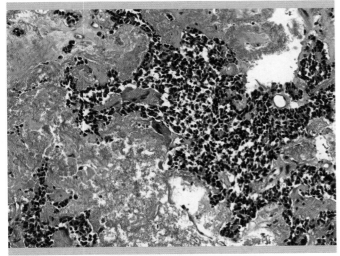

FIGURE 11-1

(A) Glucagon
(B) Insulin
(C) Pancreatic polypeptide
(D) Somatostatin
(E) Vasoactive intestinal polypeptide

2. A 75-year-old man has a large pancreatic mass on imaging. No other lesions are identified in the chest or abdomen. A biopsy is performed (see Figure 11-2). The tumor has a high mitotic rate, with over 35 mitotic figures per 10 high-power fields. Immunohistochemical staining for synaptophysin and chromogranin are positive within the neoplastic cells. What is the best diagnosis for this lesion?

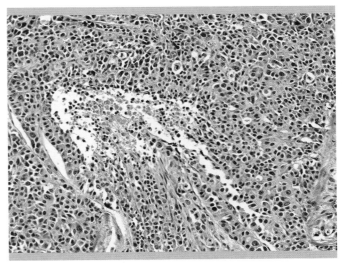

FIGURE 11-2

(A) Metastatic small cell undifferentiated carcinoma of the lung
(B) Pancreatic neuroendocrine carcinoma, large cell type
(C) Pancreatic neuroendocrine tumor, grade 1
(D) Pancreatic neuroendocrine tumor, grade 2
(E) Pancreatic neuroendocrine tumor, grade 3

3. A 55-year-old man has a 3 cm pancreatic body mass that is biopsied (see Figure 11-3). All of the following immunohistochemical stains would be positive in this tumor except

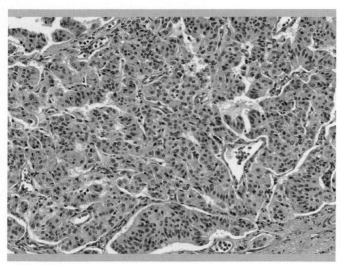

FIGURE 11-3

(A) β-catenin (nuclear)
(B) CD56
(C) Chromogranin
(D) Cytokeratin
(E) Synaptophysin

4. The photomicrograph demonstrates a section of normal adrenal gland. What is the main secretory product of the cells at the arrows (see Figure 11-4)?

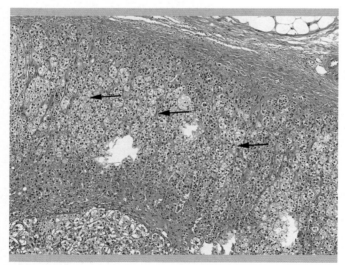

FIGURE 11-4

(A) Aldosterone
(B) Cortisol
(C) Epinephrine
(D) Estrogen
(E) Testosterone

5. A 17-year-old high school student presents with severe neck pain, photophobia, fevers, and confusion. He is hospitalized with a presumptive diagnosis of bacterial meningitis. Several hours later, he develops severe hypotension and shock, along with purpura of the skin, and dies. At autopsy, his adrenals have the following appearance (see Figure 11-5). These findings are consistent with what clinical syndrome?

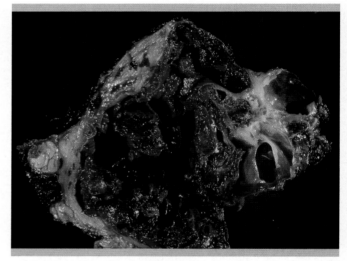

FIGURE 11-5

(A) Addison disease
(B) Beckwith–Wiedemann syndrome
(C) Cushing disease
(D) Cushing syndrome
(E) Waterhouse–Friderichsen syndrome

6. A 50-year-old woman has a computed tomography (CT) scan, and an incidental 4 cm unilateral adrenal mass is identified. Adrenalectomy is performed, and the mass has the following appearance (see Figure 11-6). What is the most likely diagnosis?

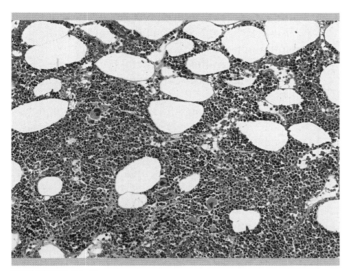

FIGURE 11-6

(A) Adrenal cortical adenoma
(B) Adrenal cortical carcinoma
(C) Angiomyolipoma
(D) Myelolipoma
(E) Pheochromocytoma

7. A 52-year-old man presents with progressive central obesity, skin striae, and a round face ("moon facies"). His adrenal gland has the following gross appearance (see Figure 11-7). What is the most likely cause of his symptoms?

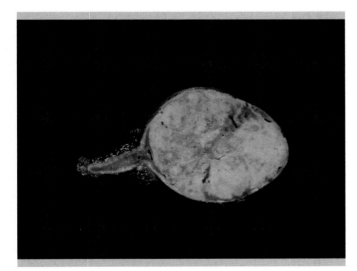

FIGURE 11-7

(A) Adrenocorticotropic hormone (ACTH)-secreting pituitary adenoma
(B) Aldosterone-secreting adrenal cortical adenoma
(C) Cortisol-secreting adrenal cortical adenoma
(D) Pheochromocytoma
(E) Primary pigmented nodular adrenocortical disease

8. A 51-year-old man with medication-resistant hypertension and hypokalemia is found to have an adrenal mass. Excision of his adrenal gland demonstrates a well-circumscribed yellow-tan nodule arising from the adrenal cortex. Microscopic examination demonstrates round, eosinophilic inclusions with the cytoplasm of the neoplastic cells (see Figure 11-8). What medication was he most likely treated with prior to surgery?

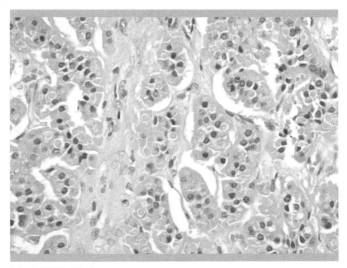

FIGURE 11-8

(A) Angiotensin-converting enzyme inhibitor
(B) β-blockers
(C) Furosemide
(D) Prednisone
(E) Spironolactone

9. A 57-year-old woman presents with flank pain, and a 12 cm left adrenal mass is found. Adrenalectomy is performed (see Figure 11-9). Which of the following findings is not a predictor of malignancy in this tumor?

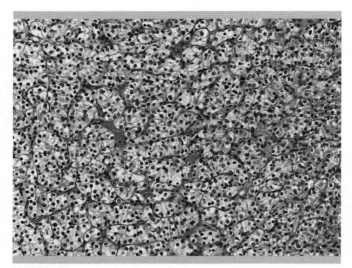

FIGURE 11-9

(A) Atypical mitotic figures
(B) Invasion of other anatomic structures (e.g., kidney)
(C) Mitotic rate >6 mitotic figures per 10 high-power fields
(D) Nuclear pleomorphism and hyperchromasia
(E) Vascular invasion

10. A 45-year-old man presents with hypertension and episodes of palpitations, headaches, and diaphoresis. An adrenal mass is discovered on imaging, and the resection has the following appearance (see Figure 11-10). All of the following statements are true regarding this lesion except

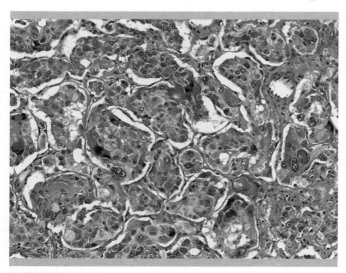

FIGURE 11-10

(A) 10% of patients will have bilateral tumors
(B) Associated with *RET* gene gain-of-function mutation
(C) Derived from the adrenal medulla
(D) Distant metastasis can occur late (>20 years after diagnosis)
(E) Vascular invasion is diagnostic of malignancy

11. A 14-year-old boy presents with double vision and headaches. CT scan demonstrates a suprasellar mass that is partially calcified. The lesion is removed, and has the following appearance (see Figure 11-11). What is the best diagnosis?

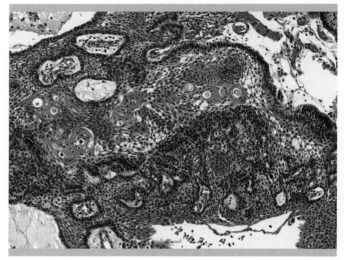

FIGURE 11-11

(A) Craniopharyngioma
(B) High-grade glioma
(C) Meningioma
(D) Metastatic squamous cell carcinoma
(E) Pituitary adenoma

12. A 32-year-old woman undergoes pituitary biopsy. A reticulin stain is performed on the biopsy specimen (see Figure 11-12). This reticulin staining pattern is most consistent with what diagnosis?

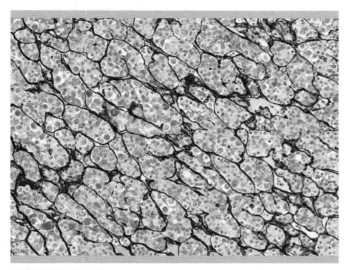

FIGURE 11-12

(A) Brain glial tissue
(B) Normal anterior pituitary
(C) Pituitary adenoma
(D) Pituitary infarction
(E) Posterior pituitary

13. A patient with elevated serum levels of parathyroid hormone is found to have four enlarged abnormal parathyroid glands at surgery, which have the following appearance (see Figure 11-13). All of the following processes are a possible cause of these changes except

FIGURE 11-13

(A) Chronic renal failure
(B) Lithium therapy
(C) Multiple endocrine neoplasia type 1
(D) Parathyroid carcinoma
(E) Vitamin D deficiency

14. A 60-year-old woman is diagnosed with primary hyperparathyroidism. At neck exploration, a 1.0 cm mass in the region of the right upper parathyroid is excised (see Figure 11-14). All of the following stains will be positive in this lesion except

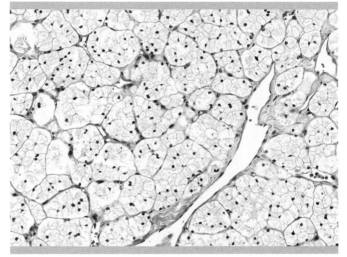

FIGURE 11-14

(A) Chromogranin
(B) Cytokeratin
(C) Parathyroid hormone
(D) Periodic acid Schiff without diastase
(E) Renal cell carcinoma (RCC) antigen

15. A 53-year-old man presents with primary hyperparathyroidism. At surgery, a single abnormal appearing parathyroid gland is found, which weighs 2.5 g and measures 1.8 cm in greatest dimension. The other three parathyroid glands are normal in size and appearance. After excision, the intraoperative parathyroid hormone levels drop within the normal range. A portion of the abnormal parathyroid gland is submitted to pathology (see Figure 11-15). What is the best diagnosis for this lesion?

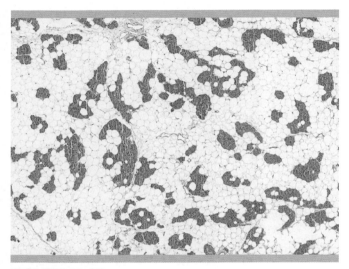

FIGURE 11-15

(A) Normal parathyroid gland
(B) Parathyroid adenoma
(C) Parathyroid hyperplasia
(D) Parathyroid lipoadenoma
(E) Water-clear cell hyperplasia

16. A 25-year-old woman presents with a midline cystic neck mass, which is excised (see Figure 11-16). All of the following statements are true regarding this lesion except

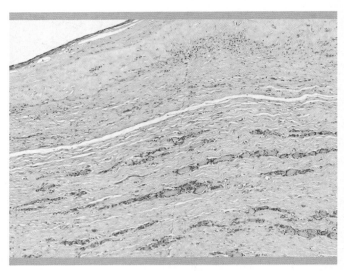

FIGURE 11-16

(A) Clinically moves upward with swallowing
(B) Contain C-cells that can undergo malignant transformation
(C) Papillary thyroid carcinoma is the most common malignancy to arise from this lesion
(D) Removal of the hyoid bone is necessary to prevent recurrence
(E) Thyroid tissue in the cyst wall is variable

17. An 18-year-old girl presents with heat intolerance, weight loss, sweating, and palpitations. Her thyroid gland is diffusely enlarged and undergoes excision, with the following appearance (see Figure 11-17). What is the underlying mechanism of her disease?

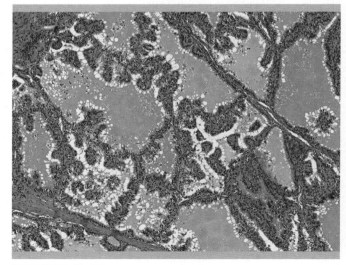

FIGURE 11-17

(A) Autonomously hyperfunctioning hyperplastic nodule
(B) Nonstimulating autoimmune antibodies against thyroid antigens
(C) Stimulating autoimmune antibodies against the thyroid-stimulating hormone (TSH) receptor
(D) T-cell mediated destruction of thyroid tissue
(E) Viral infection leading to excess thyroid hormone release

18. A 75-year-old man presents with hoarseness and a rapidly enlarging neck mass. Physical examination demonstrates an enlarged and firm thyroid gland. An incisional biopsy is performed (see Figure 11-18). Which of the following statements is true regarding this lesion?

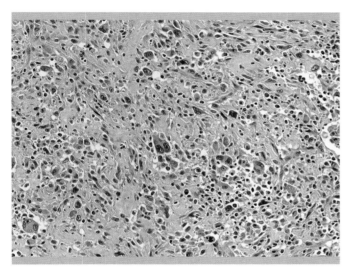

FIGURE 11-18

(A) Immunohistochemical expression of thyroglobulin is present in over 90% of cases
(B) Locally aggressive tumor but rarely develops distant metastasis
(C) Median overall survival is 20 months
(D) Most commonly arises from a preexisting medullary thyroid carcinoma
(E) Tumors confined to the thyroid gland are staged as T4a disease

19. A 34-year-old woman undergoes thyroid resection for a thyroid nodule, which has the following appearance (see Figure 11-19). What genetic syndrome is this lesion associated with?

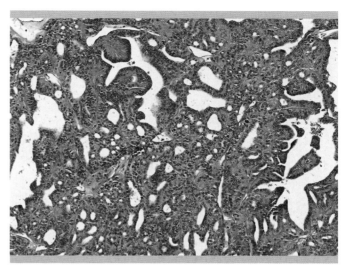

FIGURE 11-19

(A) Cowden syndrome (*PTEN* gene mutation)
(B) Familial adenomatosis polyposis (FAP)
(C) Hereditary nonpolyposis colorectal carcinoma (HNPCC) syndrome
(D) Multiple endocrine neoplasia type 1 (MEN 1)
(E) Multiple endocrine neoplasia type 2a (MEN 2a)

20. A 63-year-old woman has a 4.5 cm thyroid mass that is resected (see Figure 11-20). Examination of the capsule demonstrates lymphovascular space invasion. All of the following statements are true regarding this lesion except

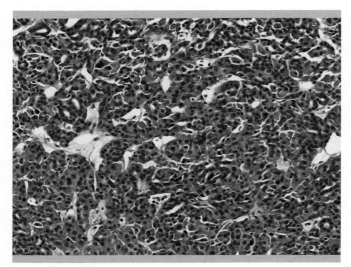

FIGURE 11-20

(A) Abundant eosinophilic cytoplasm is composed of lysosomes
(B) Calcification of colloid can mimic psammoma bodies
(C) Criteria for malignancy are similar to conventional follicular carcinoma
(D) Immunohistochemical staining for thyroid transcription factor 1 (TTF-1) will be positive
(E) More commonly develops lymph node metastasis than conventional follicular carcinoma

21. A 58-year-old man presents with a thyroid mass. At total thyroidectomy, a 3.5 cm poorly circumscribed mass involving the right thyroid lobe is identified (see Figure 11-21). What is the best diagnosis for this tumor?

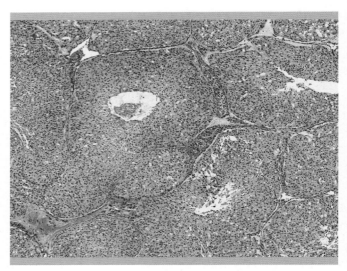

FIGURE 11-21

(A) Follicular adenoma
(B) Follicular carcinoma
(C) Papillary thyroid carcinoma, solid variant
(D) Poorly differentiated thyroid carcinoma
(E) Undifferentiated (anaplastic) thyroid carcinoma

22. A 39-year-old woman with a thyroid nodule undergoes thyroid resection, and the operative note states the thyroid was easily removed without involvement of the thyroid cartilage or recurrent laryngeal nerve. A 1.2 cm papillary thyroid carcinoma is found at histopathologic examination, with the following finding (see Figure 11-22). What is the best tumor stage for this carcinoma?

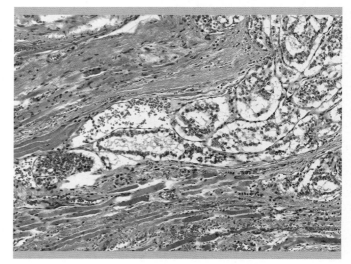

FIGURE 11-22

(A) pT1a
(B) pT1b
(C) pT2

(D) pT3
(E) pT4a

23. A thyroid mass has the following appearance
    (see Figure 11-23). Which of the following
    immunohistochemical stains will not be positive
    in the neoplastic cells?

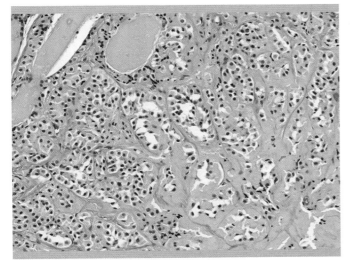

FIGURE 11-23

(A) Calcitonin
(B) Carcinoembryonic antigen (CEA)
(C) Cytokeratin
(D) Thyroglobulin
(E) TTF-1

24. A 59-year-old man presents with a 5.0 cm thyroid
    mass. Total thyroidectomy is performed (see
    Figure 11-24). What is the best diagnosis?

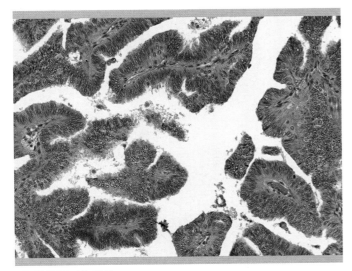

FIGURE 11-24

(A) Medullary thyroid carcinoma
(B) Metastatic endometrioid adenocarcinoma
(C) Columnar cell variant of papillary thyroid
    carcinoma
(D) Cribriform-morular variant of papillary thyroid
    carcinoma
(E) Poorly differentiated thyroid carcinoma

25. A 45-year-old woman has a thyroid gland excised
    for a solitary well-circumscribed 1.5 cm nodule that
    has the following appearance (see Figure 11-25).
    No capsular or vascular invasion is identified.
    Immunohistochemical staining for thyroglobulin is
    positive. What is the best diagnosis for this lesion?

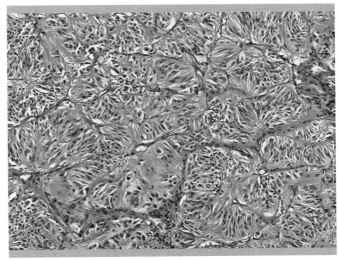

FIGURE 11-25

(A) Follicular adenoma
(B) Follicular carcinoma
(C) Hyalinizing trabecular tumor
(D) Medullary thyroid carcinoma
(E) Tall cell variant of papillary thyroid carcinoma

26. A 62-year-old woman presents with hypothyroidism.
Physical exam demonstrates an enlarged, hard,
fixed thyroid gland. At the time of surgery, the
process involving the thyroid gland extends into the
surrounding strap muscles and perithyroidal fat, so
only an incisional biopsy is performed (see Figure
11-26). What is the best diagnosis for this process?

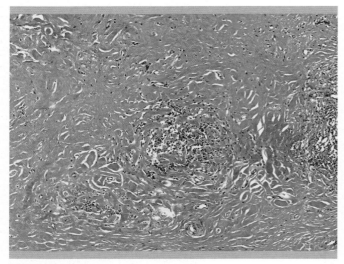

FIGURE 11-26

    (A) Anaplastic thyroid carcinoma
    (B) Graves disease
    (C) Hashimoto thyroiditis
    (D) Diffuse sclerosing variant of papillary thyroid
        carcinoma
    (E) Riedel's disease

27. A 51-year-old woman presents with a painful neck
mass, palpitations, weight loss, and heat intolerance.
Clinical exam demonstrates a diffusely enlarged and
tender thyroid gland. A biopsy is performed (see
Figure 11-27). What is the best diagnosis?

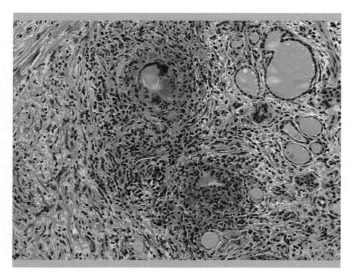

FIGURE 11-27

    (A) Chronic lymphocytic thyroiditis
    (B) Graves disease
    (C) Palpation thyroiditis
    (D) Sarcoidosis
    (E) Subacute thyroiditis

28. A 41-year-old woman has hypothyroidism. A biopsy
of her thyroid gland is shown in Figure 11-28. All
of the following statements are true regarding this
process except

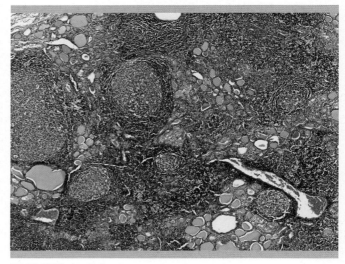

FIGURE 11-28

    (A) Associated with antithyroglobulin antibodies
    (B) More common in men than women
    (C) Oncocytic (Hürthle cell) metaplasia of follicular
        epithelium is characteristic
    (D) Patients with this disorder have an increased
        risk of other autoimmune diseases
    (E) This disease is a risk factor for the develop-
        ment of papillary thyroid carcinoma

29. A 55-year-old man undergoes radical neck dissection for squamous cell carcinoma of the tonsil. A lymph node from the right lateral level 4 shows the following finding (see Figure 11-29). What is most likely explanation for this finding?

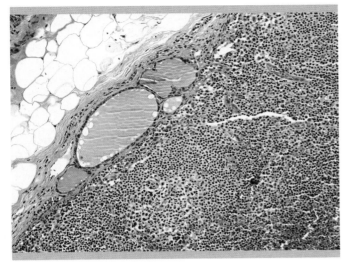

FIGURE 11-29

(A) Embryonic remnant of thyroid tissue within lymph node capsule
(B) Iatrogenic disruption of normal thyroid tissue with lymph node embolization
(C) Normal lymph node with prominent vascular structures in the hilum
(D) Occult papillary thyroid carcinoma with lymph node metastasis
(E) Squamous cell carcinoma metastasis with variant morphology

30. A 47-year-old man undergoes thyroid lobectomy for a thyroid nodule. Upon gross evaluation, a single 3.5 cm nodule with a thick fibrous capsule is present in the thyroid lobe, and a frozen section has the following appearance (see Figure 11-30). How should sections be taken to exclude malignancy?

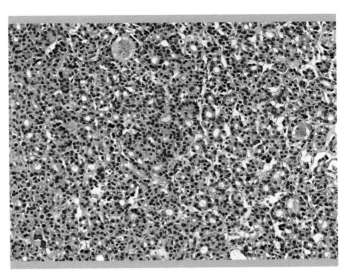

FIGURE 11-30

(A) No additional sections are needed; the frozen section is diagnostic
(B) Submit representative sections of the nodule in relationship to adjacent thyroid tissue
(C) Submit representative sections of the nodule in relationship to the margins of resection
(D) Submit the entire fibrous capsule of the nodule and random sections of uninvolved thyroid tissue
(E) Submit two random sections of nodule and the remaining uninvolved thyroid gland

31. A 19-year-old man presents with a thyroid mass. At resection, the tumor is composed of densely packed bland spindle cells that merge with gland-like structures, and are positive for cytokeratin and negative for thyroglobulin, TTF-1, and calcitonin. What is the most likely diagnosis?
(A) Carcinoma showing thymus-like differentiation (CASTLE)
(B) Papillary thyroid carcinoma, solid variant
(C) Poorly differentiated thyroid carcinoma
(D) Spindle epithelial tumor with thymus-like differentiation (SETTLE)
(E) Undifferentiated (anaplastic) thyroid carcinoma

32. A 37-year-old woman with acne undergoes thyroid resection. The thyroid cut surface is diffusely black in color. What medication was she taking?
(A) Clindamycin
(B) Isotretinoin
(C) Minocycline
(D) Oral contraceptives
(E) Salicylic acid

33. A 62-year-old man presents with diarrhea and severe peptic ulcer disease. His symptoms do not improve despite maximal medical therapy. A pancreatic tumor is found on imaging. What is the most likely hormone to be produced by this tumor?
    (A) Gastrin
    (B) Glucagon
    (C) Insulin
    (D) Somatostatin
    (E) Vasoactive intestinal peptide

34. At autopsy, examination of the pancreas demonstrates diffuse islet cell hyperplasia. Which of the following clinical scenarios is a likely cause of this finding?
    (A) A 1-week-old baby girl exposed to uncontrolled maternal diabetes
    (B) A 14-year-old girl with new diagnosis of type 1 diabetes
    (C) A 48-year-old woman with an insulin-secreting pancreatic endocrine neoplasm
    (D) A 53-year-old obese woman with a new diagnosis of type 2 diabetes
    (E) A 72-year-old woman on a short steroid taper for rheumatoid arthritis

35. A 13-year-old girl is diagnosed with type 1 diabetes. Histologic examination of her pancreas would show what pathologic change?
    (A) Acinar atrophy and fibrosis
    (B) Amyloid deposition within the islets
    (C) Dystrophic calcification and fat necrosis
    (D) Increased number of islets
    (E) Infiltration of islet cells by T-lymphocytes

36. In an experimental mouse model, a researcher is able to selectively destroy all of the α-cells within the pancreatic islet cells, but leaves all other cell types intact. What hormone will this mouse be unable to produce?
    (A) Glucagon
    (B) Insulin
    (C) Pancreatic polypeptide
    (D) Somatostatin
    (E) Vasoactive intestinal polypeptide

37. A 75-year-old man undergoes a distal pancreatectomy for a pancreatic neuroendocrine tumor. All of the following pathologic features would favor an excellent prognosis except
    (A) Confined to the pancreas
    (B) Ki-67 proliferative index of 3%
    (C) Mitotic rate of 1 mitotic figure per high-power field

    (D) No angiolymphatic invasion
    (E) Size 1.8 cm

38. A newborn baby has ambiguous genitalia, and within 2 weeks develops dehydration, hyponatremia, hyperkalemia, and vomiting. Ultrasound shows enlarged adrenal glands bilaterally. What is the most common cause of this syndrome?
    (A) 17-alpha-hydroxylase deficiency
    (B) Autoimmune adrenalitis
    (C) Cushing disease
    (D) 21-hydroxylase deficiency
    (E) X-linked congenital adrenal hypoplasia

39. A 74-year-old man with clear cell renal cell carcinoma has a nodule is present in the ipsilateral adrenal gland composed of cells with abundant clear cytoplasm. Which of the following immunohistochemical stains, if positive, would favor a diagnosis of adrenal cortical adenoma?
    (A) Calretinin
    (B) Chromogranin
    (C) Cytokeratin 7
    (D) HMB-45
    (E) Renal cell carcinoma (RCC) antigen

40. A 47-year-old man presents with slowly progressive fatigue, weakness, and skin hyperpigmentation. Serologic studies show low levels of cortisol and aldosterone, which do not increase when exogenous adrenocorticotropic hormone (ACTH) is administered. All of the following are possible causes of this disease except
    (A) Acquired immunodeficiency syndrome (AIDS)
    (B) Autoimmune adrenalitis
    (C) Disseminated tuberculosis infection
    (D) Metastasis to the adrenal glands
    (E) Pituitary infarction

41. Pheochromocytomas are highly associated with all of the following syndromes except
    (A) Hereditary paraganglioma-pheochromocytoma syndrome
    (B) Multiple endocrine neoplasia 1 (MEN 1)
    (C) Multiple endocrine neoplasia 2a (MEN 2a)
    (D) Multiple endocrine neoplasia 2b (MEN 2b)
    (E) von Hippel–Lindau disease (VHL)

42. A 42-year-old woman is diagnosed with an adrenal cortical adenoma. All of the following statements are true regarding adrenal cortical adenomas except
    (A) Are grossly well circumscribed with a smooth border
    (B) If hyperfunctional, most commonly produce aldosterone

(C) Incidentally discovered adenomas are usually not hyperfunctional
(D) Typically weigh <100 g
(E) Virilization or feminization is a good prognostic sign

43. A cross section of a large adrenal mass is soaked in a potassium dichromate solution, and turns a dark blue-black color. This color change favors what diagnosis?
(A) Adrenal cortical adenoma
(B) Adrenal cortical carcinoma
(C) Metastatic melanoma
(D) Pheochromocytoma
(E) Tuberculosis infection

44. Which of the following hormones is released from the posterior pituitary?
(A) Adrenocorticotropic hormone (ACTH)
(B) Antidiuretic hormone (ADH)
(C) Corticotropin-releasing hormone (CRH)
(D) Growth hormone (GH)
(E) Thyroid stimulating hormone (TSH)

45. A 32-year-old woman presents with amenorrhea and bilateral white breast discharge. No breast lesions are palpated, and a pregnancy test is negative. What is the most likely finding on an MRI scan of the brain?
(A) An empty sella turcica
(B) Glioblastoma
(C) Pituitary macroadenoma
(D) Pituitary microadenoma
(E) Subarachnoid hemorrhage

46. A patient on glucocorticoids for multiple medical problems dies in the intensive care unit. An autopsy is performed, and examination of the otherwise normal pituitary shows scattered cells containing a ring of cytoplasmic pale-pink amorphous material around the nucleus, which is positive for low molecular weight cytokeratin immunohistochemical stain. What hormone would these cells normally secrete?
(A) Adrenocorticotropic hormone (ACTH)
(B) Growth hormone (GH)
(C) Luteinizing hormone (LH)
(D) Prolactin (PRL)
(E) Thyroid stimulating hormone (TSH)

47. A 37-year-old pregnant woman goes through a difficult home labor and delivery, which results in significant postpartum hemorrhage. Two weeks later, she calls her midwife about problems breastfeeding, and reports that her breast milk still has not "come in." What is the most likely cause of her inability to breastfeed?
(A) Cushing syndrome
(B) Poor hydration
(C) Prior breast surgery
(D) Prolactin-secreting pituitary adenoma
(E) Sheehan syndrome

48. A 55-year old man is found to have a pituitary adenoma. Serologic studies show elevated levels of insulin-like growth factor 1 (IGF-1). What clinical symptoms did he most likely present with?
(A) Bilateral galactorrhea
(B) Changing facial features and large hands with sausage-like fingers
(C) Erectile dysfunction and fatigue
(D) Obesity and abdominal striae
(E) Very tall with disproportionately long arms and legs

49. A diagnosis of pituitary carcinoma requires which of the following findings?
(A) Direct invasion of bone or brain
(B) Discontinuous subarachnoid space deposits
(C) >10 mitotic figures per 10 high-power fields
(D) Marked nuclear pleomorphism
(E) Tumor necrosis

50. All of the following are features of an atypical pituitary adenoma except
(A) Diffuse nuclear staining for p53
(B) Increased mitotic activity
(C) Ki-67 index of >3%
(D) Microscopic bone invasion
(E) Microscopic dura invasion

51. A 52-year-old woman presents with a lytic lesion of the jaw, which on biopsy shows bone resorption and replacement by fibrous tissue and osteoclast-like giant cells. She also has recently been diagnosed with kidney stones and osteopenia. A serum calcium level is 12.4 mg/dL. What is the most likely cause of her symptoms?
(A) Four gland parathyroid hyperplasia
(B) Hypoparathyroidism
(C) Osteomalacia (vitamin D deficiency)
(D) Parathyroid adenoma
(E) Renal failure

52. A newborn baby girl with congenital heart disease develops convulsions and tetany shortly after birth. A serum calcium level is low. Chest x-ray shows an absent thymus gland. What is the most likely cause of her clinical findings?
    (A) DiGeorge syndrome
    (B) Down syndrome
    (C) Iatrogenic hypoparathyroidism
    (D) Multiple endocrine neoplasia type 1
    (E) X-linked familial hypoparathyroidism

53. A patient with hypercalcemia undergoes a neck exploration, and a parathyroid gland is excised. Which of the following features would favor a solitary adenoma over multiple gland hyperplasia?
    (A) All four glands appear abnormal
    (B) Circumscribed hypercellular nodule with a rim of atrophic parathyroid tissue
    (C) Gland weight over 0.5 g
    (D) Oil red O staining shows reduced intracellular fat
    (E) Recurrent hyperparathyroidism within 2 years

54. A 52-year-old woman presents with severe hyperparathyroidism, and a calcium of 14.8 mg/dL. In the operating room, the surgeon identifies a single, enlarged parathyroid gland that is difficult to excise. Which of the following histopathologic findings would support a diagnosis of parathyroid carcinoma?
    (A) Diffuse or solid growth pattern
    (B) Fibrosis
    (C) Increased mitotic activity
    (D) Immunohistochemical staining with para-fibromin
    (E) Vascular space invasion

55. A 45-year-old woman is undergoing parathyroid exploration for primary hyperparathyroidism. A biopsy is submitted for frozen section evaluation, and the surgeon is uncertain whether the tissue represents abnormal parathyroid gland tissue or a portion of thyroid parenchyma. Which of the following findings would only be seen in thyroid tissue?
    (A) Interspersed fibroadipose tissue
    (B) Microfollicular architecture
    (C) Oxalate crystals
    (D) Rim of normal parathyroid gland
    (E) Two cell types (oxyphil and chief cell)

56. A 32-year-old woman with severe hypothyroidism is pregnant. What disorder is her fetus at risk for developing if she is not treated?

    (A) Congenital heart disease
    (B) Limb defects
    (C) Neural tube defects
    (D) Renal agenesis
    (E) Severe mental retardation

57. A 42-year-old woman presents with fatigue, weight gain, cold intolerance, and loss of appetite. Serum laboratory testing demonstrates low T3 and T4 levels, and an elevation in thyroid stimulating hormone (TSH). All of the following are potential causes of these findings except
    (A) Chronic lymphocytic thyroiditis
    (B) History of radiation therapy to the neck
    (C) Iodine deficiency
    (D) Pituitary infarction
    (E) Total thyroidectomy

58. All of the following statements regarding diffuse sclerosing variant of papillary thyroid carcinoma are true except
    (A) Approximately 20% of patients will have lymph node metastasis at diagnosis
    (B) Associated with severe chronic lymphocytic thyroiditis
    (C) Excellent long-term prognosis despite aggressive behavior
    (D) Most common in young adults
    (E) Requires diffuse involvement of at least one thyroid lobe by carcinoma

59. All of the following histologic changes can be seen in a thyroid nodule after a previous fine-needle aspiration biopsy except
    (A) Artifactual displacement or implantation of tumor with vascular lumens
    (B) Complete infarction of the thyroid nodule
    (C) Irregular capsular contour suggestive of capsular invasion (capsular pseudoinvasion)
    (D) Nuclear enlargement, chromatin clearing, and nuclear pseudoinclusions
    (E) Proliferation of bland spindle cells with abundant mitotic figures (postoperative spindle cell nodule)

60. What is the most common primary malignant neoplasm of the thyroid gland in countries with adequate dietary iodine?
    (A) Follicular adenoma
    (B) Follicular carcinoma
    (C) Medullary thyroid carcinoma
    (D) Papillary thyroid carcinoma
    (E) Primary thyroid lymphoma

61. What is the most common molecular alteration found in tall cell variant of papillary thyroid carcinoma?
    (A) *BRAF* point mutation
    (B) *PAX8/PPAR-γ* translocation
    (C) *RAS* point mutation
    (D) *RET* point mutation
    (E) *RET/PTC* translocation

62. A minimally invasive follicular carcinoma is defined as having which of the following features?
    (A) Invasion into adjacent normal thyroid parenchyma
    (B) Invasion into large caliber vessels
    (C) Invasion into less than one-third of the tumor capsule
    (D) Invasion into perithyroidal structures
    (E) Invasion into small caliber vessels within the tumor capsule

63. All of the following are features of poorly differentiated thyroid carcinomas except
    (A) Classic nuclear features of papillary thyroid carcinoma
    (B) Convoluted nuclei
    (C) Increased mitotic activity (3 or more mitotic figures per 10 high-power fields)
    (D) Solid or insular growth pattern
    (E) Tumor necrosis

64. A 54-year-old woman presents with a diffusely enlarged and firm thyroid gland. She has a history of chronic lymphocytic thyroiditis, and the surgeon is concerned for a primary thyroid lymphoma. Which of the following pathologic features, if present, would favor a diagnosis of malignant lymphoma over chronic lymphocytic thyroiditis?
    (A) Lymphoepithelial lesions involving thyroid epithelium
    (B) Polytypic B-cells lacking kappa or lambda light chain restriction
    (C) Preserved architecture of the thyroid gland
    (D) Prominent germinal centers containing tingible body macrophages.
    (E) Sharp borders between lymphoid infiltrates and perithyroidal soft tissue

65. All of the following nuclear changes are typically seen in papillary thyroid carcinoma except
    (A) Fine chromatin
    (B) Grooves
    (C) Macronucleoli
    (D) Nuclear enlargement
    (E) Pseudoinclusions

66. Examination of a thyroid gland demonstrates an increase in C-cells. All of the following statements are true regarding nodular (neoplastic) C-cell hyperplasia except
    (A) Associated with multiple endocrine neoplasia 2 (MEN 2)
    (B) C-cells must remain confined within the basement membrane of thyroid follicles
    (C) Defined as nodular foci of C-cells filling or partially destroying thyroid follicles, usually over 50 cells
    (D) Requires immunohistochemistry with calcitonin for identification in most cases
    (E) *RET* gene mutations can be demonstrated in these cells

67. A 31-year-old woman is diagnosed with adrenocortical insufficiency, and if biopsied, her adrenal gland would likely show changes of autoimmune adrenalitis (see Figure 11-31). She notices patchy increased skin pigmentation around her knuckles and elbows. What is the cause of her skin hyperpigmentation?

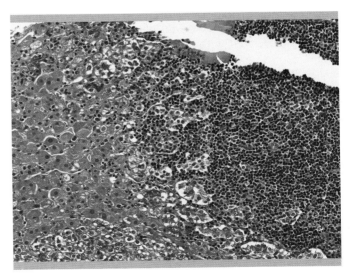

FIGURE 11-31

    (A) Excess aldosterone production
    (B) Excess melanocyte-simulating hormone
    (C) Hemochromatosis
    (D) Malignant melanoma
    (E) Melasma

68. A 61-year-old woman presents with a cold thyroid nodule. A resection is performed (see Figure 11-32). All of the following statements are true regarding this lesion except

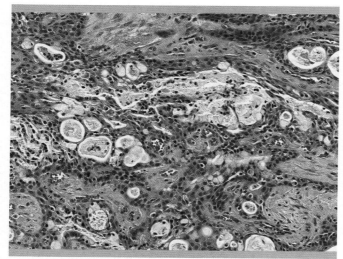

FIGURE 11-32

(A) Histologically indistinguishable from similar tumor of salivary glands
(B) Immunohistochemical staining for thyroglobulin is focally positive in the nonsclerosing type
(C) Likely derived from salivary gland inclusions within the thyroid gland
(D) Mucicarmine stain is positive in the goblet cell component
(E) The sclerosing variant with eosinophilia is associated with chronic lymphocytic thyroiditis

69. A 71-year-old man undergoes PET scan during follow-up for a diagnosis of renal cell carcinoma 12 years ago, and a thyroid mass is identified. He undergoes thyroid lobectomy, which contains a well-circumscribed nodule with the following appearance (see Figure 11-33). What is the most helpful feature in differentiating a primary thyroid neoplasm from metastatic renal cell carcinoma?

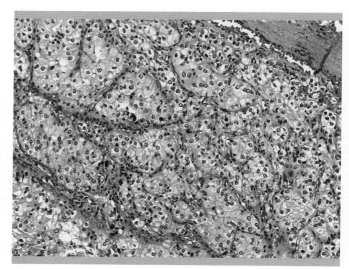

FIGURE 11-33

(A) Absence of colloid
(B) Absence of thyroglobulin staining
(C) Clear cytoplasm
(D) Papillary structures
(E) Solitary well-circumscribed nodule

70. A 23-year-old man presents with a thyroid mass. At total thyroidectomy, a 3.5 cm mass is found with the following appearance (see Figure 11-34). What genetic mutation is most likely present in the tumor cells?

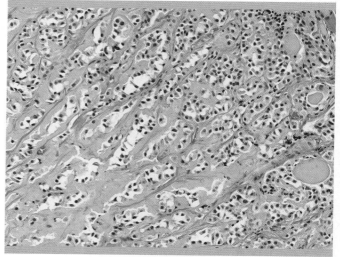

FIGURE 11-34

(A) *BRAF* point mutation
(B) *RAS* point mutation
(C) *RET* activating point mutation
(D) *RET* inactivating point mutation
(E) *RET/PTC* translocation

71. A 42-year-old woman presents with episodes of confusion and loss of consciousness, which are precipitated by exercise. Drinking orange juice results in immediate improvement. A blood glucose level during one of these episodes is 38 mg/dL, along with elevated C-peptide levels. What is the most likely cause of her fainting spells?
(A) Diabetes mellitus type 1
(B) Diffuse hyperplasia of the islets of the pancreas
(C) Factitious hypoglycemia
(D) Glucagon-secreting pancreatic endocrine neoplasm
(E) Insulin-secreting pancreatic endocrine neoplasm

72. All of the following are features of a pancreatic neuroendocrine microadenoma except
(A) Associated with multiple endocrine neoplasia type 1 when multiple microadenomas are present
(B) Clinically functional, most commonly causing hyperinsulinemia
(C) Immunohistochemical staining restricted to one or two pancreatic hormones
(D) Low mitotic rate (<10 mitotic figures per 10 high-power fields)
(E) Size <0.5 cm

73. The most common neoplasm responsible for an adrenal mass is
(A) Adrenal cortical adenoma
(B) Adrenal cortical carcinoma
(C) Metastatic carcinoma
(D) Myelolipoma
(E) Pheochromocytoma

74. The anterior pituitary is derived from what embryologic structure?
(A) First branchial arch
(B) Neural tube
(C) Notochord
(D) Rathke's pouch
(E) Second branchial cleft

75. What two anterior pituitary hormones would a mammosomatotroph cell pituitary adenoma express?
(A) Adrenocorticotropic hormone and growth hormone
(B) Adrenocorticotropic hormone and prolactin
(C) Follicle stimulating hormone and thyroid stimulating hormone
(D) Growth hormone and prolactin
(E) Prolactin and thyroid stimulating hormone

76. A 49-year-old man presents with paresthesias, tetany, convulsions, and a prolonged QT interval on electrocardiogram. He had a recent total thyroidectomy. What are serum calcium, parathyroid hormone (PTH), and phosphate levels likely to show in this patient?
(A) High calcium, high PTH level, high phosphate level
(B) High calcium, high PTH level, low phosphate level
(C) Low calcium, high PTH level, high phosphate level
(D) Low calcium, low PTH level, high phosphate level
(E) Low calcium, low PTH level, low phosphate level

77. It is common for ectopic parathyroid glands to be found in the mediastinum. This is because the inferior parathyroid glands are derived from what embryologic structure?
(A) Rathke's pouch
(B) Second branchial cleft (pharyngeal pouch)
(C) Third branchial arch (pharyngeal arch)
(D) Third branchial cleft (pharyngeal pouch)
(E) Thyroglossal duct

78. What is the most common extrathyroidal manifestation of Graves disease?
(A) Alopecia
(B) Exophthalmos
(C) Hyperpigmentation
(D) Nail pitting
(E) Pretibial myxedema

79. The foramen cecum of the tongue is a remnant of what embryologic structure?
(A) Palatoglossal duct
(B) Schneiderian membrane
(C) Second branchial cleft
(D) Third branchial arch
(E) Thyroglossal duct

80. An 8-year-old boy with deafness has a large thyroid goiter causing obstructive symptoms. He is euthyroid. A subtotal thyroidectomy is performed, and the thyroid gland is diffusely involved by multiple small nodules that show papillary hyperplasia, reduced to absent colloid, fibrosis, and marked nuclear pleomorphism. What is the most likely cause of his thyroid abnormalities?
(A) Dyshormonogenetic goiter
(B) Endemic goiter (iodine deficiency)
(C) Graves disease
(D) Hashimoto's thyroiditis
(E) Riedel's thyroiditis

81. Which of the following variants of papillary thyroid carcinoma has a worse prognosis than conventional papillary thyroid carcinoma?
    (A) Columnar cell variant of papillary thyroid carcinoma
    (B) Follicular variant of papillary thyroid carcinoma
    (C) Macrofollicular variant of papillary thyroid carcinoma
    (D) Oncocytic variant of papillary thyroid carcinoma
    (E) Warthin-like variant of papillary thyroid carcinoma

ANSWERS

1. **(B) Insulin.**
   The photomicrograph demonstrates a pancreatic endocrine neoplasm, characterized by sheets and ribbon-like arrangements of monotonous polygonal cells with salt and pepper chromatin. The stroma contains abundant amorphous pink-hyaline material, consistent with amyloid. Amyloid deposition in a pancreatic endocrine neoplasm is characteristic of an insulinoma, or insulin-secreting pancreatic endocrine neoplasm. This amyloid is composed of islet amyloid polypeptide, which is also secreted by the β-cells, and is often coexpressed in insulin-secreting pancreatic endocrine neoplasms.

2. **(B) Pancreatic neuroendocrine carcinoma, large cell type**
   According to the 2010 World Health Classification, pancreatic endocrine neoplasms are divided into pancreatic neuroendocrine tumors (grade 1 and grade 2), and pancreatic neuroendocrine carcinomas (subdivided into large cell and small cell types). Grade 1 pancreatic neuroendocrine tumors must have less than 2 mitotic figures per 10 high-power fields and a Ki-67 index of ≤3%. Grade 2 pancreatic neuroendocrine tumors have between 2 and 20 mitotic figures per 10 high-power fields and/or a Ki-67 index between 3 and 20%. Pancreatic neuroendocrine carcinomas are typically high grade tumors with extensive necrosis, mitotic activity, and atypia. By definition, pancreatic neuroendocrine carcinomas must have over 20 mitotic figures per 10 high-power fields or a Ki-67 index of >20%, but often have much higher proliferative activity (>40–50 mitotic figures per 10 high-power fields). Extent of disease is no longer incorporated into the grading of these tumors. Pancreatic neuroendocrine carcinomas are further subdivided on cell morphology; large cell subtype tumors will show large nuclei, prominent nucleoli and more abundant cytoplasm, while small cell tumors will show smaller nuclei, lack nucleoli, and have scant cytoplasm.

In this case, the photomicrograph demonstrates a pancreatic neuroendocrine carcinoma, large cell type, showing the presence of necrosis, large nuclei with prominent nucleoli and abundant cytoplasm, and which is supported by the high mitotic rate provided in the clinical history. All pancreatic neuroendocrine carcinomas have an aggressive clinical course, with frequent metastases and a poor overall survival, so they are automatically considered "carcinomas." There is no category of grade 3 pancreatic neuroendocrine tumor in the current classification system.

3. **(A) β-catenin (nuclear).**
   The photomicrograph demonstrates a well-differentiated pancreatic endocrine neoplasm, characterized by ribbon-like and acinar arrangements of monotonous polygonal cells with salt and pepper chromatin. At times, the morphologic appearance of pancreatic endocrine neoplasm will overlap with other pancreatic tumors, particularly solid pseudopapillary tumors and acinar cell carcinomas. Pancreatic endocrine tumors will be positive with immunohistochemical stains for neuroendocrine markers, such as chromogranin, synaptophysin, and CD56, and some epithelial markers, including low molecular weight cytokeratins. Nuclear staining for β-catenin is not a feature of pancreatic endocrine neoplasms. Rather, nuclear staining for β-catenin is suggestive of a solid pseudopapillary tumor, which can also be positive for neuroendocrine markers.

4. **(B) Cortisol.**
   The photomicrograph demonstrates a full thickness cross section of the adrenal cortex. The adrenal cortex is composed of three distinct layers, an outermost zona glomerulosa, a middle zona fasciculata, and an inner zona reticularis. The zona glomerulosa is a thin, often discontinuous layer of cells with less cytoplasm, and secretes mineralocorticoids, including aldosterone. The zona fasciculata is the thickest layer, composed of cells with abundant, clear cytoplasm and fine vacuoles, and secretes glucocorticoids, including cortisol. The zona reticularis is thinner than the fasciculata, the cells have more eosinophilic cytoplasm, and secrete sex steroids, including estrogen and testosterone. The medulla secretes catecholamines, including epinephrine and norepinephrine.

5. **(E) Waterhouse–Friderichsen syndrome.**
   Waterhouse–Friderichsen syndrome, or massive adrenal hemorrhage secondary to bacterial infection, was originally described in patients with *Neisseria meningitidis* septicemia, but can occur with many other highly aggressive bacterial infections. Massive bilateral adrenal hemorrhage

leads to acute adrenocortical insufficiency, with profound hypotension and shock, which is usually fatal unless rapidly treated. The gross appearance of the adrenals shows expansion by abundant clotted blood, which usually obscures any residual adrenal cortex. Addison disease is caused by chronic destruction of the adrenals, usually due to autoimmune disease or tuberculosis, resulting in chronic adrenocortical insufficiency. Beckwith–Wiedemann syndrome is an overgrowth syndrome associated with an increased risk of adrenocortical carcinoma. Cushing disease is hypercortisolism caused by excess adrenocorticotropic hormone production by a pituitary adenoma, while Cushing syndrome is defined as hypercortisolism from any cause, including exogenous and endogenous sources of glucocorticoids.

6. **(D) Myelolipoma.**
The photomicrograph demonstrates expansion of the adrenal by an admixture of mature adipose tissue and bone marrow elements, including myeloid and erythroid precursors and megakaryocytes, consistent with an adrenal myelolipoma. Adrenal myelolipomas are benign tumors of the adrenal that are almost always solitary and unilateral. These should not be confused with angiomyolipomas, which are typically of renal origin, and composed of smooth muscle, mature fat, and large irregular vessels. While adrenal cortical tumors have a high lipid content, mature fat is not a common component of these tumors.

7. **(C) Cortisol-secreting adrenal cortical adenoma.**
The photomicrograph demonstrates an adrenal gland with a discrete solitary cortical nodule with a yellow-orange cut surface. The remainder of the adrenal cortex is thin without nodularity. This gross appearance is most consistent with an adrenal cortical neoplasm, and the small size and lack of hemorrhage or necrosis would favor an adrenal cortical adenoma. The patient's clinical history of obesity, skin striae, and moon facies is highly suggestive of cortisol excess. Therefore, the best answer is a cortisol-secreting adrenal cortical adenoma. An aldosterone-secreting adenoma would cause hypertension and hypokalemia. An adrenocorticotropin hormone secreting pituitary adenoma would result in diffuse hyperplasia of the adrenal cortex. Primary pigmented nodular adrenocortical disease grossly appears as macronodular hyperplasia of the adrenal gland with brown discoloration, due to lipofuscin pigment deposition. A pheochromocytoma would expand the medulla of the adrenal gland and cause symptoms of catecholamine excess.

8. **(E) Spironolactone.**
The clinical scenario of medication-resistant hypertension and hypokalemia with an associated unilateral adrenal mass is highly suggestive of an aldosterone-secreting adrenal cortical adenoma. The most effective medical treatment for hyperaldosteronemia is spironolactone, which inhibits release of aldosterone from the adrenal cortex. Patients treated with spironolactone preoperatively will have eosinophilic intracytoplasmic inclusions within the cortical cells of the adenoma and nearby zona glomerulosa, which are called "spironolactone bodies." Electron microscopy has demonstrated that these inclusions appear as concentrically lamellated whorls that contain aldosterone.

9. **(D) Nuclear pleomorphism and hyperchromasia.**
The photomicrograph demonstrates a neoplasm composed of cells with abundant, clear cytoplasm forming cords and nests, consistent with an adrenocortical neoplasm. The original criteria for malignancy in adrenal tumors were described by Dr. Weiss in 1984. In this study, features present in metastasizing/recurring adrenocortical tumors but not in benign tumors were (1) vascular invasion, (2) increased mitotic activity (>6 mitotic figures per 10 high-power fields), and (3) atypical mitotic figures. Many authors consider direct invasion of adjacent organs sufficiently straightforward that this feature is not included in scoring systems. Other features associated with malignancy include large size and a weight >500 g. Recent studies have defined adrenocortical tumors as malignant when at least three features are present from the following list: (1) high nuclear grade, (2) mitotic rate six or more per 50 high-power fields, (3) atypical mitotic figures, (4) clear cells <25%, (5) a diffuse architecture pattern in more than one-third of the tumor, (6) confluent necrosis, (7) venous invasion, (8) sinusoidal invasion, and (9) capsular invasion. Nuclear pleomorphism and hyperchromasia are the least specific features of malignancy, as this change is frequently seen in benign adenomas, and is not sufficient for a diagnosis of carcinoma alone. It is important to remember that these criteria do not apply to adrenocortical neoplasms of childhood.

10. **(E) Vascular invasion is diagnostic of malignancy.**
The photomicrograph demonstrates a proliferation of polygonal cells arranged in nests (or zellballen groups) within a rich vascular network, which combined with the clinical history is consistent with a pheochromocytoma. Pheochromocytomas are derived from the adrenal medulla, and produce catecholamines, such as epinephrine and norepinephrine, which cause the clinical findings

of hypertension and episodic paroxysmal episodes. While many pheochromocytomas are sporadic, the most common genetic syndrome associated with pheochromocytomas is multiple endocrine neoplasia type 2, which is caused by a germline *RET* gene mutation, which causes constitutive activity. Pheochromocytomas have a 10% rule: 10% will be bilateral, 10% will be malignant, 10% extra-adrenal, and 10% occur in childhood. The only definitive feature of malignancy in pheochromocytomas is metastasis to lymph nodes or distant sites. The Pheochromocytoma of the Adrenal Gland Scoring Scale (PASS) can predict which tumors are more likely to behave in a malignant fashion, but not all tumors with a high score will ultimately develop metastasis. Distant metastasis is often discovered years after the primary presentation, and can occur >20 years later in some patients, so close clinical follow-up for an extended period is recommended.

11. **(A) Craniopharyngioma.**
The photomicrograph demonstrates a partially cystic mass composed of squamous epithelium with nuclear palisading, associated with abundant compact keratin. When present in a suprasellar location in a child, this is most consistent with a craniopharyngioma. Craniopharyngiomas are neoplasms derived from remnants of Rathke's pouch, and most commonly occur in children under 15 years of age, or in middle-aged adults. Adamantinomatous craniopharyngiomas are more common in children, and contain squamous epithelium associated with abundant compact lamellar or "wet" keratin. The squamous epithelium in adamantinomatous craniopharyngiomas is embedded within a loose matrix, or reticulum. Cyst formation and calcification is common in these tumors. Papillary craniopharyngiomas are more common in older adults, and are composed of solid sheets and papillary structures lined by well-differentiated squamous epithelium without keratinization.

12. **(B) Normal anterior pituitary.**
The photomicrograph demonstrates an intact and well-developed reticulin network surrounding each group of endocrine cells, consistent with normal anterior pituitary gland. Reticulin stain is very useful in separating normal anterior pituitary from a pituitary adenoma. In normal anterior pituitary, the glandular cells are enveloped in a supportive reticulin network that envelops each cell. In contrast, pituitary adenomas lack a complete reticulin network and will show only focal patchy reticulin fibers. Pituitary infarction would result in collapse of the normal reticulin meshwork and reticulin fibers closely packed together. The posterior pituitary contains limited reticulin, as does normal brain tissue.

13. **(D) Parathyroid carcinoma.**
The photomicrograph demonstrates a hypercellular parathyroid gland with absent intraglandular fibroadipose tissue. Since all four parathyroids are involved by this process, this likely represents secondary hyperparathyroidism, which is defined as an increase in parathyroid parenchymal mass in response to a physiologic stimulus to increase secretion of parathyroid hormone. The most common causes of secondary hyperparathyroidism include chronic renal failure, vitamin D deficiency, and malabsorption. Lithium therapy for psychiatric disorders also is known to cause multiple parathyroid gland hyperplasia by an unknown mechanism, which clinically mimics primary hyperparathyroidism. Over 90% of patients with multiple endocrine neoplasia type 1 (and type 2a) will have primary hyperparathyroidism, which typically takes the form of multiple hyperplastic glands rather than a solitary parathyroid adenoma. In contrast, parathyroid carcinomas arise from a single gland, and the excess parathyroid hormone production will cause the other three glands to atrophy.

14. **(E) Renal cell carcinoma (RCC) antigen.**
The photomicrograph shows a proliferation of cells with abundant clear cytoplasm arranged in cords and nests, with no interspersed fibroadipose tissue. This appearance, in a patient with primary hyperparathyroidism, is consistent with water-clear cell hyperplasia of the parathyroid glands. This change is typically seen in multigland hyperplasia, and rarely in solitary adenomas. It can be mistaken for renal cell carcinoma on histologic examination if this variant is not recognized. The clear appearance of the cytoplasm in water-clear cell parathyroid change is due to accumulation of glycogen, so a periodic acid Schiff without diastase will be positive. The cells will stain with other markers typical of parathyroid tissue, including cytokeratin, synaptophysin, chromogranin, and parathyroid hormone. Markers of renal cell carcinoma, such as CD10 and RCC antigen, will be negative. Metastatic renal cell carcinoma should not cause clinical and laboratory findings of hyperparathyroidism.

15. **(D) Parathyroid lipoadenoma.**
The photomicrograph demonstrates a portion of parathyroid gland with abundant intraparenchymal fat. The proportion of fat to endocrine cells is within the normal range; however, the clinical and biochemical studies clearly indicate that the parathyroid gland was abnormal, and responsible for the patient's hyperparathyroidism. This combination

is consistent with a parathyroid lipoadenoma, an unusual variant of parathyroid adenoma. Parathyroid lipoadenomas retain a normal fat to parenchyma ratio, but have an overall increase in parathyroid parenchyma that results in hyperparathyroidism. The lipoadenoma is usually well circumscribed, and may have a rim of normal parathyroid tissue, similar to other parathyroid adenomas. In contrast to parathyroid hyperplasia, the other glands are normal in size, texture, and appearance. The lipoadenoma does not show clear cell change as would be seen in water-clear cell hyperplasia.

16. **(B) Contain C-cells that can undergo malignant transformation.**
The photomicrograph demonstrates a squamous lined cyst that contains normal-appearing thyroid tissue in the cyst wall, consistent with a thyroglossal duct cyst. Thyroglossal duct cysts are remnants of the thyroglossal duct, and therefore can occur anywhere along its route in the midline of the neck, but most commonly occur near the level of the hyoid bone. Because the hyoid bone forms after the thyroglossal duct descends, it is common for thyroglossal duct cysts to be attached to or even pass through the hyoid bone. This results in the classic appearance of a thyroglossal duct cyst that moves upward with swallowing. In addition, removal of the hyoid bone along with the cyst is required to prevent recurrence, called the Sistrunk procedure. Up to 40% of thyroglossal duct cysts will lack thyroid tissue in the cyst wall, and thorough sampling is often required in order to demonstrate thyroid tissue in many of the remaining cases. Any pathologic process that involves the thyroid gland can affect the thyroid tissue in a thyroglossal duct cyst, including thyroiditis, nodular hyperplasia, or malignancy. Papillary thyroid carcinoma is the most common malignancy to arise from a thyroglossal duct cyst. C-cells are not a component of thyroglossal duct cysts, due to separate embryologic derivation. C-cells migrate with the third branchial cleft and integrate into the lateral portions of the thyroid gland.

17. **(C) Stimulating autoimmune antibodies against the thyroid stimulating hormone (TSH) receptor.**
The photomicrograph demonstrates a classic example of Graves disease (diffuse toxic goiter), which is characterized by diffuse hyperplasia of the thyroid gland with papillary architecture, tall columnar follicular epithelium, and reduced or "scalloped" colloid. Occasionally lymphoid aggregates may be seen, with or without germinal centers. The diffuse involvement of the thyroid gland and a retained lobular architecture of the thyroid are features that

differentiate Graves disease from a hyperfunctioning hyperplastic nodule (or toxic nodule). Graves disease is caused by the production of autoimmune antibodies that bind to the TSH receptor of follicular epithelium on the ligand-binding epitope and stimulate the receptor, leading to increased thyroid hormone production and release. Nonstimulating autoimmune antibodies against thyroid antigens are seen in Hashimoto's thyroiditis, which leads to T-cell mediated destruction of the thyroid epithelium. Subacute thyroiditis (or de Quervain's thyroiditis) is believed to be caused by a viral infection, which causes a granulomatous inflammatory response, and the subsequent thyroid destruction can release sufficient thyroid hormone to cause hyperthyroidism.

18. **(E) Tumors confined to the thyroid gland are staged as T4a disease.**
The photomicrograph demonstrates a spindle cell neoplasm with marked pleomorphism and mitotic activity, which in this clinical setting is most consistent with an undifferentiated (anaplastic) thyroid carcinoma. Undifferentiated thyroid carcinomas arise in elderly adults (typically older than 65 years of age), who present with a rapidly enlarging neck mass that is fixed and hard, and may cause vocal cord paralysis or airway obstruction. As these tumors are undifferentiated, immunohistochemical staining for thyroid markers is typically lost, with thyroglobulin and TTF-1 negative in the majority of cases. Undifferentiated thyroid carcinoma arises from preexisting thyroid follicular disease in almost all cases, with over 80% containing papillary thyroid carcinoma at least focally. These tumors are both locally aggressive and frequently metastasize, with over 50% of patients harboring pulmonary, bone, or brain metastasis at presentation. The median survival for patients with this carcinoma is dismal, averaging 3–6 months. Staging undifferentiated thyroid carcinoma is different from all other thyroid tumors; all undifferentiated thyroid carcinomas are automatically T4 disease, and those limited to the thyroid gland are T4a while those with gross extrathyroidal extension are T4b.

19. **(B) Familial adenomatosis polyposis (FAP).**
The photomicrograph shows an example of cribriform morular variant of papillary thyroid carcinoma, which is characterized by cribriform, solid, and spindled growth of follicular epithelium interspersed with squamous islands (morules) and follicular spaces lacking colloid. The epithelium often has optically clear nuclei with varying nuclear grooves or pseudoinclusions. This rare variant of papillary thyroid carcinoma is highly associated

with FAP. Approximately 2% patients with FAP will develop this variant of papillary thyroid carcinoma, and are almost always women with multifocal disease. These tumors contain an APC gene mutation similar to other tumors arising in FAP, and will have nuclear staining for β-catenin. Multiple endocrine neoplasia type 1 is associated with hyperparathyroidism, pancreatic islet cell tumors, and pituitary adenomas. Multiple endocrine neoplasia type 2 is associated with medullary thyroid carcinoma, pheochromocytoma, and hyperparathyroidism. Cowden syndrome is associated with follicular adenomas and follicular carcinomas of the thyroid gland, along with breast, endometrial, and colorectal carcinomas. Hereditary nonpolyposis colorectal carcinoma syndrome is associated with colon cancer and endometrial carcinomas.

20. **(A) Abundant eosinophilic cytoplasm is composed of lysosomes.**
The photomicrograph demonstrates a follicular-derived thyroid neoplasm with abundant eosinophilic granular cytoplasm and large nuclei with prominent nucleoli. When vascular or capsular invasion is present, these findings are consistent with an oncocytic (Hürthle cell) variant of follicular carcinoma. The abundant pink cytoplasm is caused by accumulation of numerous mitochondria, not lysosomes. The oncocytic variant of follicular carcinoma is often larger than conventional follicular carcinomas and present at a higher stage, but when stratified for stage the prognosis is similar for conventional and oncocytic follicular carcinomas. The criteria for malignancy are the same as for conventional follicular carcinoma, including capsular or vascular invasion. As these tumors are derived from follicular epithelium, they will be positive for TTF-1 and thyroglobulin. For some reason the colloid in these tumors has a tendency to calcify, which can mimic psammoma bodies. Location of the calcification within a follicle rather than in the interstitial fibrous septae is helpful in distinguishing them. While the oncocytic variant of follicular carcinoma primarily spreads along hematogenous routes, including lung and bone metastasis, lymph node metastases are more common in patients with these tumors compared with conventional follicular carcinomas.

21. **(D) Poorly differentiated thyroid carcinoma.**
The photomicrograph demonstrates a follicular-derived thyroid neoplasm that has insular growth and tumor necrosis in the absence of nuclear features of papillary thyroid carcinoma. These changes are consistent with a poorly differentiated thyroid carcinoma. These tumors have an increased

risk of metastasis and death compared with well-differentiated thyroid carcinomas, such as papillary thyroid carcinoma and follicular carcinoma, but not as dismal a prognosis as undifferentiated (anaplastic) thyroid carcinoma. The tumors were originally called "insular carcinomas" due to the prominent insular or solid growth patterns typical of these tumors. Strict criteria (the Turin proposal) have been proposed for the diagnosis of poorly differentiated thyroid carcinoma. These include the presence of a solid or insular growth pattern, absence of nuclear features of papillary thyroid carcinoma, and the presence of at least one of the following findings: convoluted nuclei, 3 or more mitotic figures per 10 high-power fields, or tumor necrosis.

22. **(D) pT3.**
The photomicrograph demonstrates papillary thyroid carcinoma invading perithyroidal skeletal muscle, which is diagnostic of extrathyroidal extension. It is important to recognize extrathyroidal extension histopathologically, as it directly affects tumor staging. In the absence of involvement of major neck structures (thyroid cartilage, trachea, esophagus, recurrent laryngeal nerve), invasion of muscle or perithyroidal fat is considered minimal extrathyroidal extension. Any tumor with minimal extrathyroidal extension, regardless of size, is staged as pT3 disease. Tumors ≤1.0 cm in size, which are confined to the thyroid gland, are pT1a disease. Tumors >1.0 cm but <2.0 cm in size confined to the thyroid gland are pT1b disease. Tumors between 2.0 cm and 4.0 cm confined to the thyroid gland are pT2 disease. Tumors over 4.0 cm in size are pT3 disease as well as tumors with minimal extrathyroidal extension. Tumors invading the thyroid cartilage, trachea, esophagus, skin, or recurrent laryngeal nerve are pT4a disease, while tumors invading the prevertebral fascia or encasing carotid and/or mediastinal vessels are pT4b disease. Of note, anaplastic thyroid carcinomas are automatically pT4 disease, regardless of size, and are subdivided into pT4a if confined to the thyroid gland and pT4b disease if extending beyond the thyroid gland.

23. **(D) Thyroglobulin.**
The photomicrograph demonstrates a classic medullary thyroid carcinoma, which is characterized by plasmacytoid cells with salt and pepper chromatin arranged in nests and trabeculae within amorphous eosinophilic material consistent with amyloid. Medullary thyroid carcinoma is a neuroendocrine neoplasm, and therefore is positive for low molecular weight cytokeratins, synaptophysin, and chromogranin. Medullary thyroid carcinoma is also positive for calcitonin and carcinoembryonic antigen

(CEA), which are often produced in such quantities that serum monitoring of CEA and calcitonin is one of the most effective methods for identification of recurrent/persistent disease. Interestingly, despite the fact that medullary thyroid carcinoma is derived from C-cells and not from thyroid follicular epithelium, it is positive for TTF-1 in nearly all cases, although the nuclear staining is often weak and patchy compared with follicular-derived neoplasms. Thyroglobulin is not positive in medullary thyroid carcinoma, and expression of this marker is restricted to follicular epithelium-derived tumors such as follicular carcinoma and papillary thyroid carcinoma.

24. **(C) Columnar cell variant of papillary thyroid carcinoma.**

The photomicrograph demonstrates a neoplasm composed of tall columnar cells with nuclear stratification, hyperchromasia, and papillary growth. This appearance in a thyroid mass is most consistent with the columnar cell variant of papillary thyroid carcinoma (PTC). Columnar cell variant of PTC is a rare tumor that more commonly occurs in older men. Histologically, it is characterized by tall columnar cells with elongated, oval, hyperchromatic nuclei that are stratified. Classical nuclear changes of papillary thyroid carcinoma are typically patchy and focal. Other common findings are parallel epithelial strips ("railroad tracks"), squamous metaplasia forming "morules," and cytoplasmic vacuolization (often subnuclear). The combination of these features often gives this tumor an appearance similar to metastatic endometrioid adenocarcinoma. Immunohistochemical staining for TTF-1 and thyroglobulin are positive. Columnar cell variant of PTC is typically more aggressive than conventional PTC with higher mortality rates, and is often diagnosed at higher stage with larger tumors and extrathyroidal extension common.

25. **(C) Hyalinizing trabecular tumor.**

The photomicrograph demonstrates an example of hyalinizing trabecular tumor (HTT), which is characterized by elongated cells with an organoid or trabecular growth pattern within a hyalinized eosinophilic stroma. The cells are fusiform, and have oval nuclei with nuclear grooves, nuclear pseudoinclusions, and perinuclear halos. Follicular growth with colloid formation is not seen. HTTs are typically well circumscribed without capsular or vascular invasion; HTT-like tumors that show vascular invasion may be best classified as papillary thyroid carcinoma. HTTs are most likely related to papillary thyroid carcinomas, as HTTs occasionally contain a *RET/PTC* translocation, and have similar nuclear

changes. However, unlike most papillary thyroid carcinomas, the long-term prognosis is excellent with almost no reports of lymph node or distant metastasis. The main differential diagnoses of HTT include papillary thyroid carcinoma and medullary thyroid carcinoma, both of which can have nuclear pseudoinclusions and trabecular or solid growth. The presence of any follicular or papillary growth and an invasive growth pattern is more consistent with papillary thyroid carcinoma. Medullary thyroid carcinoma is differentiated from HTT by the absence of staining with thyroglobulin and positive staining for CEA and calcitonin.

26. **(E) Riedel's disease.**

The photomicrograph demonstrates thyroid gland tissue, which has been extensively replaced by dense fibrous tissue and chronic inflammation. This appearance, combined with the clinical history of extension into the surrounding soft tissue, is consistent with Riedel's disease (invasive fibrosing thyroiditis). The etiology of Riedel's disease remains unclear, but recent studies suggest it is part of the spectrum of IgG4-related sclerosing disease, such as autoimmune pancreatitis and sclerosing sialadenitis. Another common feature of Riedel's disease is the presence of phlebitis that can result in vascular thrombosis, similar to other IgG4-related diseases. The clinical appearance often mimics malignancy, which needs to be excluded at biopsy. The major histopathologic differential diagnosis is the fibrosing variant of Hashimoto's thyroiditis. Features that favor Riedel's disease over Hashimoto's thyroiditis include absence of antithyroid antibodies, extension beyond the capsule of the thyroid gland, and lack of Hürthle cell metaplasia. Graves disease will show diffuse thyroid papillary hyperplasia and colloid scalloping. Anaplastic thyroid carcinoma will show infiltrating pleomorphic malignant cells that may be spindled, squamoid, or giant cell type. Diffuse sclerosing variant of papillary thyroid carcinoma would have abundant thyroid fibrosis with interspersed nests of malignant cells showing nuclear changes of papillary thyroid carcinoma and psammoma bodies.

27. **(E) Subacute thyroiditis.**

The photomicrograph demonstrates thyroid tissue that is largely destroyed by acute and chronic inflammation, multinucleated giant cells, and histiocytes (granulomatous inflammation). This morphologic appearance, along with the clinical presentation of a painful enlarged thyroid gland, is most consistent with subacute thyroiditis, or de Quervain's thyroiditis. Subacute thyroiditis most commonly affects women between 20 and 60 years of age, and can cause symptoms of hyperthyroidism or hypothyroidism depending on the phase of the disease. Early destruction of thyroid follicles releases substantial thyroid hormone, causing hyperthyroidism, while later significant parenchymal loss results in hypothyroidism. Patients with subacute thyroiditis often present with neck pain, weight loss, myalgias, and fever, and have a thyroid gland that is tender to palpation. Treatment with corticosteroids and nonsteroidal anti-inflammatory medications will resolve most symptoms quickly. Although patients may become hypothyroid, most patients will eventually return to a euthyroid state after resolution of the disease.

28. **(B) More common in men than women.**
The photomicrograph demonstrates thyroid tissue infiltrated by chronic inflammation that forms germinal centers along with follicular epithelial atrophy and oncocytic (Hürthle cell) metaplasia. These findings are consistent with chronic lymphocytic thyroiditis, which in the appropriate clinical setting is called Hashimoto's thyroiditis. Chronic lymphocytic thyroiditis is an autoimmune disorder associated with antithyroid antibodies, such as antithyroglobulin or antimicrosomal antibodies. Patients with this autoimmune process are much more likely to develop other autoimmune diseases, such as autoimmune adrenalitis, Sjögren's disease, or myasthenia gravis. Chronic lymphocytic thyroiditis occurs nearly 10 times more frequently in women than in men. The presence of chronic lymphocytic thyroiditis is considered a risk factor for the development of papillary thyroid carcinoma, due to chronic stimulation of the epithelium.

29. **(D) Occult papillary thyroid carcinoma with lymph node metastasis.**
The presence of thyroid follicles within a lymph node in the lateral neck is highly concerning for metastatic papillary thyroid carcinoma. Metastatic thyroid carcinoma can appear bland and lack nuclear features of papillary thyroid carcinoma. Whenever thyroid epithelium is identified in lymph nodes from the lateral neck (lateral to the jugular vein, including levels 2 through 5), the presumptive diagnosis is metastatic papillary thyroid carcinoma, as embryologic remnants of thyroid tissue should be confined to the central neck. In addition, regardless of location, if the thyroid epithelium shows nuclear changes of papillary thyroid carcinoma, it should be diagnosed as metastatic disease. It is not uncommon for papillary thyroid carcinoma to be clinically occult. Some authors contend that all thyroid epithelium within a lymph node is derived from metastatic thyroid cancer, but most thyroid experts accept benign thyroid inclusions (embryologic remnants)

within a lymph node when strict criteria are met. These criteria include location in the central neck, thyroid epithelium in only one lymph node capsule, no features of papillary thyroid carcinoma, and a primary papillary thyroid carcinoma is not present in the thyroid gland.

30. **(D) Submit the entire fibrous capsule of the nodule and random sections of uninvolved thyroid tissue.**
The frozen section photomicrograph demonstrates a highly cellular nodule composed of follicular epithelium lacking nuclear changes of papillary thyroid carcinoma. The differential diagnosis of a solitary nodule with this histologic appearance includes follicular adenoma and follicular carcinoma. The diagnosis of follicular adenoma requires examination of the entire fibrous capsule of the nodule to exclude capsular or vascular invasion, which if present would be diagnostic of follicular carcinoma. Therefore, the most appropriate way to process this specimen would be to submit the entire capsule of the nodule, along with at least one section of uninvolved thyroid gland tissue for comparison.

31. **(D) Spindle epithelial tumor with thymus-like differentiation (SETTLE).**
The histologic description is consistent with SETTLE of the thyroid gland. SETTLE tumors are seen in young patients, typically under 20, and are believed to be derived from remnants of intrathyroidal ectopic thymus tissue or branchial clefts. SETTLE tumors are characterized by a biphasic tumor containing a highly cellular proliferation of bland spindle cells with scant cytoplasm along with areas of glandular and tubulopapillary structures that may be mucinous. Pleomorphism, increased mitotic activity, and necrosis are not typical of this tumor. SETTLE tumors have an excellent 5-year survival (over 90%), but are prone to delayed distant metastasis up to 20 years after diagnosis; therefore prolonged follow-up is required. In contrast, carcinoma showing thymus-like differentiation (CASTLE), which has a similar name, has a radically different histopathologic appearance. CASTLE tumors occur in older adults, typically over 50 years of age, and are high-grade neoplasms, often with an undifferentiated lymphoepithelial-like carcinoma appearance, similar to thymic carcinoma or undifferentiated nasopharyngeal carcinoma. Overt squamous differentiation in CASTLE tumors is not typically seen by routine stains, but immunohistochemistry will show staining for p63 and cytokeratin 5/6, and an absence of staining for thyroid transcription factor 1 (TTF-1), thyroglobulin, calcitonin, and Epstein–

Barr virus RNA. CASTLE tumors typically present at high stage with extrathyroidal extension, and lymph node metastasis develops in close to 30% of patients. However, patients with CASTLE generally have a good long-term prognosis with 82% overall survival at 10 years. Undifferentiated (anaplastic) thyroid carcinoma would have a higher grade appearance with necrosis and increased mitotic activity, and is seen in older adults. Poorly differentiated thyroid carcinoma and papillary thyroid carcinoma of any variant would retain TTF-1 and thyroglobulin expression, and generally do not have a significant spindle cell component.

32. **(C) Minocycline.**
"Black thyroid" is caused by minocycline therapy. Minocycline is an antibiotic, related to tetracycline, which is used to treat a variety of conditions, including acne. The pigment deposited in the thyroid gland is believed to be a combination of degradation products of the drug combined with lipofuscin. Minocycline pigment deposition in the thyroid gland does not affect thyroid function, and this finding is usually incidental at thyroid resection for other causes. The additional medications listed above are possible treatments for acne, but do not affect thyroid appearance.

33. **(A) Gastrin.**
The clinical history provided is classic for Zollinger–Ellison syndrome, which is caused by hypersecretion of gastrin by a pancreatic endocrine tumor. The excess gastrin production causes hypersecretion of gastric acid, which leads to severe peptic ulcer disease that does not respond to medical therapy. Over 50% of patients with hypergastrinemia will also have diarrhea. Gastrinomas are more likely to behave in a malignant fashion than islet cell secreting tumors. They are also unusual, in that the primary tumor location is as commonly duodenal wall and peripancreatic soft tissue, as it is pancreatic. An insulinoma will cause hypoglycemic episodes, and a glucagonoma will cause a mild diabetes mellitus-like syndrome along with a skin rash. VIPomas (vasoactive intestinal peptide secreting tumors) cause a syndrome of severe watery diarrhea and hypokalemia. Somatostatinomas rarely cause a clinical syndrome, but can be associated with a diabetes mellitus-like picture.

34. **(A) A 1-week-old baby girl exposed to uncontrolled maternal diabetes.**
Diffuse islet cell hyperplasia is seen in patients exposed to prolonged high serum glucose levels in the absence of other metabolic disorders. The classic example of islet cell hyperplasia is a baby born to a woman with uncontrolled diabetes; the

mother's high glucose levels cross the placenta, and the fetal islet cells undergo hyperplasia in response. Islet cells are expected to decrease in a patient with type 1 diabetes, as autoimmune destruction leads to insulin loss. A patient with an insulin-secreting islet cell tumor would have normal or slightly decreased numbers of islet cells depending on the duration of the tumor, as the excess insulin from the tumor will cause hypoglycemia. Type 2 diabetes is primarily caused by insulin resistance and an inability of the endocrine pancreas to increase production of insulin in the face of this demand; therefore, the islet cells are usually normal in number or only slightly decreased as islets begin to fail. Long-term steroid use can result in hyperglycemia and a concurrent mild hyperplasia of islet cells, but a short taper will not have any effect on the morphologic appearance of the pancreas.

35. **(E) Infiltration of islet cells by T-lymphocytes.**
Type 1 diabetes is most commonly diagnosed in children, and is caused by autoimmune destruction of the pancreatic islet cells. This autoimmune destruction of the islets manifests on histologic examination as a reduction in the number of islet cells and T-lymphocytes within residual islets. In contrast, type 2 diabetes is primarily caused by end-organ insulin resistance, with insufficient production of insulin to overcome this resistance. Histopathologically, the pancreas in type 2 diabetes appears relatively normal, or has a slightly reduced islet cell mass, along with amyloid deposition in and around islet cells. Dystrophic calcification and fat necrosis are associated with chronic pancreatitis, which can lead to acinar atrophy and fibrosis.

36. **(A) Glucagon.**
The islets of Langerhans are composed of four major and two minor cell types, each of which secretes a unique endocrine hormone. The α-cells produce glucagon, which increases serum glucose levels. The β-cells produce insulin, the major regulatory hormone responsible for serum glucose level homeostasis, which decreases glucose levels. The δ-cells produce somatostatin, which suppresses both insulin and glucagon release. PP cells produce pancreatic polypeptide, which affects gastric and intestinal enzyme secretion and intestinal motility. The minor cells are the D1 cells and the enterochromaffin cells, which produce vasoactive intestinal polypeptide and serotonin, respectively.

37. **(B) Ki-67 proliferative index of 3%.**
According to the 2010 World Health Classification, pancreatic endocrine neoplasms are divided into pancreatic neuroendocrine tumors (grade 1 and grade 2), and pancreatic neuroendocrine

carcinomas (subdivided into large cell and small cell types). Grade 1 pancreatic neuroendocrine tumors must have less than 2 mitotic figures per 10 high-power fields and a Ki-67 index of ≤3%. Grade 2 pancreatic neuroendocrine tumors have between 2 and 20 mitotic figures per 10 high-power fields and/ or a Ki-67 index between 3 and 20%. Pancreatic neuroendocrine carcinomas are typically high grade tumors with extensive necrosis, mitotic activity, and atypia. By definition, pancreatic neuroendocrine carcinomas must have over 20 mitotic figures per 10 high-power fields or a Ki-67 index of >20%, but often have much higher proliferative activity (>40–50 mitotic figures per 10 high-power fields). Good prognostic features of pancreatic neuroendocrine tumors include low stage (confined to the pancreas, small size of <2 cm), and absence of angiolymphatic invasion or lymph node metastasis. Grade 1 pancreatic neuroendocrine tumors have a better prognosis than grade 2 pancreatic neuroendocrine tumors. A mitotic rate of 1 per 10 high-power fields would be compatible with a grade 1 tumor. However, a Ki-67 rate of 3% (choice B) would be consistent with a grade 2 tumor, which implies a potentially worse prognosis.

38. **(D) 21-hydroxylase deficiency.**
Any newborn with ambiguous genitalia should be evaluated for the presence of congenital adrenal hyperplasia. Congenital adrenal hyperplasia is caused by a variety of inherited metabolic enzyme deficiencies, which result in reduced or absent production of cortisol. 21-Hydroxylase deficiency accounts for over 90% of all infants with congenital adrenal hyperplasia. This enzyme is necessary for synthesis of cortisol and aldosterone, and the precursor steroids are converted into excess androgens. The reduction in aldosterone leads to salt wasting, which presents with dehydration, hyponatremia, hyperkalemia, and vomiting, usually within 2 weeks of birth. The excess androgens cause virilization and ambiguous genitalia in baby girls. The absence of cortisol drives the pituitary to produce more adrenocorticotropic hormone (ACTH), resulting in hyperplasia of both adrenal glands, which may be up to 10 times larger than a normal adrenal gland. 17-Alpha hydroxylase deficiency is a rare cause of congenital adrenal hyperplasia, which leads to excess aldosterone, with hypertension and hypokalemia as presenting syndromes. X-liked congenital adrenal hypoplasia is a disorder where the adrenal cortex fails to develop. Autoimmune adrenalitis is a cause of adrenocortical insufficiency (or Addison's disease), which typically affects adults. Cushing disease is caused by excess ACTH production by a pituitary adenoma.

39. **(A) Calretinin.**
Differentiating clear cell renal cell carcinoma from an adrenal cortical neoplasm with clear cell change can be difficult on morphology alone. Immunohistochemical staining is helpful in this differential. Adrenal cortical tumors (and normal adrenal cortex) are positive for inhibin, melan-A, and calretinin, and are typically negative for cytokeratin. Chromogranin and synaptophysin are typically positive in adrenal medullary tissue and pheochromocytomas. RCC antigen is negative in adrenal cortical and medullary lesions, and positive in many renal cell carcinomas. While adrenal cortical tumors are positive for melan-A, they are negative for other melanoma markers, including HMB-45 and S-100.

40. **(E) Pituitary infarction.**
The clinical symptoms of progressive fatigue and weakness, combined with low cortisol and aldosterone levels, are consistent with chronic adrenocortical insufficiency, or Addison's disease. Primary adrenocortical insufficiency occurs when the adrenal glands are damaged and unable to secrete sufficient glucocorticoids and mineralocorticoids. This results in increased production of ACTH by the pituitary. As a secondary effect, high levels of the precursor protein pro-opiomelanocortin (POMC) are produced, which results in increased skin pigmentation. In developed countries, the most common cause of primary adrenocortical insufficiency is autoimmune adrenalitis, while in underdeveloped countries the most common cause is disseminated tuberculosis infection. Other common causes are metastatic tumor involving the adrenals and destructive opportunistic infections in the setting of AIDS. In contrast, secondary adrenocortical insufficiency occurs when the pituitary fails to produce sufficient ACTH. This can occur after pituitary infarction, metastasis, or infection. A key feature of secondary adrenocortical insufficiency is a rise in cortisol and aldosterone levels with the administration of exogenous ACTH.

41. **(B) Multiple endocrine neoplasia 1 (MEN 1).**
Pheochromocytomas are found in many different inherited neoplastic syndromes. Pheochromocytomas are most commonly associated with MEN syndromes 2a and 2b, which are caused by *RET* gene mutations, leading to medullary thyroid carcinoma, pheochromocytomas, and parathyroid hyperplasia. The hereditary paraganglioma-pheochromocytoma syndrome, which is due to mutations in succinate dehydrogenase subunits, is associated with the development of pheochromocytomas and extra-adrenal paragangliomas. VHL syndrome is due to a mutation in the *VHL* gene, and is primarily

associated with the development of renal cell carcinoma and hemangioblastomas, but up to 20% of patients will develop pheochromocytomas. In contrast, MEN 1 is caused by mutations in the *MENIN* gene, which leads to pituitary adenomas, pancreatic endocrine neoplasms, and hyperparathyroidism.

42. **(E) Virilization or feminization is a good prognostic sign.**

Adrenal cortical adenomas are more common in women, and are typically solitary nodules that are grossly well circumscribed with a smooth border. They are smaller than adrenal cortical carcinomas, with most adenomas weighing <100 g. Adrenal cortical adenomas are divided into nonhyperfunctional and hyperfunctional tumors. Most incidentally discovered adrenal adenomas are nonhyperfunctional. The most common clinical syndrome associated with a hyperfunctional adrenal cortical adenoma is hyperaldosteronism or Conn syndrome, followed by hypercortisolism, or Cushing syndrome. In contrast, presenting with clinical signs and symptoms of virilization or feminization is extremely worrisome for malignancy; in one study over 70% of virilizing or feminizing tumors were malignant.

43. **(D) Pheochromocytoma.**

The chromaffin reaction is rarely used in modern pathology, but is of historical significance, as it predated the use of immunohistochemistry to distinguish adrenal cortical tumors from adrenal medullary tumors. The chromaffin reaction uses a potassium dichromate solution that oxidizes catecholamines, when present, into adrenochrome pigments that are blue-black. As pheochromocytomas produce catecholamines, such as epinephrine and norepinephrine, pheochromocytomas are the only primary adrenal tumor to have a positive chromaffin reaction.

44. **(B) Antidiuretic hormone (ADH).**

The posterior pituitary consists of axonal processes originating from the hypothalamus and extending adjacent to the anterior pituitary. Two hormones are synthesized in the hypothalamus and are released from these specialized axons: ADH and oxytocin. Several other hormones synthesized in the hypothalamus are released into the pituitary portal circulation from the hypothalamus directly. These hormones include CRH, thyrotropin-releasing hormone, GH-releasing hormone, and gonadotropin-releasing hormone. The anterior pituitary is composed of ectodermal-derived endocrine cells that secrete a variety of hormones, including ACTH, GH, and TSH.

45. **(D) Pituitary microadenoma.**

The clinical signs and symptoms (amenorrhea and bilateral breast discharge) in the absence of

pregnancy are highly suggestive of hyperprolactinemia. Hyperprolactinemia is most commonly caused by a prolactin-secreting pituitary adenoma. In fact, prolactin-secreting pituitary adenomas make up over 80% of functional pituitary adenomas. In young women, even small amounts of excess prolactin can result in significant signs and symptoms, so these tumors are almost always <1 cm in size at diagnosis (microadenomas). In contrast, men and postmenopausal women more commonly present with macroadenomas, due to limited effects of the excess prolactin. An empty sella turcica is seen in women who have infarcted their anterior pituitary, and will present with symptoms of hypopituitarism. Subarachnoid hemorrhage can also cause hypopituitarism due to mass effect and interference with the normal blood supply to the pituitary. Lesions causing significant mass effect on the hypothalamus (such as a glioblastoma) can inhibit dopamine release. As dopamine is an inhibitor of prolactin, this can result in excess prolactin expression, but in this woman would most likely be causing other symptoms as well, such as headache, visual changes, and seizures.

46. **(A) Adrenocorticotropic hormone (ACTH).**

The morphologic change described (amorphous light pink material accumulating in the cytoplasm) in a subset of anterior pituitary cells is called Crooke's hyaline, and occurs in corticotroph cells that have been exposed to high glucocorticosteroid levels. The corticotroph cells secrete ACTH, which regulates endogenous glucocorticosteroid production. Electron microscopy studies have demonstrated that this change is due to an accumulation of intermediate filaments that displace the normal neurosecretory granules. This explains the immunoreactivity with low molecular weight keratins in this cytoplasmic material. This change is usually seen in non-neoplastic pituitary tissue, but rarely is seen in ACTH-secreting pituitary adenomas (so-called Crooke's cell adenomas).

47. **(E) Sheehan syndrome.**

Sheehan syndrome, or postpartum necrosis of the anterior pituitary, occurs when women lose a significant amount of blood or have a hypoxic event during childbirth. This is rare in modern medical settings, but is more common in areas with poor medical access. The anterior pituitary almost doubles in size during pregnancy to accommodate physiologic needs. However, the vascular supply to the anterior pituitary does not increase, which makes this structure more vulnerable to ischemic events. The clinical symptoms and signs of Sheehan syndrome are subtle, but the first and most common sign is trouble with breastfeeding. This is due to the absence of prolactin needed to start milk production. Women with Sheehan syndrome will fail to make any breast milk. Over the course of months and years, other symptoms related to loss of other anterior pituitary hormones will develop, such as hypothyroidism (loss of thyrotropin-stimulating hormone), low blood pressure (loss of adrenocorticotropic hormone), and loss of secondary sex characteristics such as pubic and axillary hair (loss of follicle-stimulating hormone and luteinizing hormone). A prolactin-secreting pituitary adenoma usually causes excess breast discharge (galactorrhea). While Cushing syndrome (excess adrenocorticotropic hormone) can cause prolactin deficiency if the adenoma destroys all normal anterior pituitary tissue, in this setting a woman would likely be unable to get pregnant. Prior breast surgery and poor hydration are other causes of poor lactation, but are not associated with a large postpartum hemorrhage.

48. **(B) Changing facial features and large hands with sausage-like fingers.**
Growth hormone-secreting pituitary adenomas stimulate production of IGF-1, which results in many of the clinical manifestations of excess growth hormone. In young patients without epiphyseal closure, giantism will occur, with an increase in overall body size and disproportionally long arms and legs. In older patients, excess growth hormone results in acromegaly, an increase in size of skin, soft tissue, viscera, and bones of the face, hands, and feet. These changes occur slowly over time, and can be subtle. Most commonly changes in the shape of the face are noticed by family members, and enlargement of feet is noticed due to shoe size changes. In this patient, who is 55, a growth hormone-secreting pituitary adenoma would be expected to cause acromegaly. Bilateral galactorrhea is a symptom of excess prolactin. Erectile dysfunction and fatigue is often seen in gonadotropin-secreting adenomas (excess follicle-stimulating hormone and luteinizing hormone cause reduced testosterone in men). Obesity and abdominal striae are seen in Cushing syndrome, due to excess adrenocorticotropin hormone.

49. **(B) Discontinuous subarachnoid space deposits.**
The only diagnostic feature of pituitary carcinoma is metastasis. This can take the form of systemic metastasis (to cervical lymph nodes, lungs, or distant bone) or cerebrospinal dissemination (with discontinuous subarachnoid space deposits most common). Atypical pituitary adenomas can show extensive local invasion, including into bone of the skull base and brain. Tumor necrosis, high mitotic figures, and pleomorphism are frequently seen in pituitary carcinomas, but are not considered sufficient alone for the diagnosis of malignancy.

50. **(E) Microscopic dura invasion.**
Atypical pituitary adenomas show features suggestive of more aggressive behavior than usual pituitary adenomas. These features include invasive growth (into bone, vessels, and nerves), increased mitotic activity (a normal pituitary adenoma should have essentially no mitotic figures), an increased Ki-67 growth fraction (>3%), and diffuse nuclear staining for p53. Dural invasion, particularly microscopic dura invasion, is frequently seen in otherwise typical pituitary adenomas, and is not considered a reliable marker of more aggressive behavior.

51. **(D) Parathyroid adenoma.**
The clinical presentation is classic for primary hyperparathyroidism, with hypercalcemia, renal stones, and osteopenia. The jaw tumor is typical of metabolic bone disease secondary to hyperparathyroidism, or a "brown tumor" of bone. Brown tumors most commonly occur in the jaw, ribs, and long bones, and are composed of fibrovascular marrow replacement and increased osteoclast-like giant cells, which can have the appearance of a reparative giant cell granuloma. Over 85% of patients with primary hyperparathyroidism have a parathyroid adenoma. In addition, brown tumors of bone associated with hyperparathyroidism are almost always associated with parathyroid adenoma, and less commonly parathyroid carcinomas. Multigland parathyroid hyperplasia is the cause of hyperparathyroidism in 10–15% of patients, and is rarely associated with brown tumors. Hypoparathyroidism, osteomalacia, and renal failure are causes of hypocalcemia.

52. **(A) DiGeorge syndrome.**
DiGeorge syndrome is characterized by failure of migration and development of the third and fourth branchial clefts and midline structures. This results in the classic finding of congenital heart disease (most commonly tetralogy of Fallot), failure of thymus gland development leading to immune defects, and failure of parathyroid development leading to hypocalcemia. DiGeorge syndrome is caused by a deletion on chromosome 22q11. Other causes of hypoparathyroidism include iatrogenic (usually after thyroid or parathyroid surgery), familial (X-linked recessive syndrome), and autoimmune disorders (rarely involved in Addison's disease). Down's syndrome (trisomy 21) is the most common cause of congenital heart defects, but is not associated with hypoparathyroidism or branchial cleft anomalies. Multiple endocrine neoplasia type 1

is associated with hyperparathyroidism and is not associated with heart defects.

53. **(B) Circumscribed hypercellular nodule with a rim of atrophic parathyroid tissue.**

The diagnosis of a parathyroid adenoma requires a combination of clinical and pathologic findings. Some authors suggest that a definitive diagnosis of parathyroid adenoma cannot be made until 5 years have passed without recurrent hyperparathyroidism, as diffuse hyperplasia can be asymmetric and mimic the appearance of a solitary adenoma at first presentation. Both parathyroid adenomas and glands from diffuse hyperplasia will weigh more than a typical gland. In fact, glands from hyperplasia often weigh more than adenomas. Since the parathyroid parenchyma is hyperfunctioning in both adenomas and hyperplasia, oil red O staining will show reduced intracellular fat in both processes. The most helpful findings at the time of surgery are normal appearance of the other three glands, a significant drop in intraoperative parathyroid hormone levels after excision of the presumed adenoma, and a rim of atrophic parathyroid tissue around the adenoma on histologic examination. Unfortunately, a rim of atrophic tissue is found in only 50% of parathyroid adenomas.

54. **(E) Vascular space invasion.**

The diagnosis of parathyroid carcinoma is difficult. The only histologic feature that alone is definitive for parathyroid carcinoma is metastasis; however, in the appropriate clinical setting the presence of several features can support the diagnosis. The classic clinical presentation of parathyroid carcinoma is primary hyperparathyroidism with excessively high serum calcium levels (>13 mg/dL) and serum parathyroid hormone levels (>1000 ng/L). During surgery, one of the first clues is difficulty in removing the parathyroid gland, as it often invades nearby structures or induces a desmoplastic stromal response. The two histopathologic features (other than metastasis) specific for parathyroid carcinoma are invasion into nearby structures (thyroid, muscle, etc.) and vascular invasion. Other features that should prompt careful evaluation for malignancy, but are not specific for carcinoma, are broad fibrous bands, increased mitotic activity, a trabecular or solid/diffuse growth pattern, and macronucleoli. Parathyroid neoplasms that lack local infiltration or vascular invasion, but have additional atypical features, are diagnosed as atypical parathyroid adenomas. Immunohistochemical staining for parafibromin can be useful in the diagnosis of parathyroid carcinoma. Parathyroid adenomas and hyperplasias will show retained nuclear staining

for parafibromin, while the majority of parathyroid carcinomas will show complete or partial loss of nuclear staining.

55. **(C) Oxalate crystals.**

Differentiating parathyroid from thyroid tissue on frozen section evaluation can be challenging, particularly for parathyroid adenomas that lack the typical nested growth pattern with focal residual intraparenchymal fat. Parathyroid adenomas can have a microfollicular growth pattern with colloid-like material within the follicles. The most helpful features at frozen section are the presence of two or more cell types (oxyphil and chief cell), residual intraparenchymal fat, and a rim of normal parathyroid tissue. Oxalate crystals occur within the colloid of thyroid tissue, and are not seen in the colloid-like material of hypercellular parathyroids. Unfortunately, this finding is not frequently seen in normal thyroid gland tissue, and in some cases definitive differentiation of parathyroid from thyroid tissue cannot be made at the time of frozen section.

56. **(E) Severe mental retardation.**

The thyroid hormones T3 and T4 are critical for normal brain development. The earlier a deficiency in thyroid hormone is present, the more severe the mental retardation. The developing fetus relies upon maternal T3 and T4 crossing the placenta during early embryogenesis, until the fetal thyroid develops and can start independently making hormone. Therefore, mothers with severe hypothyroidism before conception are at the highest risk of fetal mental retardation. This form of mental retardation is called cretinism, and is seen in undeveloped countries with profound iodine deficiency, a rare occurrence in the modern world. Other features of cretinism include short stature, coarse facial features, a protruding tongue, and umbilical hernias. Simple replacement of T3 and T4 in the mother can prevent the development of cretinism.

57. **(D) Pituitary infarction.**

The patient's symptoms are suggestive of hypothyroidism, which is confirmed by the reduced levels of T3 and T4. The elevated TSH levels would be consistent with primary hypothyroidism, which is caused by insufficient thyroid hormone production due to a disease or process of the thyroid gland. Examples of diseases or conditions that can cause primary hypothyroidism include chronic lymphocytic thyroiditis, prior radiation of the thyroid gland, iodine deficiency, and thyroid agenesis or surgical removal. In contrast, pituitary infarction is a cause of secondary hypothyroidism, which is due to insufficient production of TSH by the pituitary, leading to reduced T3 and T4 levels. The laboratory findings in secondary hypothyroidism would include low T3, low T4, and low TSH levels.

58. **(A) Approximately 20% of patients will have lymph node metastasis at diagnosis.**
The diffuse sclerosing variant of papillary thyroid carcinoma is important to recognize because of its more aggressive behavior and unique histopathologic appearance. This variant invariably involves at least one entire lobe of the thyroid gland by dense fibrosis, infiltrating papillary thyroid carcinoma epithelium that may show solid growth or squamous morules, and innumerable psammoma bodies. This tumor is highly associated with chronic lymphocytic thyroiditis, and prominent lymphoid infiltrates are frequently seen admixed with the neoplastic cells. It occurs in young adults, with a mean age of 18 at diagnosis. Nearly 100% of patients with this variant of papillary thyroid carcinoma will have lymph node metastases at presentation, and pulmonary metastases are common. However, with appropriate therapy, these patients have an excellent long-term prognosis with a very low tumor death rate. This may be due to the beneficial effect of younger age at diagnosis.

59. **(D) Nuclear enlargement, chromatin clearing, nuclear grooves, and nuclear pseudoinclusions.**
Fine-needle aspiration biopsy is the single best test to triage patients with thyroid nodules to surgery or conservative follow-up. However, fine-needle aspiration biopsies have been well documented to produce worrisome changes in thyroid nodules on histologic resection, and pathologists should be aware of the potential pitfalls. These worrisome histologic alterations following fine-needle aspiration of thyroid, or WHAAFT lesions, include capsular irregularities mimicking capsular invasion (or capsular pseudoinvasion), displacement of tumor cells into vascular lumens mimicking vascular invasion, and rarely sufficient proliferation of reactive myofibroblasts (bland spindle cells) with abundant mitotic activity to mimic a sarcoma or anaplastic thyroid carcinoma. Complete infarction of the nodule can occur, leaving little if any epithelium for histologic diagnosis; this occurs more commonly in oncocytic (Hürthle cell) lesions. Nuclear atypia can be seen, including nuclear enlargement and chromatin clearing in cells immediately adjacent to the biopsy tract, but nuclear pseudoinclusions should not be seen and are highly suggestive of a papillary thyroid carcinoma.

60. **(D) Papillary thyroid carcinoma.**
Papillary thyroid carcinoma is the most common malignant neoplasm of the thyroid gland in iodine-replete countries, and represents close to 80% of all thyroid malignancies. In contrast, the rate of follicular carcinoma is nearly equal to or surpasses the rate of papillary thyroid carcinoma in iodine-deficient regions of the world. When iodine supplementation is introduced to these areas, the rate of follicular carcinoma drops over time. Follicular adenoma is a benign neoplasm of the thyroid gland. Primary thyroid lymphoma and medullary thyroid carcinoma are uncommon malignancies of the thyroid gland in both iodine-deficient and iodine-replete regions of the world.

61. **(A) *BRAF* point mutation.**
The most common molecular alteration or mutation found in PTC is *BRAF* gene point mutation, which alters the amino acid structure of the protein from a valine to a glutamate at amino acid 600 (V600E). This mutation is present in over 50% of all PTC, and in up to 80% of tall cell variant of PTC. The *RET/PTC* translocation is found in a significant subset of PTCs, particularly patients with exposure to ionizing radiation (e.g., Chernobyl accident) and childhood PTCs. *RAS* point mutations are most commonly seen in follicular adenomas and follicular carcinomas, and a small subset of follicular variant of PTCs. The *PAX8/PPAR-γ* translocation is found exclusively in follicular adenomas and follicular carcinomas. *RET* point mutations are seen in medullary thyroid carcinomas and multiple endocrine neoplasia type 2.

62. **(E) Invasion into small caliber vessels within the tumor capsule.**
The diagnosis of follicular carcinoma of the thyroid requires demonstration of either vascular or capsular invasion. Most authors require penetration of more than one half of the tumor capsule to identify capsular invasion from capsular irregularities seen in benign disease (excluding choice C). Minimally invasive follicular carcinoma of the thyroid was originally defined as follicular carcinoma that invades into the tumor capsule or intracapsular small vessels, but does not penetrate beyond the tumor capsule. Follicular carcinomas that invade beyond the contour of the tumor capsule, and into normal thyroid parenchyma, perithyroidal soft tissue, or large caliber vessels (intrathyroidal or extrathyroidal) are considered widely invasive tumors. Within minimally invasive follicular carcinomas, the presence of vascular invasion within the capsule, particularly if involving 4 or more vascular profiles, is the most important risk factor for overall survival. Therefore, some authors recommend reporting minimally invasive follicular carcinomas with small vessel invasion in the capsule as angioinvasive follicular carcinomas.

63. **(A) Classic nuclear features of papillary thyroid carcinoma.**

Poorly differentiated thyroid carcinomas are follicular-derived thyroid neoplasms, which have an increased risk of metastasis and death compared with well-differentiated thyroid carcinomas, such as papillary thyroid carcinoma and follicular carcinoma, but not as dismal a prognosis as undifferentiated (anaplastic) thyroid carcinoma. The tumors were originally called "insular carcinomas" due to the prominent insular or solid growth patterns typical of these tumors. Strict criteria (the Turin proposal) have been proposed for the diagnosis of poorly differentiated thyroid carcinoma. These include the presence of a solid or insular growth pattern, absence of nuclear features of papillary thyroid carcinoma, and the presence of at least one of the following findings: convoluted nuclei, 3 or more mitotic figures per 10 high-power fields, or tumor necrosis. The presence of well-developed nuclear features of papillary thyroid carcinoma is not permitted in poorly differentiated thyroid carcinomas, as the solid variant of papillary thyroid carcinoma can have solid/insular growth and increased mitotic activity, but does not have a prognosis as bad as poorly differentiated thyroid carcinoma.

64. **(A) Lymphoepithelial lesions involving thyroid epithelium.**

The most common primary thyroid lymphoma is diffuse large B-cell lymphoma (DLBCL), followed closely by extranodal marginal zone B-cell lymphoma (EMZBCL) of mucosal-associated lymphoid tissue (MALT). Almost all thyroid lymphomas arise in the setting of chronic lymphocytic thyroiditis, so it is important to recognize features that distinguish these tumors from non-neoplastic lymphoid infiltrates. Malignant thyroid lymphomas will cause effacement of the normal thyroid gland architecture, and wipe out large areas of thyroid epithelium. Almost all thyroid lymphomas (except follicular lymphoma) will lack germinal centers, and follicular lymphomas will have poorly formed germinal centers that lack tingible body macrophages. Malignant lymphomas of the thyroid gland also classically extend beyond the thyroid capsule into perithyroidal structures (fibroadipose tissue, skeletal muscle, etc.) that usually cause the thyroid gland to adhere to surrounding structures at the time of surgery. Lymphoepithelial lesions, which in the thyroid gland appear as atypical lymphocytes colonizing and filling thyroid follicles, are not seen in chronic lymphocytic thyroiditis, but they are seen with greatest frequency in EMZBCL-type thyroid lymphomas. As most primary thyroid lymphomas are of B-cell origin, immunohistochemical staining for kappa and lambda light chains can be helpful in determining monoclonality. Chronic lymphocytic thyroiditis will show a polytypic population of B-cells and plasma cells that lack light chain restriction.

65. **(C) Macronucleoli.**

The diagnosis of papillary thyroid carcinoma is largely based on the recognition of nuclear changes of papillary thyroid carcinoma. These include nuclear enlargement compared with adjacent non-neoplastic thyroid epithelium, nuclear irregularity that results in grooves and nuclear pseudoinclusions, and fine pale chromatin. Other helpful features include nuclear crowding and overlap, Orphan Annie nuclei (optically clear nuclei due to formalin fixation artifact), and small eccentrically or peripherally located nucleoli. Macronucleoli are not typically seen in papillary thyroid carcinoma, and are more commonly seen in oncocytic (Hürthle cell) neoplasms. Architectural features, including papillary structures, are helpful but not required.

66. **(D) Requires immunohistochemistry with calcitonin for identification in most cases.**

C-cell hyperplasia can be divided into physiologic and nodular (neoplastic) types. Physiologic C-cell hyperplasia is typically seen in older patients with nonmedullary thyroid disease (e.g., lymphocytic thyroiditis) and is exceedingly difficult to detect by routine staining. Physiologic C-cell hyperplasia is defined as >50 C-cells per low-power field (100× magnification), but this increase in C-cells is largely seen as single C-cells interspersed with normal thyroid follicles. Because of the subtle increase in C-cells in physiologic C-cell hyperplasia, it almost always requires immunohistochemistry with calcitonin or carcinoembryonic antigen (CEA) for recognition and diagnosis. Physiologic C-cell hyperplasia is not associated with MEN 2 or medullary thyroid carcinoma. In contrast, nodular (or neoplastic) C-cell hyperplasia is characterized by aggregates of C-cells filling and/or partially destroying thyroid follicles, often as clusters of 50 or more C-cells, which form nodular lesions that are easily recognized on routine stains. Nodular C-cell hyperplasia is almost always seen in association with MEN 2 patients or adjacent to medullary thyroid carcinoma, and is considered neoplastic, as the C-cells harbor *RET* gene mutations. The C-cells must remain within the basement membrane of thyroid follicles. If the basement membrane is breached, identified histologically as fibrosis, a desmoplastic stromal response, and/or loss of association with thyroid follicles, a diagnosis of medullary thyroid carcinoma is made.

67. **(B) Excess melanocyte-stimulating hormone.**
The photomicrograph demonstrates an adrenal gland involved by autoimmune adrenalitis, characterized by significant adrenal cortex loss replaced by lymphoid infiltrates. Autoimmune adrenalitis is the most common cause of primary adrenocortical insufficiency in developed countries. The reduction in cortisol and aldosterone production leads to increased production of adrenocorticotropic hormone (ACTH) by the pituitary. The precursor molecule of ACTH is proopiomelanocortin (POMC), which is cleaved into ACTH and melanocyte stimulating hormone (MSH). Therefore, the increased demand for ACTH results in higher levels of MSH, leading to increased skin pigmentation, which characteristically affects the skin around joints. Hemochromatosis can cause increased skin pigmentation due to iron deposition. Melasma is patchy increased skin pigmentation, usually on the face, seen in a subset of pregnant women. Malignant melanoma usually results in localized abnormal skin pigmentation at the primary tumor site. Aldosterone is reduced in most cases of adrenocortical insufficiency.

68. **(C) Likely to be derived from salivary gland inclusions within the thyroid gland.**
The photomicrograph demonstrates a mucoepidermoid carcinoma of thyroid (MECT) origin, that is characterized by squamous or epidermoid cells admixed with mucus cells forming cysts and infiltrative nests. MECT is histologically indistinguishable from mucoepidermoid carcinoma of salivary gland origin. Mucicarmine stains will highlight intracytoplasmic and extracellular mucin. MECT has been subdivided into two types: classical type and sclerosing mucoepidermoid carcinoma with eosinophilia. The origin of these tumors remains somewhat controversial, but most authors agree that the classical type of MECT is likely derived from metaplastic thyroid follicular epithelium, as most cases will show immunohistochemical staining with thyroid transcription factor 1 (TTF-1) and thyroglobulin, and thyroid-specific mRNAs have been demonstrated in these tumors by polymerase chain reaction. The sclerosing MECT with eosinophilia is seen almost exclusively in patients with chronic lymphocytic thyroiditis, and is negative for TTF-1 and thyroglobulin. Therefore, this variant is favored to arise from hyperplastic branchial cleft remnants (ultimobranchial body) that proliferate in the setting of lymphocytic thyroiditis, although some authors think this tumor also arises from metaplastic thyroid follicular epithelium. Although ectopic salivary glands are rarely seen in thyroid tissue, most authors do not believe they are the source of these tumors.

69. **(B) Absence of thyroglobulin staining.**
The thyroid gland is a highly vascular organ that frequently is the site of metastatic tumor deposits. Interestingly, metastatic tumors have a propensity to involve thyroid lesions, such as hyperplastic nodules and follicular adenomas. Renal cell carcinoma is the most common tumor to metastasize to the thyroid gland, and is notorious for mimicking a primary thyroid neoplasm. This is because many thyroid tumors can have clear cell change (hyperplastic nodules, follicular adenomas, follicular carcinomas, and papillary thyroid carcinomas), have papillary structures, and may contain minimal to no colloid. Multifocality is a helpful general feature of metastasis to the thyroid gland, but metastatic renal cell carcinoma can present as a solitary well-circumscribed nodule in as many as 80% of patients. The most useful feature in differentiating primary thyroid neoplasms from metastatic renal cell carcinoma is immunohistochemical staining, as renal cell carcinomas are uniformly negative for thyroglobulin and thyroid transcription factor 1, and variably positive for CD10 and renal cell carcinoma (RCC) antigen. PAX8 is not useful, as follicular epithelium-derived tumors and clear cell renal cell carcinomas are both positive for this marker.

70. **(C) *RET* activating point mutation.**
The photomicrograph demonstrates a classic medullary thyroid carcinoma, which is characterized by plasmacytoid cells with salt and pepper chromatin arranged in nests and trabeculae within amorphous eosinophilic material consistent with amyloid. *RET* activating gene mutations are present in all patients with hereditary medullary thyroid carcinoma (multiple endocrine neoplasia 2 or familial medullary thyroid carcinoma syndrome) and over 60% of all sporadic medullary thyroid carcinomas. Inactivating mutations of *RET* are seen in patients with Hirschsprung disease, and *RET/PTC* translocations are found in a subset of PTCs. *BRAF* mutations are common in PTC, while *RAS* mutations are found in follicular neoplasms.

71. **(E) Insulin-secreting pancreatic endocrine neoplasm.**
The clinical presentation of episodic hypoglycemia, which is precipitated by exercise or fasting, is classic for an insulin-secreting pancreatic endocrine neoplasm (insulinoma). The typical clinical symptoms of hypoglycemia include confusion, stupor, and loss of consciousness. Diffuse islet cell hyperplasia is another cause of hyperinsulinemia, but is very rare in adults, and is most commonly seen

in neonatal infants born to mothers with uncontrolled diabetes. Factitious hypoglycemia is caused by self-administration of insulin resulting in episodes of hypoglycemia, and is differentiated from insulin-secreting tumors by low levels of C-peptide. C-peptide is produced from the β-cells of pancreatic islets, and insulin-secreting pancreatic endocrine neoplasms produce high levels of this protein. In contrast, C-peptide is not found in commercial preparations of insulin for therapeutic use. Diabetes mellitus type 1 results in a deficit of insulin, with resulting hyperglycemia and diabetic ketoacidosis. Glucagon-secreting pancreatic endocrine neoplasms cause hyperglycemia and a diabetes mellitus-like clinical picture.

72. **(B) Clinically functional, most commonly causing hyperinsulinemia.**
    Pancreatic neuroendocrine microadenomas are almost always incidentally found at autopsy or in a pancreatic resection for another process. They are defined as small (<0.5 cm) proliferations of neuroendocrine cells that are well circumscribed, and have a low mitotic rate (<10 mitotic figures per 10 high-power fields). By definition, the lesion must be clinically nonfunctional, although immunohistochemical staining will show restriction to one, or at most two, hormones, most commonly insulin and glucagon. If the patient presents with a clinical syndrome due to hormone oversecretion, the lesion is considered a well-differentiated pancreatic neuroendocrine tumor. While most sporadic pancreatic neuroendocrine microadenomas are solitary, patients with multiple endocrine neoplasia 1 (MEN1) will develop multiple microadenomas, as well as functional endocrine tumors over time. Pancreatic neuroendocrine microadenomas are differentiated from islet cell hyperplasia by the presence of a solitary nodule, and restriction to only one or at most two hormones by immunohistochemistry. Islet cell hyperplasia will typically show diffuse islet cell enlargement, and at least focal staining for four or more islet cell hormones in each group.

73. **(C) Metastatic carcinoma.**
    Metastasis to the adrenal gland is far more common than any primary adrenal neoplasms. Adrenal glands are the fourth most common site of metastasis, following lung, liver, and bone. The most common tumors to metastasize to the adrenal glands are breast carcinoma, lung carcinoma, renal cell carcinoma, and upper gastrointestinal carcinomas. Up to 40% of patients with adrenal metastasis will have bilateral involvement. Adrenal metastasis is one of the most common causes of adrenocortical insufficiency in older patient populations.

74. **(D) Rathke's pouch.**
    The anterior pituitary is derived from an invagination of the oral ectoderm during early embryogenesis, which breaks off and forms Rathke's pouch. This ectodermal-derived tissue then differentiates into specialized endocrine epithelium capable of secreting critical hormones for the developing body. The migration of Rathke's pouch can result in ectopic pituitary tissue within the sinonasal cavity, most commonly the sphenoid sinus. In contrast, the posterior pituitary is derived from neuroepithelium of the neural tube, as it is composed of axons from the hypothalamus. The notochord regresses during human development, and remnants can be found in the center of the intervertebral discs of humans. The branchial arches develop into musculature of the head and neck, while the branchial clefts largely regress, with the exception of the first branchial cleft that forms the ear canal.

75. **(D) Growth hormone and prolactin.**
    Mammosomatotroph cell adenomas express both growth hormone and prolactin. This unusual variant pituitary adenoma has been increasingly recognized with the use of immunohistochemical stains to subtype pituitary adenomas by hormone expression. In a mammosomatotroph cell adenoma, the neoplastic cells express both growth hormone and prolactin simultaneously. In contrast, a mixed growth hormone and prolactin-secreting adenoma will demonstrate two distinct cell populations that have different hormone expression. Mammosomatotroph cell adenomas most commonly present with symptoms of growth hormone excess, with or without clinical signs of prolactin secretion. Morphologically, they resemble densely granulated growth hormone adenomas.

76. **(D) Low calcium, low PTH level, high phosphate level.**
    The parathyroid glands produce PTH, an important part of calcium homeostasis. Calcium is important in nerve signal transmission, muscle contraction, and cardiac conduction. PTH stimulates bone resorption to release calcium into the bloodstream, and increases kidney reabsorption of calcium and secretion of phosphate into the urine. High levels of PTH result in hypercalcemia and low serum phosphate levels, while low levels of PTH result in hypocalcemia and high phosphate levels. The patient in this clinical scenario is demonstrating classic symptoms of hypocalcemia, which leads to muscular contractions (tetany), nerve transmission abnormalities (paresthesias), and a prolonged QT interval (cardiac conduction abnormality). With his history of recent thyroid surgery, he most likely has

developed iatrogenic hypoparathyroidism due to parathyroid injury or removal at the time of surgery. Therefore, the most likely laboratory findings would be choice D: low calcium, low PTH, and high phosphate. Choice B would be typical for a patient with hyperparathyroidism. Choice C would be typical for a patient with chronic renal failure, who has chronic hypocalcemia, which stimulates excess PTH.

77. **(D) Third branchial cleft (pharyngeal pouch).**
The parathyroid glands are derived from the third and fourth branchial clefts. The superior parathyroid glands are derived from the fourth branchial cleft, along with the ultimobranchial body and C-cells of the thyroid gland. The inferior parathyroid glands are derived from the third branchial cleft, along with the thymus gland that migrates into the mediastinum. The third branchial arch forms the muscles and cartilage of the neck, in particular the hyoid bone and supraglottic larynx. The thyroglossal duct is formed by the descent of the thyroid mesenchyme from the base of tongue ectoderm, which migrates along the midline of the anterior neck. Rathke's pouch migrates from the oral ectoderm to form the anterior pituitary.

78. **(B) Exophthalmos.**
The most common extrathyroidal manifestation of Graves disease is Graves ophthalmopathy, which leads to protrusion of the eyeball forward (exophthalmos) and can interfere with extraocular muscle function causing diplopia and visual disturbances. Graves ophthalmopathy is caused by autoantibodies stimulating orbital fibroblasts, leading to marked inflammation, edema, and fatty infiltration of the orbital apex and extraocular muscles. Graves ophthalmopathy occurs in approximately 25% of patients with Graves disease. The second most common extrathyroidal manifestation of Graves disease is pretibial myxedema, characterized by a scaly thickening and induration of the skin of the shin. Pretibial myxedema occurs in <5% of patients with Graves disease. Alopecia, hyperpigmentation, and nail pitting are not a part of the spectrum of Graves disease.

79. **(E) Thyroglossal duct.**
The foramen cecum is a remnant of the thyroglossal duct. The thyroglossal duct outpouches from the oral cavity during embryogenesis, and descends along the midline of the neck to eventually form the thyroid gland. This connection is typically lost during later fetal development, until a depression at the foramen cecum is all that is left. There is no palatoglossal duct. The Schneiderian membrane eventually forms the mucosa of the nasal cavity. The second branchial cleft largely

involutes, but can leave behind remnants that can result in branchial cleft cysts. The third branchial arch is important in development of the hyoid bone, muscle, and cartilaginous structure of the neck.

80. **(A) Dyshormonogenetic goiter.**
Dyshormonogenetic goiter is caused by a congenital inborn error of thyroid metabolism that results in reduced or absent production of circulating thyroid hormones. This causes increased secretion of thyroid stimulating hormone (TSH) by the pituitary gland, which stimulates the thyroid parenchyma to proliferate and be hyperactive. Depending on the severity of the inborn error of metabolism, patients may present as neonates with severe mental retardation and cretinism, or later in life with goiter and few other symptoms. Regardless of which inborn error of metabolism present, the pathologic changes are similar. The thyroid gland is diffusely involved by multiple nodules, fibrosis, and marked epithelial hyperplasia that often is papillary or solid/trabecular. Reduced to absent colloid within follicles is typical, and marked nuclear pleomorphism is frequently seen. Pendred syndrome occurs in patients with deficient hydrogen peroxide activity; these patients also present with deafness and develop a goiter in late childhood or young adulthood. While Graves disease shares some histopathologic features with dyshormonogenetic disorder, patients with Graves disease would be hyperthyroid and have diffuse enlargement without nodules. Endemic goiter due to iodine deficiency is uncommon in developed countries, and would contain larger hyperplastic nodules interspersed with normal thyroid gland tissue. Hashimoto's thyroiditis is characterized by chronic inflammation, germinal center formation, and oncocytic (Hürthle cell) metaplasia. Riedel's thyroiditis is characterized by dense fibrous obliteration of the thyroid gland that extends into the surrounding soft tissues.

81. **(A) Columnar cell variant of papillary thyroid carcinoma.**
Many variants of papillary thyroid carcinoma have been described, some to aid in histopathologic recognition and diagnosis, and others because the variant is associated with more aggressive clinical behavior. The variants of papillary thyroid carcinoma that behave more aggressively include tall cell variant, columnar cell variant, and diffuse sclerosing variant. Variants of papillary thyroid carcinoma that behave similar to conventional papillary thyroid carcinoma include follicular variant, oncocytic variant, Warthin-like variant, cribriform morular variant, solid variant, and

clear cell variant. Variants of papillary thyroid carcinoma that may have a better prognosis than conventional papillary thyroid carcinoma include encapsulated variant, macrofollicular variant, and papillary microcarcinoma (papillary thyroid carcinoma <1.0 cm in greatest dimension).

SUGGESTED READING

1. Albores-Saavedra J, Wu J. The many faces and mimics of papillary thyroid carcinoma. *Endocr Pathol.* 2006;17(1):1-18.
2. Are C, Shaha AR. Anaplastic thyroid carcinoma: biology, pathogenesis, prognostic factors, and treatment approaches. *Ann Surg Oncol.* 2006;13(4):453-464.
3. Asa SL. My approach to oncocytic tumours of the thyroid. *J Clin Pathol.* 2004;57(3):225-232.
4. Baloch ZW, Solomon AC, LiVolsi VA. Primary mucoepidermoid carcinoma and sclerosing mucoepidermoid carcinoma with eosinophilia of the thyroid gland: a report of nine cases. *Mod Pathol.* 2000;13(7):802-807.
5. Bejarano PA, Nikiforov YE, Swenson ES, Biddinger PW. Thyroid transcription factor-1, thyroglobulin, cytokeratin 7, and cytokeratin 20 in thyroid neoplasms. *Appl Immunohistochem Mol Morphol.* 2000;8(3):189-194.
6. Bell CD, Kovacs K, Horvath E, Rotondo F. Histologic, immunohistochemical, and ultrastructural findings in a case of minocycline-associated "black thyroid". *Endocr Pathol.* 2001;12(4):443-451.
7. Cameselle-Teijeiro J, Chan JK. Cribriform-morular variant of papillary carcinoma: a distinctive variant representing the sporadic counterpart of familial adenomatous polyposis-associated thyroid carcinoma? *Mod Pathol.* 1999;12(4):400-411.
8. Carcangiu ML, Bianchi S. Diffuse sclerosing variant of papillary thyroid carcinoma. Clinicopathologic study of 15 cases. *Am J Surg Pathol.* 1989;13(12):1041-1049.
9. Carney JA, Hirokawa M, Lloyd RV, Papotti M, Sebo TJ. Hyalinizing trabecular tumors of the thyroid gland are almost all benign. *Am J Surg Pathol.* 2008;32(12):1877-1889.
10. Chung AY, Tran TB, Brumund KT, Weisman RA, Bouvet M. Metastases to the thyroid: a review of the literature from the last decade. *Thyroid.* 2012;22(3):258-268.
11. Cryer PE, Axelrod L, Grossman AB, et al. Evaluation and management of adult hypoglycemic disorders: an Endocrine Society Clinical Practice Guideline. *J Clin Endocrinol Metab.* 2009;94(3):709-728.
12. Dedivitis RA, Camargo DL, Peixoto GL, Weissman L, Guimaraes AV. Thyroglossal duct: a review of 55 cases. *J Am Coll Surg.* 2002;194(3):274-277.
13. Del Gaudio AD, Del Gaudio GA. Virilizing adrenocortical tumors in adult women. Report of 10 patients, 2 of whom each had a tumor secreting only testosterone. *Cancer.* 1993;72(6):1997-2003.
14. DeLellis DA, LR, Heitz PU (ed.). *Pathology and Genetics of Tumours of Endocrine Organs. WHO Classification of Tumours.* Lyon, France: IARC Press; 2004.
15. Delellis RA. Challenging lesions in the differential diagnosis of endocrine tumors: parathyroid carcinoma. *Endocr Pathol.* 2008;19(4):221-225.
16. DeLellis RA, Mazzaglia P, Mangray S. Primary hyperparathyroidism: a current perspective. *Arch Pathol Lab Med.* 2008;132(8):1251-1262.
17. Derringer GA, Thompson LD, Frommelt RA, Bijwaard KE, Heffess CS, Abbondanzo SL. Malignant lymphoma of the thyroid gland: a clinicopathologic study of 108 cases. *Am J Surg Pathol.* 2000;24(5):623-639.
18. Edge SB BD, Carducci MA, Compton CC (ed.). *AJCC Cancer Staging Manual.* 7th ed. New York, NY: Springer; 2009.
19. Folpe AL, Lloyd RV, Bacchi CE, Rosai J. Spindle epithelial tumor with thymus-like differentiation: a morphologic, immunohistochemical, and molecular genetic study of 11 cases. *Am J Surg Pathol.* 2009;33(8):1179-1186.
20. Gerard-Marchant R, Caillou B. Thyroid inclusions in cervical lymph nodes. *Clin Endocrinol Metab.* 1981;10(2):337-349.
21. Ghossein RA, Rosai J, Heffess C. Dyshormonogenetic goiter: a clinicopathologic study of 56 cases. *Endocr Pathol.* 1997;8(4):283-292.
22. Heffess CS, Thompson LD. Minimally invasive follicular thyroid carcinoma. *Endocr Pathol.* 2001;12(4):417-422.
23. Heffess CS, Wenig BM, Thompson LD. Metastatic renal cell carcinoma to the thyroid gland: a clinicopathologic study of 36 cases. *Cancer.* 2002;95(9):1869-1878.
24. Hruban RH, Huvos AG, Traganos F, Reuter V, Lieberman PH, Melamed MR. Follicular neoplasms of the thyroid in men older than 50 years of age. A DNA flow cytometric study. *Am J Clin Pathol.* 1990;94(5):527-532.
25. Isotalo PA, Lloyd RV. Presence of birefringent crystals is useful in distinguishing thyroid from parathyroid gland tissues. *Am J Surg Pathol.* 2002;26(6):813-814.
26. Katoh R, Miyagi E, Nakamura N, et al. Expression of thyroid transcription factor-1 (TTF-1) in human C cells and medullary thyroid carcinomas. *Hum Pathol,* 2000;31(3):386-393.
27. Klimstra DS. Nonductal neoplasms of the pancreas. *Mod Pathol.* 2007;20 Suppl 1:S94-S112.
28. Kung IT. Distinction between colloid nodules and follicular neoplasms of the thyroid. Further observations on cell blocks. *Acta Cytol.* 1990;34(3):345-351.
29. LiVolsi VA, Baloch ZW. Follicular neoplasms of the thyroid: view, biases, and experiences. *Adv Anat Pathol.* 2004;11(6):279-287.
30. LiVolsi VA, Merino MJ. Worrisome histologic alterations following fine-needle aspiration of the thyroid (WHAFFT). *Pathol Annu.* 1994;29 (Pt 2):99-120.
31. New MI. An update of congenital adrenal hyperplasia. *Ann N Y Acad Sci.* 2004;1038:14-43.
32. Nikiforov YE, Erickson LA, Nikiforova MN, Caudill CM, Lloyd RV. Solid variant of papillary thyroid carcinoma: incidence, clinical-pathologic characteristics, molecular analysis, and biologic behavior. *Am J Surg Pathol.* 2001;25(12):1478-1484.
33. Perry A, Molberg K, Albores-Saavedra J. Physiologic versus neoplastic C-cell hyperplasia of the thyroid: separation of distinct histologic and biologic entities. *Cancer.* 1996;77(4):750-756.

34. Polyzos SA, Patsiaoura K, Zachou K. Histological alterations following thyroid fine needle biopsy: a systematic review. *Diagn Cytopathol.* 2009;37(6):455-465.

35. Pusztaszeri M, Triponez F, Pache JC, Bongiovanni M. Riedel's thyroiditis with increased IgG4 plasma cells: evidence for an underlying IgG4-related sclerosing disease? *Thyroid.* 2012.

36. Reimann JD, Dorfman DM, Nose V. Carcinoma showing thymus-like differentiation of the thyroid (CASTLE): a comparative study: evidence of thymic differentiation and solid cell nest origin. *Am J Surg Pathol.* 2006;30(8):994-1001.

37. Sasano H, Suzuki T, Moriya T. Recent advances in histopathology and immunohistochemistry of adrenocortical carcinoma. *Endocr Pathol.* 2006;17(4):345-354.

38. Sporny S, Lewinski A. Diagnosis and differentiation of follicular neoplasms of the thyroid gland. *Pol Tyg Lek.* 1990;45(25-26):525-529.

39. Thompson LD. Pheochromocytoma of the Adrenal gland Scaled Score (PASS) to separate benign from malignant neoplasms: a clinicopathologic and immunophenotypic study of 100 cases. *Am J Surg Pathol.* 2002;26(5):551-566.

40. Thompson LD, Wieneke JA, Heffess CS. Diffuse sclerosing variant of papillary thyroid carcinoma: a clinicopathologic and immunophenotypic analysis of 22 cases. *Endocr Pathol.* 2005;16(4):331-348.

41. Thompson LD, Wieneke JA, Paal E, Frommelt RA, Adair CF, Heffess CS. A clinicopathologic study of minimally invasive follicular carcinoma of the thyroid gland with a review of the English literature. *Cancer.* 2001;91(3):505-524.

42. Toshimori H, Narita R, Nakazato M, et al. Islet amyloid polypeptide in insulinoma and in the islets of the pancreas of non-diabetic and diabetic subjects. *Virchows Arch A Pathol Anat Histopathol.* 1991;418(5):411-417.

43. Turner WJ, Baergen RN, Pellitteri PK, Orloff LA. Parathyroid lipoadenoma: case report and review of the literature. *Otolaryngol Head Neck Surg.* 1996;114(2):313-316.

44. Volante M, Collini P, Nikiforov YE, et al. Poorly differentiated thyroid carcinoma: the Turin proposal for the use of uniform diagnostic criteria and an algorithmic diagnostic approach. *Am J Surg Pathol.* 2007;31(8):1256-1264.

45. Wall J. Extrathyroidal manifestations of Graves' disease. *J Clin Endocrinol Metab.* 1995;80(12):3427-3429.

46. Weiss LM. Comparative histologic study of 43 metastasizing and nonmetastasizing adrenocortical tumors. *Am J Surg Pathol.* 1984;8(3):163-169.

47. Wenig BM, Adair CF, Heffess CS. Primary mucoepidermoid carcinoma of the thyroid gland: a report of six cases and a review of the literature of a follicular epithelial-derived tumor. *Hum Pathol.* 1995;26(10):1099-1108.

48. Wenig BM, Thompson LD, Adair CF, Shmookler B, Heffess CS. Thyroid papillary carcinoma of columnar cell type: a clinicopathologic study of 16 cases. *Cancer.* 1998;82(4):740-753.

49. Wick MR, Ritter JH, Humphrey PA, Nappi O. Clear cell neoplasms of the endocrine system and thymus. *Semin Diagn Pathol,* 1997;14(3):183-202.

50. Yamashina M. Follicular neoplasms of the thyroid. Total circumferential evaluation of the fibrous capsule. *Am J Surg Pathol.* 1992;16(4):392-400.

51. Bosman F, Carneiro F, Hruban R, Theise N. *WHO Classification of Tumours of the Digestive System.* Lyon, France: IARC Press, 2010.

52. Rindi G, Kloppel G, Alhman H, et al. TNM staging of foregut (neuro)endocrine tumors: a consensus proposal including a grading system. *Virchows Arch.* 2006;449:395-401.

CHAPTER 12

FORENSIC PATHOLOGY

1. A 72-year-old woman had not been seen by her neighbors for 3 days. She was found supine in the kitchen on the floor in her locked apartment. Contusions and abrasions were noted on her face, torso, and extremities. White foamy fluid was draining from her nose. The radio cord was loosely wrapped around her head. Two chairs were knocked over and several drinking glasses were broken. The cause of death was ruled to be atherosclerotic heart disease with an acute myocardial infarct. The most likely cause of the contusions and abrasions are
   (A) Due to falling off a chair
   (B) Due to hypoxia causing confusion terminally
   (C) Self-inflicted, as attempt at committing suicide
   (D) The result of assault
   (E) The result of postmortem-related decomposition

2. An elderly woman was found naked at home. A large pool of blood was on the bedroom floor close to the body. Blood was noted on the top of her feet and on the soles of her feet. There was no evidence of foul play. All of the following are possible causes of death except
   (A) Esophageal varices
   (B) Hemodialysis shunt-related bleed
   (C) Lung carcinoma
   (D) Ovarian carcinoma
   (E) Pulmonary tuberculosis

3. All of the following are manners of death except
   (A) Accidental
   (B) Deliberate
   (C) Natural
   (D) Suicidal
   (E) Undetermined

4. Which of the following causes of death is a scene-dependent diagnosis?
   (A) Drowning
   (B) Heroin overdose
   (C) Myocardial infarct
   (D) Positional asphyxia
   (E) Suicide-jumping from a high bridge

5. The least desirable autopsy specimen for DNA studies would be from which of the following?
   (A) Blood
   (B) Bone
   (C) Hair
   (D) Liver
   (E) Skeletal muscle

6. In suspected arson cases, clothing should be stored in sealed metal containers for what reason?
   (A) To prevent contamination by environmental fungi and molds
   (B) To prevent contamination by fingerprints
   (C) To prevent disintegration of the clothing
   (D) To prevent DNA contamination
   (E) To prevent possible volatiles (accelerants) from evaporating

7. A 19-year-old woman with an unremarkable medical history collapses and dies suddenly after a 4-day history of chest pain. At autopsy, she is noted to be tall (185 cm) with a long arm span. She had arachnodactyly, a high arched palate, and mild pectus excavatum. She had a hemopericardium due to an aortic dissection. The most likely underlying condition that resulted in her death was
   (A) Atherosclerotic cardiovascular disease
   (B) Hypertension
   (C) Infective endocarditis
   (D) Marfan syndrome
   (E) Mitral valve prolapse

8. A 20-year-old college student had been feeling unwell for the last 4–5 days. While walking to class, he collapsed and died. At autopsy, he was noted to have cardiomegaly with subendocardial pallor. Microscopically, he had a marked lymphocytic interstitial inflammatory cell infiltrate with myofiber necrosis. The most likely cause of death is due to which organism?
   (A) Coxsackie A
   (B) Group B streptococcus
   (C) Herpes virus
   (D) *Staphylococcus aureus*
   (E) West Nile virus

9. The setting of blood to dependent portions of the vascular system is referred to as
   (A) Contusion
   (B) Ecchymosis
   (C) Hematoma
   (D) Livor mortis
   (E) Petechiae

10. A 1-year-old male child died suddenly after presenting with an episode of vomiting. A small contusion was noted on the abdomen. At autopsy, the small bowel showed evidence of near transection. There were multifocal omental lacerations and 200 mL of intraabdominal blood. The most likely cause of death was
    (A) Blunt trauma
    (B) Fall from the bed
    (C) Food poisoning
    (D) Repeated abdominal abrasions
    (E) Petechiae

11. Periorbital ecchymoses are usually indicative of which of the following?
    (A) Basilar artery tear
    (B) Basilar skull fracture
    (C) Hemorrhage into mastoid air cells
    (D) Linear occipital skull fracture
    (E) Shaken baby syndrome

12. A 64-year-old pedestrian was struck by a car. A large area of soft tissue was torn from her right leg and buttock region. This pattern of injury is best characterized as representing a(n)
    (A) Abrasion
    (B) Avulsion
    (C) Contusion
    (D) Crush injury
    (E) Laceration

13. A 32-year-old man was found in a building that was severely damaged in a fire and explosion. Which of the following findings would suggest that the person was alive at the time of the explosion?
    (A) Burned horizontal creases on the forehead
    (B) Pieces of wire embedded in the skin
    (C) Relative sparing of the earlobes
    (D) Ruptured tympanic membranes
    (E) Unburned skin at the outer edges of the eye

14. The most common complication of blunt force traumatic injury is
    (A) Acute respiratory distress syndrome
    (B) Acute tubular necrosis
    (C) Disseminated intravascular coagulopathy
    (D) Infection
    (E) Pulmonary embolus

15. Incisions of the legs to identify deep leg bruises could be important in which of the following?
    (A) A 62-year-old alcoholic found in bed at home
    (B) A 32-year-old diabetic who was found in the bathtub
    (C) A 26-year-old IV drug abuser found in his car
    (D) A 14-year-old pedestrian found by the side of the road
    (E) A 72-year-old who had fallen from a barstool right before he died

16. All of the following can affect the size and shape of a knife stab wound except
    (A) Angle of withdrawal
    (B) Body region stabbed
    (C) Depth of insertion
    (D) Metal composition of the blade
    (E) Shape of blade

17. A 19-year-old man is noted to have a stab wound on his left chest. Which of the following findings indicate that the knife had been inserted up to the crossguard?
    (A) Abrasion around the stab wound
    (B) Bruised tissue around the stab wound
    (C) A wound that is more broad than deep
    (D) There is no finding that would suggest this
    (E) V-shaped wound

18. The handedness (right versus left hand) of the assailant in a knife stab wound can be determined by which of the following?
    (A) It cannot be determined by examination of the wound alone
    (B) The depth of the stab wound
    (C) The direction of the incised wound

(D) The location of ecchymoses adjacent to the wound

(E) The wound track

19. Injuries on which part of the body least likely represent defensive injuries?
(A) Back
(B) Feet
(C) Forearm
(D) Hands
(E) Upper arm

20. The most common cause of homicidal death in an urban setting in the United States is
(A) Asphyxia
(B) Blunt force trauma
(C) Gunshot wounds
(D) Stab wounds
(E) Vehicular

21. All of the following are indicative of an entrance contact range gunshot wound except
(A) Gunpowder residue
(B) Muzzle imprint
(C) Soot in the wound
(D) Stellate wound shape
(E) Stretch lacerations along the bullet path

22. A 52-year-old man had a history of diabetes, hypertension, and a gunshot wound to the back 15 years ago that left him paraplegic. He subsequently developed decubitus ulcers and osteomyelitis, requiring a left above the knee amputation. He also developed neurogenic bladder. At autopsy, he was found to have purulent meningitis associated with acute sacral osteomyelitis. The manner of death is
(A) Accidental
(B) Homicide
(C) Indeterminate
(D) Natural
(E) Suicide

23. The distribution and concentration of a bloodstain pattern may suggest which of the following?
(A) The distance between the origin of blood and the surface upon which it is deposited
(B) The impact angle of the blood as it falls onto a surface
(C) The kind of energy available for bloodstain productions (in the setting of an impact)
(D) The origin of the blood
(E) The volume of blood lost

24. All of the following represent transient evidence at a crime scene except
(A) Body odor
(B) Body temperature
(C) Color of a contusion
(D) Color of bloodstains
(E) Livor mortis

25. Stomach contents found in a 72-year-old would represent which type of physical evidence in a forensic case?
(A) Associative
(B) Conditional
(C) Transfer
(D) Transient
(E) Pattern

26. A 23-year-old woman is suspected of being raped prior to being beaten to death. Which of the following tests would be most useful in evaluating a vaginal swab?
(A) Acid phosphatase test
(B) Amylase test
(C) Jaffe test
(D) Kastle–Meyer test
(E) Pepsin test

27. An 80-year-old woman dies of a pulmonary embolus after being confined in bed for 2 months following a hip fracture from a fall. Which of the following is the manner of death?
(A) Accidental
(B) Homicide
(C) Indeterminate
(D) Natural
(E) Suicide

28. In a body embalmed 4 days prior to autopsy, which of the following chemical compounds can be most reliably qualitatively tested for?
(A) Barbiturates
(B) Carbon monoxide
(C) Cyanide
(D) Ethanol
(E) Opiates

29. A 62-year-old man is found dead at home. Which of the following would be least useful in determining the time of death?
(A) Body temperature
(B) Gastric contents
(C) Postmortem reactivity of muscles to electrical stimulation
(D) Rigor mortis
(E) Serum glucose level

30. Postmortem cooling may be affected by all of the following factors except
    (A) Clothing
    (B) Environmental temperature
    (C) Relative humidity
    (D) Skin color
    (E) Temperature of body at death

31. A 16-year-old woman's body is found and is marked by cherry-pink livor mortis. This finding suggests which of the following as the most likely cause of death?
    (A) Drowning
    (B) Gunshot wound
    (C) Hydrogen sulfide poisoning
    (D) Sodium chlorate poisoning
    (E) Waterhouse–Friderichsen syndrome

32. In a body found at room temperature, onset of rigor mortis would occur how long after death?
    (A) 1 hour
    (B) 2 hours
    (C) 5 hours
    (D) 12 hours
    (E) 24 hours

33. All of the following findings at autopsy are consistent with rigor mortis-associated changes except
    (A) Bile staining of the stomach
    (B) Collapsed lung
    (C) Cutis anserina
    (D) Difference in pupil diameter
    (E) Semen on the penis tip

34. All of the following are true regarding adipocere except
    (A) Forms in high environmental temperature
    (B) Forms in low-humidity environment
    (C) Gray-white coloration
    (D) Preferentially involves buttocks and extremities
    (E) Results from bacterial conversion of unsaturated fats to saturated fats

35. A diagnosis of diabetic ketoacidosis at autopsy can be best made postmortem by measuring elevated glucose levels in which of the following?
    (A) Cerebrospinal fluid
    (B) Serum
    (C) Urine
    (D) Vitreous fluid
    (E) Whole blood

36. Forensic entomology may be least useful in establishing which of the following?
    (A) Areas of trauma on the remains
    (B) Geographic location of death
    (C) Manner of death
    (D) Time of death
    (E) Toxicological determination

37. A decomposed body is found in the woods. All of the following would serve as scientific methods of definitive identification except
    (A) Birthmark
    (B) Dental records
    (C) DNA analysis
    (D) Fingerprints
    (E) Radiographs

38. Which of the following features of mitochondrial DNA makes it potentially useful in forensic science?
    (A) Allows for individualization of a sample
    (B) It has low copy number
    (C) It is inherited maternally
    (D) It is over 2 billion base pairs in length
    (E) It is unique to the individual

39. Skeletal remains are found in the woods. In determining the gender of the skeleton, which of the following would be least useful?
    (A) Bone buildup on the sacroiliac bone
    (B) Examination of the skull
    (C) Length of the pubic bone
    (D) Measurements of the teeth
    (E) Width of the sciatic notch

40. A 69-year-old man was at home when two intruders broke into his house. There was no sign of trauma and no obvious cause of death at autopsy. It is concluded that he died from the emotional stress of the event. The underlying cause is most likely which of the following?
    (A) Lev disease
    (B) Long QT syndrome
    (C) Sick sinus syndrome
    (D) Spontaneous ventricular fibrillation
    (E) Wolf–Parkinson–White syndrome

41. The typical profile of a mother who murders or abandons a newborn child includes all of the following except
    (A) Age of mother usually over 40 years
    (B) No help is obtained during labor and delivery

(C) Pregnancy often concealed from friends and relatives

(D) Usually conceals the infant's body

(E) When confronted with the death, most claim the baby was stillborn

42. In determining if a baby found dead was born alive, which of the following findings would be most useful?
(A) Empty stomach
(B) Eyes closed
(C) Maceration
(D) Open alveoli on lung examination
(E) Skin sloughing

43. A 3-year-old child is suspected to have died of child abuse. All of the following brain findings may be the result of child abuse except
(A) Basal ganglia bleed
(B) Cerebral contusion
(C) Chronic subdural hematoma
(D) Diffuse axonal injury
(E) Retinal hemorrhages

44. Bruises in which location are most suspicious for potential child abuse?
(A) Abdomen
(B) Elbows
(C) Forehead
(D) Knees
(E) Shins

45. All of the following are characteristic of Münchausen syndrome by proxy except
(A) Knowledge about the cause of the child's illness is freely admitted by the perpetrator
(B) The child is repetitively taken to a doctor or hospital
(C) The child is subjected to multiple unnecessary procedures
(D) The child's acute symptoms improve when the child is separated from the perpetrator
(E) The illness and symptoms of the child are fabricated or produced by the parent or caregiver

46. All of the following are epidemiological factors associated with Sudden Infant Death Syndrome (SIDS) except
(A) Age 2–4 months
(B) Female gender of the infant
(C) History of smoking
(D) Low birth weight infant
(E) Young maternal age

47. A 22-year-old man jumps from his apartment balcony and lands on his feet. Which of the following types of skull base fractures would be expected?
(A) Diagonal
(B) Hinge
(C) Longitudinal
(D) Ring
(E) Transverse

48. Fat embolism is most commonly identified in association with which of the following?
(A) Blunt trauma to the face
(B) Cellulitis of a proximal extremity
(C) Fracture of the femur
(D) Pulmonary embolus
(E) Stab wound to the chest

49. Intravascular air is least likely to be encountered in which of the following situations?
(A) Chest trauma
(B) Decompression sickness
(C) Obstetric procedure
(D) Open neck injury
(E) Strangulation

50. A 69-year-old man sustained a gunshot wound to the head. Homicide is suspected. An entrance wound in what location would provide the most support for a homicide?
(A) Back of the head
(B) In the mouth
(C) Side of the head
(D) Temple
(E) Under the chin

51. Which of the following terms is used in reference to small fragments of metal derived from the bullet?
(A) Fouling
(B) Full metal jacket
(C) Powder burns
(D) Powder stippling
(E) Tattooing

52. Pseudotattooing may be produced by all the following except
(A) .22 caliber handgun
(B) Fragmented tempered glass
(C) Postmortem insect bite
(D) Spattered grease burns
(E) Wood slivers

53. All of the following may affect the pattern of injury observed on the victim made by a shotgun fired from a distance of 5 feet except
    (A) Choke
    (B) Gauge of gun
    (C) Metal composition of the shot
    (D) Powder load
    (E) Size of shot

54. A 6-year-old female child has burns over most of her lower body. On examination, both the epidermis and dermis show damage. The underlying soft tissues appear intact. Which of the following best characterizes the injury observed?
    (A) Fifth-degree burns
    (B) First-degree burns
    (C) Fourth-degree burns
    (D) Second-degree burns
    (E) Third-degree burns

55. The extent of burns should be estimated at autopsy in a burn victim. Burns covering most of the head in an infant account for approximately what percent of the body surface area?
    (A) <5%
    (B) 9%
    (C) 15%
    (D) 18%
    (E) 27%

56. Remnants of a burn victim found in a house fire are examined. Which of the following bone lesions are characteristic of heat fractures encountered in the setting?
    (A) Bones are reduced to ash
    (B) Curved fracture
    (C) Depressed fracture
    (D) Fractures are not seen secondary to heat; bones look normal
    (E) Jagged fractures

57. All of the following may be encountered in 32-year-old man who committed suicide by hanging himself by the neck (semi-suspended) except
    (A) Bulging eyes
    (B) Face is purple
    (C) Petechiae on the chest
    (D) Subconjunctival petechiae
    (E) Swollen face

58. A 29-year-old woman was found submerged in a bathtub. An initial examination of the body at the scene showed only two small whitish scar-like areas on the side of the neck. At autopsy, after the body was dried, fingernail marks were observed on all sides of the neck. The most likely cause of death was
    (A) Accidental drowning
    (B) Accidentally slipped and hit her head on the tub
    (C) Homicidal strangulation
    (D) Suicidal hanging
    (E) Suicidal strangulation

59. A 62-year-old woman was involved in a car accident. It is thought that her neck struck the rim of the steering wheel at the time of impact. All of the following findings would support this theory except
    (A) Battle sign
    (B) Fracture of cricoid cartilage
    (C) Fracture of hyoid bone
    (D) Thyroid cartilage tear
    (E) Thyroid gland hemorrhage

60. In a 16-year-old suspected of dying via hanging, which of the following findings would be most supportive of the diagnosis?
    (A) Cricoid cartilage fracture
    (B) Horizontal mark on the neck
    (C) Hyoid bone fracture
    (D) Mark on neck above the thyroid cartilage
    (E) Thyroid cartilage fracture

61. A 62-year-old man is found dead in the garage with his car running. The cause of death is suspected to be carbon monoxide poisoning. Which of the following findings is most consistent with this diagnosis?
    (A) Cherry-red discolorations of the skeletal musculature
    (B) Foaming at the mouth
    (C) Oral hemorrhage
    (D) Swelling of the nasopharynx
    (E) None of the above

62. The most common cause of death in the coroner's office in a 6-year-old would be which of the following?
    (A) Burns
    (B) Drowning
    (C) Electrocution
    (D) Gunshot wound
    (E) Motor vehicle accident

63. Which of the following scenarios would be most commonly encountered in a 6-month-old drowning victim?
    (A) Drowning in a backyard pool
    (B) Drowning in a bathtub
    (C) Drowning in a community pool
    (D) Drowning in a lake
    (E) Drowning in an industrial bucket

64. All of the following are expected findings in a body found completely submerged in water except
    (A) Body shows extensive mummification.
    (B) Fungi growth may be seen on the body.
    (C) Postmortem loss of facial soft tissue due to fish feeding.
    (D) Putrefaction is slower in saltwater versus freshwater.
    (E) Putrefaction proceeds more slowly in water than on land.

65. Which of the following findings is suggestive of an electrical burn?
    (A) Brain white matter petechiae
    (B) Epidermal microblisters with nuclear streaming
    (C) Fern-like discoloration of the skin
    (D) Liver hemorrhage
    (E) Red-brown discoloration of the cerebral cortex

66. All of the following are true regarding bumper injuries sustained by a pedestrian struck by a car except
    (A) Amount of clothing does not affect degree of injury
    (B) Calf region should be examined for injury
    (C) Injury sustained depends on speed of the vehicle
    (D) Leg bone fractures are a common finding
    (E) Severity of injury depends on the shape of the bumper

67. Which of the following injuries is least likely the result of air bag deployment?
    (A) Facial fracture
    (B) Forearm fracture
    (C) Hemothorax
    (D) Laceration of the brain stem
    (E) Skull fracture

68. Which of the following factors is least important in determining survivability following an aircraft crash?
    (A) Design of aircraft
    (B) Number of individuals in the aircraft
    (C) Post-crash environment
    (D) Restraints in the aircraft
    (E) Use of energy absorptive material

69. All of the following are findings associated with uncal herniation except
    (A) Cranial nerve III compression
    (B) Duret hemorrhage
    (C) Ipsilateral cerebral peduncle compressed
    (D) Ipsilateral fixed, dilated pupil
    (E) Posterior cerebral artery compression

70. With complete loss of cerebral circulation, how long does it take to develop loss of consciousness?
    (A) Immediately
    (B) 5 seconds
    (C) 10 seconds
    (D) 15 seconds
    (E) 30 seconds

71. A 41-year-old man was found unconscious at the scene of a car accident where he was a passenger. An MRI study showed only small hemorrhages in the corpus callosum and fornices. He remained in a coma for 4 days with decerebrate and decorticate posturing. He expired on day 4. Which of the following is an expected pathologic finding that might explain his neurologic status?
    (A) Anoxic encephalopathy
    (B) Development of cerebral contusions
    (C) Diffuse axonal injury
    (D) Subdural hematoma
    (E) Vascular malformation rupture

72. All of the following are true regarding epidural hematoma except
    (A) A common finding in head trauma cases in children less than 1-year-old
    (B) Most cases are associated with a skull fracture
    (C) Most cases are due to tearing of the middle meningeal artery
    (D) Most occur overlying the cerebral hemispheres
    (E) The hematoma is typically shaped like a biconcave lens

73. The beginning development of a yellow neomembrane on the dural aspect of a subdural hematoma with invasion of the clot by thin-walled capillaries along with fibroblasts allows one to date a subdural hematoma to which of the following time periods?
    (A) 24 hours
    (B) 2–4 days
    (C) 1 week
    (D) 3 weeks
    (E) Over 1 month

74. Which of the following is the most likely site of a contrecoup contusion?
    (A) Basal ganglia
    (B) Cerebellar hemisphere
    (C) Frontal lobe
    (D) Occipital lobe
    (E) Pons

75. A pattern of numerous bilateral white matter petechiae in a 72-year-old woman found dead at home is a characteristic pathologic finding suggestive of which of the following?
    (A) Anoxic encephalopathy
    (B) Brain lacerations sustained in a fall
    (C) Fat emboli syndrome
    (D) Posttraumatic seizures
    (E) White matter contusions

76. Which of the following pathologic findings is least consistent with a history of chronic alcoholism?
    (A) Acute and chronic pancreatitis
    (B) Loss of Purkinje cells with cerebellar atrophy
    (C) Macrovesicular steatosis
    (D) Neuronal loss, gliosis, and blood vessel hyperplasia of the mamillary bodies
    (E) Testicular hypertrophy

77. Which of the following findings would be least expected in a patient who died of heat stroke?
    (A) Centrilobular hepatic necrosis
    (B) Myocardial necrosis
    (C) Pulmonary hemorrhage and necrosis
    (D) Purkinje cell shrinkage and necrosis
    (E) Rhabdomyolysis

78. Which of the following is least likely to be encountered in an individual suspected of dying of cocaine use?
    (A) Cardiac arrhythmia
    (B) Cardiac crossband necrosis
    (C) Hypertensive crisis
    (D) Pancreatic hemorrhagic necrosis
    (E) Sudden death due to coronary artery vasospasm

79. Three individuals, all man ranging from 18 to 23 years, were found dead in the living room of a house. There is no evidence of trauma on any of the bodies. No drug paraphernalia is found in the house. Which of the following is the most likely cause of death?
    (A) Aspirin use
    (B) Carbon monoxide poisoning
    (C) Cyanide poisoning
    (D) Freebase cocaine use
    (E) Meningitis

80. A marginal abrasion around an exit gunshot wound would suggest which of the following?
    (A) Body was leaning against a wall when shot
    (B) The bullet disintegrated and numerous fragments exited the body
    (C) The bullet entered the body at an angle (tangential)
    (D) The gun was fired at least 10 feet away
    (E) The gun was fired less than 1 foot from the victim

81. A 49-year-old man was swimming in the ocean on vacation in Australia. He was reported to have staggered from the water and collapsed dead on the beach. This finding was observed on his chest. The most likely cause of death is which of the following? (See Figure 12-1.)

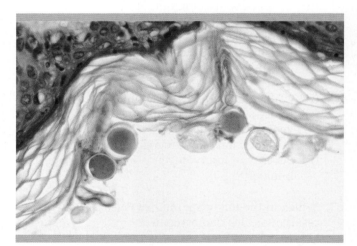

FIGURE 12-1

    (A) Allergic reaction to algae
    (B) Cannot tell from this figure
    (C) Fungal infection
    (D) Parasitic infection
    (E) Portuguese man-of-war sting

82. The most likely manner of death in this 39-year-old man is (Figure 12-2)

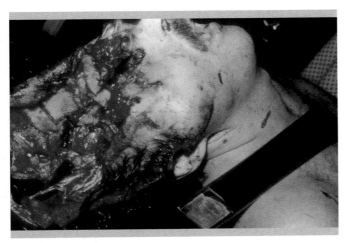

FIGURE 12-2

(A) Accidental
(B) Homicide
(C) Natural
(D) Suicide
(E) None of the above

83. The injury shown in Figure 12-3 in this 52-year-old woman represents which of the following?

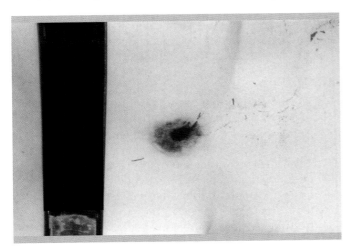

FIGURE 12-3

(A) Electrical burn
(B) Gunshot entrance wound
(C) Gunshot exit wound
(D) Knife wound
(E) Result of blunt trauma

84. On examination of the lung in a 28-year-old man, this finding was observed. The most likely cause of this finding is (Figure 12-4)

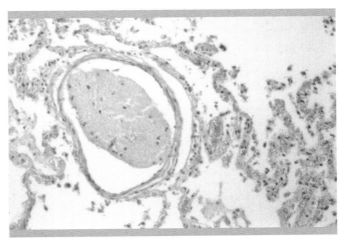

FIGURE 12-4

(A) Aspiration
(B) Fall from a high-level bridge
(C) Gunshot wound to the head
(D) Multiple bone fractures
(E) Strangulation

85. The most likely underlying pathophysiologic factor for the pathology shown in Figure 12-5 is which of the following?

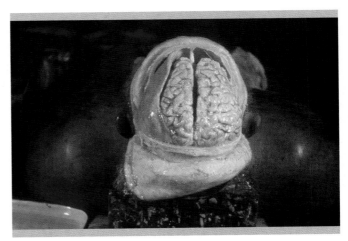

FIGURE 12-5

(A) Metastatic spread of a pulmonary carcinoma
(B) Neoplastic transformation of meningothelial (arachnoidal cap) cells
(C) Penetrating wound (gunshot)
(D) Rotational movement of the brain in the skull
(E) Sudden acceleration or deceleration of the skull relative to the brain

86. A 36-year-old man died of a gunshot wound to the chest. No other objects are found at the scene. At autopsy, you notice this injury on the scalp. The most likely etiology would be which of the following? (Figure 12-6)

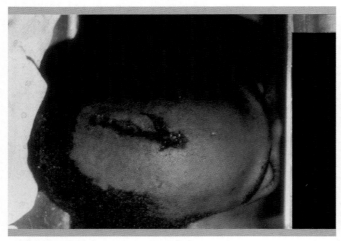

FIGURE 12-6

(A) Blunt trauma wound
(B) Defense wound
(C) Knife wound
(D) Laceration due to fall
(E) Superficial gunshot wound

87. A 34-year-old anesthesiologist was found dead in his car in a parking lot. His pants were down at his ankles and his head was leaning back on the top of the seat. At autopsy, needle puncture marks were found in his genital and inguinal region. A syringe was found on the floor of the car. Figure 12-7 shows a section taken from the lung and supports which of the following?

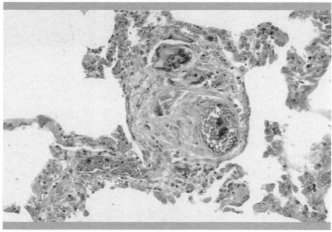

FIGURE 12-7

(A) Amphetamine overdose
(B) Aspiration
(C) Autoerotic asphyxia
(D) Blunt trauma to the chest
(E) Ventricular arrhythmia

88. The finding illustrated (in Figure 12-8) in this 56-year-old man is most likely associated with which of these findings?

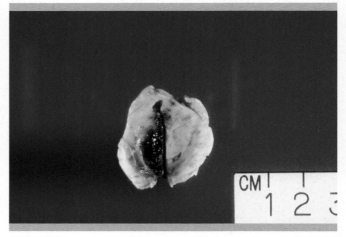

FIGURE 12-8

(A) Bifrontal contusion
(B) Diffuse axonal injury
(C) Infarct in the posterior cerebral artery distribution
(D) Right occipital lobe metastatic melanoma
(E) Vertebral artery aneurysm

ANSWERS

1. **(B) Due to hypoxia causing confusion terminally.** The most likely cause of contusions and abrasions in this woman was hypoxia causing confusion terminally. The presence of abrasions and contusions raises a suspicion for foul play. Those dying from natural causes may become hypoxic and confused in the endstages of life. They frequently fall and items are knocked over. In the process of falling, they may sustain contusions and abrasions.

2. **(D) Ovarian carcinoma.** The presence of blood at the scene of death does not always indicate trauma. There are a variety of natural diseases that may account for bleeding including esophageal varices, pulmonary tuberculosis, and pulmonary carcinomas with hematemesis or hemoptysis. Large tumors under the skin may erode and cause hemorrhage externally. Patients on hemodialysis may have vascular shunts that can erode through the skin and bleed. An ovarian carcinoma may cause hemorrhage internally, but the likelihood of

finding hemorrhage externally at the scene of death is less likely than the other options listed.

3. **(B) Deliberate.**

Forensic autopsies are performed with the goal of determining the cause and manner of death in people. The manner of death is defined as the circumstance under which the person died. The designations that are commonly used to describe the manner of death include natural, accidental, suicidal, homicidal, or undetermined. Deliberate does not indicate a manner of death; the term may imply either a suicidal or homicidal manner.

4. **(D) Positional asphyxia.**

In some forensic autopsy cases, investigation of the scene of injury or death is important in arriving at the correct cause of death. Positional asphyxia is an example where the position of the body in relationship to its surroundings is critical for making the correct diagnosis.

5. **(D) Liver.**

For certain cases, it may be important to be able to extract DNA for purposes of identification. Certain tissue types are better utilized to this end. Available blood adequately serves this purpose. The blood standard can be obtained by placing several drops of an individual's blood on a prepackaged filter paper and then allowing it to dry. The blood in this form does not need to be refrigerated. Skeletal muscle also can provide a good source of DNA. Liver and spleen generally are less desirable organs because they have high levels of autolytic enzymes. In bodies that have undergone more advanced decomposition, teeth, ribs, and femurs are good specimens for DNA. If hair is utilized, it should be pulled and not cut, because much of the valuable DNA is located in the roots of the hair.

6. **(E) To prevent possible volatiles (accelerants) from evaporating.**

In cases of suspected arson, it is important to store clothing in sealed metal containers. If the clothing is allowed to air-dry before an analysis is preformed, important volatiles that may have served as accelerants might evaporate and will not be detectable. Likewise, bloody clothing from cases of injury should be allowed to dry in a secure place and then packaged in a breathable paper bag before delivery to the crime laboratory.

7. **(D) Marfan syndrome.**

In younger patients with a history of aortic dissection, Marfan syndrome should be considered in the differential diagnosis. Marfan syndrome is inherited as an autosomal-dominant condition in many cases, and there is a potential genetic implication for surviving family members. This particular patient has many of the typical features of a Marfan patient including tall stature and long arm span, arachnosyndactyly, pectus excavatum, and a high arched palate.

8. **(A) Coxsackie A.**

In an individual who has prodromal systems of fever and flu-like illness followed by sudden death, a diagnosis of myocarditis should be entertained. In North America and Western Europe, most cases of myocarditis are caused by viral organisms, with Coxsackie A and Coxsackie B viruses being the most commonly encountered viral culprits.

9. **(D) Livor mortis.**

Livor mortis involves the settling of blood in dependent portions of the vascular system and not the surrounding tissues. Incised areas of livor mortis will not appear hemorrhagic. Livor mortis needs to be distinguished from a contusion or bruise, which usually results from blunt trauma due to the tearing of capillaries and larger blood vessels and an extravasation of blood into extravascular spaces.

10. **(A) Blunt trauma.**

The scenario represents an example of blunt trauma injury. In external examination, there is very little evidence of trauma. One needs to remember that the appearance of contusion may not be in line with the degree of force used to cause the injury. Individuals on systemic steroids or blood thinning medications may often have prominent numbers of ecchymoses related to bleeding secondary to trauma of relatively little force or in some cases spontaneous hemorrhage. In this child, the internal injuries are severe and are suggestive of trauma, possibly related to abuse.

11. **(B) Basilar skull fracture.**

Basilar skull fractures are characteristically associated with leakage of cerebrospinal fluid from the nasal cavity and periorbital or postauricular ecchymoses or bruises.

12. **(B) Avulsion.**

An avulsion represents a tearing away of tissues from their attachments. In this particular case, a large area of soft tissue is torn from her right leg and buttock region.

13. **(E) Unburned skin at the outer edges of the eye.**

Injury related to explosions often consists of blunt force injury, often caused by physical objects, and concussive pressure wave or shock wave injuries. In cases of explosion-related injury, the body may be burned in part in the process. If one sees linear streaks of unburned skin at the outer edges of the eyes, similar to crow's feet, and unburned horizontal creases in the forehead, these findings suggest that the individual was squinting and hence was alive at the time of the explosion.

14. **(D) Infection.**
    Infection is the most common complication of trau-
    matic injuries leading to morbidity and mortality.

15. **(D) A 14-year-old pedestrian found by the side of
    the road.**
    In cases of a pedestrian found in or around a road, it is
    appropriate to consider making incisions in the legs in
    order to identify deep leg bruises that may have been
    the result of impact of the vehicle on a pedestrian.

16. **(D) Metal composition of the blade.**
    The size and shape of a knife stab wound is depen-
    dent on a variety of factors including the type of
    blade used, the body region stabbed, the depth of
    insertion of the knife blade, and the angle of with-
    drawal of the knife. Composition of the metal mak-
    ing up the knife blade does not significantly impact
    on the size and shape of the stab wound.

17. **(A) Abrasion around the stab wound.**
    The crossguard of a knife is the flared area of pro-
    tection between the handle and the blade. When
    the knife is inserted up to the crossguard, there is
    often evidence of abrasion around the stab wound
    that is the result of the crossguard making contact
    with the skin.

18. **(A) It cannot be determined be examination of
    the wound alone.**
    The handedness of an assailant in a knife stab
    wound cannot be determined by examination of the
    wounds alone. If the relative positions of the assail-
    ant and the victim are known at the time of the
    stabbing, an opinion can potentially be generated
    that suggests that the wound is more consistent
    with right or left handed assailant.

19. **(A) Back.**
    Defense injuries or wounds are the result of the
    victim trying to protect himself or herself from an
    assailant. The labeling of a wound as a defense
    injury is generally circumstance dependent. Clas-
    sically, defense injuries involve the hands, arms,
    and upper arms. The feet may be a site of a defense
    injury if a victim is on the ground and kicking in
    an attempt to protect himself or herself from an
    assailant. Back injury is generally not considered a
    common defense injury site.

20. **(C) Gunshot wounds.**
    The most common cause of death in homicides in
    an urban setting in the United States is gunshot
    wounds.

21. **(E) Stretch lacerations along the bullet path.**
    Findings that are suggestive of an entrance contact
    range gunshot wound include a muzzle imprint,
    gunpowder residue staining the wound edges dark
    gray or black, or evidence of soot in the wound.
    Hard contact gunshot wounds, where the muzzle is

pressed firmly against the skin, can result in a
stellate-shaped wound (tear). Stretch lacerations
along the bullet path are less specific and are not
necessarily seen exclusively with contact range
gunshot wounds.

22. **(B) Homicide.**
    This case raises the issue of delayed gunshot would
    death. The gunshot wound in this case started a
    series of events that ultimately culminated in the
    patient's death. The death can be attributed to the
    gunshot wound. In this case, the gunshot wound
    resulted in paraplegia. The paraplegia predisposed
    the patient to the development of decubitus ulcers
    that are prone to infection and an increased risk of
    developing osteomyelitis. Infection spreading then to
    the central nervous system resulted in the proximal
    death of the patient. This sequence of events can
    be traced back to the original gunshot wound. The
    death in this case is appropriately ruled a homicide.

23. **(A) The distance between the origin of blood and
    the surface upon which it is deposited.**
    In evaluating bloodstain patterns, a number of
    features can be important in their interpretation.
    The shape of the individual bloodstains, the size
    of the individual bloodstains, and the distribution
    and concentration of a bloodstain pattern may all
    provide useful information. The distribution and
    concentration of a bloodstain pattern, in particular,
    may suggest the distance between the origin of
    blood and the surface upon which it was deposited.
    This can be important in differentiating between
    impact spatter, expired blood, and arterial pat-
    terns. The size of individual bloodstains may sug-
    gest the kind of energy available for their produc-
    tion, if they were the result of an impact. The shape
    of the individual bloodstains may allow delineation
    of their origin to be determined in 3 dimensions.

24. **(E) Livor mortis.**
    Transient evidence is physical evidence that is tem-
    porary and can be easily changed or altered. Com-
    monly encountered transient evidence may include
    the color of bloodstains, temperature of the room,
    and the color of the flame in a fire. Transient evi-
    dence found on a body may include body tempera-
    ture, body odor, color of contusions, the wetness of
    a bloodstain or body fluids, and the size of insect
    larvae. Livor mortis and rigor mortis are examples
    of conditional evidence, that is, physical evidence
    that results from an event or action.

25. **(B) Conditional.**
    Conditional evidence is a type of physical evidence
    that results from an event or action. Common types
    of conditional evidence found at a crime scene may
    include lighting of an area or room, the condition of

the doors or windows, the condition of television or radio, or furniture positions. Conditional evidence found on a body may include livor mortis and rigor mortis, the condition of clothing, the condition of bullet entrance and exit wounds, degree of decomposition, and stomach contents including types of food and the degree of digestion of that food. Pattern evidence is generally produced by physical contact between persons, vehicles, weapons, and other objects. Transfer evidence is produced by physical contact between persons, objects, or both and includes such things as paint chips, hairs, soil, and glass particles. Associative evidence is defined as evidence that can associate a victim or suspect with a crime scene and may include things such as a wallet or identification card, jewelry, photographs, money, or clothing that belong to a victim or suspect.

26. **(A) Acid phosphatase test.**
A useful screening test for the presence of semen is the acid phosphatase test. Acid phosphatase is present in high levels in semen, but may be present in low levels in other fluid samples such as feces, saliva, or vaginal secretions. A confirmatory test for semen is the immunological human seminal fluid protein test. Pepsin represents a digestive enzyme found in stomach contents. Kastle–Meyer or phenolphthalein can be used to assess for the presence of blood. Amylase is an enzyme found in saliva and in certain other body fluids. The Jaffe test is a presumptive test for urine that detects creatinine.

27. **(A) Accidental.**
Since there is no indication of foul play in this case, the hip fracture, which resulted from the fall, was considered accidental. A pulmonary embolus that resulted from confinement to the bed likely ensued from the hip fracture and is part of the accidental manner of death.

28. **(A) Barbiturates.**
Embalming a body can interfere with chemical analysis of many compounds including ethanol, carbon monoxide, cyanide, and opiates. Other chemicals such as tricyclic compounds, benzodiazepines, and barbiturates can be qualitatively tested, if testing is performed within a few weeks or months of the embalming. Quantitative evaluation of these compounds may be unreliable due to dilution by the embalming fluid and other factors. Metallic compounds and metalloids, such as arsenic, can be recovered from an embalmed body several years after death.

29. **(E) Serum glucose level.**
A variety of parameters can be used in the determination of time of death. Changes in body temperature, livor mortis, rigor mortis, and decomposition

may be useful. Changes in the chemical composition of body fluids or tissues such as postmortem potassium concentration in the vitreous fluid may be helpful. Postmortem residual reactivity of muscles to electrical or chemical stimuli has been reported by some to be useful. The assessment of physiological processes with known start time or progression rate such as the presence of gastric contents or gastric emptying time can be accessed. Survival time after injury, especially when the time of infliction is unknown, can provide information in this regard as well. Serum glucose levels are not terribly reliable in the determination time of death.

30. **(D) Skin color.**
Postmortem cooling of the body can be affected by a variety of factors including the clothing on the body, state of nutrition of the individual, environmental temperature and wind, relative humidity, whether or not the body is in contact with hot or cold objects, and the temperature of the body at death. Skin color does not play a significant role in postmortem body cooling rates.

31. **(A) Drowning.**
Cherry-pink livor may be seen in bodies recovered from water or bodies covered in wet clothes. Moisture on the body's surface prevents the escape of oxygen, causing retention of an excess of bright red oxyhemoglobin in the skin, accounting for the color. Carbon monoxide poisoning, cyanide poisoning, and fluoroacetate exposure (found in insecticides and rodenticides) can also account for cherry-pink or red discoloration. A hemorrhagic rash may be noted in association with livor mortis in patient dying of fulminate sepsis or Waterhouse–Friderichsen syndrome. Sodium chlorate poisoning may result in a brownish coloration to the livor due to methemoglobin. Hydrogen sulfide can result in a greenish coloration to the livor due to sulfhemoglobin.

32. **(A) 1 hour.**
At room temperature, rigor mortis may develop as soon as 30 minutes to 1 hour after death and may progress over the next 12 hours. Rigor usually begins to disappear about 24 hours.

33. **(B) Collapsed lung.**
Rigor mortis associated changes involving involuntary musculature may include differences in pupil diameter, cutis anserina or gooseflesh, rigidity of facial arrectores pilorum resulting in apparent beard growth, semen at or near the tip of the penis, and bile staining of the stomach. A collapsed lung usually is not the result of rigor mortis.

34. **(B) Forms in low-humidity environment.**
Adipocere or waxy fat develops under conditions of high (not low) humidity and high environmental

temperature. These findings typically involve subcutaneous tissues on the female breast, extremities,
buttocks, and face. The formation of adipocere is
the result of hydration and dehydrogenation of body
fats, which result in a gray-white coloration and a
soft greasy, clay-like consistency. Bacterial enzymes
from organisms such as Clostridia may be involved
in the process.

35. **(D) Vitreous fluid.**
Vitreous fluid levels of glucose and the presence of
ketones are useful in the confirmation of a diagnosis of diabetic ketoacidosis.

36. **(C) Manner of death.**
Forensic entomology is the application of the study
of insects and arthropods in legal proceedings.
Examination of insect larvae and egg stages can be
useful in determining how long a patient has been
dead, geographic location of the death, areas of
trauma of the remains (which tend to be preferentially involved), and toxicological determination.
Manner of death cannot be definitively established
utilizing forensic entomology.

37. **(A) Birthmark.**
Identification of human remains can be classified
as definitive, presumptive, or speculative. Definitive identification is a legally sufficient identification, usually based on objective comparison
of perimortem and postmortem information. A
presumptive identification describes a situation
in which positive identification has more likely
than not been established; however, all other possibilities cannot be excluded. Speculative identification carries the lowest degree of certainty and
essentially means the decedent is unidentified.
The most common method of definitive identification is visual recognition of the decedent's
face or body by someone who is knowledgeable.
Scientific methods of definitive identification
include comparison of fingerprints, radiographs,
DNA analysis, dental records, unique anthropo-
morphic features, and physical evidence such as
fingernails or hair. Birthmarks, tattoos, scars, and
clothing represent methods of presumptive identification.

38. **(C) It is inherited maternally.**
Mitochondrial DNA analysis may be helpful in
many cases in the identification of human remains.
Mitochondrial DNA is inherited maternally. It is
approximately 16,000–17,000 base pairs in length
(not over 2 billion base pairs in length like regular
DNA). Mitochondrial DNA has a high copy number and is not unique to the individual. It does
not allow for individualization of a sample. It can
be efficiently amplified. Mitochondrial testing can

establish that a deceased individual is a biological
relative of living family members.

39. **(D) Measurements of the teeth.**
Forensic anthropology focuses on the examination
of skeletal remains in order to obtain information regarding the decedent. In order to determine gender of the skeleton, there are a variety of
parameters that can be utilized including length of
the pubic bone, width of the sciatic notch, bone
buildup on the sacroiliac joint, and examination of
the skull. It is difficult to determine gender from
measurements of teeth size.

40. **(D) Spontaneous ventricular fibrillation.**
In the scenario presented in this question, the cause
of death is supposedly related to the emotional
stress of the event. This is most commonly the
result of a lethal ventricular arrhythmia.

41. **(A) Age of mother usually over 40 years.**
A typical profile of mother who murders or abandons her newborn child is that she is young,
unmarried, and has received little or no prenatal
care. The pregnancy has often been concealed
from friends and relatives; she obtained no help
during the labor and delivery process. She usually
conceals the infant's body and placenta and when
confronted with the death, typically claims the baby
was stillborn.

42. **(D) Open alveoli on lung examination.**
In determining if a baby found dead was born alive,
a variety of factors can be useful to assess. Open
alveoli imply that the lungs have been expanded
by breathing. Food in the stomach implies ante-
mortem swallowing. Vital reaction of the umbilical
cord stump associated with injury is also proof of
a live birth, in that a dead body cannot elicit an
inflammatory response. The other options listed are
not useful in the determination of whether a baby
found dead was born alive.

43. **(A) Basal ganglia bleed.**
A variety of injuries to the central nervous system
may be seen in association with child abuse. These
findings may include chronic subdural hematomas,
retinal hemorrhages, subarachnoid hemorrhages,
cerebral contusions, and diffuse axonal injury.
Basal ganglia bleeds are not usually encountered
in this setting and are often the site of bleeding in
hypertension-associated hemorrhages or with
certain toxicities.

44. **(A) Abdomen.**
Bruising caused by accidental injury in a child is
most typically found on the forehead, knees, shins,
and elbows. These are areas that are more likely
subject to low-level trauma, resulting from falls
or aggressive play. Bruises found in other parts,

including the chest, abdomen, buttock, and low back regions, are more likely to be the result of child abuse.

45. **(A) Knowledge about the cause of the child's illness is freely admitted by the perpetrator.**
Münchausen syndrome by proxy is a form of child abuse characterized by illness and symptoms of a child that are made up or produced by a parent or caregiver. The child is repeatedly taken to a doctor or hospital for medical attention and is subjected to numerous unnecessary medical procedures. The cause of the child's illness is typically denied by the parent or caregiver. The child's acute symptoms usually abate when the child is separated from the caregiver.

46. **(B) Female gender of the infant.**
Epidemiological factors that have been associated with SIDS include young maternal age, low socioeconomic group, history of smoking and drug abuse, overcrowded home, a minority group, unmarried mother, and inadequate prenatal care. Infant risk factors include prematurity and low birth weight, male gender, multiple births, brain and skeletal growth retardation, age of 2–4 months, and body found in the prone position.

47. **(D) Ring.**
A ring fracture occurs when the base of the skull separates the rim of the foramen magnum from the remainder of the base. This form of fracture usually occurs in a fall from a height, when the victim lands on his/her buttocks or feet, thereby driving the skull downward onto the vertebral column. The findings in a fall from a height include the tibias being driven through the soles of the feet. Major blood vessels at the base of the heart may be torn and small horizontal tears of the inner lining of the carotid artery may be seen. Hearts may be forced through the pericardial sac and the diaphragm. The aorta may be partially torn at the ligamentum arteriosum. A longitudinal fracture divides the base of the skull into two halves: a right and left half. This commonly occurs as a result of blunt impact to the face, forehead, and back of the head or in crushing injuries. Transverse fractures divide the skull into a front and rear half. Transverse fractures often occur from an impact on either side of the head or as a result of side-to-side compression. Hinge fracture represents a type of transverse fracture, which results in the independent movement of the front and rear halves of the base of the skull.

48. **(C) Fracture of the femur.**
Fat embolism is defined by the presence of fat droplets in the bloodstream. Commonly, these are detected in small blood vessels in the lung. The most common injuries that are associated with the development of fat emboli are crushing and tearing injuries involving subcutaneous fat and skeletal fractures, typically involving the femur, vertebrae, and pelvis. These bony sites contain abundant bone marrow contents and lipid.

49. **(E) Strangulation.**
Intravascular air or air embolism may be encountered in a variety of conditions including open neck injuries, complications of obstetric procedures, chest trauma, and decompression sickness as observed in divers. Strangulation typically does not result in air embolism.

50. **(A) Back of the head.**
Gunshot wounds in the temple, under the chin, in the mouth, and the side of the head are more commonly associated with suicides. Since it is logistically more difficult to aim and fire a gun at the back of one's own head, such an injury would be more suspect for a homicide.

51. **(A) Fouling.**
The term fouling is used in reference to small fragments of metal derived from the bullet. Tattooing, powder stippling, and powder burns are usually terms used to describe the dispersed grains of gunpowder and primer around the bullet wound. A full metal jacket is a bullet consisting of a soft core, usually made of lead, encased in a shell of harder metal.

52. **(A) .22 caliber handgun.**
The term pseudotattooing is used to describe tattooing produced by something other than gunpowder. A variety of causes for pseudotattooing can be found and include postmortem insect bites, spattered grease burns, superficial pinpoint-sized wounds from fragmented glass, and slivers of wood. A handgun would not directly be responsible for producing pseudotattooing and would be able to do so only if fired through wood or glass.

53. **(C) Metal composition of the shot.**
The pattern of injury observed on a victim of a shotgun fired from a distance of 5 feet away would vary based on the choke (constriction at the end of the barrel that is used to tailor the pattern of resulting pellets as they disperse, exiting the barrel), gauge of the gun, length of the barrel, powder load, and the size of the shot. The metal composition of the shot generally does not have a significant impact on the pattern of injury observed.

54. **(E) Third-degree burns.**
In this individual, both the epidermis and dermis show damage with sparing of the underlying soft tissues. These findings are characteristic of a third-degree burn that involves the entire thickness of the skin (full thickness burn). First-degree burns are usually superficial and are marked by reddish

discoloration and increased temperature in the burned areas. Blisters generally do not form in association with first-degree burns. Second-degree burns are marked by blister formations and destruction of the upper layers of the skin. Fourth-degree burns are marked by severe thermal injury, resulting in charring and complete destruction of the skin and underlying soft tissues. A fifth-degree burn does not exist.

55. **(D) 18%.**
The body surface area estimates of burns follow the rule of nines. In an adult, the head area covers approximately 9% of the total surface area of the body. In an infant, the head area covers a larger percentage of the body's total surface area at 18%.

56. **(B) Curved fracture.**
Fractures associated with high temperatures are characteristically curved fractures. Straight fractures may also be at times seen in association with high temperatures. The fracturing results from the heat causing bones to become brittle and break. Typically, temperatures of 900–1200 °F are required to accomplish fracturing.

57. **(C) Petechiae on the chest.**
In the setting of hanging (semi-suspension hanging), arterial blood flow to the head persists while the venous return is interrupted. This causes purplish discoloration of the face with swelling, bulging of the eyes, subconjunctival and facial petechiae, and hemorrhages in the skin above the area of the noose. Petechiae on the chest below the noose are not a typical feature of this scenario.

58. **(C) Homicidal strangulation.**
Fingernail marks in a strangulation case may appear as small superficial gouges or parallel linear scratches. Underlying hemorrhage is usually limited to the superficial layers of the skin. In a wet body, such as this case where the body was submerged in a bathtub, the fingernail marks may not be as evident until the skin has dried. The fingernail marks around the neck area suggest strangulation and homicide. It is virtually impossible for an individual to self-strangulate themselves (manual strangulation) in a suicide.

59. **(A) Battle sign.**
Blunt trauma in the neck region may result in fractures of the larynx including hyoid bone, thyroid cartilage, and cricoid cartilage. The underlying thyroid gland may show evidence of hemorrhage. The Battle sign is associated with a basilar skull fracture, which is usually associated with head and not neck trauma.

60. **(D) Mark on neck above the thyroid cartilage.**
In a strangulation death due to hanging, the mark typically presses upward toward the knot. The mark on the neck is usually above the thyroid cartilage. The hyoid bone and thyroid cartilage are usually intact, except in hanging cases, where there is a long drop or in elderly individuals. In a strangulation case by ligature, the mark on the neck is typically horizontal in orientation and is usually below the level of thyroid cartilage. The hyoid bone and thyroid cartilage are often fractured and occasionally the cricoid cartilage may also be fractured.

61. **(A) Cherry-red discolorations of the skeletal musculature.**
A variety of finding may be seen in association with carbon monoxide poisoning. Among these findings are cherry-red discoloration of the blood, skeletal musculature, and livor mortis. The nail beds may also show a bright red or pink coloration. Oral hemorrhages, swelling of the nasopharynx, and foaming at the mouth are not typical features of carbon monoxide poisoning.

62. **(E) Motor vehicle accident.**
The most common cause of death in a 6-year-old in the forensic setting is a motor vehicle accident followed by drowning.

63. **(B) Drowning in a bathtub.**
In an infant drowning victim, the most likely scenario is drowning in a bathtub. Industrial buckets are a common mechanism of drowning of toddlers, who grab the edge of the bucket for support and fall forward and become trapped inside. In preschool age children, drowning in pools either in the backyard or community is more common. In adolescents and young adults, most drowning accidents tend to occur in association with larger bodies of water, such as lakes or oceans.

64. **(A) Body shows extensive mummification.**
In most cases, putrefaction of the body occurs at a slower rate in water than on land. Upon removal from the water, putrefaction in a previously submerged body may be accelerated. As a general rule of thumb, putrefaction of a body exposed in the air for 1 week equals about 2 weeks in the water and 8 weeks in the ground. Putrefaction generally occurs more slowly in saltwater versus freshwater. Mummification is not a typical finding in the setting of a submerged body. Fungi growth may be seen on the outer surface of the body, and loss of facial soft tissue may also be encountered due to fish feeding on the body. Likewise, algae growth may also be present on the skin.

65. **(B) Epidermal microblisters with nuclear streaming.**
In the case of an electrical burn, the findings are similar to what is encountered in surgery-related cautery artifact, which includes a streaming of

nuclei and epidermal microblistering. Fern-like discoloration of the skin may be seen in the setting of lightning strike. The other findings are not typical features of electrical burns.

66. **(A) Amount of clothing does not affect degree of injury.**
The severity of injury sustained due to a pedestrian being struck by the bumper of a vehicle can be related to a variety of factors including the age of the pedestrian, the speed the vehicle was moving at when striking the pedestrian, the shape of the bumper, and the amount of clothing overlying the area. In suspected cases, the skin in the calf area should be examined for injury and careful attention should be paid to leg bone fractures, which is a fairly common finding in this setting.

67. **(E) Skull fracture.**
A variety of injuries have been attributed to air bag deployment including fractures of the forearm, facial bruises and abrasions, lacerations of the brain stem and cervical dislocations, and hemithorax accompanied by rib fractures. Air bag deployment does not usually result in a skull fracture.

68. **(B) Number of individuals in the aircraft.**
A variety of fractures are important in determining the survivability of an individual following an aircraft crash. Among these findings are the restraints in the aircraft, the use of energy absorptive materials in building the aircraft, the design of the aircraft, and the environment in which the crash occurs (post-crash environment). The number of individuals in the aircraft usually does not impact significantly on survivability.

69. **(C) Ipsilateral cerebral peduncle compressed.**
Uncal or parahippocampal herniation is associated with a constellation of concomitant findings including posterior cerebral artery compression and infarcts of the visual cortex, cranial nerve III compressions, ipsilateral fixed, dilated pupil, and Duret hemorrhage. Uncal herniation is also associated with contralateral (not ipsilateral) cerebral peduncle compression or Kernohan notch.

70. **(C) 10 seconds.**
With complete disruption of cerebral circulation, loss of consciousness usually occurs within 10 seconds, with permanent ischemic damage resulting when the ischemia lasts for about 4–5 minutes.

71. **(C) Diffuse axonal injury.**
Diffuse axonal injury is usually the result of a lateral rotational acceleration injury, resulting in a shearing of axons. Patients with severe diffuse axonal injury are often rendered immediately unconscious. Imaging studies typically show little in the way of abnormalities except possible evidence of small hemorrhages in the subcortical white matter, corpus callosum, and fornices. A ruptured vascular malformation or subdural hematoma should be evident on an MRI study. Cerebral contusions or infarct secondary to trauma would also be evident on imaging studies. Given the clinical scenario of a car accident, a rotational injury pattern such as diffuse axonal injury would be a more viable explanation as compared with anoxic encephalopathy (unless there was some explanation for the low oxygen state in the brain or significant loss of blood).

72. **(A) A common finding in head trauma cases in children less than 1-year-old.**
Epidural hemorrhages occur in the space between the inner table of the skull and the dura. Most cases are due to a tearing of the middle meningeal artery and are associated with skull fractures. Most commonly, these hemorrhages occur overlying the cerebral hemispheres. Because of the compartment in which the hemorrhage develops, the hematoma typically has biconcave lens shape. Epidural hematomas are rare before the age of 2 years because the dura is more firmly attached to inner table of the skull and less likely provides a space for the hematoma to accumulate in when the middle meningeal artery is ruptured.

73. **(C) 1 week.**
During the first 24 hours, a subdural hematoma consists of liquid and fragments of blood clot. There is no cellular reaction to the hemorrhage at this point. By 2–4 days, clots start to stick loosely to the dura. The blood is black-brown in coloration. Scattered macrophages may be evident and occasional spindle cells may be invading the clot from the dura. By 1 week, a yellow neomembrane begins to form at the dural aspect of the hematoma with invasion of the clot by thin-walled capillaries and fibroblasts. By the end of the second and third weeks, the dural neomembrane thickens and becomes more vascular. It begins to partially cover the inner surface of the clot, which begins to liquify. The clot acquires an orange to yellow-brown coloration. Macrophages with hemosiderin deposition are prominently noted. By 1 month, the outer dural and inner arachnoidal membranes are complete and grossly visible. Most of the blood is semiliquid and orange-brown in color.

74. **(C) Frontal lobe.**
Contusions are described as being coup, occurring at the site of impact, and contrecoup, occurring at a point opposite the site of impact. The most common sites for contrecoup contusions include the inferior frontal and temporal lobes; these contusions result

from areas of the brain being traumatically pushed up against the skull.

75. **(C) Fat emboli syndrome.**
The presence of numerous, bilateral, white matter petechiae suggests skeletal trauma and fat emboli syndrome.

76. **(E) Testicular hypertrophy.**
A variety of pathologies are well documented to be associated with chronic alcoholism. Among these changes include macrovesicular steatosis, development of alcoholic hepatitis and alcoholic cirrhosis, acute and chronic pancreatitis, degeneration of the mamillary bodies associated with Wernicke–Korsakoff syndrome, rare demyelination of the corpus callosum (Marchia-fava–Bignami syndrome), central pontine myelinoly-sis, cerebellar atrophy, peripheral neuropathy, car-diomyopathy, peripheral myopathy, gastritis, gastric ulcers, and testicular atrophy (not hypertrophy).

77. **(C) Pulmonary hemorrhage and necrosis.**
Heat stroke results from persistently high environ-mental temperatures coupled with endogenous heat production resulting in a failure of the body's ability to regulate temperature. A variety of pathologic find-ings may be observed in patients who succumb to heat stroke including rhabdomyolysis, centrilobular hepatic necrosis, myocardial necrosis, and Purkinje cell shrinkage and necrosis. Pulmonary hemorrhage and necrosis are not typical features of heat stroke.

78. **(D) Pancreatic hemorrhagic necrosis.**
Cocaine use may be associated with a variety of pathologies including sudden death due to coro-nary artery vasospasm, hypertensive crises, cardiac crossband necrosis, and cardiac arrhythmias. Pan-creatic hemorrhagic necrosis is not a common finding in patients dying of cocaine toxicity.

79. **(B) Carbon monoxide poisoning.**
In this scenario with the three presumably healthy young men found dead in the living room of a house with no trace of trauma and no evidence of drug use or paraphernalia, the most likely cause of death would be carbon monoxide poisoning.

80. **(A) Body was leaning against a wall when shot.**
Marginal abrasions around an exit wound are an infrequent finding and usually occur when there is a firm object against the body at the site of an exit-ing bullet. Such objects may include tight clothing such as a belt or brassiere, or a hard surface such as the ground, pavement, or a wall.

81. **(E) Portuguese man-of-war sting.**
Jellyfish stings are an uncommon cause of fatal death. Waters in certain part of the world, includ-ing the Australian shore, are rich in these potentially dangerous jellyfish. Portuguese man-of-war is one of the potentially dangerous types. The organism gener-ates a neurotoxin that can be fatal. This section from the victim shows several round nematocysts on the surface of the skin that corroborate the diagnosis.

82. **(D) Suicide.**
Findings in this figure are suggestive of a gunshot wound fired in the mouth and aimed toward the top of the head. This is most consistent with a suicidal gunshot wound.

83. **(B) Gunshot entrance wound.**
The wound shown here shows black discoloration corresponding to soot and gunpowder, suggesting a relatively close- range gunshot entrance wound.

84. **(C) Gunshot wound to the head.**
This figure shows a piece of brain parenchyma within a pulmonary blood vessel. A gunshot wound can sometime force pieces of brain parenchyma into vessels that can embolize to the lung, as in this case.

85. **(E) Sudden acceleration or deceleration of the skull relative to the brain.**
The finding illustrated in this figure is that of an organized subdural hematoma. These occur as a result of tearing of bridging of veins, resulting from a sudden acceleration or deceleration of the skull relative to the brain and a tearing injury.

86. **(E) Superficial gunshot wound.**
The injury shown on the scalp represents a linear laceration, which is rather long, and most consis-tent with a superficial gunshot wound. The site of injury would be unusual for a laceration due to a fall related to the gunshot wound to the chest. The injury is not in the usual site for a defense wound (more typically arms, hands, and sometimes feet). There is no evidence of a knife in addition to a gun in this case, which would not support a knife wound injury as the etiology.

87. **(A) Amphetamine overdose.**
The presence of a syringe and needle tract marks sug-gests that this individual has a history of IV drug abuse. The figure shows a talc granuloma. These can occur as a result of talcum powder being pushed into a blood vessel by a needle. Granulomas in the subcutaneous tissues at the sites of injection may also be evident.

88. **(C) Infarct in the posterior cerebral artery distri-bution.**
The slit-like midline hemorrhage observed in the brain stem section, shown in the figure, is consis-tent with Duret hemorrhage. These bleeds result from a tearing of perforating vessels coming off the basilar artery. This finding is most commonly asso-ciated with uncal or parahippocampal herniation. Other findings associated with uncal herniation include compression of the posterior cerebral artery, which may result in an infarct in the occipital cortex supplied by that vessel.

SUGGESTED READING

1. Bouchama A, Knochel JP. Heat stroke. *N Engl J Med*. 2002; 346:1978-1988.

2. Byers S. *Introduction to Forensic Anthropology: A Textbook*. Boston, MA:Allyn & Bacon; 2002.

3. Catts EP, Goff ML. Forensic entomology in criminal investigations. *Annu Rev Entomol*. 1992;37:253-272.

4. Dawson SL, Hirsch CS, Lucas FV, et al. The contrecoup phenomenon. Reappraisal of a classic problem. *Hum Pathol*. 1980;11:155-166.

5. DiMaio VJ. Homicidal asphyxia. *Am J Forensic Med Pathol*. 2000;21:1-4.

6. Dolinak D, Matshes E, Law E. *Forensic Pathology*. Oxford, UK: Elsevier Academic Press; 2005.

7. Duhaime AC, Gennarelli TA, Thibault LE, et al. The shaken baby syndrome. A clinical, pathological, and biomechanical study. *J Neurosurg*. 1987;66:409-415.

8. Ernst A, Zibrak JD. Carbon monoxide poisoning. *N Engl J Med*. 1998;339:1603-1608.

9. Fackler ML. Gunshot wound review. *Ann Emerg Med*. 1996; 28:194-203.

10. Fackler ML. Wound ballistics. A review of common misconceptions. *JAMA*. 1988;259:2730-2736.

11. France D. Observational and metric analysis of sex in the skeleton. In: Reichs K, ed. *Forensic Osteology: Advances in the Identification of Human Remains*. Springfield, IL: Charles C. Thomas; 1998.

12. Geddes JF, Hackshaw AK, Vowles GH, et al. Neuropathology of inflicted head injury in children. I. Patterns of brain damage. *Brain*. 2001;124(Pt 7):1290-1298.

13. Geddes JF, Vowles GH, Hachshaw AK, et al. Neuropathology of inflicted head injury in children. II. Microscopic brain injury in infants. *Brain*. 2001;124(Pt 7):1299-1306.

14. Geddes JF, Whitwell HL, Graham DI. Traumatic axonal injury: practical issues for diagnosis in medicolegal cases. *Neuropathol Appl Neurobiol*. 2000;26:448-453.

15. Jentzen JM. Forensic toxicology. An overview and an algorithmic approach. *Am J Clin Pathol*. 1989;92(4 suppl 1): S48-S55.

16. Karger B. Penetrating gunshots to the head and lack of immediate incapacitation. I. Wound ballistics and mechanisms of incapacitation. *Int J Legal Med*. 1995;108: 53-61.

17. Krous HF, Beckwith JB, Byard RW, et al. Sudden infant death syndrome and unclassified sudden infant deaths: a definitional and diagnostic approach. *Pediatrics*. 2004;11: 234-238.

18. Meyersohn J. Putrefaction: a difficulty in forensic medicine. *J Forensic Med*. 1971;18:114-117.

19. Moar JJ. Drowning–postmortem appearances and forensic significance. *South Afr Med J*. 1983;64:792-795.

20. Moritz AR. Classical mistakes in forensic pathology. *Am J Forensic Med Pathol*. 1981;2:299-308.

21. Nikolic S, Micic J, Atanasijevic T, et al. Analysis of neck injuries in hanging. *Am J Forensic Med Pathol*. 2003;24: 179-182.

22. Scheuer L. Application of osteology to forensic medicine. *Clin Anat*. 2002;15:297-312.

23. Shkrum MJ, McClafferty KJ, Nowak ES, et al. Driver and front seat passenger fatalities associated with air bag deployment. Part 2: a review of injury patterns and investigative issues. *J Forensics Sci*. 2002;47:1035-1040.

24. Simonsen J. Patho-anatomic findings in neck structures in asphyxiation due to hanging: a survey of 80 cases. *Forensic Sci Int*. 1988;38:83-91.

25. Spitz WU, Spitz DJ. *Spitz and Fisher's Medicolegal Investigation of Death*. 4th ed. Springfield, IL: Charles C. Thomas Publisher LTD; 2006.

26. Stephenson T, Bialas Y. Estimation of the age of bruising. *Arch Dis Child*. 1996;74:53-55.

27. Sturner WQ. Common errors in forensic pediatric pathology. *Am J Forensic Med Pathol*. 1998;19:317-320.

28. Weedn VW. Postmortem identifications of remains. *Clin Lab Med*. 1998;18:115-137.

29. Wright RK, Davis JH. The investigation of electrical deaths: a report of 220 fatalities. *J Forensic Sci*. 1980;25: 514-521.

CHAPTER 13

GASTROINTESTINAL, HEPATOBILIARY, AND PANCREATIC PATHOLOGY

1. All the following histologic changes can be related to bowel-preparation, except
   (A) Crypt abscess
   (B) Edema
   (C) Epithelial sloughing
   (D) Hemorrhage
   (E) Mucin depletion

2. The phenomenon of duplication of muscularis mucosae is associated with which of the following conditions?
   (A) Achalasia
   (B) Barrett's esophagus
   (C) Diverticular disease
   (D) Eosinophilic esophagitis
   (E) Reflux esophagitis

3. Chief cells of the stomach are characterized by all of the following, except
   (A) They are concentrated in the upper half of oxyntic glands
   (B) They are most abundant in the fundus and body of stomach
   (C) They demonstrate basophilic granular cytoplasm
   (D) They have extensive subnuclear rough endoplasmic reticulum
   (E) They secrete pepsinogen

4. Enterochromaffin-like cells are predominantly found in which part of the upper gastrointestinal tract?
   (A) Esophagus
   (B) Gastric antrum
   (C) Gastric body
   (D) Gastric fundus
   (E) Gastroesophageal junction

5. In addition to crypt architectural distortion, Paneth cell metaplasia serves as an indicator of chronic mucosal injury in all the following parts of the colon, except
   (A) Cecum
   (B) Descending
   (C) Distal transverse
   (D) Rectum
   (E) Sigmoid

6. The portion of colon that is entirely suspended by mesentery, and therefore prone to volvulus, is
   (A) Ascending colon
   (B) Cecum
   (C) Descending colon
   (D) Rectum
   (E) Sigmoid colon

7. Which part of the colon has the widest diameter?
   (A) Ascending colon
   (B) Cecum
   (C) Descending colon
   (D) Rectum
   (E) Transverse colon

8. What are the normal surface undulations of the colonic mucosa known as?
   (A) Anthemic folds
   (B) Epiploic appendages
   (C) Haustral folds
   (D) Taenia coli
   (E) Valves of Kerckring

9. Which of the following choices is not considered to be a significant risk factor for development of gastric cancer?
   (A) African American descent
   (B) Family history of gastric cancer
   (C) Hispanic descent
   (D) History of idiopathic inflammatory bowel disease
   (E) Immigration from high-risk geographic location

10. Per the 2011 American Gastroenterology Association guidelines, which of the following therapy is not recommended for focal Barrett's esophagus-related high-grade dysplasia?
    (A) Continued endoscopic surveillance
    (B) Endoscopic mucosal resection
    (C) Esophagectomy
    (D) Photodynamic therapy
    (E) Radiofrequency ablation

11. Per the Crohn's and Colitis Foundation of America consensus group guidelines, after how many years following an initial diagnosis of pancolitis or left-sided colitis should a patient undergo colonoscopic surveillance?
    (A) 1 year
    (B) 2–3 years
    (C) 5 years
    (D) 8–10 years
    (E) 15 years

12. In the setting of idiopathic inflammatory bowel disease, all the following are attributes of a non-adenoma-like dysplasia-associated lesion/mass (DALM), except
    (A) Endoscopically resectable lesion
    (B) Indistinct borders
    (C) Irregular surface
    (D) Plaque-like appearance
    (E) Poor circumscription

13. In evaluating a malignant colorectal polyp, which of the following features is not categorized as "unfavorable histology"?
    (A) Cancer is poorly differentiated
    (B) Cancer is <2 mm from deep margin
    (C) Lymphovascular invasion is present
    (D) Pedunculated polyp
    (E) Polyp is incompletely excised

14. Cytomegalovirus colitis is least likely to present as
    (A) Mucosal hemorrhage
    (B) Obstructive inflammatory mass
    (C) Pseudomembranes
    (D) Stricture
    (E) Ulcers

15. A 4-year-old boy presents with symptoms of acute intestinal obstruction and is found to have an intussusception located at the ileocecal region. A section from his small bowel resection is shown in Figure 13-1. What is the most likely etiology for his intestinal obstruction?

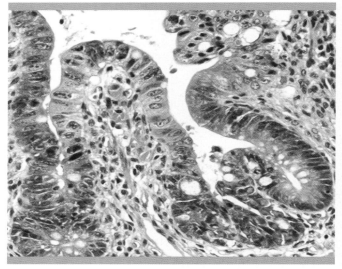

FIGURE 13-1

    (A) Adenovirus infection
    (B) Cytomegalovirus infection
    (C) Herpes simplex infection
    (D) Rotavirus infection
    (E) Norwalk virus infection

16. Human papilloma virus infection is implicated in the pathogenesis of all of the following entities, except
    (A) Anal squamous cell carcinoma
    (B) Condyloma
    (C) Esophageal squamous cell carcinoma
    (D) Kaposi's sarcoma
    (E) Squamous papilloma

17. Which of the following infections is least likely to induce a granulomatous pattern of injury?
    (A) *Actinomyces israelii*
    (B) *Clostridium difficile*
    (C) *Mycobacterium tuberculosis*
    (D) *Mycobacterium avium–intracellulare*
    (E) *Yersinia pseudotuberculosis*

18. All the following conditions are associated with pseudomembrane formation, except
    (A) *Campylobacter jejuni colitis*
    (B) *Clostridium difficile colitis*
    (C) Collagenous colitis
    (D) *Enterohemorrhagic E. coli*
    (E) Ischemia

19. Which of the following infections is not associated with acute self-limited pattern of colitis?
    (A) *Aeromonas*
    (B) *Campylobacter jejuni*
    (C) *Enterohemorrhagic E. coli*
    (D) *Salmonella*
    (E) *Shigella*

20. A colonic biopsy from a 70-year-old woman with history of cardiovascular disease shows a pseudo-membranous pattern of mucosal injury. Which of the following histologic features is considered to be specific for ischemic colitis?
    (A) Ballooned crypts
    (B) Cryptitis and crypt abscesses
    (C) Degenerating goblet cells "pseudo signet-ring cells"
    (D) Hyalinized lamina propria
    (E) Mucosal necrosis

21. Which region of the gastrointestinal tract is most commonly affected by tuberculosis?
    (A) Anal canal
    (B) Colon
    (C) Esophagus
    (D) Ileocecal valve
    (E) Stomach

22. All the following pathologic features favor a diagnosis of Crohn's disease over intestinal tuberculosis, except
    (A) Chronic mucosal injury in adjacent mucosa
    (B) Circumferential ulcers
    (C) Deep fistulas
    (D) Mucosal cobblestoning
    (E) Transmural lymphoid aggregates

23. The special stain of choice for confirming the pathologic finding shown in this figure is (Figure 13-2)

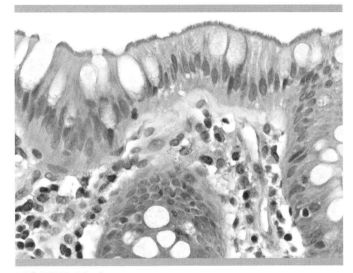

FIGURE 13-2

    (A) Brown–Hopps stain
    (B) Giemsa stain
    (C) Trichrome stain
    (D) Von Kossa stain
    (E) Warthin-Starry stain

24. A 45-year-old man presents with malabsorption, arthritis, and lymphadenopathy. A duodenal biopsy obtained from this patient is shown in Figure 13-3. He does not have hepatosplenomegaly. A PAS with diastase stain is found to be positive and diagnostic of this condition. The most likely etiology for this patient's symptoms is

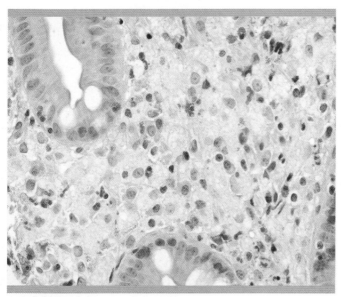

FIGURE 13-3

  (A) Crushed Brunner's glands
  (B) Gaucher's disease
  (C) Malakoplakia
  (D) *Mycobacterium avium–intracellulare* infection
  (E) Whipple's disease

25. Which protozoal organism causes dysentery, flask-shaped cecal ulcers, and resembles macrophages on histologic examination?
  (A) *Entamoeba histolytica*
  (B) *Cryptococcus neoformans*
  (C) *Giardia lamblia*
  (D) *Leishmania donovani*
  (E) *Trypanosoma cruzi*

26. Which of the following features is not typically associated with the finding shown in this duodenal biopsy? (Figure 13-4)

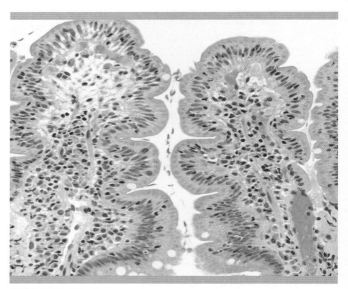

FIGURE 13-4

  (A) Foul-smelling watery diarrhea
  (B) Minimal inflammation
  (C) Normal endoscopy
  (D) Tissue invasion
  (E) Underlying immunodeficiency disorder

27. Which of the following flagellate organisms is implicated in the pathogenesis of megaesophagus and megacolon?
  (A) *Cryptosporidium parvum*
  (B) *Giardia lamblia*
  (C) *Leishmania donovani*
  (D) *Toxoplasma gondii*
  (E) *Trypanosoma cruzi*

28. A 20-year-old woman with history of biliary dyskinesia undergoes cholecystectomy (see Figure 13-5). Which of the following infectious organisms is highlighted by the PAS stain?

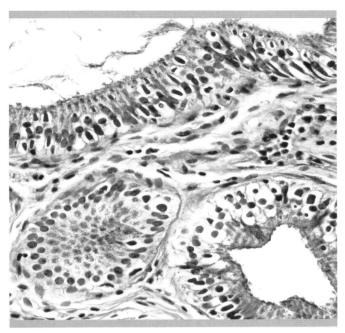

FIGURE 13-5

(A) *Cryptosporidium parvum*
(B) *Cyclospora cayetanensis*
(C) *Enterocytozoon bieneusi* (microsporidia)
(D) *Isospora belli*
(E) *Toxoplasma gondii*

29. A duodenal biopsy from a patient with history of diarrhea is shown in Figure 13-6. Which of the following nematodes is responsible for the patient's symptom and will most likely result in a stage of autoinfection?

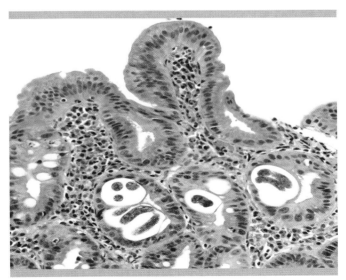

FIGURE 13-6

(A) *Ascaris lumbricoides*
(B) *Ancylostoma duodenale*
(C) *Enterobius vermicularis*
(D) *Strongyloides stercoralis*
(E) *Trichuris trichiura*

30. A 30-year-old man presents with epigastric pain, nausea, and vomiting within 12 hours of consuming sushi. Endoscopic examination shows mucosal edema, hemorrhage, and slightly thickened gastric folds. Which of the following nematodes is most likely to be seen in the tissue sections from his stomach?
(A) *Anisakis simplex*
(B) *Ascaris lumbricoides*
(C) *Enterobius vermicularis*
(D) *Strongyloides stercoralis*
(E) *Trichuris trichiura*

31. Which primary immunodeficiency disorder results from mutation in the *TNFRSF13B* gene and is associated with celiac disease as its most common noninfectious GI complication?
(A) Common variable immunodeficiency
(B) Hyper-IgM syndrome
(C) Selective IgA deficiency
(D) Severe combined immunodeficiency
(E) X-linked agammaglobulinemia

32. Adult patients of common variable immunodeficiency are at risk for all of the following disorders, except
(A) B-cell non-Hodgkin lymphoma
(B) Colonic adenocarcinoma
(C) Gastric adenocarcinoma
(D) Small bowel adenocarcinoma
(E) Nodular lymphoid hyperplasia

33. Which chronic relapsing vasculitis is associated with oral aphthous ulcers, perianal disease, and ulcerative lesions of the GI tract that mimic Crohn's disease?
(A) Behçet's disease
(B) Churg-Strauss syndrome
(C) Microscopic polyangiitis
(D) Polyarteritis nodosa
(E) Wegener's granulomatosis

34. Brown bowel syndrome is characterized by all the following clinicopathologic features, except
    (A) Accumulation of lipofuscin within muscularis propria
    (B) It is a congenital disorder
    (C) It is commonly associated with Vitamin E deficiency
    (D) It most commonly involves the small bowel
    (E) The accumulated pigment is Periodic acid Schiff positive

35. In which part of the colon are muciphages most commonly found?
    (A) Ascending colon
    (B) Ileocecal valve
    (C) Rectum
    (D) Sigmoid colon
    (E) Transverse colon

36. Figure 13-7 shows a submucosal tumor resected from a 40-year-old man. What is its most common location in the GI tract?

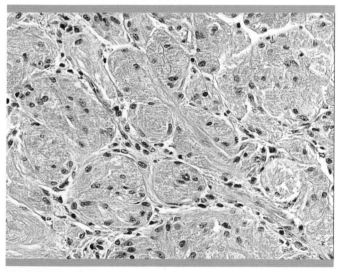

FIGURE 13-7

    (A) Esophagus
    (B) Colon
    (C) Rectum
    (D) Small bowel
    (E) Stomach

37. Which of the following cells are increased in biopsies obtained from patients with irritable bowel syndrome and diarrhea?
    (A) Eosinophils
    (B) Lymphocytes
    (C) Mast cells

    (D) Neutrophils
    (E) Plasma cells

38. Which of the following findings is not associated with achalasia?
    (A) Cytoplasmic vacuolation of myocytes
    (B) Inflammatory infiltrate composed of CD20-positive lymphocytes
    (C) Lymphocytic ganglionitis
    (D) Near total absence of myenteric ganglion cells
    (E) Squamous epithelial hyperplasia and intraepithelial lymphocytosis

39. All the listed conditions have an association with Hirschsprung's disease, except
    (A) Down syndrome
    (B) Multiple endocrine neoplasia
    (C) Neurofibromatosis
    (D) Neuroblastoma
    (E) Turner syndrome

40. In a rectal suction biopsy, which of the following histologic findings supports a diagnosis of Hirschsprung's disease?
    (A) Lack of ganglion cells
    (B) Lack of interstitial cells of Cajal
    (C) Lack of neural plexuses
    (D) Lymphocytic ganglionitis
    (E) Submucosal fibrosis

41. Which of the following findings represents the most commonly encountered variation of the omphalomesenteric (vitelline) duct remnant?
    (A) Meckel's diverticulum
    (B) Omphalomesenteric cyst
    (C) Omphalomesenteric fistula
    (D) Umbilical polyp
    (E) Umbilical sinus

42. What is the most common type of heterotopic mucosa/epithelium found in a Meckel's diverticulum?
    (A) Biliary
    (B) Colonic
    (C) Duodenal
    (D) Gastric
    (E) Pancreatic

43. A 3-week-old boy with history of refractory diarrhea undergoes a duodenal biopsy that shows severe villous atrophy without crypt hyperplasia, increased apoptosis, or inflammation. There is no evidence of intraepithelial lymphocytosis. A PAS stain shows absence of a distinct brush border. What is the diagnostic test of choice?

(A) Electron microscopy
(B) Serum anti-enterocyte antibody
(C) Serum gastrin
(D) Serum IgA
(E) Serum tissue transglutaminase

44. A 15-year-old boy with malabsorption is suspected to have autoimmune enteropathy. All the following findings are associated with this entity, except
(A) Anti-enterocyte antibodies
(B) Anti-goblet cell antibodies
(C) Increased crypt apoptosis
(D) Marked surface intraepithelial lymphocytosis
(E) Minimal response to gluten-free diet

45. An infant with very low birth weight is admitted with lethargy, abdominal distention, and absent bowel sounds. Imaging studies reveal changes consistent with pneumatosis. Which part of the bowel is most frequently involved by the condition described here?
(A) Descending colon
(B) Jejunum
(C) Ileocecal region
(D) Ileum
(E) Rectum

46. All the choices listed below are categorized as secondary causes of intestinal lymphangiectasia, except
(A) Constrictive pericarditis
(B) Lymphangioma
(C) Mesenteric tuberculosis
(D) Milroy disease
(E) Neuroblastoma

47. Which of the following choices describes a bleeding ulcer that is caused when an ulcer erodes into a single, unusually large submucosal mural arteriole?
(A) Cameron's ulcer
(B) Chemical injury-induced ulcer
(C) Dieulafoy's lesion
(D) Stress ulcer
(E) Variceal ulcer

48. A patient with cirrhosis undergoes endoscopic evaluation for gastrointestinal bleeding. The stomach shows a mosaic mucosal pattern and the biopsy reveals numerous ectatic capillaries and venules within the lamina propria, without evidence of vascular thrombi. What is the most likely cause of the gastrointestinal bleeding?

(A) Chronic gastritis
(B) Gastric antral vascular ectasia
(C) Ischemia
(D) Peptic ulcer disease
(E) Portal hypertensive gastropathy

49. A gastric biopsy from a 45-year-old man with iron deficiency anemia and an endoscopic appearance of linear mucosal hyperemia is shown in Figure 13-8. What is the most likely cause of patient's anemia?

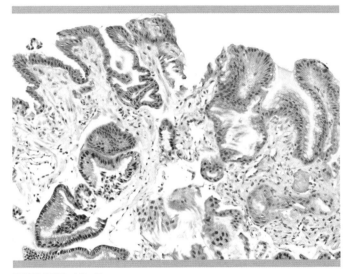

FIGURE 13-8

(A) Chronic gastritis
(B) Gastric antral vascular ectasia
(C) Hereditary hemorrhagic telangiectasia
(D) Portal hypertensive gastropathy
(E) Reactive gastropathy

50. What is the most common cause of lower gastrointestinal tract bleeding?
(A) Angiodysplasia
(B) Arteriovenous malformation
(C) Diverticular disease
(D) Hemorrhoids
(E) Ulcerative colitis

51. All of the features listed below are associated with angiodysplasia, except
(A) It is a developmental disorder
(B) It primarily affects elderly patients
(C) It is often located in the right colon
(D) It is characterized by dilated submucosal blood vessels
(E) It is a common source of bleeding in patients with renal failure

52. Which of the following drugs/medications causes "diaphragm disease"?
    (A) Iron pills
    (B) Laxatives
    (C) Non-steroidal anti-inflammatory drugs
    (D) Oral contraceptives
    (E) Proton pump inhibitors

53. Which of the following etiologies would be categorized as an arterial cause of gastrointestinal ischemia?
    (A) Buerger's disease
    (B) Behçet's disease
    (C) Chronic radiation injury
    (D) Idiopathic myointimal hyperplasia of mesenteric veins
    (E) Portal hypertension

54. Which of the listed histologic features favors squamous dysplasia over reactive squamous hyperplasia?
    (A) Irregular papillae
    (B) Lack of atypical mitosis
    (C) Maintenance of nuclear polarity
    (D) Non-overlapping nuclei
    (E) Regular nuclear membranes

55. A mid-esophageal biopsy from a 30-year-old man with history of dysphagia is shown in Figure 13-9. What is the characteristic endoscopic finding associated with this entity?

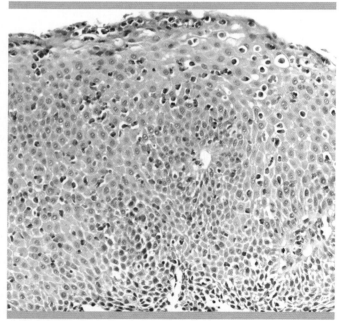

FIGURE 13-9

(A) Erosions
(B) Mass
(C) Rings and furrows
(D) Salmon-colored mucosa
(E) Ulcer

56. In evaluating biopsy from a patient suspected to have Barrett's esophagus, which of the following histologic findings favors the presence of pseudo-goblet cells over true goblet cells?
    (A) Alcian-blue reactivity at pH 2.5
    (B) Blue cytoplasm
    (C) Continuous distribution
    (D) Eccentric, compressed nuclei
    (E) Rounded shape of the cell

57. The esophageal biopsy shown in Figure 13-10 was obtained from a patient with chronic reflux and ulcerated salmon-colored mucosa on endoscopy. What is the best diagnosis?

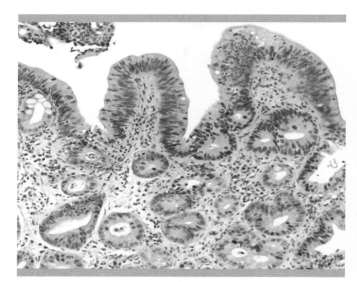

FIGURE 13-10

(A) Barrett's esophagus, negative for dysplasia
(B) Barrett's esophagus, indefinite for dysplasia
(C) Barrett's esophagus with high-grade dysplasia
(D) Barrett's esophagus with low-grade dysplasia
(E) Intramucosal adenocarcinoma

58. Which of the following drugs/chemicals is associated with changes shown in this biopsy? (Figure 13-11)

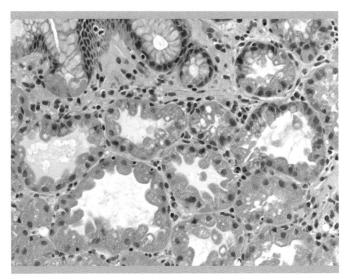

FIGURE 13-11

(A) Alcohol
(B) Colchicine
(C) Iron
(D) Non-steroidal anti-inflammatory drugs
(E) Proton pump inhibitor

59. Which of the following etiologies is least likely to cause acute hemorrhagic gastritis?
(A) Alcohol
(B) Allergy
(C) Burns
(D) Non-steroidal anti-inflammatory drugs
(E) Stress

60. The campylobacter organism-like (CLO) test detects which of the following enzymes produced by *Helicobacter pylori*?
(A) Ammonia
(B) cag A toxin
(C) Phospholipase
(D) Urease
(E) vac A toxin

61. In the setting of *Helicobacter pylori* gastritis, the presence of which of the following histologic findings suggests therapy failure and antibiotic resistance?
(A) Granulomas
(B) Intestinal metaplasia

(C) Lymphocytes
(D) Neutrophils
(E) Plasma cells

62. Which of the following histologic findings in a gastric biopsy is considered to be specific for *Helicobacter pylori* infection?
(A) Intraepithelial lymphocytes
(B) Intestinal metaplasia
(C) Lymphoid follicle formation
(D) Neutrophils
(E) Superficial lamina propria inflammation

63. In the setting of *Helicobacter pylori* gastritis, all of the listed findings are highly suspicious for the presence of extranodal marginal zone B-cell lymphoma, except
(A) Active gastritis with intestinal metaplasia
(B) Endoscopic evidence of a mass/nodule
(C) Expansile inflammatory infiltrate of uniform-appearing cells
(D) Lymphoepithelial lesions with glandular disruption
(E) Monocytoid appearance of lymphocytes

64. Which specific pattern of *Helicobacter pylori* gastritis is associated with a high risk for development of intestinal-type dysplasia and gastric adenocarcinoma?
(A) Antral-predominant nonatrophic *Helicobacter pylori* gastritis
(B) Antrum-restricted atrophic *Helicobacter pylori* gastritis
(C) Corpus-predominant *Helicobacter pylori* gastritis
(D) Multifocal atrophic *Helicobacter pylori* gastritis
(E) Non-atrophic pangastritis

65. A gastric antral biopsy obtained from a 72-year-old woman shows superficial lymphoplasmacytic inflammatory infiltrate with focal active gastritis and intestinal metaplasia. All the following are possible explanations for the inability to demonstrate *Helicobacter pylori*, except
(A) Low bacterial load
(B) Presence of intestinal metaplasia
(C) Proton pump inhibitor use
(D) Recent antibiotic use
(E) Use of immunohistochemical stain for *H. pylori*

66. A 10-year-old boy with history of nausea and vomiting undergoes a gastric biopsy, which is depicted in Figure 13-12. He loves to play with his pets that include dogs, cats, and parakeets. All the following statements are true regarding this organism, except

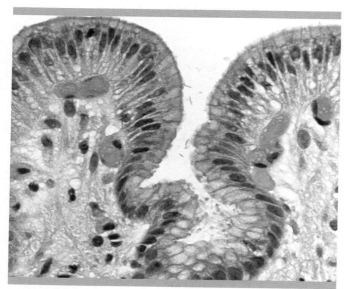

FIGURE 13-12

(A) It causes severe gastritis
(B) It has a patchy pattern of mucosal involvement
(C) It has 5–7 spirals
(D) It is difficult to culture
(E) It measures 5–9 microns in length

67. A gastric ulcer is more likely to be benign when the following features are present, except
(A) Located close to the incisura angularis
(B) Located on the lesser curvature of the antrum
(C) Ranges in size from 0.5 to 2.0 cm in diameter
(D) Shows heaped up mucosal borders with irregular rugal folds
(E) Shows sharply demarcated boundaries

68. A 70-year-old woman presents with long-standing anemia and early satiety. A biopsy from the gastric body is shown in Figure 13-13. The gastric antrum was completely normal. No *Helicobacter pylori* organisms were identified. Which of the following serologic abnormalities is least likely to be present in this patient?

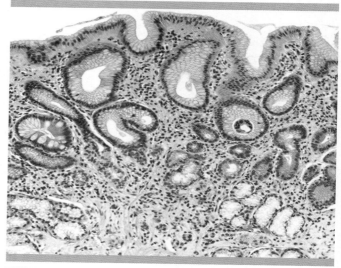

FIGURE 13-13

(A) Achlorhydria
(B) Hypochlorhydria
(C) Hypergastrinemia
(D) Hypogastrinemia
(E) Low serum pepsinogen I level

69. Enterochromaffin cell-like hyperplasia is least likely to be associated with which of the following conditions?
(A) Autoimmune gastritis
(B) Multifocal atrophic *Helicobacter pylori* gastritis
(C) Multiple endocrine neoplasia
(D) Non-steroidal anti-inflammatory drug-related gastritis
(E) Zollinger-Ellison syndrome

70. The pattern of mucosal injury depicted in Figure 13-14 is least likely to be associated with which of the following conditions?

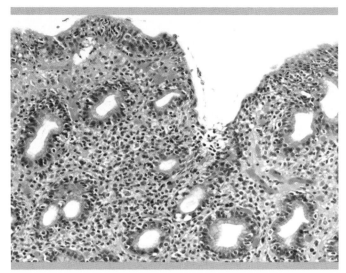

FIGURE 13-14

(A) Celiac disease
(B) Extranodal marginal zone B-cell lymphoma
(C) *Helicobacter pylori* gastritis
(D) Ménétrier's disease
(E) Non-steroidal anti-inflammatory drug-related gastritis

71. A gastric biopsy from a 70-year-old man with osteoarthritis and chronic non-steroidal anti-inflammatory drug use is shown in Figure 13-15. All the following pathologic features are helpful in diagnosing this pattern of injury, except

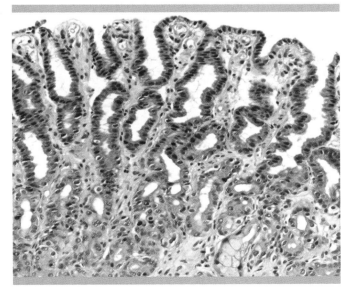

FIGURE 13-15

(A) Crowded glands with angulated profiles
(B) Foveolar hyperplasia
(C) Mucin depletion
(D) Nuclear hyperchromasia
(E) Smooth muscle proliferation within lamina propria

72. Toxic level of which of the following drugs is associated with this biopsy finding? (Figure 13-16)

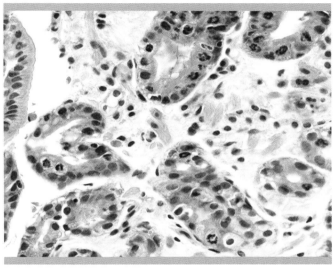

FIGURE 13-16

(A) Alcohol
(B) Colchicine
(C) 5-FU
(D) Non-steroidal anti-inflammatory drugs
(E) Proton pump inhibitors

73. All the following pathologic findings favor chemo-radiation atypia over a neoplastic process, except
(A) Angulated and crowded glandular architecture
(B) Cytoplasmic vacuolation
(C) Large, irregular nuclei with smudged chromatin pattern and low N:C ratio
(D) Presence of surface epithelial maturation
(E) Stromal atypia

74. Which of these features is not helpful in distinguishing esophageal columnar metaplasia from gastric carditis?
(A) Active inflammation
(B) Hybrid glands
(C) Multilayered epithelium
(D) Presence of esophageal glands and ducts
(E) Squamous mucosa overlying intestinalized glands

75. In a patient suspected to have gluten-sensitive enteropathy, which of the listed endoscopic and pathologic findings would argue against this diagnosis?
    (A) Expansion of the lamina propria by plasma cells and lymphocytes
    (B) Increased CD20-positive lymphocytes within the surface epithelium
    (C) Involvement of proximal jejunum
    (D) Scalloped appearance of the duodenal mucosa
    (E) Villous blunting

76. In a duodenal biopsy, which of the following entities is not associated with the findings of villous blunting and intraepithelial lymphocytosis?
    (A) Autoimmune enteropathy
    (B) *Helicobacter pylori* gastritis
    (C) Primary intestinal lymphangiectasia
    (D) Protein intolerance
    (E) Tropical sprue

77. Which of the following segments of gastrointestinal tract is most commonly involved by eosinophilic gastroenteritis?
    (A) Colon
    (B) Duodenum
    (C) Esophagus
    (D) Ileum
    (E) Stomach

78. A small bowel resection specimen from a patient suspected to have Crohn's disease would show all the following features, except
    (A) Circumferential ulcers
    (B) Cobblestone appearance of the mucosa
    (C) Fat wrapping
    (D) Fistula formation
    (E) Strictures

79. Which of the following histologic findings would be very unusual for a diagnosis of Crohn's disease?
    (A) Epithelioid granulomas
    (B) Fissuring ulcers
    (C) Lymphocytic phlebitis
    (D) Transmural lymphoid aggregates
    (E) Neural hypertrophy and thickening of the muscularis mucosae

80. A 24-year-old man with history of peripheral edema and steatorrhea undergoes small bowel resection for symptoms of obstruction. Based on Figure 13-17, what is the most likely diagnosis?

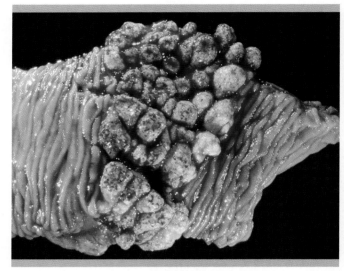

FIGURE 13-17

(A) Adenocarcinoma
(B) Cavernous lymphangioma
(C) Crohn's disease
(D) Diaphragm disease
(E) Intestinal tuberculosis

81. The pathologic finding depicted in Figure 13-18 occurs in the setting of all the following underlying intestinal diseases, except

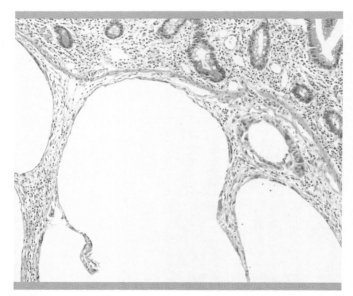

FIGURE 13-18

(A) Adenocarcinoma
(B) Diverticular disease
(C) Infectious colitis
(D) Idiopathic inflammatory bowel disease
(E) Neonatal necrotizing enterocolitis

82. Which of the following histologic findings is the most reliable marker of chronic mucosal injury/chronic colitis?
   (A) Crypt abscess formation
   (B) Crypt architectural distortion
   (C) Cryptitis
   (D) Granulomas
   (E) Superficial-predominant lymphoplasmacytic infiltrate

83. Which of the following pathologic features is not typical for untreated ulcerative colitis?
   (A) Backwash ileitis
   (B) Chronic active colitis
   (C) Crypt rupture-associated granulomas
   (D) Patchy and segmental involvement
   (E) Rectal involvement

84. In patients with ulcerative colitis, which of the following risk factors is considered to be the strongest risk factor for development of dysplasia/carcinoma?
   (A) Alcohol use
   (B) Extent and severity of disease
   (C) Family history of sporadic colon cancer
   (D) Primary sclerosing cholangitis
   (E) Smoking

85. Per 2010 American Gastroenterological Association (AGA) guidelines, the duration of disease after which patients with ulcerative colitis need to be enrolled in an endoscopic surveillance program is
   (A) 1 year
   (B) 2 years
   (C) 5 years
   (D) 8 years
   (E) 10 years

86. A 70-year-old woman with refractory diarrhea undergoes colonoscopic examination that shows no mucosal abnormalities. A biopsy from left colon is shown in Figure 13-19. All the following features are diagnostic of this entity, except

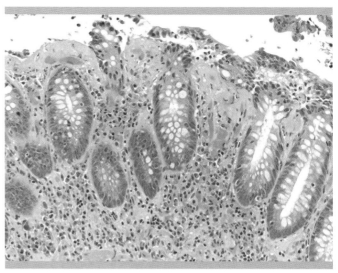

FIGURE 13-19

   (A) Basal lymphoplasmacytosis
   (B) Increased intraepithelial lymphocytes
   (C) Normal to slightly distorted crypt architecture
   (D) Pseudomembrane formation and linear mucosal breaks
   (E) Thickening of subepithelial collagen table

87. Which of the following pathologic findings favors a diagnosis of diverticular disease-associated colitis over idiopathic inflammatory bowel disease?
   (A) Bearclaw-like ulcers
   (B) Fistula formation
   (C) Segmental disease with fat wrapping
   (D) Rectal sparing
   (E) Transmural lymphoid aggregates

88. A patient with a history of bone marrow transplant (8 months ago) undergoes colonoscopy for evaluation of diarrhea. A biopsy obtained from the sigmoid colon shows increased numbers of eosinophils within the lamina propria and prominent crypt apoptotic activity. The patient has been compliant with his medications. What is the most likely cause of his symptoms?
   (A) Antibiotics
   (B) Chemotherapy
   (C) Graft-versus-host disease
   (D) Mycophenolate mofetil-associated colitis
   (E) Non-steroidal anti-inflammatory drugs

89. All the following histologic features are pathognomonic of mucosal prolapse syndrome/solitary rectal ulcer syndrome, except
    (A) Always associated with an ulcer
    (B) History of excessive straining
    (C) Mass lesions may mimic carcinoma
    (D) More common in females
    (E) Usually located in the rectum

90. Which of the following pathologic findings favors a diagnosis of adenocarcinoma over colitis cystica profunda?
    (A) Discrete rim of lamina propria around the glands
    (B) Evidence of previous injury such as radiation vasculopathy, hemosiderin-laden macrophages
    (C) Irregular and infiltrative glandular contours lined by dysplastic epithelium
    (D) Mucin-filled cysts
    (E) Polypoid configuration

91. Fibrous obliteration of the appendiceal lumen results from replacement of the entire lumen and underlying crypts by spindle cells. Which immunohistochemical marker is often expressed by this spindle cell proliferation?
    (A) Caldesmon
    (B) Cytokeratin
    (C) Desmin
    (D) S-100 protein
    (E) Synaptophysin

92. What is the most common parasitic infection of vermiform appendix?
    (A) *Ancylostoma duodenale*
    (B) *Ascaris lumbricoides*
    (C) *Enterobius vermicularis*
    (D) *Strongyloides stercoralis*
    (E) *Trichuris trichiura*

93. An appendectomy specimen from a patient with history of rupture 4 weeks ago, and subsequent antibiotic therapy, is most likely to show which of the following histologic findings?
    (A) Cryptitis
    (B) Eosinophilic inflammatory infiltrate
    (C) Granulomatous inflammation
    (D) Lymphoid hyperplasia
    (E) Periappendicitis

94. Histologic evaluation of one of several nodular esophageal lesions shows prominent intracytoplasmic glycogen. Based on this finding, which of the following syndromes should be suspected?

    (A) Cowden syndrome
    (B) Familial adenomatous polyposis
    (C) Gardner syndrome
    (D) Neurofibromatosis
    (E) Turcot syndrome

95. The gastric polyp shown here (Figure 13-20) is least likely to be associated with which of the following conditions?

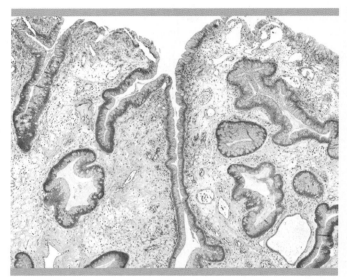

FIGURE 13-20

    (A) Autoimmune gastritis
    (B) Familial adenomatous polyposis
    (C) *Helicobacter pylori* gastritis
    (D) Non-steroidal anti-inflammatory drug-induced gastritis
    (E) Post-Billroth II gastrectomy

96. Which of the following causes of enlarged gastric folds is associated with protein-losing enteropathy, foveolar hyperplasia, and excessive secretion of transforming growth factor-alpha?
    (A) Chronic gastritis
    (B) Lymphoma
    (C) Ménétrier's disease
    (D) Signet ring cell carcinoma
    (E) Zollinger-Ellison syndrome

97. Which of the following clinicopathologic features is not associated with fundic gland polyps arising in the setting of familial adenomatous polyposis?
    (A) *APC* gene mutation
    (B) Equal male:female ratio
    (C) Less than 1% risk of developing dysplasia
    (D) Often associated with multiple polyps
    (E) Younger age at presentation

98. What is the best diagnosis for the submucosal gastric lesion depicted in Figure 13-21?

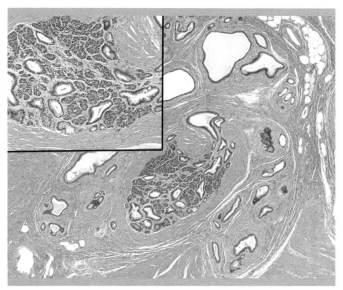

FIGURE 13-21

(A) Carcinoid tumor
(B) Gastritis cystica profunda
(C) Lymphangioma
(D) Pancreatic heterotopia
(E) Well-differentiated adenocarcinoma

99. A 65-year-old woman undergoes resection of a gastric polyp shown in Figure 13-22. Which of the following features is not typical of this entity?

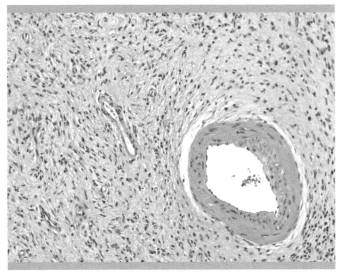

FIGURE 13-22

(A) Antrum is the most common location for this lesion
(B) A subset of these lesions may show *KIT* mutation
(C) The lesional cells express CD34 and vimentin
(D) They are often submucosal in location
(E) They may occasionally arise in the small bowel

100. Gastric mucosal calcinosis most commonly occurs in which of the following disease settings?
(A) Acute myeloid leukemia
(B) End-stage renal disease
(C) *Helicobacter pylori* gastritis
(D) Liver failure
(E) Proton pump inhibitor use

101. In gastric mucosal hemosiderosis, what is the pattern of iron deposition observed in patients with systemic iron overload or hemochromatosis?
(A) Luminal
(B) Predominantly extracellular
(C) Predominantly glandular, diffuse
(D) Predominantly stromal, patchy
(E) Vascular

102. Hamartomatous polyps of the small intestine are most commonly associated with which of the following syndrome/condition?
(A) Cowden syndrome
(B) Cronkhite-Canada syndrome
(C) Inflammatory diseases such as Crohn's disease
(D) Juvenile polyposis syndrome
(E) Peutz-Jeghers syndrome

103. A 14-year-old boy presents with small bowel obstruction and undergoes resection of an obstructing polypoid mass shown in Figure 13-23. He has numerous polyps within the small bowel. Which genetic mutation is associated with this condition?

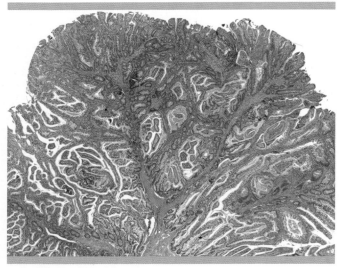

FIGURE 13-23

   (A) *APC*
   (B) *BMBR1A*
   (C) *PTEN*
   (D) *SMAD4*
   (E) *STK11*

104. Type-1 neurofibromatosis is associated with all of the following gastrointestinal neoplasms, except
   (A) Ampullary adenocarcinoma
   (B) Gangliocytic paraganglioma
   (C) Gastrointestinal stromal tumor
   (D) Inflammatory fibroid polyp
   (E) Somatostatinoma

105. Which type of lymphoma most commonly presents as lymphomatous polyposis within the GI tract?
   (A) Diffuse large B-cell lymphoma
   (B) Follicular lymphoma
   (C) Hodgkin lymphoma
   (D) Mantle cell lymphoma
   (E) Marginal zone lymphoma

106. Based on histologic features alone, which of the following findings favors a primary small bowel adenocarcinoma over metastatic adenocarcinoma involving the small bowel?

   (A) Extensive angiolymphatic space invasion
   (B) Extensive mural disease with minimal mucosal involvement
   (C) Presence of a precursor lesion
   (D) Signet ring cell morphology and a diffuse growth pattern
   (E) Tumor multifocality

107. All the following statements regarding inflammatory polyps are true, except
   (A) The stroma may harbor bizarre atypical cells that resemble a sarcomatous proliferation
   (B) They are composed of mixture of inflamed lamina propria and dilated glandular elements
   (C) They are exclusively associated with idiopathic inflammatory bowel disease (pseudopolyps)
   (D) They may be histologically indistinguishable from juvenile polyps
   (E) They usually do not have a tendency toward neoplastic progression

108. A 20-year-old man presents with multiple colonic hamartomatous polyps and is confirmed to have a mutation in the *PTEN* gene. He also has facial trichilemmomas. Besides hamartomatous polyps, which of the following colonic lesions is common in these patients?
   (A) Adenomyoma
   (B) Carcinoid
   (C) Ganglioneuroma
   (D) Inflammatory fibroid polyp
   (E) Leiomyoma

109. A patient with multiple colonic polyps is clinically suspected to have Cronkhite-Canada syndrome. Which of the following features is least likely to be associated with this syndrome?
   (A) Autosomal-dominant inheritance pattern
   (B) Death resulting from malnutrition and bleeding
   (C) Ectodermal abnormalities such as alopecia and nail dystrophy
   (D) Esophageal sparing
   (E) Presence of polyps that resemble juvenile polyps

110. During a routine colonoscopy, a 53-year-old man is found to have this 1.5 cm sessile polyp in the ascending colon (see Figure 13-24). Which of the following molecular alterations is most commonly associated with this lesion?

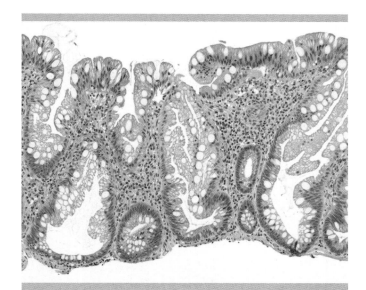

FIGURE 13-24

(A) *APC* mutation
(B) *BRAF* mutation
(C) *KRAS* mutation
(D) *MSH2* mutation
(E) *SMAD4* mutation

111. Resection of an esophageal cyst shows a unilocular cyst lined by ciliated columnar epithelium, with evidence of cartilage, smooth muscle, and mucous glands within the cyst wall. The cyst does not communicate with the esophageal lumen. What is the best designation for this cyst?
(A) Bronchogenic cyst
(B) Diverticulum
(C) Dorsal enteric cyst
(D) Duplication cyst
(E) Intramural cyst

112. Of the choices listed below, which is the most common type of heterotopic tissue found in the esophagus?
(A) Gastric
(B) Pancreatic
(C) Parathyroid
(D) Sebaceous
(E) Thyroid

113. Verrucous carcinoma of the esophagus is usually associated with all of the following features, except
(A) Accompanied by minimal cytologic atypia
(B) Locally aggressive neoplasm
(C) More common in males than females
(D) Often presents as a very large lesion
(E) Often present with distant metastasis

114. Which of the following features is not associated with *CDH1* mutated gastric adenocarcinoma?
(A) Adjacent gastric mucosa is non-atrophic
(B) Age of presentation is 3rd–4th decade
(C) Gene penetrance varies from 70% to 80%
(D) Increased risk of lobular breast carcinoma
(E) Intestinal-type morphology

115. Which of the tumors listed below is the most common extracolonic malignancy arising in the setting of familial adenomatous polyposis?
(A) Anal squamous cell carcinoma
(B) Barrett's adenocarcinoma
(C) Esophageal squamous cell carcinoma
(D) Gastric adenocarcinoma arising in fundic gland polyp
(E) Periampullary adenocarcinoma

116. All the following conditions are considered to be a significant risk factor for development of small intestinal adenocarcinoma, except
(A) Celiac disease
(B) Crohn's disease
(C) Cronkhite-Canada syndrome
(D) Familial adenomatous polyposis
(E) Hereditary nonpolyposis colon cancer syndrome

117. What percentage of colon cancers arises as a result of chromosomal instability?
(A) 2%
(B) 15%
(C) 30%
(D) 50%
(E) 85%

118. Which of the following histologic types of colorectal cancer is more common in patients with long-standing ulcerative colitis?
(A) Adenosquamous carcinoma
(B) Medullary carcinoma
(C) Mucinous carcinoma
(D) Signet ring cell carcinoma
(E) Small cell carcinoma

119. All the listed pathologic features are associated with this colonic adenocarcinoma (see Figure 13-25) resected from a 40-year-old man, except

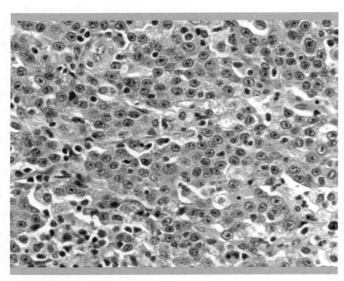

FIGURE 13-25

    (A) Crohn's-like lymphoid response
    (B) Exophytic/polypoid configuration
    (C) Located in the descending colon
    (D) Mucinous differentiation in other areas
    (E) Tumor heterogeneity

120. All the following statements regarding *KRAS* mutation analysis of colorectal neoplasms are true, except
    (A) Codon 12 and 13 mutations are the most common activating mutations
    (B) Presence of a *KRAS* mutation indicates response to cetuximab
    (C) Sanger sequencing, pyrosequencing, and melt curve analysis are common techniques of analysis
    (D) The test is performed on stage IV colorectal cancers
    (E) The test may be performed on biopsy samples as well as cytology specimens

121. An appendectomy specimen from a 42-year-old man reveals a carcinoid tumor. Which of the following pathologic features is not considered to be an indication for right hemicolectomy?
    (A) Extensive angiolymphatic space invasion
    (B) Mesoappendiceal involvement
    (C) Regional lymph node metastasis

    (D) Size of 1.0 cm
    (E) Rupture with presence of extraappendiceal tumor

122. What percentage of gastrointestinal tumors is known to harbor *KIT* mutations?
    (A) 5%
    (B) 10%
    (C) 25%
    (D) 50%
    (E) 85%

123. The submucosal tumor shown in Figure 13-26 is diffusely positive for DOG1. The tumor most likely originates from which part of the GI tract?

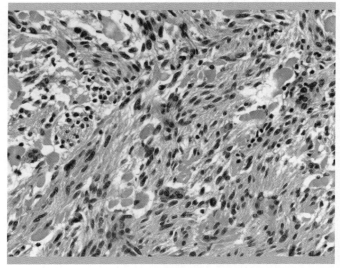

FIGURE 13-26

    (A) Esophagus
    (B) Ileum
    (C) Omentum
    (D) Rectum
    (E) Stomach

124. The gastric tumor shown in this figure (Figure 13-27) was resected from a 52-year-old man. What is the most likely diagnosis?

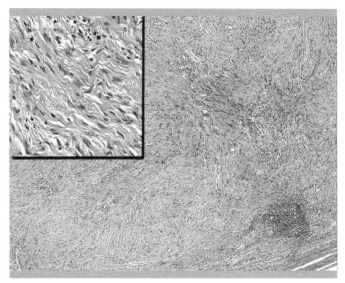

FIGURE 13-27

(A) Fibromatosis
(B) Gastrointestinal stromal tumor
(C) Inflammatory fibroid polyp
(D) Leiomyoma
(E) Schwannoma

125. A mesenteric nodule resected from a 40-year-old woman is shown in Figure 13-28. The lesion was immunoreactive for β-catenin. Which of the following clinicopathologic features is not associated with this entity?

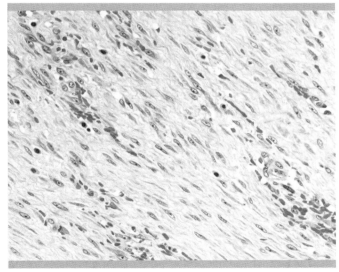

FIGURE 13-28

(A) Commonly associated with Turcot syndrome
(B) Composed of bland spindle/stellate cells with scattered dilated, thin-walled vessels
(C) Patients are usually asymptomatic
(D) They commonly arise in the mesentery and pelvis
(E) They typically infiltrate into adjacent soft tissue and bowel wall

126. During a Whipple procedure for a pancreatic head mass, the surgeon notices this 2.0 cm lesion in the fundus of the gallbladder (see Figure 13-29). The surgeon is very worried about this lesion and requests a frozen section. What is your diagnosis?

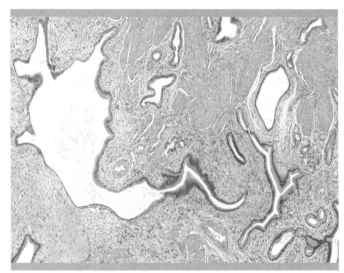

FIGURE 13-29

(A) Adenomyoma
(B) Chronic cholecystitis
(C) Gallbladder adenocarcinoma
(D) Hyperplastic Luschka's ducts
(E) Metastatic pancreatic adenocarcinoma

127. All the following histologic features on a pancreatic resection margin sample favor a diagnosis of adenocarcinoma, except
(A) Incomplete glandular lumens
(B) Irregular and angulated growth pattern
(C) Nuclear size variation of 2:1
(D) Presence of atypical glands adjacent to muscular arteries and fat
(E) Presence of perineural invasion

128. A 65-year-old woman undergoes resection of this pancreatic mass (Figure 13-30). What is the best diagnosis?

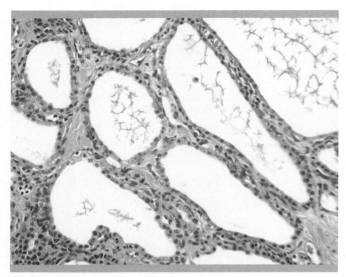

FIGURE 13-30

(A) Intraductal papillary mucinous neoplasm
(B) Lymphoepithelial cyst
(C) Microcystic serous cystadenoma
(D) Mucinous cystic neoplasm
(E) Pancreatic adenocarcinoma with cystic degeneration

129. An incidental histologic lesion characterized by tall columnar mucinous cells with well-polarized nuclei, slight nuclear stratification, and papillary formation, is encountered in a Whipple resection specimen. What is the best classification for this lesion?
(A) Pancreatic intraepithelial neoplasia IA
(B) Pancreatic intraepithelial neoplasia IB
(C) Pancreatic intraepithelial neoplasia II
(D) Pancreatic intraepithelial neoplasia III
(E) Intraductal papillary mucinous neoplasm

130. A 50-year-old woman undergoes resection of a cystic lesion located in the tail of pancreas. Microscopically, the cyst wall is lined by mucinous epithelium and shows variable amount of ovarian-type subepithelial stroma. What is the best diagnosis for this cystic lesion?
(A) Cystic neuroendocrine tumor
(B) Cystic pancreatic adenocarcinoma
(C) Intraductal papillary mucinous neoplasm
(D) Microcystic serous cystadenoma
(E) Mucinous cystic neoplasm

131. Based on (Figure 13-31), what would be this patient's demographic profile and gross appearance of this lesion?

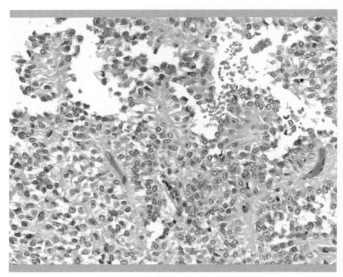

FIGURE 13-31

(A) A 2-year-old boy with pancreatic body mass
(B) A 30-year-old woman with a well-circumscribed hemorrhagic and cystic lesion in the body of pancreas
(C) A 50-year-old man with tan-white lesion in the body of pancreas
(D) A 62-year-old woman with a cystic pancreatic tail mass
(E) A 75-year-old man with a solid pancreatic head mass

132. A liver biopsy from a 20-year-old man shows extensive parenchymal necrosis involving approximately 80% of the parenchyma. Which of the following is the least likely etiology for this histologic finding?
(A) Acute viral hepatitis E infection
(B) Autoimmune hepatitis
(C) Drug toxicity
(D) Primary biliary cirrhosis
(E) Wilson's disease

133. Based on the findings shown in Figure 13-32, what is the most likely etiology for this histologic change?

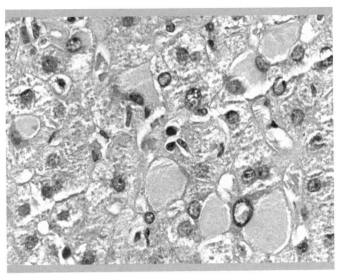

FIGURE 13-32

(A) Cytomegalovirus infection
(B) Epstein-Barr virus infection
(C) Hepatitis B infection
(D) Hepatitis E infection
(E) Yellow fever

134. Which histologic finding distinguishes chronic hepatitis due to primary biliary cirrhosis from chronic viral hepatitis C-induced disease?
(A) Ductopenia
(B) Lobular activity
(C) Lobular granulomas
(D) Portal interface activity
(E) Steatosis

135. A 10-year-old boy presents with recent onset fever and increased serum aminotransferases. Which of the following histologic findings would support the clinical impression of Epstein-Barr virus hepatitis?
(A) Apoptotic hepatocytes
(B) Cholestasis
(C) Granulomas
(D) Sinusoidal lymphocytosis
(E) Steatosis

136. A 40-year-old man presents with recent onset abdominal pain, fever, and hepatomegaly. Imaging studies reveal a multiloculated cyst with rounded densities. A histologic section from this lesion is shown in Figure 13-33. Which parasitic organism causes this condition?

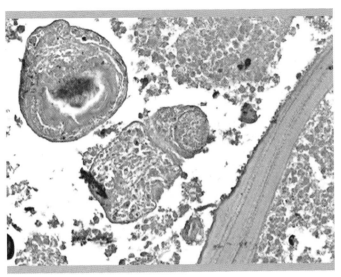

FIGURE 13-33

(A) *Clonorchis sinensis*
(B) *Echinococcus granulosus*
(C) *Entamoeba histolytica*
(D) *Enterobius vermicularis*
(E) *Escherichia coli*

137. A 45-year-old woman complains of recent onset jaundice and abdominal pain. Lab investigations show elevated levels of AST and ALT, and slightly elevated total bilirubin with normal serum alkaline phosphatase. Additional investigations reveal elevated serum ANA titer and negative viral hepatitis serologies. Which of the following clinicopathologic features is not associated with this form of hepatic injury?
(A) Brisk interface activity
(B) Dramatic clinical response to steroid therapy
(C) Elevated serum anti-smooth muscle antibodies
(D) Hypogammaglobulinemia
(E) Patchy bile duct damage

138. A 40-year-old woman presents to the hepatology clinic with vague abdominal pain over a period of 1 month. Investigations reveal elevated levels of serum alkaline phosphatase, gamma-glutamyl transferase, cholesterol, and normal levels of serum ALT, AST, and bilirubin. Additional studies show that she also tests positive for an antibody targeted against the E2 component of pyruvate dehydrogenase at a titer of 1:160. Which of the following findings would be expected in her liver biopsy?
(A) Florid duct lesion
(B) Intrahepatic and canalicular cholestasis
(C) Marked lobular inflammation
(D) Parenchymal necrosis
(E) Sinusoidal dilatation

139. An early ductal lesion in primary sclerosing cholangitis is typified by concentric periductal fibrosis with epithelial atrophy. Which part of the biliary tree is least likely to be involved by these lesions?
(A) Canals of Hering
(B) Common bile duct
(C) Interlobular bile duct
(D) Right hepatic duct
(E) Segmental bile duct

140. Which of the following drugs/toxins/medications causes bland cholestasis?
(A) Alcohol
(B) Amiodarone
(C) Cocaine
(D) Methotrexate
(E) Oral contraceptive pills

141. A 19-year-old man treated with chemotherapy for osteosarcoma undergoes a liver biopsy that demonstrates occlusion of the terminal hepatic vein and sinusoidal dilatation. These histologic changes are diagnostic of which of the following entities?
(A) Budd-Chiari syndrome
(B) Hepatic vein thrombosis
(C) Nodular regenerative hyperplasia
(D) Peliosis
(E) Sinusoidal obstruction syndrome

142. Macrovesicular steatosis is caused by all the following conditions, except
(A) Acute fatty liver of pregnancy
(B) Alcohol
(C) Obesity
(D) Type II diabetes mellitus
(E) Wilson disease

143. Which of the following statements is not applicable to the intracytoplasmic inclusions shown in Figure 13-34?

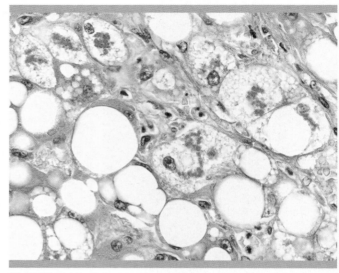

FIGURE 13-34

(A) Depending on their age they may stain red or blue with trichrome stain
(B) They are most commonly seen in ballooned hepatocytes
(C) They can be highlighted by cytokeratin 7 immunohistochemical stain
(D) They can occur in two forms – ropy and globular
(E) They may be observed in renal cell carcinoma and pulmonary adenocarcinoma

144. A 20-year-old woman with history of oral contraceptive use is investigated for vague abdominal pain and is found to have a large liver lesion shown in Figure 13-35. According to the surgeon, the adjacent liver was completely normal in appearance. What is the most likely diagnosis?

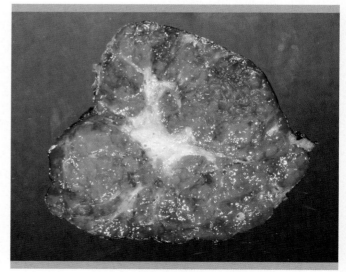

FIGURE 13-35

(A) Cholangiocarcinoma
(B) Focal nodular hyperplasia
(C) Hepatic adenoma
(D) Hepatocellular carcinoma
(E) Metastatic adenocarcinoma

145. In a liver biopsy, until what age is it normal to find intracytoplasmic copper-binding proteins and copper?
(A) 1-week-old
(B) 1-month-old
(C) 3-month-old
(D) 6-month-old
(E) 1-year-old

146. A 5-week-old baby boy with a normal birth weight and gestational age presents with progressively rising serum bilirubin levels, mildly elevated serum aspartate transaminase and alanine transaminase, and a marked increase in serum gamma-glutamyl transferase. An ultrasound examination of the abdomen is unremarkable. All the listed histologic findings would support the clinical diagnosis of extrahepatic biliary atresia, except
(A) Arterial hypertrophy
(B) Bile ductular proliferation
(C) Hepatocanalicular cholestasis
(D) Parenchymal necrosis
(E) Portal edema

147. A 16-month-old baby is found to be severely jaundiced with high unconjugated serum bilirubin levels. This hereditary disorder of bilirubin metabolism that lacks the conjugating enzyme is a result of mutation of which of the following genes?
(A) *ATP7B*
(B) *BSEP*
(C) *CFTR*
(D) *MDR3*
(E) *UGT1*

148. A 32-year-old man, who is otherwise healthy, is found to be icteric with conjugated hyperbilirubinemia. He has never taken any herbal medications. A liver biopsy on gross and microscopic examination shows the presence of dark brown pigment. What is the most likely diagnosis?
(A) Crigler-Najjar syndrome type I
(B) Crigler-Najjar syndrome type II
(C) Dubin-Johnson syndrome
(D) Gilbert's syndrome
(E) Wilson's disease

149. In a patient with C282Y *HFE* gene mutation, which component of the liver parenchyma is the first to demonstrate intracytoplasmic hemosiderin granules?
(A) Biliary epithelium
(B) Kupffer cells
(C) Zone 1 hepatocytes
(D) Zone 2 hepatocytes
(E) Zone 3 hepatocytes

150. A 14-year-old boy with neuropsychiatric symptoms presents with recent onset transaminitis. His liver biopsy shows chronic hepatitis with steatosis, Mallory's hyaline inclusions, cholestasis, and portal fibrosis. Serological evaluation shows low serum ceruloplasmin levels. Which special stain would be helpful in evaluating this biopsy?
(A) Oil Red-O
(B) Periodic Acid-Schiff
(C) Periodic Acid-Schiff with diastase
(D) Perls
(E) Rhodanine

151. A liver explant specimen from a 52-year-old man is shown in Figure 13-36. Which of the following statements is not applicable to this condition?

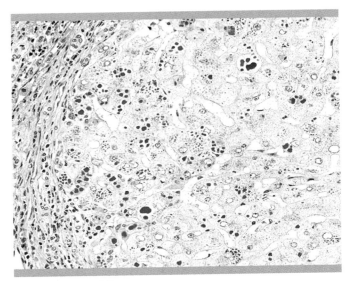

FIGURE 13-36

(A) It is an autosomal-dominant disorder
(B) It is characterized by low levels of protease inhibitor
(C) In neonates, this disease may present as cholestatic hepatitis
(D) PiZZ genotype is associated with the most severe form of the disease
(E) These patients are at risk for developing pulmonary emphysema and cirrhosis

152. Which of the listed conditions would not be classified as a developmental abnormality of the intrahepatic biliary tree?
    (A) Alagille syndrome
    (B) Bile duct adenoma
    (C) Caroli's disease
    (D) Congenital hepatic fibrosis
    (E) Von Meyenburg complex

153. All these clinicopathologic features favor a diagnosis of biliary hamartoma over a bile duct adenoma, except
    (A) Commonly located in the subscapular region
    (B) Commonly observed in patients with congenital hepatic fibrosis and polycystic liver disease
    (C) The duct lumens often contain inspissated bile
    (D) The lesion is composed of dilated and tortuous bile ducts embedded in a hyalinized stroma
    (E) The lesion is typically found in expanded and edematous-appearing portal tracts

154. A 32-year-old man with a history of anabolic steroid use undergoes resection of a 5.0 cm liver lesion shown in Figure 13-37. Which of the listed finding, if present, significantly increases the risk of progression to hepatocellular carcinoma?

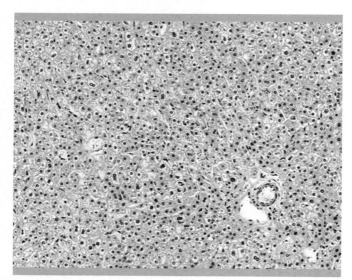

FIGURE 13-37

    (A) *APC* gene mutation
    (B) β-catenin mutation
    (C) HNF1-α mutation
    (D) Presence of inflammatory cell infiltrate and sinusoidal dilatation
    (E) Presence of steatosis

155. Which of the following lesions is least likely to arise in a non-cirrhotic background?
    (A) Cholangiocarcinoma
    (B) Conventional hepatocellular carcinoma
    (C) Fibrolamellar carcinoma
    (D) Focal nodular hyperplasia
    (E) Hepatic adenoma

156. Differentiating hepatic adenoma from a well-differentiated hepatocellular carcinoma can be quite challenging. Which of the following features is least helpful?
    (A) Hepatocyte trabecular thickness of >3 cell layers
    (B) Increased nuclear density
    (C) Loss of reticulin framework
    (D) Mitotic activity with atypical mitoses
    (E) Presence of unpaired arteries

157. A 70-year-old man presents with multiple liver lesions. Which immunohistochemical marker is most helpful in supporting a diagnosis of metastatic pulmonary adenocarcinoma over hepatocellular carcinoma?
    (A) Cytokeratin AE1/AE3
    (B) Cytokeratin 7
    (C) Cytokeratin 8/18
    (D) Cytokeratin 20
    (E) MOC-31

158. What is the most common primary tumor of the liver?
    (A) Cholangiocarcinoma
    (B) Focal nodular hyperplasia
    (C) Hemangioma
    (D) Hepatic adenoma
    (E) Hepatocellular carcinoma

159. A 45-year-old woman was found to have multiple liver lesions involving both the right and the left lobe of the liver. Based on Figure 13-38, what would be the best immunohistochemical marker to highlight the cells of interest?

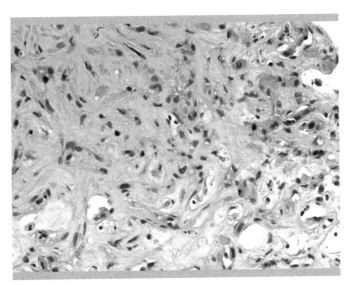

FIGURE 13-38

(A) CD31
(B) Cytokeratin AE1/AE3
(C) Cytokeratin 7
(D) Heppar-1
(E) MOC-31

160. A 2-year-old boy was found to have a palpable liver mass that is shown in Figure 13-39. What is the best diagnosis?

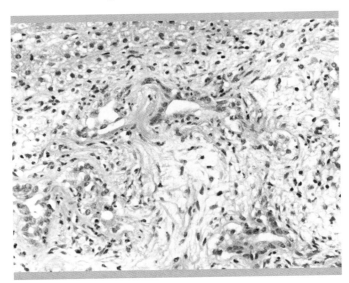

FIGURE 13-39

(A) Cholangiocarcinoma
(B) Embryonal sarcoma
(C) Hepatoblastoma
(D) Infantile hemangioendothelioma
(E) Mesenchymal hamartoma

ANSWERS

1. **(A) Crypt abscess.**
   While clumping of neutrophils or focal neutro-philic infiltration can be associated with bowel preparation agents, crypt abscess formation is very unusual. The most common mucosal changes include lamina propria edema and hemorrhage. Occasionally, mucosal erosion and influx of air into the tissue (pseudolipomatosis) may also be seen.

2. **(B) Barrett's esophagus.**
   Duplicated muscularis mucosae is associated with Barrett's esophagus. The superficial layer, which is usually irregular and thin, lies in close proximity to the metaplastic glands and represents the new duplicated layer. The importance of recognizing this phenomenon is in assessing the depth of invasion, especially in mucosal biopsy specimens and endoscopic mucosal resections. Infiltration of dysplastic glands into or between the two layers of duplicated muscularis mucosae should not be interpreted as submucosal invasion.

3. **(A) They are concentrated in the upper half of oxyntic glands.**
   The chief cells are concentrated in the lower half of the oxyntic glands. The parietal cells populate most of the upper half of the oxyntic glands.

4. **(C) Gastric body.**
   While most endocrine cells in gastric antral mucosa consist of gastrin-producing G cells, in the gastric body, the endocrine cells produce histamine, and are known as the enterochromaffin-like cells. Histamine binds the H_2 receptor on parietal cells that leads to increased acid production. Other enterochromaffin-like cells in the body include D cells (produce somatostatin) and X cells (produce endothelin).

5. **(A) Cecum.**
   Paneth cells, recognized by their bright eosinophilic apical granules, contain growth factors and a variety of antimicrobial proteins. They are normally absent in the left colon and, therefore, serve as an indicator of previous or chronic mucosal injury.

6. **(E) Sigmoid colon.**
   The ascending colon, cecum, and descending colon are anchored to the posterior abdominal wall. Similarly, rectum is adherent to the pelvic wall. The transverse colon is suspended by lesser omentum. As the sigmoid colon is suspended by mesentery, complications related to volvulus may occasionally affect this part of the colon.

7. **(B) Cecum.**
   The cecum has the widest diameter and the highest bowel wall tension within the gastrointestinal tract.

8. **(A) Anthemic folds.**

Because of the presence of anthemic folds, the crypts arising at the base of these folds appear to branch into the upper third of the mucosal layer. The importance of recognizing this variation in normal histology is that this finding may be interpreted as crypt architectural distortion associated with chronic colitis. Thus, crypt branching is only significant when found at the base of the crypts.

9. **(D) History of idiopathic inflammatory bowel disease.**

The incidence of gastric cancer in United States is low. Therefore, surveillance of patients with intestinal metaplasia or any of the above risk factors, except choice D (history of idiopathic inflammatory bowel disease), is not recommended. Patients with documented gastric dysplasia, however, should be placed in a surveillance program.

10. **(C) Esophagectomy.**

Esophagectomy is associated with significant morbidity and mortality compared to the currently available endoscopic therapy options. The 2011 American College of Gastroenterology (ACG) guidelines propose that esophagectomy is no longer a necessary treatment modality for Barrett's esophagus-related high-grade dysplasia (HGD). They propose that surgical intervention should be restricted to cases with multifocal HGD, while HGD identified in a flat mucosa may be followed endoscopically at 3-month intervals, and HGD with mucosal irregularity could be managed by endoscopic mucosal resection.

11. **(D) 8–10 years.**

The risk of colorectal cancer is increased in patients with long-standing and extensive ulcerative colitis. Per 2010 Crohn's and Colitis Foundation of America consensus group guidelines, this surveillance should begin at 8–10 years following an initial diagnosis of pancolitis or left-sided colitis. A repeat colonoscopy should be performed within 1–2 years. After two negative exams, colonoscopy is performed every 1–3 years, provided the duration of disease does not exceed 20 years. Current guidelines also recommend that for an adequate surveillance, a minimum of 33 biopsies should be obtained using jumbo forceps.

12. **(A) Endoscopically resectable lesion.**

Raised, endoscopically visible, dysplastic lesions in idiopathic inflammatory bowel disease (IBD) have been referred to as "DALM" or dysplasia-associated lesion or mass. DALMs can be broadly categorized as those that resemble a sporadic adenoma (adenoma-like DALM) and those that do not (non-adenoma-like DALM). Adenoma-like DALMs represent well-circumscribed, smooth or papillary, non-necrotic, sessile or pedunculated polyps that are can be resected by routine endoscopic methods. Other synonyms used to describe these lesions include adenoma-like low-grade dysplasia, adenoma-like dysplastic polyp, polypoid dysplasia, and adenoma-like mass. Non-adenoma-like DALMs present as velvety patches, plaques, irregular bumps and nodules, wart-like thickenings, stricturing lesions, and broad-based masses. Non-adenoma-like and adenoma-like DALMs are best differentiated on the basis of their endoscopic features because there is much overlap in the histologic, immunohistochemical, and molecular features between these two types of lesions. Treatment decisions, therefore, should not be based on histologic grounds alone. There is good evidence to support the concept that non-surgical treatment of adenoma-like DALMs in IBD by polypectomy, followed by continued surveillance, is a safe approach if there is no evidence of flat dysplasia elsewhere in the colon.

13. **(D) Pedunculated polyp.**

All the listed features, except choice D, are categorized as malignant polyp with unfavorable histology. These features predict risk of relapse or residual lesions. In polyps with these features, this risk ranges between 10–39%. Endoscopic polypectomy rather than surgery seems to be sufficient for malignant polyps with "favorable" features, which include well-to moderately differentiated adenocarcinoma, presence of carcinoma at least 2 mm from the cauterized margin of resection, and absence of lymphovascular invasion.

14. **(D) Stricture.**

Cytomegalovirus infection can cause a variety of gross lesions, the most common being an ulcer. Segmental lesions and linear ulcers may mimic Crohn's disease. Stricture formation is very unusual. Histologically, the changes range from minimal inflammation to deep ulcers with cryptitis, crypt apoptosis, and mucosal hemorrhage.

15. **(A) Adenovirus infection.**

The figure shows numerous intranuclear basophilic inclusions that are diagnostic of adenovirus infection. Cytomegalovirus inclusions typically occur in enlarged cells, and can either be intranuclear or intracytoplasmic in location. They are eosinophilic to amphophilic in color. Herpes simplex viral inclusions are characterized by multinucleation, margination of chromatin, and molding. Viral infections often induce marked lymphoid hyperplasia that may form a leading point for intussusception of the bowel.

16. **(D) Kaposi's sarcoma.**
   Kaposi's sarcoma is associated with Human Herpes Virus-8 (HHV-8) infection, and an immunohistochemical stain targeted against HHV-8 antigen is often used to confirm a diagnosis of Kaposi's sarcoma.

17. **(B) *Clostridium difficile*.**
   Clostridium difficile infection is typically associated with active colitis with ulcers and pseudomembrane formation. *Actinomycosis israelii* is a filamentous anaerobic gram-positive bacterium that causes diverticular disease, perianal fistulas, and appendicitis. Yersinia species can cause both suppurative and granulomatous inflammation.

18. **(A) *Campylobacter jejuni* colitis.**
   Pseudomembranes are composed of fibrin, mucin, and neutrophils. While *Clostridium difficile* is the most common cause of pseudomembranous colitis, other etiologies include ischemia, *Enterohemorrhagic E. coli,* and rarely collagenous colitis. *Campylobacter jejuni* colitis is a common cause of acute self-limited colitis. It is associated with cryptitis and crypt abscess formation, but rarely causes pseudomembrane formation.

19. **(C) *Enterohemorrhagic E. coli*.**
   Enterohemorrhagic E. coli is typically associated with marked edema and hemorrhage within the lamina propria and submucosa. Mucosal necrosis is common. Microthrombi as well as pseudomembrane formation may also be seen. Acute self-limited pattern of colitis is characterized by neutrophils in the lamina propria, with or without crypt abscesses and cryptitis, preservation of crypt architecture, and lack of basal lymphoplasmacytosis.

20. **(D) Hyalinized lamina propria.**
   All other features including ballooned crypts with cryptitis, crypt abscesses, degenerating goblet cells, and mucosal necrosis, may be seen in *Clostridium difficile* colitis. Hyalinization of lamina propria, lamina propria hemorrhage, and withered/atrophic crypts are typically associated with an ischemic etiology.

21. **(D) Ileocecal valve.**
   The ileocecal valve and jejunoileal segments of gastrointestinal tract are most commonly affected by tuberculosis. This disease is more common in developing countries and immigrant population. Mesenteric adenopathy is common. Both typical and atypical mycobacteria (especially *Mycobacterium kansasii* and *Mycobacterium bovis*) present with similar histologic findings.

22. **(B) Circumferential ulcers.**
   Crohn's disease typically gives rise to linear ulcers rather than circumferential ulcers. Mycobacterial infection spreads via lymphatics that usually run in a circumferential manner, and hence the circumferential ulcers. Mucosal cobblestoning is not associated with tuberculosis. Granulomas in Crohn's disease are typically well-formed, often perivascular, and lack atypical features, such as, large size and central areas of caseating necrosis.

23. **(E) Warthin-Starry stain.**
   The figure shows colonic mucosa with a fuzzy, "fringed", basophilic, luminal border that is characteristic of spirochetosis. The organisms are highlighted by silver stain such as Warthin-Starry stain. Intestinal spirochetosis is commonly seen in immunocompromised individuals who are HIV-positive. The infection may also be seen in patients with diverticular disease, ulcerative colitis, etc. Patients typically present with diarrhea. The differential diagnosis includes prominent glycocalyx. *Enteroadherent E. coli* may also give rise to a similar morphology. These bacteria are gram-negative and lack the characteristic spiral morphology of intestinal spirochetosis.

24. **(E) Whipple's disease.**
   The duodenal biopsy shows expansion of lamina propria by histiocytes, the differential diagnosis for which includes Whipple's disease, *Mycobacterium avium-intracellulare* infection, metabolic storage disorders such as Gaucher's disease and Niemann-Picks disease, and malakoplakia. Crushed Brunner's glands can sometimes mimic foamy histiocytes. Storage disorders are usually associated with hepatosplenomegaly. *Tropheryma whippelii* is the causative agent for Whipple's disease. It usually affects middle-aged white men. Patients sometimes present only with arthritic or neuropsychiatric symptoms. Small bowel is most commonly involved. In addition to aggregates of foamy histiocytes, the lamina propria may show foci of adipose tissue.

25. **(A) *Entamoeba histolytica*.**
   Entamoeba histolytica causes deep flask-shaped ulcers that often erode through mucosal blood vessels giving rise to bloody diarrhea. The presence of parasitic organisms (trophozoites) with intracytoplasmic erythrocytes is pathognomonic of amoebic infection. Another clue is that the nuclear chromatin of trophozoites is much more open and paler compared to the basophilic human chromatin. Cecum is commonly involved. The deep ulcers of amebiasis may mimic ulcers associated with idiopathic inflammatory bowel disease.

26. **(D) Tissue invasion.**
   The figure shows numerous "kite-shaped" and "pear-shaped" organisms layered between the villi, diagnostic of *Giardia lamblia*. Giardiasis is the

leading protozoal disease in United States. Patients usually present with explosive foul-smelling watery diarrhea. The cyst, which is the infective form of the organism, is resistant to chlorine. Endoscopic examination is usually unremarkable. Biopsy changes range from minimal inflammation to villous blunting and increased lamina propria inflammation. The trophozoites are pear-shaped forms with two ovoid nuclei and a central karyosome. The trophozoite forms are typically found in between the villi towards the luminal surface of the mucosa. Tissue invasion is not a feature of this infection. Giardiasis is frequently seen in association with immunodeficiency disorders such as CVID.

27. **(E) *Trypanosoma cruzi*.**
Infection by *Trypanosoma cruzi* (Chagas disease) targets the enteric nervous system and leads to achalasia-like megaesophagus and megacolon due to inflammatory destruction of the myenteric plexus. *Giardia lamblia* does not invade the tissues. The amastigote forms of *Leishmania donovani* are usually found within the lamina propria and do not involve the myenteric plexus. *Cryptosporidium parvum* and *Toxoplasma gondii* are classified as ciliates, and typically involve the surface/crypt epithelium and ulcer bases, respectively.

28. **(D) *Isospora belli*.**
The figure shows PAS-positive banana-shaped parasites surrounded by a parasitophorous vacuole, characteristic of *Isospora belli*. Although small bowel is the more commonly involved, rarely, the parasite may involve gallbladder parenchyma as well. Their morphology can be confused with goblet cells/intracytoplasmic mucin. However, their large size and intracellular location help in this distinction.

29. **(D) *Strongyloides stercoralis*.**
Of the listed nematodes, the female worm of *Strongyloides stercoralis* resides and lays eggs in the small bowel. This allows the parasite to stay in an autoinfective stage. The infection typically occurs in hospitalized or chronically ill and immunosuppressed patients. Both adult worms and larvae can be found in histologic sections. The figure shows cross section of the female worm and larvae within the lamina propria.

30. **(A) *Anisakis simplex*.**
Anisakis simplex is a nematode that parasitizes fish and sea mammals. Ingestion of raw fish or pickled fish leads to acute gastric anisakiasis that is characterized by symptoms that mimic peptic ulcer disease. Rarely, the clinical manifestations are those of a hypersensitivity reaction. The stomach is the most frequent site of involvement. Worms as well as larvae can be seen in tissue sections.

The parasites are often surrounded by an eosinophilic inflammatory reaction. The other nematodes enlisted are transmitted via food or water that has been contaminated by nematode eggs.

31. **(C) Selective IgA deficiency.**
While both common variable immunodeficiency (CVID) and selective IgA deficiency show mutations in the *TNFRSF13B* gene in select cases, celiac disease is the most common non-infectious GI complication associated with selective IgA deficiency. It is important to remember that serologies for celiac disease are often IgA based, and therefore, antigliadin IgA and antiendomysial IgA antibodies cannot be used as screening tools in these patients. The morphology of celiac disease in patients with selective IgA deficiency is identical to that in immunocompetent individuals.

32. **(D) Small bowel adenocarcinoma.**
Of the listed entities, patients with common variable immunodeficiency (CVID) do not have an increased risk for developing small bowel adenocarcinoma. CVID is characterized by impaired B-cell maturation, and may present at any age. Pernicious anemia, autoimmune hemolytic anemia, granulomatous involvement of skin, and chronic GI disorders, are some of the common clinical manifestations. In a patient with malabsorption, the finding of a marked decrease or absence of plasma cells within the lamina propria should prompt a workup for CVID.

33. **(A) Behçet's disease.**
Behçet's disease commonly involves the ileocecal valve region and causes mucosal ulcerations that mimic Crohn's disease. The diagnostic feature is the presence of lymphocytic inflammatory infiltrate within the walls of medium to small arteries and veins. The classic stigmata of Crohn's disease such as transmural lymphoid aggregates and deep fissuring ulcers are helpful in distinguishing the two entities.

34. **(B) It is a congenital disorder.**
Brown bowel syndrome is a rare acquired disorder and not a congenital disorder. It is associated with conditions that lead to malabsorption and vitamin E deficiency. Lipofuscin pigment accumulation within the smooth muscle cells of the muscularis propria and muscularis mucosae gives a brown color to the bowel. Clinically, the pigment deposition does not seem to have much effect on bowel function; however, defects in contractility, intussusception, and toxic megacolon have been reported.

35. **(C) Rectum.**
Phagocytes that engulf mucin are known as muciphages. They are commonly associated with

mucosal damage and are most numerous within the lamina propria of the rectum. They demonstrate fine cytoplasmic vacuolations and bland nuclei. They may occasionally form endoscopically visible nodules and mimic signet ring cell carcinoma. The immunoreactivity for CD68 helps in differentiating them from signet ring cell carcinoma, which should be positive for cytokeratin.

36. **(A) Esophagus.**
The figure shows a neoplasm composed of epithelioid or histiocytic cells with abundant granular eosinophilic cytoplasm, diagnostic of a granular cell tumor. The lesion is believed to be of neurogenic origin. Esophagus is the most common location. However, it can occur in any part of the GI tract. The cells are positive S-100 protein. Electron microscopic examination shows that the cells are filled with large autophagic vacuoles (lysosomes) that contain myelin-like debris.

37. **(C) Mast cells.**
Studies have demonstrated increased numbers of mast cells in patients with irritable bowel syndrome. The term mastocytic enterocolitis has been recommended for this condition. Studies suggest that >20 mast cells per high-power field indicate a pathologically increased mast cell number. The cells can be highlighted using CD117 or tryptase immunohistochemistry.

38. **(B) Inflammatory infiltrate composed of CD20-positive lymphocytes.**
Achalasia is a motor disorder of the esophagus characterized by failure of the lower esophageal sphincter to relax in response to swallowing. The pathologic hallmark of this disease is loss of myenteric ganglion cells. The other findings include hypertrophy of muscularis propria, eosinophilia of myocytes, and degenerative features, such as, cytoplasmic vacuolation. The mucosal changes include squamous hyperplasia, papillomatosis, and intraepithelial lymphocytosis. These patients have a long-term risk for developing squamous cell carcinoma.

39. **(E) Turner syndrome.**
Hirschsprung's disease is a congenital disorder with a striking male predominance. It is associated with many conditions, including those listed above, except Turner syndrome.

40. **(A) Lack of ganglion cells.**
Hirschsprung's disease (HD) is characterized by a complete lack of ganglion cells in all neural plexuses and relative hypertrophy of nerves. Rectal suction biopsies are most commonly used to establish a pre-operative diagnosis. An adequate biopsy should contain at least one-third submucosa and two-third mucosa. The biopsy must be obtained more than 2 cm above the pectinate line to avoid sampling of the physiologic aganglionic/hypoganglionic zone. Acetylcholinesterase-positive nerves within the lamina propria and muscularis mucosae support a diagnosis of HD. Calretinin immunohistochemistry can also be employed to evaluate for the presence of nerve fibers within lamina propria and muscularis mucosae. The lack of nerve fiber staining is typical of HD.

41. **(A) Meckel's diverticulum.**
Omphalomesenteric duct connects the intestine with the yolk sac. It usually closes by 10th week of embryonic life. Meckel's diverticulum is the most common variation of omphalomesenteric duct remnant. It is located immediately adjacent to the bowel wall. The other variations are rarely encountered.

42. **(D) Gastric.**
Meckel's diverticulum is a true diverticulum that is composed of all layers of the normal intestinal wall. Normally, the diverticulum is lined by ileal mucosa. The most common type of heterotopic mucosa found in Meckels' diverticulum is gastric, followed by the pancreatic type. Gastric fundic-type mucosa causes ulcers and patients may present with abdominal pain, intestinal hemorrhage, or perforation. Other complications include Meckel's diverticulitis, intussusception, and volvulus.

43. **(A) Electron microscopy.**
The condition described here is microvillous inclusion disease. This is a primary enterocyte abnormality with an autosomal- recessive pattern of inheritance. In contrast to celiac disease and autoimmune enteropathy, microvillous inclusion disease is usually not associated with intraepithelial lymphocytosis. The pathognomonic findings are present on electron microscopy, which include absent or small stubby microvilli, vesicular structures located towards the apex of the enterocytes with microvilli, and granules containing dense amorphous material. Similar inclusions may be also be seen in the colonic, gallbladder, and renal tubular epithelium. Medical therapy is generally ineffective. Small bowel transplantation is the best form of treatment for these patients.

44. **(D) Marked surface intraepithelial lymphocytosis.**
Autoimmune enteropathy (AIE) was first described as a syndrome of protracted diarrhea with the presence of autoantibodies directed against the gut epithelium. The biopsy findings include the presence of marked villous atrophy, crypt hyperplasia, and expansion of the lamina propria by a mixed inflammatory cell infiltrate. In contrast to celiac disease, AIE is notably associated with

crypt apoptosis without significant intraepithelial lymphocytosis. Some cases may show complete absence of Paneth cells, or goblet cells or both.

45. **(C) Ileocecal region.**
The condition described here is neonatal necrotizing enterocolitis. It is the most common cause of intestinal perforation in neonatal intensive care unit patients. The ileocecal region is a vascular watershed area and, therefore, is frequently affected by this condition. The affected bowel is distended, gray-purple, and shows marked thinning of the wall. Histologically, it is characterized by ischemic hemorrhagic necrosis of the bowel wall. Intestinal pneumatosis occurs as a result of bacterial overgrowth and fermentation luminal contents.

46. **(D) Milroy disease.**
All the listed conditions, except Milroy disease, are causes of secondary intestinal lymphangiectasia. Milroy disease (hereditary lymphedema) results from congenital obstruction of lymphatic flow or presence of abnormal lymphatics. It can involve multiple organs. Patients usually present with protein-losing enteropathy, malabsorption, and secondary immunodeficiency. In general, secondary lymphangiectasia occurs due to cardiovascular disorders or from conditions leading to lymphatic obstruction.

47. **(C) Dieulafoy's lesion.**
Dieulafoy's lesion, also known as caliber-persistent artery, is the type of ulcer described in this question. It causes massive arterial bleeding, and is most commonly encountered in the stomach, followed by small intestine and colon. Cameron's ulcers are linear ulcers that arise in the setting of sliding hiatal hernia.

48. **(E) Portal hypertensive gastropathy.**
Portal hypertensive gastropathy occurs in nearly 90% of patients with cirrhosis. It is a common cause of chronic gastrointestinal bleeding. The characteristic mucosal findings described here usually involve the fundus and body of the stomach. Duodenal involvement is referred to as portal hypertensive duodenopathy.

49. **(B) Gastric antral vascular ectasia.**
The figure shows foveolar hyperplasia with dilated capillaries and microthrombi. In conjunction with the endoscopic appearance of linear mucosal hyperemia ("watermelon" stomach), these features are diagnostic of gastric antral vascular ectasia (GAVE). The other associated features are fibromuscular hyperplasia, hyalinosis, edema, and congestion of lamina propria. This condition mainly affects the gastric antral mucosa of middle-aged women and is associated with portal hypertension in about 40% of cases.

50. **(C) Diverticular disease.**
Diverticular disease accounts for 30–40% of cases with significant gastrointestinal tract bleeding. Sigmoid colon is most commonly affected. The process is characterized by mucosal outpouchings located within weak points of the bowel wall, where vasa recta enter the muscularis propria. Inflammation leads to vascular erosion and bleeding.

51. **(A) It is a developmental disorder.**
Angiodysplasia is an acquired disorder associated with aging. It is the second most common cause of GI bleeding. The abnormality is marked by the presence of dilated, tortuous, thin-walled submucosal vessels, and secondary dilatation of the capillaries in the lamina propria. As the abnormality is predominantly present in the deeper blood vessels, diagnosing angiodysplasia in mucosal biopsy samples is often challenging.

52. **(C) Non-steroidal anti-inflammatory drugs.**
Chronic use of non-steroidal anti-inflammatory drugs (NSAIDs) can cause GI bleeding and symptoms related to obstruction. This form of NSAIDs-related injury is marked by the presence of circumferential ulcers, followed by mucosal regeneration, and "diaphragm" formation involving the mucosa and submucosa. This circumferential tent-like projection causes reduction in the diameter of bowel lumen. The submucosa is typically fibrotic, and shows a disorderly arrangement of vessels, nerves, and smooth muscle fibers (so called neuromuscular and vascular hamartoma).

53. **(C) Chronic radiation injury.**
Of the listed options, chronic radiation injury usually causes arterial ischemia. Buerger's disease and Behçet's disease cause mesenteric phlebitis. Buerger's disease very rarely affects the GI tract. Idiopathic myointimal hyperplasia of mesenteric veins is a rare condition affecting young and middle-aged men. It usually affects the left colon and is characterized by myointimal hyperplasia of the veins without an associated inflammatory infiltrate.

54. **(A) Irregular papillae.**
Reactive epithelial changes due to reflux esophagitis may be difficult to distinguish from squamous dysplasia. The architectural uniformity of reactive hyperplasia is reflected in the uniform height and width of papillae. The individual cells may show hyperchromasia and prominent nucleoli. However, they lack nuclear overlapping, irregular nuclear membranes, loss of polarity, and variation in the size and shape of the nuclei; features that are associated with dysplasia.

55. **(C) Rings and furrows.**
The findings depicted in this figure are those of eosinophilic esophagitis (EoE), which is

characterized by increased intraepithelial eosinophils (≥15 per high-power field) accompanied by basal cell hyperplasia, spongiosis, superficial eosinophilic microabscesses, and submucosal fibrosis. By definition, these patients have normal intraluminal pH and fail to respond to anti-reflux therapy. Most patients are young, white males, who have some form of atopy. In contrast to reflux esophagitis, which can also show intramucosal eosinophilia, EoE typically affects both the proximal and distal esophagus. Rings, furrows, strictures, and plaques, are some of the endoscopic findings characteristically associated with EoE. Other causes of mucosal eosinophilia include eosinophilic gastroenteritis, collagen vascular disease, infectious esophagitis, and pill-induced esophagitis.

56. **(C) Continuous distribution.**
Mucinous cells in Barrett's esophagus (pseudogoblet cells or distended foveolar cells) have a barrel-shaped appearance and show cytoplasmic vacuoles that may mimic a goblet cell. Although Alcian-blue is a time-honored stain to distinguish true goblet cells (stains dark blue), pseudogoblet cells can show light blue staining, depending on the quality of the stain. H&E stain is the best way to distinguish these two cell types. True goblet cells are arranged in a discontinuous fashion within the surface and glandular epithelium. They are round in shape and contain blue-staining intracytoplasmic mucin.

57. **(D) Barrett's esophagus with low-grade dysplasia.**
The biopsy shows intestinal metaplasia that is diagnostic of Barrett's esophagus. In addition, the surface epithelium shows nuclear hyperchromasia, stratification, and loss of surface maturation, changes that are consistent with low-grade dysplasia. The cells also show preservation of nuclear polarity. High-grade dysplasia is associated with significant cytologic atypia with loss of nuclear polarity. In addition, there is architectural atypia in the form of crowded, back-to-back or cribriform arrangement of glands. Intramucosal adenocarcinoma is marked by the presence of one of the following patterns: single cell infiltration into the lamina propria, sheets of dysplastic glands replacing the lamina propria, angulated glandular profiles, and a never-ending glandular pattern.

58. **(E) Proton pump inhibitor.**
The biopsy shows dilated gastric oxyntic glands with parietal cell hypertrophy and cytoplasmic vacuolation. In addition to this, chronic proton pump inhibitor use is also associated with increased cellular apoptosis and development of fundic gland polyps.

59. **(B) Allergy.**
Acute hemorrhagic gastritis is characterized by the presence of diffuse mucosal hyperemia along with erosions and ulcers. Histologically, the findings include dilatation and congestion of mucosal capillaries, edema, and interstitial hemorrhage. The injured epithelium shows regenerative changes such as mucin loss, nuclear hyperchromasia, and mitotic activity, changes that may be misinterpreted as dysplasia.

60. **(D) Urease.**
The CLO test is a rapid test used for detection of *Helicobacter pylori*. The basis of this test is the ability of the organism to secrete urease enzyme, which catalyzes the conversion of urea to ammonia and bicarbonate. This process also helps the organism to survive the harsh acidic environment of the stomach.

61. **(D) Neutrophils.**
Recent studies have shown that *Helicobacter pylori* organisms are developing resistance to standard antibiotic therapy. Following treatment, lymphocytes and plasma cells can be evident in biopsy samples for up to a period of 6 months or more. Activity in the form of neutrophilic cryptitis usually resolves promptly following antibiotic therapy, and thus its presence is indicative of therapy failure.

62. **(C) Lymphoid follicle formation.**
In a gastric biopsy, especially from the antrum, *Helicobacter pylori* infection causes a specific pattern of injury that is characterized by superficial chronic lymphoplasmacytic inflammation with neutrophilic cryptitis and abscesses. Occasionally, one may encounter prominent intraepithelial lymphocytosis as well as intestinal metaplasia. The presence of lymphoid aggregates with germinal centers, however, is considered to be the most specific finding for *Helicobacter pylori*-associated gastritis.

63. **(A) Active gastritis with intestinal metaplasia.**
The histologic findings that should prompt a workup for extranodal marginal zone B-cell lymphoma, a known complication of chronic *Helicobacter pylori* gastritis, include the presence of an expansile, monotypic inflammatory infiltrate that destroys the glandular architecture, and is present deep within the lamina propria and upper submucosa. The cells usually have a monocytoid appearance with a moderate amount of pale eosinophilic cytoplasm. Rarely, they may appear plasmacytoid. Lymphoepithelial lesions with epithelial injury and glandular disruption are almost always present. Active gastritis, with or without intestinal metaplasia, may be variably present in these biopsies, and

does not necessarily suggest the presence of concurrent lymphoma.

64. **(D) Multifocal atrophic *Helicobacter pylori* gastritis.**

Atrophic gastritis is a significant risk factor for gastric ulceration, intestinal-type dysplasia, and adenocarcinoma. While antrum is the most common site for *Helicobacter pylori* gastritis, the infection can show a multifocal pattern of involvement. This pattern carries the highest risk for development of dysplasia and carcinoma.

65. **(E) Use of immunohistochemical stain for *H. pylori*.**

In a biopsy that is highly suspicious for *H. pylori* infection, the inability to demonstrate the organisms could be due to several reasons such as presence of low bacterial load, presence of intestinal metaplasia, and recent antibiotic use. The use of proton pump inhibitors causes the organisms to migrate towards the gastric body and fundus and, therefore, the antral biopsies may be negative. Immunohistochemical stain for *H. pylori* is a highly sensitive and specific technique to highlight these organisms and should be employed in biopsies that show chronic active gastritis.

66. **(A) It causes severe gastritis.**

The figure shows *Helicobacter heilmannii* gastritis caused by an organism with a tightly spiraled structure that is at least twice as long, and considerably thicker than, *Helicobacter pylori* (*H. pylori*). The pattern of gastritis is slightly different from *H. pylori* gastritis. This infection is patchy in distribution and is usually associated with less active inflammation. *Helicobacter heilmannii* gastritis is more common in children. It is transmitted via animals. The distinction between *Helicobacter heilmannii* gastritis and *H. pylori* gastritis may not be of much clinical significance since the treatment for both conditions is similar. The organisms can be highlighted by immunohistochemical stain used for *H. pylori*.

67. **(D) Shows heaped up mucosal borders with irregular rugal folds.**

Gastric ulcers are characterized by loss of mucosa and often extend deep into the submucosa and superficial muscularis propria. The vast majority of peptic ulcers occur in the stomach and duodenum. In the stomach, they usually present as chronic ulcers with sharply demarcated boundaries, and are only slightly elevated compared to the surrounding mucosa. The presence of heaped up borders with irregular mucosal folds and size >3.0 cm are findings more commonly associated with a malignant gastric ulcer.

68. **(D) Hypogastrinemia.**

The gastric body biopsy shows near total absence of specialized glands (parietal cells and chief cells) and replacement of the glands by pseudo-pyloric and intestinalized glands. In the presence of normal antrum and lack of *Helicobacter pylori*, these changes are highly suggestive of autoimmune gastritis. The diagnosis is clinically confirmed by the presence of anti-intrinsic factor and anti-parietal cell antibodies, pernicious anemia (lack of intrinsic factor prevents absorption of vitamin B12), and hypergastrinemia (an attempt to stimulate acid production from residual parietal cells).

69. **(D) Non-steroidal anti-inflammatory drug-related gastritis.**

Both autoimmune and multifocal atrophic gastritis cause depletion of parietal cells leading to hypergastrinemia. Gastrin acts as a trophic hormone for enterochromaffin-like cells present in the gastric body and fundus. Therefore, it is not uncommon to see neuroendocrine proliferation in these settings. Most cases of Zollinger-Ellison syndrome are due to a functioning pancreatic endocrine tumor. Multiple endocrine neoplasia (especially type I) may also be associated with enterochromaffin-like cell hyperplasia.

70. **(B) Extranodal marginal zone B-cell lymphoma.**

The biopsy shows expansion of lamina propria by lymphocytes and plasma cells. In addition, there is prominent intraepithelial lymphocytosis, consistent with lymphocytic gastritis-pattern of injury. The intraepithelial lymphocytes are CD8-positive T lymphocytes, similar to those found in celiac disease. All the listed conditions can show this pattern of mucosal injury, except extranodal marginal zone B-cell lymphoma, wherein the intraepithelial lymphocytes are of B-cell phenotype.

71. **(A) Crowded glands with angulated profiles.**

The biopsy shows findings that are diagnostic of reactive gastropathy, or in this case, chemical gastropathy. By definition, this entity usually lacks inflammatory cells within the lamina propria. Other findings include foveolar hyperplasia with smooth muscle hyperplasia within the lamina propria, and a corkscrew configuration of the glands, as opposed to crowded and angulated glands that are typically associated with a neoplastic process. The surface epithelium often demonstrates the so-called "purple cell change," wherein the mucin depletion imparts a hyperchromatic appearance to the epithelium. The cells display a normal nucleus to cytoplasmic ratio and this is helpful in distinguishing reactive gastropathy from dysplasia. Bile reflux, medications, and alcohol are some of the common causes of reactive gastropathy.

72. **(B) Colchicine.**
The figure shows gastric epithelium with mitotic figures in metaphase, arranged in a characteristic ring-like configuration. These changes are consistent with colchicine toxicity. The other histologic changes include loss of nuclear polarity, increased apoptosis, and nuclear pseudostratification. These changes are most common in the duodenum and antrum. Colchicine binds to tubulin and prevents its polymerization, thus interfering with several cellular processes, such as, degranulation, chemotaxis, and mitosis.

73. **(A) Angulated and crowded glandular architecture.**
Ulcers due to chemoradiation therapy can demonstrate atypical glandular changes that mimic carcinoma. All the listed choices favor a diagnosis of reactive atypia, except choice A. In the post-therapy setting, the glands maintain a parallel arrangement with respect to each other. They do not show an infiltrative or angulated profile that is usually associated with a neoplastic process.

74. **(A) Active inflammation.**
In evaluating biopsies obtained from the gastro-esophageal junction, certain histologic features can help in determining if the biopsy was obtained from the tubular esophagus or gastric cardia. The presence of hybrid glands (glands that show incomplete intestinal metaplasia and mucinous columnar epithelium), multilayered epithelium (squamoid cells at the base and mucinous columnar cells on the surface), esophageal ducts and glands, and squamous mucosa overlying intestinalized glands, suggests that the biopsy has been obtained from tubular esophagus. Presence of neutrophilic inflammation is not helpful.

75. **(B) Increased CD20-positive lymphocytes within the surface epithelium.**
Gluten-sensitive enteropathy is associated with a distinct scalloped appearance of the mucosa, and is histologically characterized by villous blunting and intraepithelial lymphocytosis. Villous blunting is accompanied by expansion of the lamina propria by a lymphoplasmacytic infiltrate and crypt hyperplasia. The intraepithelial lymphocytes are CD3-positive and CD8-positive T-lymphocytes. While the duodenal bulb and second portion of the duodenum are the best locations to obtain a diagnostic biopsy, proximal jejunum may also be biopsied to confirm this diagnosis.

76. **(C) Primary intestinal lymphangiectasia.**
The finding of villous blunting and intraepithelial lymphocytosis is associated not only with celiac disease, but also with a variety of clinical conditions such as tropical sprue, protein intolerance, autoimmune enteropathy, and infections such as *Helicobacter pylori* gastritis. While primary intestinal lymphangiectasia can be associated with patchy villous blunting, the finding of intra-epithelial lymphocytosis is unusual.

77. **(E) Stomach.**
Eosinophilic gastroenteritis is characterized by eosinophilic infiltration within one or more segments of the gastrointestinal tract along with peripheral blood eosinophilia. Most patients also have a clinical history of allergies or asthma. Stomach is the most common site of involvement. Based on the layer of bowel wall involved, three subtypes have been described: mucosal, mural, and subserosal. The differential diagnosis of eosinophilia in GI tract includes parasitic infections, vasculitis, collagen vascular disease, drugs/medications, and Crohn's disease.

78. **(A) Circumferential ulcers.**
A segmental resection specimen from a patient suspected to have Crohn's disease typically shows linear, bear claw-type ulcers with intervening edematous mucosa, giving rise to the characteristic cobblestone appearance of the mucosal surface. Circumferential ulcers are usually seen in intestinal tuberculosis. The presence of fat wrapping or "creeping fat" on the serosal surface is associated with transmural inflammation of the underlying bowel segment. Fistula formation and strictures are known complications of Crohn's disease.

79. **(C) Lymphocytic phlebitis.**
Histologic stigmata of Crohn's disease include patchy chronic active enteritis with fissuring ulcers, transmural lymphoid aggregates, and epithelioid granulomas. Secondary changes include neural hypertrophy, muscle hypertrophy and submucosal fibrosis. Vascular changes are typically restricted to arterioles and consist of intimal hyperplasia, thrombosis, and rarely, granulomatous or fibrinoid vasculitis.

80. **(B) Cavernous lymphangioma.**
The figure shows an intraluminal mass composed of nodular areas. The surface of these nodules shows pin-point white to hemorrhagic areas. Given the history of edema and steatorrhea, the lesion most likely represents cavernous hemangioma. Intestinal tuberculosis, diaphragm disease (due to NSAID use), and Crohn's disease are usually associated with mucosal ulcers. Adenocarcinoma of the small bowel usually arises in the setting of Crohn's disease, celiac disease, FAP, or Lynch syndrome. The lack of any specific background mucosal

pathology makes this diagnosis unlikely. Patients with intestinal lymphangiectasia present with protein-losing enteropathy and malabsorption. In addition to primary (congenital obstruction of lymph flow) and secondary causes of lymphangiectasia (cardiac conditions such as constrictive pericarditis, cardiomyopathy), volvulus, lymphangioma, retroperitoneal fibrosis, radiation therapy, and lymphoproliferative disorders may be associated with lymphangiectasia as well.

81. **(A) Adenocarcinoma.**
The figure shows gas-filled cysts within the bowel wall, a condition referred to as pneumatosis cystoides intestinalis. It frequently occurs in the setting of an underlying intestinal disease, such as those listed in the question, except choice A (adenocarcinoma). The other clinical associations include pulmonary diseases such as cystic fibrosis and chronic obstructive pulmonary disease. The gas-filled cysts may be found throughout the bowel wall and are characteristically surrounded by macrophages and multinucleated giant cells.

82. **(B) Crypt architectural distortion.**
Chronic mucosal injury is characterized by the presence of crypt architectural distortion in the form of variation in the size and shape of the crypts, bifid crypts, irregular spacing in between the crypts, and crypt foreshortening (base of the crypt does not reach the muscularis mucosae). In addition, idiopathic inflammatory bowel disease is usually associated with prominent basal lymphoplasmacytosis. In biopsies obtained from the descending colon, sigmoid colon, and rectum, the finding of Paneth cell metaplasia indicates previous or chronic mucosal injury. Cryptitis and crypt abscess formation are markers of activity and do not indicate chronic mucosal injury.

83. **(D) Patchy and segmental involvement.**
Ulcerative colitis (UC) is a mucosal-based disease characterized by diffuse chronic active colitis. In the setting of severe pancolitis, the distal terminal ileum shows active inflammation, with or without architectural distortion, termed backwash ileitis. Injured crypts are associated with mucin rupture granulomas. Studies have shown that in treated UC, the disease may demonstrate patchy and segmental distribution, similar to Crohn's disease. Rectal involvement or ulcerative proctitis is more common in UC than in Crohn's disease.

84. **(B) Extent and severity of disease.**
Patients with long-standing disease are at risk of developing dysplasia or carcinoma and should therefore be enrolled in an endoscopic surveillance program. Among the listed risk factors, extent and

severity of disease is the strongest risk factor for development of dysplasia. The other risk factors are family history of sporadic colon cancer and primary sclerosing cholangitis. There is no direct association between neoplastic progression and alcohol use or smoking.

85. **(D) 8 years.**
Studies have shown that patients with a disease duration of at least 8 years have a significantly increased risk for development of dysplasia/carcinoma. Ideally, at least 33 four-quadrant biopsies should be obtained at a distance of every 10 cm throughout the colon. In addition, any suspicious lesions or masses should also be biopsied.

86. **(A) Basal lymphoplasmacytosis.**
The findings illustrated in the figure are diagnostic of collagenous colitis. The condition is characterized by the presence of thickened subepithelial collagen table along with superficial lymphoplasmacytic inflammatory infiltrate and lymphocyte-mediated epithelial injury. Occasionally, collagenous colitis is associated with a pseudomembranous colitis pattern of injury and patients may rarely present with colonic perforation. The collagen table typically entraps inflammatory cells, stromal cells, as well as capillaries. A trichrome stain may be employed to highlight the thickened collagen table that typically ranges from 10 to 30 microns in collagenous colitis (normal basement membrane is 2–3 microns thick).

87. **(D) Rectal sparing.**
Idiopathic inflammatory bowel disease, especially Crohn's disease, may be difficult to distinguish from diverticular disease-associated colitis. Both these entities cause deep ulcers, chronic active colitis, transmural lymphoid aggregates, granulomas (predominantly foreign-body type in diverticular disease), mural fibrosis, and fistulas. The lack of chronic mucosal injury in a segment of colon unaffected by diverticular disease, and rectal sparing, are helpful in excluding idiopathic inflammatory bowel disease.

88. **(D) Mycophenolate mofetil-associated colitis.**
Patients who have undergone bone marrow transplantation often receive several medications that include a bone marrow conditioning regimen, prophylactic antibiotics, and immunosuppressive therapy, espcially mycophenolate mofetil (Cellcept). Mycophenolate mofetil-associated colitis has histologic features that overlap with acute graft-versushost disease. Prominent crypt apoptosis with crypt dropout and regenerative epithelial changes may be seen in both these settings. In this case, the patient has been compliant with his medications,

and thus acute graft-versus-host disease is less likely.

89. **(A) Always associated with an ulcer.**
Mucosal prolapse syndrome is a spectrum of changes related to excessive straining during defecation, and encompasses entities such as solitary rectal ulcer syndrome, inflammatory cloacogenic polyp, and polypoid mucosal prolapse. It usually involves the anterior rectal wall, within 4–10 cm from the anal verge. The lesions may present as solitary ulcers, polyps, or masses. Polypoid masses may mimic a malignant neoplasm.

90. **(C) Irregular and infiltrative glandular contours lined by dysplastic epithelium.**
Colitis cystica profunda represents a reactive change secondary to prior episodes of injury related to mucosal prolapse, radiation, chronic idiopathic inflammatory bowel disease, and surgery. The hallmark of this process includes the presence of mucin-filled cysts lined by benign colonic epithelium that are surrounded by lamina propria. They usually show rounded glandular configuration. Presence of complex glandular architecture, irregular glandular profiles with variation in the size and shape of glands, and cytologic atypia, support a diagnosis of adenocarcinoma over colitis cystic profunda.

91. **(D) S-100 protein.**
Fibrous obliteration of the appendiceal tip as well as lumen occurs with advancing age. The bland spindle cells often show wavy nuclei amidst myxoid stroma. S-100 protein highlights these spindle cells and, therefore, this process has also been referred to as neural hyperplasia or neuroma.

92. **(C) *Enterobius vermicularis.***
Enterobius vermicularis is the most common parasite involving the appendix. It is found within the lumen and often does not incite much of an inflammatory response. The cross section of a worm typically shows lateral cuticular crests.

93. **(C) Granulomatous inflammation.**
Some patients with history of appendicitis and rupture are empirically treated with antibiotics and undergo appendectomy once the inflammation subsides. This procedure is called interval appendectomy. Non-necrotizing epithelioid granulomas are very common in such specimens. Other histologic findings include mural fibrosis, transmural chronic inflammation, and crypt architectural distortion. These changes can mimic Crohn's disease.

94. **(A) Cowden syndrome.**
The esophageal lesions represent glycogen acanthosis. These are commonly seen in patients with Cowden syndrome or tuberous sclerosis.

95. **(B) Familial adenomatous polyposis.**
The polyp illustrated in this figure is a gastric hyperplastic polyp characterized by irregular cystically dilated glands lined by foveolar epithelium. The surrounding lamina propria is inflamed, edematous, and congested. Majority of the gastric hyperplastic polyps arise in the background of chronic gastritis (choices A, C, D, and E). Rarely, hyperplastic polyps may show dysplasia. Familial adenomatous polyposis is usually associated with tubular adenomas and fundic gland polyps in the stomach.

96. **(C) Ménétrier's disease.**
Ménétrier's disease is a rare condition that is characteristized by diffuse foveolar hyperplasia of the gastric body and fundus and hypoproteinemia. It is a type of hyperplastic gastropathy that results from excessive secretion of transforming growth factor-alpha. Some cases are associated with intraepithelial lymphocytosis, glandular atrophy, or atrophy of the parietal and chief cells.

97. **(C) Less than 1% risk of developing dysplasia.**
Fundic gland polyps can either be sporadic in nature or arise in the setting of familial adenomatous polyposis (FAP). Sporadic fundic gland polyps are more common in women. As they are associated with proton pump inhibitor use, their incidence has dramatically increased over the past few years. Those arising in the setting of FAP have an increased risk of developing dysplasia (up to 48%).

98. **(D) Pancreatic heterotopia.**
The figure shows a lesion composed of variably sized ducts and pancreatic acini (inset) amidst fibromuscular stroma, consistent with pancreatic heterotopia. Ectopic pancreatic tissue is most commonly found in the stomach, and often presents as a submucosal nodule. The nodule may have a central dimple representing opening of the pancreatic duct. Histologically, the lesion shows a variable admixture of pancreatic ducts, acini, and islets. The lobular arrangment, and the lack of cytologic atypia or atypical mitoses, is helpful when trying to distinguish this lesion from an invasive well-differentiated adenocarcinoma.

99. **(B) A subset of these lesions may show *KIT* mutation.**
The lesion depicted in this figure is an inflammatory fibroid polyp that is composed of a proliferation of bland spindle cells admixed with an inflammatory cell infiltrate that is rich in eosinophils. Small thin-walled blood vessels are scattered throughout this lesion. The spindle cells often show a characteristic concentric arrangement around these vessels. The cells express CD34 and

vimentin and are negative for CD117. A subset of these lesions harbors *PDGFRA* mutation. Stomach and small bowel are common sites of involvement in the GI tract.

100. **(B) End-stage renal disease.**

Gastric mucosal calcinosis is characterized by deposition of calcium compounds within the lamina propria. Interstitial calcium deposition is most frequently associated with end-stage renal disease. This finding may be seen in other conditions that cause hypercalcemia or hyperphosphatemia, such as, primary hyperparathyroidism, sarcoidosis, lymphoma, and multiple myeloma. Patients undergoing organ transplantation and those who consume aluminum-containing antacids may also show this finding.

101. **(C) Predominantly glandular, diffuse.**

Gastric mucosal hemosiderosis occurs in patients with hemochromatosis, alcoholics, or in those who take oral iron pills. The biopsy shows refractile yellow-brown deposits that are highlighted by Prussian blue stain. Three distinct patterns of iron deposition have been described. The stromal, patchy pattern is most commonly seen with gastric inflammation, and possibly represents iron deposition due to prior mucosal hemorrhage. Extracellular iron deposition is associated with history of oral iron intake, and the glandular and diffuse pattern is predominantly seen in patients with hemochromatosis or systemic iron overload.

102. **(E) Peutz-Jeghers syndrome.**

Hamartomatous polyps are characterized by the presence of a variable admixture of epithelial and stromal elements indigenous to the anatomic location. Peutz-Jeghers polyps are the most common hamartomatous polyps of the small intestine. They are typically irregular, multilobulated polypoid lesions. They may rarely arise in a sporadic setting.

103. **(E) *STK11.***

The polypoid lesion shown in this figure represents a hamartomatous polyp with a prominent arborizing muscularis mucosae, typically associated with Peutz-Jeghers syndrome. These individuals usually harbor mutations in the *LKB1/STK11* gene located on chromosome 19p13.3. The syndrome is associated with mucocutaneous pigmentation and an increased risk for malignancies in other organs (ovarian sex cord stromal tumor with annular tubules, testicular large cell calcifying Sertoli cell tumor, adenoma malignum of the cervix, breast, colon, and pancreatic cancers). Dysplasia and/or carcinoma has been reported in 2–6% of Peutz–Jeghers polyps. *APC*

mutation (chromosome 5q) is associated with familial adenomatous polyposis. *BMBR1A* (chromosome 10q) and *SMAD4* (chromosome 18q21.1) mutations have been associated with juvenile polyposis syndrome. *PTEN* mutation (chromosome 10q23) is commonly found in patients with Cowden syndrome and rarely in patients with juvenile polyposis syndrome.

104. **(D) Inflammatory fibroid polyp.**

Type-1 Neurofibromatosis (NF1) is associated with a variety of gastrointestinal (GI) tract neoplasms including ampullary adenocarcinoma, gangliocytic paraganglioma, gastrointestinal stromal tumor, somatostatinoma, and neurofibromas. Inflammatory fibroid polyp is not associated with NF1. Patients with NF1 have germline mutations of the neurofibromatosis 1 tumor suppressor gene located on chromosome 17q11.2. NF2 usually does not affect the GI tract.

105. **(D) Mantle cell lymphoma.**

Of the listed choices, mantle cell lymphoma most commonly presents as multiple polypoid lesions. This presentation has been referred to as lymphomatous polyposis. Rarely, follicular lymphoma, marginal zone lymphoma, and even T-cell lymphoma may produce a similar pattern. Histologically, mantle cell lymphoma is composed of nodules of neoplastic B-cells with small to medium lymphocytes with irregular nuclear membranes. The cells have scant cytoplasm and indistinct nucleoli. True lymphoepithelial lesions are generally absent. Immunophenotypically, mantle cell lymphoma shows positive staining with CD20, CD5, CD43, and cyclin D1. The cells are negative for CD10 and CD23. Most patients are >50 years of age. The ileocecal region tends to contain the largest number of polyps.

106. **(C) Presence of a precursor lesion.**

Primary small bowel adenocarcinomas are less frequent than colonic adenocarcinomas. In the presence of a clinical history, a diagnosis of a secondary malignancy involving the small bowel is fairly simple. Secondary involvement may occur by direct extension, serosal seeding, or via hematogenous or lymphovascular spread. Tumor multifocality, high cytologic grade, presence of extensive mural disease with minimal mucosal disease, and extensive angiolymphatic space invasion are findings that favor a metastatic adenocarcinoma over a primary. Similarly, signet ring cell differentiation and a diffuse growth pattern are quite unusual for a primary small bowel adenocarcinoma. Presence of an adenoma is a good clue that the lesion is primary in origin.

107. **(C) They are exclusively associated with idiopathic inflammatory bowel disease (pseudopolyps).**
Inflammatory polyps can arise a result of mucosal injury due to several etiologies including idiopathic inflammatory bowel disease, ischemia, drugs/medication-related injury, and infections. They may be sessile or pedunculated. Occasionally, they may have a filiform appearance, and the presence of many such polyps has been referred to as filiform polyposis. In the active phase, they show extensive neutrophilic cryptitis, crypt abscesses, mucosal erosions, granulation tissue, and stromal atypical cells that mimic sarcoma. In the later stages, the surface epithelium may be normal and the core may contain slightly fibrotic submucosal tissue.

108. **(C) Ganglioneuroma.**
The patient's clinical profile is consistent with Cowden syndrome. Besides hamartomatous polyps, patients may show colonic lipomas, fibrolipomas, fibromas, ganglioneuromas, and adenomas.

109. **(A) Autosomal-dominant inheritance pattern.**
Cronkhite-Canada syndrome is a non-hereditary polyposis syndrome with no known etiology. Most patients are middle-aged. The polyps are characterized by inflamed lamina propria with cystically dilated crypts and can occur anywhere in the GI tract except the esophagus. As they are indistinguishable from juvenile polyps, sampling of the intervening mucosa is critical. The intervening mucosa in Cronkhite-Canada syndrome shows edema, cystically dilated glands, and increased inflammatory cells, while the mucosa in juvenile polyposis syndrome is normal.

110. **(B) *BRAF* mutation.**
The lesion shown in this figure is a polyp with serrated epithelium accompanied by crypt dilatation, horizontal configuration of the crypts, and hypermucinous cells, consistent with a sessile serrated polyp without evidence of cytologic dysplasia. These are usually located on the right side and lack a readily identifiable proliferative zone. Most of them harbor *BRAF* mutations and show a high rate of DNA methylation. Microsatellite instability is usually not associated with these lesions, unless they develop epithelial dysplasia or carcinoma.

111. **(A) Bronchogenic cyst.**
The cyst described here is best classified as a bronchogenic cyst. Bronchogenic cyst results from anomalous budding of bronchial structures that are derived from the foregut. These cysts do not communicate with the esophageal lumen and may be located in the mediastinum or esophageal wall. Dorsal enteric cysts (neurenteric cysts) occur in the posterior mediastinum and are thought to result from incomplete closure of notochordal remnant. They are lined by gastric, intestinal, squamous, or respiratory epithelium and are covered by all the layers of the bowel wall. Duplication cysts are lined by squamous, gastric, ciliated columnar, or pancreatic tissue, and the wall typically does not contain organized layers of muscle or cartilage. Intramural cysts likely develop from a defect in the recanalization of the esophageal lumen and are lined by respiratory, cuboidal, or squamous epithelium with smooth muscle or ganglia in the cyst wall.

112. **(A) Gastric.**
Gastric heterotopia ("inlet patch") is the most common type of heterotopic tissue found in the esophagus. Most heterotopias occur in the upper one-third of the esophagus. The patients may complain of heartburn and dysphagia related to acid production. Rarely, adenocarcinoma may arise from this inlet patch. Heterotopic sebaceous glands are the second most common type of heterotopic tissue.

113. **(E) Often present with distant metastasis.**
Verrucous carcinoma of the esophagus is a rare neoplasm that characteristically shows a very well-differentiated, verrucoid or papillary proliferation of squamous cells with minimal cytologic atypia, marked acanthosis, and bulbous rete pegs. The invasive front of the neoplasm typically shows broad pushing margins. Repeated biopsies are often diagnosed as hyperplastic squamous proliferation and, therefore, these lesions grow very large until they are confidently diagnosed on a resection specimen. Lymph node metastasis is rare; distant metastasis has never been reported.

114. **(E) Intestinal-type morphology.**
Germline mutations in the *CDH1*/E-cadherin gene have been linked to a familial form of diffuse gastric carcinoma (signet ring cell carcinoma). These patients are at an increased risk for developing lobular carcinoma of the breast. The tumor is not associated with any background gastritis or precursor lesions. Genetic counseling and testing for E-cadherin mutation is recommended for patients with a positive family history. Most patients are offered the option of undergoing prophylactic gastrectomy.

115. **(E) Periampullary adenocarcinoma.**
Patients with familial adenomatous polyposis (FAP) syndrome and multiple duodenal adenomas have a 100- to 300-fold lifetime risk of developing duodenal or periampullary carcinomas. In general, periampullary adenocarcinoma is the most common extracolonic neoplasm in this setting of FAP.

116. **(C) Cronkhite-Canada syndrome.**
Small intestinal adenocarcinomas are very rare compared to colorectal adenocarcinomas. The risk factors for small bowel cancers include Crohn's disease, celiac disease, familial adenomatous polyposis, and hereditary nonpolyposis colon cancer syndrome. Cronkhite-Canada syndrome is not considered to be a risk factor for development of small bowel cancers.

117. **(E) 85%.**
A variety of molecular alterations have been implicated in colorectal carcinogenesis. The most common pathway is the chromosomal instability pathway that results from aneuploidy, gains and losses of chromosomal material, and translocations. Nearly 10–15% of tumors occur as a result of microsatellite instability (MSI), of which approximately 2–5% are related to Lynch syndrome and the remainder arise due to hypermethylation of *MLH1* gene. CpG island methylation (CIMP) pathway is another molecular pathway that gives rise to colorectal cancers. It encompasses some of the sporadic MSI-H cancers and about 10% of chromosomal instability pathway-related cancers.

118. **(D) Signet ring cell carcinoma.**
Signet ring cell carcinoma is more common in patients with ulcerative colitis. Like mucinous carcinomas, they usually present at an advanced stage. Medullary carcinomas are composed of sheets of cells with abundant eosinophilic cytoplasm with vesicular nuclei and prominent nucleoli. They are associated with a prominent lymphocytic response. This morphology is quite predictive of microsatellite instability. Adenosquamous carcinomas are extremely rare in the colon. They are associated with paraneoplastic hypercalcemia and often present at a higher stage.

119. **(C) Located in the descending colon.**
The colonic tumor shown in this figure shows a "medullary" phenotype with large neoplastic cells containing abundant eosinophilic cytoplasm, vesicular nuclei, and prominent nucleoli. In addition, there are prominent tumor-infiltrating lymphocytes. These morphologic features are very suggestive of a microsatellite unstable cancer. These tumors are often located on the right side and show a distinct Crohn's like lymphoid reaction, mucinous morphology, as well as tumor heterogeneity (e.g., poorly differentiated areas admixed with mucinous areas).

120. **(B) Presence of a *KRAS* mutation indicates response to cetuximab.**
Cetuximab and panitumumab are monoclonal antibodies that bind to EGFR and inhibit EGFR-mediated cell signaling. KRAS encodes a small G-protein that is downstream of EGFR. As a result of *KRAS* mutation, this protein is in a permanently active phase, and thus leads to ineffectiveness of anti-EGFR therapy such as cetuximab and panitumumab. Thus, presence of a *KRAS* mutation indicates resistance to these biologic agents. These mutations are most common in codons 12 and 13 of the *KRAS* gene. The diagnostic techniques typically target these regions and employ a nuclei acid amplification process followed by DNA sequencing. The high sensitivity of these techniques allows this test to be performed on limited samples such as biopsies and cytology specimens.

121. **(D) Size of 1.0 cm.**
Of the listed features, tumor size of 1.0 cm is not an indication for right hemicolectomy. Appendiceal carcinoid tumors are the most common incidental neoplasms of the appendix. In fact, the incidence of this lesion is very high in older patients undergoing appendectomy for appendicitis. The indications for additional surgery are controversial. Some of the suggested pathologic factors that are considered to be indications for right hemicolectomy include size >2.0 cm, presence of angiolymphatic space invasion, regional lymph node metastasis, rupture with extraappendiceal tumor, high mitotic count, and presence of mesoappendiceal involvement.

122. **(E) 85%.**
Approximately 85% of sporadic gastrointestinal stromal tumors (GISTs) harbor *KIT* gene mutation. The common mutation involves the juxtamembrane domain of exon 11. Other less common mutations involve exons 9, 13, and 17. Some GISTs have been found to harbor mutations in *PDGFRA* gene (exon 18). Mutations in the *KIT* and *PDGFRA* genes are mutually exclusive events. *PDGFRA* mutations occur in 10% of all GISTs and are most common in gastric GISTs. These tumors often demonstrate an epithelioid morphology. Majority of the patients who harbor *KIT* mutation and develop metastatic GIST respond to targeted therapy with imatinib mesylate, a small-molecule inhibitor that binds to the intracellular portion of *KIT*, thereby inhibiting intracellular signaling.

123. **(B) Ileum.**
The tumor shown in this figure is composed of fascicles of spindle cells admixed with dense collagen fibers (skenoid fibers). Spindle cell GISTs account for nearly 70% of all GISTs. Discovered on GIST 1 (DOG1) is a relatively new immunohistochemical marker that is expressed by GISTs. It has a higher sensitivity in detecting KIT-positive as well as KIT-negative tumors. Tumors arising in the small bowel are often associated with this peculiar stromal change referred to as skenoid fibers.

124. **(E) Schwannoma.**
The tumor nodule is surrounded by a cuff of lymphoid aggregates and is composed of short fascicles of bland spindle cells with wavy nuclei, characteristic of a schwannoma. Schwannomas of the GI tract are common in the stomach, followed by the colon, and rectum. Compared with peripheral schwannomas, GI tract schwannomas typically show a discontinuous cuff of lymphoid aggregates, lack the characteristic Antoni A and Antoni B areas, and often do not harbor the thick-walled hyalinized blood vessels. They are strongly positive for S-100 protein and GFAP.

125. **(A) Commonly associated with Turcot syndrome.**
The mesenteric nodule is composed of long fascicles of bland spindle cells with scattered dilated thin-walled blood vessels, diagnostic of mesenteric fibromatosis. Pelvic and mesenteric fibromatosis is associated with familial adenomatous polyposis (FAP) and Gardner syndrome. The tumors often reach a large size by the time they are resected. They frequently express β-catenin and are negative for CD117.

126. **(A) Adenomyoma.**
The picture illustrates a lesion composed of dilated glands lined by low columnar to cuboidal epithelium, admixed with smooth muscle bundles. These glands represent exaggerated Rokitansky-Aschoff sinuses, and these findings are diagnostic of adenomyoma or adenomyomatous hyperplasia. The lesion presents as a thickening or a nodule located in the fundus of the gallbladder. The uniform architecture and lobular configuration of the glands without cytologic atypia helps in distinguishing these lesions from invasive adenocarcinoma. Rarely, high-grade dysplasia as well as adenocarcinoma is known to arise in the background of adenomyomatous hyperplasia.

127. **(C) Nuclear size variation of 2:1.**
Pancreatic resection margins, especially in the setting of chronic pancreatitis, can pose a significant diagnostic challenge during intraoperative consultation. The presence of lobular architecture, minimal cytologic atypia, lack of necrosis, lack of atypical mitosis, regular glandular lumens, and lack of perineural or vascular invasion favor reactive glandular proliferation. Malignant ducts are usually larger, are more irregularly distributed, show partial lumens, and are cytologically characterized by a greater variation in nuclear size (rule of 4:1 or greater).

128. **(C) Microcystic serous cystadenoma.**
The lesion shown in this figure shows variably sized cysts that are lined by cuboidal epithelium with clear cytoplasm and well-defined cytoplasmic borders. These histologic features are diagnostic of microcystic serous cystadenoma, a lesion that commonly arises in the body or tail of the pancreas. Grossly, they show numerous tiny cysts that have a honeycomb appearance. The tumors often have a central scar. The individual cells have abundant intracytoplasmic glycogen. The other variants include macrocystic serous cystadenomas (common in males) and solid serous adenoma. The differential diagnosis includes lymphangioma, metastatic renal cell carcinoma, and cystic neuroendocrine tumor.

129. **(B) Pancreatic intraepithelial neoplasia IB.**
Pancreatic intraepithelial neoplasia (PanIN) lesions are a spectrum of ductal proliferative lesions that are believed to be the precursors of pancreatic ductal adenocarcinoma. They are classified using a three-tiered system as PanIN IA, IB, II, and III. PanIN IA is composed of small ductules lined by mucinous epithelium without evidence of cytologic atypia or loss of nuclear polarity. The histologic changes described in this question are categorized as PanIN IB. PanIN II lesions show tall columnar cells with full-thickness nuclear stratification and mild-to-moderate cytologic atypia. PanIN III lesions show loss of nuclear polarity with marked cytoarchitectural atypia (similar to carcinoma in situ). PanIN shares many cytologic features with intraductal papillary mucinous neoplasms (IPMN). Most IPMNs, however, are macroscopically visible cystic lesions that are >1 cm in diameter.

130. **(E) Mucinous cystic neoplasm.**
Mucinous cystic neoplasm almost exclusively occurs in women. It tends to be located in the tail of pancreas. The lesion is composed of unilocular or multilocular cysts containing mucoid fluid. The cyst wall is lined by tall, mucinous epithelium with characteristic subepithelial ovarian-type stroma that can be highlighted by immunohistochemistry with progesterone receptor. Dysplasia arising in the setting of mucinous cystic neoplasm is graded as low, moderate, or high grade. Careful sampling of these lesions, especially the solid-appearing areas, is important, as occasionally, they may harbor foci of invasive adenocarcinoma. The lack of communication with main pancreatic duct is helpful in its distinction from intraductal papillary mucinous neoplasm.

131. **(B) A 30-year-old woman with a well-circumscribed hemorrhagic and cystic lesion in the body of pancreas.**
The photomicrograph shows a solid pseudopapillary neoplasm composed of tumor cells arranged between numerous small vessels. They show a

discohesive appearance, resulting in the formation of pseudopapillae. The individual cells show uniform, bland nuclei, which often contain nuclear grooves. Intracytoplasmic eosinophilic hyaline globules are a common finding. The neoplastic cells are positive for CD56, synaptophysin, vimentin, CD10, nuclear β-catenin, and cytokeratin (in about 50% of the cases). They do not express chromogranin.The tumor usually affects young women.

132. **(D) Primary biliary cirrhosis.**
The differential diagnosis for extensive hepatic parenchymal necrosis includes acute viral hepatitis (especially Hepatitis E), autoimmune hepatitis, and drug toxicity (Tylenol). In younger individuals, Wilson's disease is also in the differential. Primary biliary cirrhosis typically presents with chronic hepatitis-pattern of injury and is often associated with granulomatous bile duct injury. Lobular inflammation is usually minimal.

133. **(C) Hepatitis B infection.**
The figure shows ground-glass appearance of hepatocytes characterized by homogenous eosinophilic cytoplasmic inclusions that are usually encountered in chronic Hepatitis B viral infection. This change, however, is not specific for Hepatitis B infection, and may be seen in other conditions such as Lafora's disease, drug intake (phenobarbital, phenytoin, cyanamide), and renal transplant patients. Ground-glass hepatocytes in Hepatitis B infection reflects the presence of abundant HBsAg within the smooth endoplasmic reticulum. Special stains such as Victoria blue, orcein, aldehyde fuchsin, or immunohistochemistry for HBsAg can be used to highlight these inclusions. Intranuclear HBcAg accumulation produces the characteristic "sanded" appearance of the hepatocyte nuclei.

134. **(A) Ductopenia.**
Of the listed features, both primary biliary cirrhosis (PBC) and chronic hepatitis C infection can show lobular granulomas, lobular activity, portal interface activity, and steatosis. Ductopenia, however, is typically associated with advanced PBC. Although granulomas can be seen in both these entities, granulomatous bile duct injury is a hallmark feature of PBC.

135. **(D) Sinusoidal lymphocytosis.**
The findings of acute viral hepatitis include lobular inflammation with apoptotic hepatocytes (acidophil bodies), hepatocyte disarray, and occasionally, intrahepatic cholestasis. Kupffer cell aggregates are often present throughout the parenchyma. Epstein-Barr virus infection shows a specific pattern of lobular inflammation characterized by sinusoidal lymphocytosis.

136. **(B) *Echinococcus granulosus*.**
The figure shows a multilayered wall (germinal layer) with amorphous basophilic cyst contents. In addition, brood capsules containing protoscolex (head of an immature adult worm) are also seen. The head typically shows a rostellum with hooks (also seen in this figure). These histologic findings are characteristic of a hydatid cyst, a parasitic infestation caused by the tapeworm *Echinococcus granulosus*.

137. **(D) Hypogammaglobulinemia.**
The clinical profile of a patient with hepatitic serologies (elevated transaminases), negative viral serologies, and elevated serum ANA, is highly suggestive of autoimmune hepatitis (AIH). Histologically, AIH is characterized by prominent portal inflammation composed of lymphocytes and plasma cells with spillage of inflammatory cells into the periportal parenchyma (interface activity or piecemeal necrosis). Patchy bile duct injury is not uncommon. Patients may also have elevated serum anti-smooth muscle antibodies and anti-liver kidney microsomal antibodies. In addition, serum hypergammaglobulinemia is also present. AIH is a clinicopathologic diagnosis and confirmation of this diagnosis is achieved by observing dramatic response to steroid therapy with rapid normalization of serum aminotransferase levels.

138. **(A) Florid duct lesion.**
The clinical scenario described in this question is consistent with a diagnosis of primary biliary cirrhosis (PBC). PBC is characterized by cholestatic serologies and the presence of anti-mitochondrial antibody. This antibody is targeted against the E2 component of pyruvate dehydrogenase complex present within the mitochondria. Granulomatous bile duct injury, so characteristic of PBC, is also referred to as florid duct lesion. Cholestasis, prominent lobular activity, parenchymal necrosis, and sinusoidal dilatation are not common in biopsies from patients with PBC.

139. **(A) Canals of Hering.**
Primary sclerosing cholangitis (PSC) primarily affects medium- to large-sized bile ducts that are usually not sampled in a needle core biopsy. By definition, "small duct PSC" involves ducts that are not readily identified by endoscopic retrograde cholangiopancreatography (ERCP). Canals of Hering, which drain bile from the biliary canaliculi, do not show the classic "onion skinning" fibrosis seen in PSC. The diagnosis of PSC requires the presence of cholestatic serologies, cholangiographic findings of multifocal strictures and beading of the extrahepatic and intrahepatic larger bile ducts, and

exclusion of all other causes of secondary cholangitis (surgery, trauma, stones, infections, ischemia).

140. **(E) Oral contraceptive pills.**
Of the listed choices, oral contraceptive pills cause intrahepatic and canalicular cholestasis, without an accompanying inflammatory response (bland cholestasis). Alcohol and amiodarone cause a steatohepatitis-pattern of injury. In addition, amiodarone also causes phospholipidosis. Cocaine leads to microvascular injury and parenchymal necrosis. Methotrexate causes steatosis and manifests as chronic hepatitis-pattern of injury.

141. **(E) Sinusoidal obstruction syndrome.**
The histologic findings in this liver biopsy are diagnostic of veno-occlusive disease, which is now considered to be a part of sinusoidal obstruction syndrome. This syndrome often occurs secondary to chemotherapy and radiation therapy. The sinusoidal injury eventually injury results in non-thrombotic occlusion of the terminal hepatic vein. Budd-Chiari syndrome occurs as a result of thrombotic obstruction of the large or small hepatic veins, which leads to centrilobular hepatocyte necrosis. Alkaloids, irradiation, oral contraceptives, and myeloproliferative disorders are commonly associated with Budd-Chiari syndrome. Nodular regenerative hyperplasia (NRH) is defined by the presence of multiple 1- to 2-mm nodules, separated by hepatocyte atrophy, without accompanying fibrosis. Multiple clinical conditions, including rheumatoid arthritis, colon cancer chemotherapy, and polyarteritis nodosa, have been implicated in the pathogenesis of NRH. Microscopically, the condensation or collapse of reticulin fibers around the nodular parenchyma is considered to be diagnostic of this entity.

142. **(A) Acute fatty liver of pregnancy.**
All the listed conditions, except acute fatty liver of pregnancy, cause macrovesicular steatosis, wherein large intracytoplasmic fat droplets push the nucleus toward the periphery of the hepatocyte. Microvesicular steatosis is believed to be a result of mitochondrial injury and is characterized by the presence of multiple small fat vacuoles within the cytoplasm of the hepatocyte. The nucleus remains within the center of the cell. It is considered to be a harbinger of liver failure. Reye's syndrome and drug toxicity (tetracycline, valproic acid) are some other conditions that may cause microvesicular steatosis.

143. **(C) They can be highlighted by cytokeratin 7 immunohistochemical stain.**
The figure shows ropy, eosinophilic, intracytoplasmic inclusions that are refered to as Mallory's hyaline inclusions or Mallory-Denk bodies. They

are often seen in injured hepatocytes and represent aggregates of ubiquitinated and cross-linked cytokeratin intermediate filaments. Thus, immunohistochemical markers that may be used to highlight these inclusions include CAM5.2 (cytokeratin 8/18), p62, and heat shock protein-70. Cytokeratin 7 is a biliary epithelial marker and does not stain these inclusions. With trichrome stain, the early forms stain red, while the advanced forms stain grayish-blue. Mallory's hyaline inclusions are not specific for alcoholic steatohepatitis, and may be observed in non-alcoholic steatohepatitis, primary biliary cirrhosis, Wilson's disease, drug toxicity (amiodarone), benign tumors (focal nodular hyperplasia, hepatic adenoma), as well as malignancies (hepatocellular carcinoma, renal cell carcinoma, and pulmonary adenocarcinoma).

144. **(B) Focal nodular hyperplasia.**
The figure shows a well-circumscribed, tan-brown, solid tumor with a central fibrous scar. The differential diagnosis of a solitary liver lesion with central scar in a non-cirrhotic liver includes focal nodular hyperplasia and fibrolamellar carcinoma. Cholangiocarcinoma typically has a tan-white appearance due to the presence of extensive desmoplastic stroma. Hepatic adenoma is usually well circumscribed and has a soft consistency. It does not show a central scar. Hepatocellular carcinoma (HCC) is the only primary hepatic tumor that produces bile, and, therefore, appears greenish-brown on gross examination. Nearly 80% of HCCs arise in a background of cirrhosis. Metastatic adenocarcinomas are usually multifocal, subcapsular, and often demonstrate foci of central necrosis leading to surface umbilication.

145. **(C) 3-month-old.**
Until a postnatal age of approximately 3 months, hepatocytes normally contain copper-binding protein and copper that can be highlighted by special stains such as orcein and rhodanine.

146. **(D) Parenchymal necrosis.**
Extrahepatic biliary atresia accounts for approximately 30% of cases of neonatal cholestasis. The exact pathogenesis is still unclear, but the possible mechanisms include defective hepatic morphogenesis, defective prenatal hepatic circulation, and immune dysregulation. The findings of bile ductular proliferation, cholestasis, and portal edema reflect an obstructive process. Parenchymal necrosis is usually associated with acute hepatic injury. Other findings of extrahepatic biliary atresia include arterial hypertrophy, giant cell transformation of hepatocytes, and lobular inflammation. Hepatoportal enterostomy procedure (Kasai procedure) is the therapy of choice for these patients.

147. **(E)** *UGT1.*

The disorder described here is Crigler-Najjar syndrome, which results from deficiency of a conjugation enzyme UDP-glucuronosyl transferase 1A1 (UGT1A1). In the type I syndrome, the enzyme is completely absent, and without liver transplantation, this condition is fatal. The type II form is less severe, and results from reduced levels of UGT1A1 enzyme. Phenobarbital therapy promotes bilirubin glucuronidation by inducing hypertrophy of endoplasmic reticulum, and is thus useful in treating the type II form of this syndrome.

148. **(C) Dubin-Johnson syndrome.**

Dubin-Johnson syndrome is a disorder of bilirubin metabolism that causes conjugated hyperbilirubinemia. It results from a defect in the canalicular transport protein called multidrug resistance protein-2 (MRP-2). The liver parenchyma shows black-brown discoloration due to the accumulation of a chemical polymer in lysosomes that resembles epinephrine. Microscopic evaluation shows globular brown intracellular inclusions within the hepatocytes.

149. **(C) Zone 1 hepatocytes.**

Hereditary hemochromatosis results from mutations in the *HFE* gene, and the most common mutation is the C282Y mutation, followed by the H63D mutation. The periportal hepatocytes are the first to be exposed to excess iron deposition and, therefore, zone 1 hepatocytes are the first to be affected by this disorder. Hepatocyte iron deposition is semiquantitatively graded on a scale of 0–4 using the iron stain. The most accurate way of estimating iron overload is quantifying the amount of iron per gram dry weight of liver. Adults with hemochromatosis usually demonstrate over 10,000 µg iron/g dry weight of liver. Fibrosis is associated with a hepatic iron concentration of over 22,000 µg iron/g dry weight of liver.

150. **(E) Rhodanine.**

The condition described here is Wilson's disease, which is an autosomal-recessive disorder marked by the accumulation of toxic levels of copper due to mutations in the *ATP7B* gene. While advanced liver disease is the most common presentation, rarely patients may present with acute form of transient hepatitis or even fulminant hepatitis. Elevation of hepatic copper content (>250 µg/g dry weight of liver), low serum ceruloplasmin level, and intracytoplasmic copper deposition are helpful in establishing a diagnosis of Wilson's disease. The copper content of the protein complexes stains redbrown with rhodanine stain and the sulfhydryl-rich copper-binding proteins stain black-brown with orcein stain.

151. **(A) It is an autosomal-dominant disorder.**

The figure demonstrates a PAS with diastase stain with numerous intracytoplasmic hyaline globules located within the periportal hepatocytes, consistent with alpha-1 antitrypsin deficiency. This disorder is an autosomal-recessive condition. The most common mutation is the PiZ mutation. The mutation leads to defective hepatocellular secretion of alpha-1 antitrypsin and excessive accumulation of this abnormal polypeptide within the hepatocyte. PiZZ is the homozygous form of disease while PiMZ is the heterozygous form. Both these forms may demonstrate PAS-positive diastase resistant inclusions.

152. **(B) Bile duct adenoma.**

Alagille syndrome, von Meyenburg complexes, congenital hepatic fibrosis, polycystic liver disease, and Caroli's disease/syndrome are conditions that fall under the rubric of ductal plate malformations. They affect the intrahepatic biliary tree and represent embryologic arrest of ductal plate development. Bile duct adenoma is a localized ductular proliferation that develops as a response to previous injury. It typically presents as an incidental finding, and is often biopsied intraoperatively to exclude metastatic disease.

153. **(A) Commonly located in the subscapular region.**

Bile duct adenomas tend to be subcapsular in location. They are usually composed of uniform bile ductules without dilatation and very little intervening fibrous stroma. Biliary hamartoma (von Meyenburg complex) represents a form of ductal plate malformation and usually shows all the features (except choice A) listed in the question. The presence of well-defined borders, bland cytologic features, and lack of mitotic activity helps in distinguishing biliary hamartoma and bile duct adenoma from a metastatic adenocarcinoma.

154. **(B) β-catenin mutation.**

The lesion depicted in this figure is a hepatic adenoma, which is composed entirely of hepatocytes without significant cytologic atypia, mitotic activity, or necrosis. The cells are arranged in 1–2 cell thick cords. The lesion does not contain normal portal tracts. Instead, there are numerous unpaired arteries. Based on recent molecular studies, hepatic adenomas are genotypically classified into three subtypes: β-catenin mutated adenomas, inflammatory adenomas, and HNF1-α-mutated adenomas. It has been shown that adenomas that harbor β-catenin mutation have a higher risk for transformation to hepatocellular carcinoma. Although more common in women with history of oral contraceptive use, hepatic adenomas are also associated with anabolic steroid use, tyrosinemia, and glycogen storage disorders.

155. **(B) Conventional hepatocellular carcinoma.**
Nearly 80% of conventional hepatocellular carcinomas arise in a background of cirrhosis due to chronic viral hepatitis, metabolic disease, chronic biliary diseases, autoimmune hepatitis, and drugs/toxin-induced hepatic injury.

156. **(E) Presence of unpaired arteries.**
The presence of increased nuclear density, >3 cell thick hepatocyte cords, loss of reticulin framework, and increased mitotic activity with atypical mitoses, favors a diagnosis of well-differentiated hepatocellular carcinoma. Absence of portal tracts and the finding of unpaired arteries is not very helpful, since they can be observed in both these lesions.

157. **(E) MOC-31.**
Hepatocellular carcinomas are usually positive for cytokeratin 8/18 and can express cytokeratin AE1/AE3 and cytokeratin 7. Cytokeratin 20 is usually negative in both hepatocellular carcinoma and pulmonary adenocarcinoma. MOC-31 is rarely expressed (<2%) by neoplastic hepatocytes and, thus, can be helpful in distinguishing the two tumors.

158. **(C) Hemangioma.**
Hemangioma (cavernous hemangioma) is the most common primary tumor of the liver. It is composed of cavernous vascular channels separated by fibrous stromal bands lined by a single layer of flattened endothelial cells. Large lesions are often resected to avoid complications such as rupture and massive abdominal hemorrhage.

159. **(A) CD31.**
The figure shows a proliferation of neoplastic cells with an epithelioid morphology in a background of fibrous to fibromyxoid stroma. Some cells show intracytoplasmic lumens that mimic signet ring cells. One may often find red blood cells within these lumens. These histologic findings are diagnostic of an epithelioid hemangioendothelioma, and the choice of immunohistochemical stain is CD31. Other vascular markers such as CD34 (less specific) and ERG (nuclear stain) can also be used. Epithelioid hemangioendotheliomas tend to be more common in women. They are tan-white with irregular borders. Venous invasion as well as entrapment of surrounding normal tissues is fairly common. In the presence of multiple lesions, it is important to differentiate this lesion from metastatic signet ring cell carcinoma.

160. **(E) Mesenchymal hamartoma.**
The lesion shown in the figure is composed of a mixture of epithelial and stromal components. The epithelial component consists of relatively normal-appearing hepatocytes and bile ducts, surrounded by fibromyxoid stroma. These features are consistent with a diagnosis of mesenchymal hamartoma. The hepatocytes are arranged in the form of small clusters and retain their normal trabecular thickness. The ducts often show some degree of branching and dilatation, and are accompanied by inflammatory cells. The tumor may show cystic change, wherein the cysts are lined by bland flattened to cuboidal epithelium.

SUGGESTED READING

1. Meisel JL, Bergman D, Graney D, et al. Human rectal mucosa: proctoscopic and morphological changes caused by laxatives. *Gastroenterology.* 1977;72:1274-1279.
2. Takubo K, Sasajima K, Yamashita K, et al. Double muscularis mucosae in Barrett's esophagus. *Hum Pathol.* 1991;22:1158-1161.
3. Hirota WK, Zuckerman MJ, Adler DG, et al. ASGE guideline: the role of endoscopy in the surveillance of premalignant conditions of the upper GI tract. *Gastrointest Endosc.* 2006;63:570-580.
4. Spechler SJ, Sharma P, Souza RF, et al. American Gastroenterological Association medical position statement on the management of Barrett's esophagus. *Gastroenterology.* 2011;140:1084-1091.
5. Wang KK, Sampliner RE. Practice Parameters Committee of the American College of Gastroenterology. Updated guidelines 2008 for the diagnosis, surveillance and therapy of Barrett's esophagus. *Am J Gastroenterol.* 2008;103:788-797.
6. Rodriguez SA, Collins JM, Knigge KL, Eisen GM. Surveillance and management of dysplasia in ulcerative colitis. *Gastrointest Endosc.* 2007;65:432-439.
7. Farraye FA, Odze RD, Eaden J, et al. AGA Institute Medical Position Panel on Diagnosis and Management of Colorectal Neoplasia in Inflammatory Bowel Disease. AGA Medical Position Statement on the Diagnosis and Management of Colorectal Neoplasia in Inflammatory Bowel Disease. *Gastroenterology.* 2010;138(2):738-745.
8. Bond JH. Polyp guideline: diagnosis, treatment, and surveillance for patients with colorectal polyps. Practice Parameters Committee of the American College of Gastroenterology. *Am J Gastroenterol.* 2000;95(11):3053-3063.
9. Greenson JK, Stern RA, Carpenter SL, Barnett JL. The clinical significance of focal active colitis. *Hum Pathol.* 1997;28:729-733.
10. Dignan CR, Greenson JK. Can ischemic colitis be differentiated from C. difficile colitis in biopsy specimens? *Am J Surg Pathol.* 1997;21:706-710.
11. Horvath KD, Whelan RL. Intestinal tuberculosis: return of an old disease. *Am J Gastroenterol.* 1998;93:692-696.
12. Pulimood AB, Peter S, Ramakrishna BS, et al. Segmental colonoscopic biopsies in the differentiation of ileocolonic tuberculosis from Crohn's disease. *J Gastroenterol Hepatol.* 2005;20:688-696.

13. Drake WM, Winter TA, Price SK, et al. Small bowel intussusception and brown bowel syndrome in association with severe malnutrition. *Am J Gastroenterol.* 1996;91:1450-1452.

14. Jakate S, Demeo M, John R, et al. Mastocytic enterocolitis: increased mucosal mast cells in chronic intractable diarrhea. *Arch Pathol Lab Med.* 2006;130:362-367.

15. Goldblum JR, Whyte RI, Orringer MB, Appelman HD. Achalasia: a morphologic study of 42 resected specimens. *Am J Surg Pathol.* 1994;18:327-337.

16. Reyes-Mugica M. Hirschsprung disease. *Path Case Rev.* 2000;5:51-59.

17. Cutz E, Sherman PM, Davidson GP. Enteropathies associated with protracted diarrhea of infancy: Clinicopathological features, cellular and molecular mechanisms. *Pediatr Pathol Lab Med.* 1997;17:335-368.

18. Akram S, Murray JA, Pardi DS, et al. Adult autoimmune enteropathy: Mayo Clinic Rochester experience. *Clin Gastroenterol Hepatol.* 2007;5(11):1282-1290; quiz 1245.

19. Hsueh W, Caplan MS, Qu XW, et al. Neonatal necrotizing enterocolitis: clinical considerations and pathogenetic concepts. *Pediatr Dev Pathol.* 2003;6:6-23.

20. Burak KW, Lee SS, Beck PL. Portal hypertensive gastropathy and gastric antral vascular ectasia (GAVE) syndrome. *Gut.* 2001;49:866-872.

21. Suit PF, Petras RE, Bauer TW, et al. Gastric antral vascular ectasia: a histologic and morphometric study of "the watermelon stomach. *Am J Surg Pathol.* 1987;11:750-757.

22. Peura DA, Lanza FL, Gostout CJ, et al. The American College of Gastroenterology Bleeding Registry: preliminary findings. *Am J Gastroenterol.* 1997;92:924-928.

23. Boley SJ, Brandt LJ. Vascular ectasias of the colon. *Dig Dis Sci.* 1986;31:26S-42S.

24. Bjarnason I, Price AB, Zanelli G, et al. Clinicopathological features of nonsteroidal antiinflammatory drug-induced small intestinal strictures. *Gastroenterology.* 1988;94:1070-1074.

25. Liacouras CA, Furuta GT, Hirano I, et al. Eosinophilic esophagitis: updated consensus recommendations for children and adults. *J Allergy Clin Immunol.* 2011;128(1):3-20.e6; quiz 21-2.

26. Pusztaszeri MP, Genta RM, Cryer BL. Drug-induced injury in the gastrointestinal tract: clinical and pathologic considerations. *Nat Clin Pract Gastroenterol Hepatol.* 2007;4:442-453.

27. Genta RM, Lew GM, Graham DY. Changes in the gastric mucosa following eradication of Helicobacter pylori. *Mod Pathol.* 1993;6:281-289.

28. Ferrucci PF, Zucca E. Primary gastric lymphoma pathogenesis and treatment: what has changed over the past 10 years? *Br J Haematol.* 2007;136:521-538.

29. Correa P, Houghton J. Carcinogenesis of Helicobacter pylori. *Gastroenterology.* 2007;133:659-672.

30. Leung WK, Chan FK, Graham DY. Ulcers and gastritis. *Endoscopy.* 2006;38:2-4.

31. Wu TT, Hamilton SR. Lymphocytic gastritis: association with etiology and topology. *Am J Surg Pathol.* 1999;23:153-158.

32. Genta RM. Differential diagnosis of reactive gastropathy. *Semin Diagn Pathol.* 2005;22:273-283.

33. Iacobuzio-Donahue CA, Lee EL, Abraham SC, et al. Colchicine toxicity: distinct morphologic findings in gastrointestinal biopsies. *Am J Surg Pathol.* 2001;25:1067-1073.

34. Brien TP, Farraye FA, Odze RD. Gastric dysplasia-like epithelial atypia associated with chemoradiotherapy for esophageal cancer: a clinicopathologic and immunohistochemical study of 15 cases. *Mod Pathol.* 2001;14:389-396.

35. Odze RD. Unraveling the mystery of the gastroesophageal junction: a pathologist's perspective. *Am J Gastroenterol.* 2005;100:1853-1867.

36. Rothenberg ME, Mishra A, Brandt EB, Hogan SP. Gastrointestinal eosinophils in health and disease. *Adv Immunol.* 2001;78:291-328.

37. Geller SA, Cohen A. Arterial inflammatory cell infiltrate in Crohn's disease. *Arch Pathol Lab Med.* 1983;107:473-475.

38. Kleer CG, Appelman HD. Ulcerative colitis: patterns of involvement in colorectal biopsies and changes with time. *Am J Surg Pathol.* 1998;22:983-989.

39. Nugent FW, Haggitt RC, Gilpin PA. Cancer surveillance in ulcerative colitis. *Gastroenterology.* 1991;100:1241-1248.

40. Makapugay LM, Dean PJ. Diverticular disease-associated chronic colitis. *Am J Surg Pathol.* 1996;20:94-102.

41. Papadimitriou JC, Cangro CB, Lustberg A, et al. Histologic features of mycophenolate mofetil-related colitis: a graft-versus-host disease-like pattern. *Int J Surg Pathol.* 2003;11:295-302.

42. Magidson JG, Lewin KJ. Diffuse colitis cystica profunda: report of a case. *Am J Surg Pathol.* 1981;5:393-399.

43. Stanley MW, Cherwitz D, Hagen K, Snover DC. Neuromas of the appendix: a light-microscopic, immunohistochemical and electron-microscopic study of 20 cases. *Am J Surg Pathol.* 1986;10:801-815.

44. Guo G, Greenson JK. Histopathology of interval (delayed) appendectomy specimens: strong association with granulomatous and xanthogranulomatous appendicitis. *Am J Surg Pathol.* 2003;27:1147-1151.

45. Hizawa K, Iida M, Matsumoto T, et al. Gastrointestinal manifestations of Cowden's disease. Report of four cases. *J Clin Gastroenterol.* 1994;18:13-18.

46. Abraham SC, Singh VK, Yardley JH, et al. Hyperplastic polyps of the stomach: associations with histologic patterns of gastritis and gastric atrophy. *Am J Surg Pathol.* 2001;25:500-507.

47. Coffey RJ, Washington MK, Corless CL, et al. Ménétrier disease and gastrointestinal stromal tumors: hyperproliferative disorders of the stomach. *J Clin Invest.* 2007;117:70-80.

48. Wu TT, Kornacki S, Rashid A, et al. Dysplasia and dysregulation of proliferation in foveolar and surface epithelia of fundic gland polyps from patients with familial adenomatous polyposis. *Am J Surg Pathol.* 1998;22:293-298.

49. Gorospe M, Fadare O. Gastric mucosal calcinosis: clinicopathologic considerations. *Adv Anat Pathol.* 2007;14(3):224-228.

50. Marginean EC, Bennick M, Cyczk J, et al. Gastric siderosis: patterns and significance. *Am J Surg Pathol.* 2006;30:514-520.

51. McGarrity TJ, Kulin HE, Zaino RJ. Peutz-Jeghers syndrome. *Am J Gastroenterol.* 2000;95:596-604.

52. Kodama T, Ohshima K, Nomura K, et al. Lymphomatous polyposis of the gastrointestinal tract, including mantle cell lymphoma, follicular lymphoma and mucosa-associated lymphoid tissue lymphoma. *Histopathology*. 2005;47:467-478.

53. Ward EM, Wolfsen HD. The non-inherited gastrointestinal polyposis syndromes. *Aliment Pharmacol Ther*. 2002;16:333-342

54. Torlakovic E, Skuvlund E, Snover D, et al. Morphologic reappraisal of serrated colorectal polyps. *Am J Surg Pathol*. 2003;27:65-81.

55. Snover DC. Serrated polyps of the large intestine. *Semin Diagn Pathol*. 2005;22:301-308.

56. Huntsman DG, Carneiro F, Lewis FR, et al. Early gastric cancer in young, asymptomatic carriers of germ-line E-cadherin mutations. *N Engl J Med*. 2001;344:1904-1909.

57. Offerhaus GJA, Giardiello FM, Krush AJ, et al. The risk of upper gastrointestinal cancer in familial adenomatous polyposis. *Gastroenterology*. 1992;102:1980-1982.

58. Tung SY, Wu CS, Chen PC. Primary signet ring cell carcinoma of colorectum: an age- and sex-matched controlled study. *Am J Gastroenterol*. 1996;91:2195-2199.

59. Smyrk TC, Watson P, Kaul K, Lynch HT. Tumor-infiltrating lymphocytes are a marker for microsatellite instability in colorectal carcinoma. *Cancer*. 2001;91:2417-2422.

60. Patil DT, Rubin BP. Gastrointestinal stromal tumor: advances in diagnosis and management. *Arch Pathol Lab Med*. 2011;135(10):1298-1310.

61. Miettinen M, Shekitka KM, Sobin LH. Schwannomas in the colon and rectum: a clinicopathologic and immunohistochemical study of 20 cases. *Am J Surg Pathol*. 2001;25:846-855.

62. Jutras JA, Levesque HP. Adenomyoma and adenomyomatosis of gallbladder: radiologic and pathologic correlations. *Radiol Clin North Am*. 1966;4:483-500.

63. Charatcharoenwitthaya P, Lindor KD. Primary sclerosing cholangitis: diagnosis and management. *Curr Gastroenterol Rep*. 2006;8:75-82.

64. Vierling JM. Diagnosis and treatment of autoimmune hepatitis. *Curr Gastroenterol Rep*. 2012;14(1):25-36.

65. Hirschfield GM. Diagnosis of primary biliary cirrhosis. *Best Pract Res Clin Gastroenterol*. 2011;25(6):701-712.

66. LaRusso NF, Shneider BL, Black D, et al. Primary sclerosing cholangitis: summary of a workshop. *Hepatology*. 2006;44(3):746-764.

67. Zatloukal K, French SW, Stumptner C, et al. From Mallory to Mallory-Denk bodies: what, how and why? *Exp Cell Res*. 2007;313(10):2033-2049.

68. Santos JL, Choquette M, Bezerra JA. Cholestatic liver disease in children. *Curr Gastroenterol Rep*. 2010;12(1):30-39.

69. Servedio V, d'Apolito M, Maiorano N, et al. Spectrum of UGT1A1 mutations in Crigler-Najjar (CN) syndrome patients: identification of twelve novel alleles and genotype-phenotype correlation. *Hum Mutat*. 2005;25:325.

70. Kartenbeck J, Leuschner U, Mayer R, et al. Absence of the canalicular isoform of the MRP gene-encoded conjugate export pump from the hepatocytes in Dubin-Johnson syndrome. *Hepatology*. 1996;23:1061-1066.

71. Brunt EM, Olynyk JK, Britton RS, et al. Histological evaluation of iron in liver biopsies: relationship to HFE mutations. *Am J Gastroenterol*. 2000;95:1788-1793.

72. Bioulac-Sage P, Cubel G, Balabaud C, Zucman-Rossi J. Revisiting the pathology of resected benign hepatocellular nodules using new immunohistochemical markers. *Semin Liver Dis*. 2011;31(1):91-103.

73. Goodman ZD. Neoplasms of the liver. *Mod Pathol*. 2007;20(suppl 1):S49-S60.

74. Siddiqui MA, McKenna BJ. Hepatic mesenchymal hamartoma: a short review. *Arch Pathol Lab Med*. 2006;130(10):1567-1569.

CHAPTER 14

GENITOURINARY PATHOLOGY

1. Which part of the normal prostatic parenchyma is composed of glands that may histologically mimic high-grade prostatic intraepithelial neoplasia?
   (A) Anterior fibromuscular stroma
   (B) Central zone
   (C) Peripheral zone
   (D) Periurethral tissue
   (E) Transitional zone

2. Which of the following statements does not apply to basal cells of the prostatic glands?
   (A) They are inconspicuous in benign glands
   (B) They do not stain with PSA
   (C) They have a contractile function
   (D) They lie beneath the secretory cells
   (E) They react with antibodies to high molecular weight cytokeratin and p63

3. Which of the following lesions is composed of a localized proliferation of small- to medium-size glands embedded in a cellular, edematous stroma, with a thick hyalinized basement membrane around some of the glands, and basal cells that co-express high molecular weight cytokeratin, S-100, and muscle-specific actin?
   (A) Atypical adenomatous hyperplasia
   (B) Cystic atrophy
   (C) Postatrophic hyperplasia
   (D) Sclerosing adenosis
   (E) Simple atrophy

4. All the following are associated with the finding shown in this bladder biopsy (Figure 14-1), except

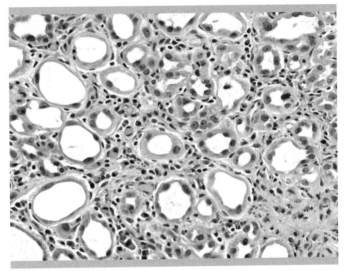

FIGURE 14-1

   (A) Associated with radiation, stones, and renal transplantation
   (B) Lacks AMACR expression
   (C) Most commonly found in bladder and prostatic urethra
   (D) Often an incidental lesion
   (E) Tubules are surrounded by a thickened hyaline sheath

5. Which of the following histologic features is considered to be cancer-specific and has not been described in benign glands?
   (A) Collagenous micronodules
   (B) Haphazard glandular arrangement
   (C) Intraluminal crystalloids
   (D) Nuclear hyperchromasia
   (E) Small glands with straight luminal borders

6. How would you classify the Gleason pattern of prostatic adenocarcinoma shown in Figure 14-2?

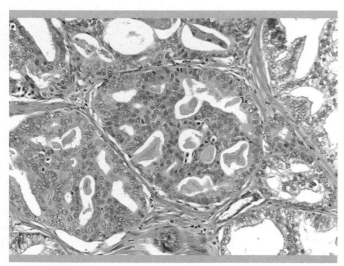

FIGURE 14-2

(A) Pattern 1
(B) Pattern 2
(C) Pattern 3
(D) Pattern 4
(E) Pattern 5

7. On an average, how long does it take for prostatic adenocarcinoma to show complete therapeutic response to radiation therapy?
(A) 6 months
(B) 10 months
(C) 12 months
(D) 24 months
(E) 30 months

8. Androgen deprivation causes all of the following changes in benign prostatic tissue, except
(A) Cytoplasmic clearing
(B) Glandular atrophy
(C) Loss of basal cells
(D) Nuclear pyknosis
(E) Stromal predominance

9. A 64-year-old man undergoes prostate biopsy, which is shown in Figure 14-3. Which of the following statements does not apply to this finding?

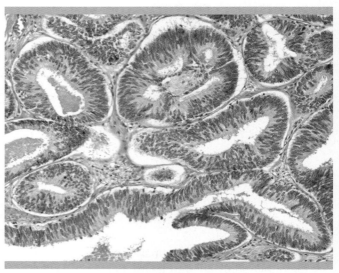

FIGURE 14-3

(A) Better prognosis than acinar carcinoma
(B) In its pure form, it comprises <2% of all prostate cancers
(C) Histology is equivalent of Gleason pattern 4
(D) Presenting symptoms include hematuria and urinary obstruction
(E) Variable cytologic atypia

10. Which of the listed histologic patterns is least likely to be associated with prostatic stromal proliferation of uncertain malignant potential (STUMP)?
(A) Cytologic atypia and necrosis
(B) Hypercellular stroma with atypical cells and normal glandular elements
(C) Hypercellular stroma without atypical cells and normal glandular elements
(D) Hypercellular stroma without glandular elements
(E) Phylloides-like pattern

11. Which of the following compartments comprise majority of the prostatic parenchymal volume?
(A) Anterior fibromuscular stroma
(B) Central zone
(C) Peripheral zone
(D) Periurethral tissue
(E) Transitional zone

12. A 60-year-old man was noted to have irregular nodular elevations of the bladder mucosa. The findings present in his bladder biopsy (see Figure 14-4) are diagnostic of

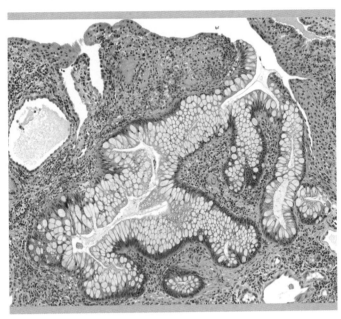

FIGURE 14-4

(A) Adenocarcinoma
(B) Cystitis glandularis
(C) Inverted papilloma
(D) Nested variant of urothelial carcinoma
(E) Urothelial carcinoma in-situ

13. Which of the following clinicopathologic features is least likely to be associated with interstitial cystitis?
(A) Common in elderly women
(B) Essentially incurable disease
(C) Hematuria and pyuria
(D) Mucosal rupture and submucosal hemorrhage
(E) Mural fibrosis and inflammation

14. Which of the following entities is characterized by deposition of inorganic salts within injured urothelial mucosa due to the action of urea-splitting bacteria?
(A) Emphysematous cystitis
(B) Encrusted cystitis
(C) Eosinophilic cystitis
(D) Interstitial cystitis
(E) Malakoplakia

15. All the following statements regarding assessment of renal sinus invasion in a case of clear cell renal cell carcinoma are true, except
(A) The renal sinus is the central fatty compartment that invests the collecting system and abuts the cortical columns of Bertin without a connective tissue interface
(B) Invasion of the renal sinus is staged as pT1
(C) Renal sinus invasion is associated with a poor prognosis
(D) Intravenous extension is the first step in extrarenal spread of clear cell renal cell carcinoma
(E) Most nodules within the renal sinus represent venous involvement

16. Which of the following injurious agents is associated with hemorrhagic cystitis?
(A) BCG
(B) Cytoxan
(C) Mitomycin C
(D) Radiation
(E) Thiotepa

17. A 5-year-old boy presents with leakage of urine from the umbilicus and recurrent episodes of urinary tract infection. Which of the following anomalies is the likely cause of patient's clinical symptoms?
(A) Bladder exstrophy
(B) Infected umbilical vessels
(C) Omphalitis
(D) Patent omphalomesenteric duct
(E) Patent urachus/urachal cyst

18. In which of the following locations within the bladder is ectopic prostate tissue most likely to be found?
(A) Anterior wall
(B) Dome
(C) Periurethral
(D) Posterior wall
(E) Trigone

19. What is the best classification for a urothelial lesion that shows normal mucosal thickness with loss of cell polarity, irregular nuclear borders, mild cytologic atypia, and rare mitoses?
(A) Flat urothelial hyperplasia
(B) Normal urothelium
(C) Reactive atypia
(D) Urothelial carcinoma in-situ
(E) Urothelial dysplasia

20. A bladder biopsy from a 56-year-old man is shown in Figure 14-5. This diagnostic entity is characterized by all of the following pathologic features, except

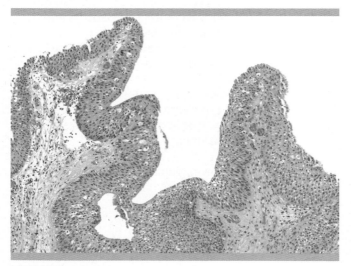

FIGURE 14-5

(A) Arborization of papillae
(B) Cytologic findings resembling normal urothelium
(C) Lack of detached-appearing papillae
(D) Thicker than normal urothelium
(E) Undulating papillary folds

21. Which of the following risk factors is least likely to cause bladder cancer?
(A) Alcohol
(B) Aniline dyes
(C) Aromatic amines
(D) Cigarette smoking
(E) Phenacetin

22. Which of the following statements is incorrect regarding staging urothelial tumors?
(A) Invasion into adipose tissue indicates extravesical extension and constitutes pT3
(B) Invasion into adjacent organs constitutes pT4
(C) Invasion into muscularis propria constitutes pT2
(D) Invasion into subepithelial connective constitutes pT1
(E) Stage T2-T4 are treated with total cystectomy or cystoprostatectomy

23. A 75-year-old man of Egyptian origin undergoes resection of a bladder tumor (see Figure 14-6). Which of the following risk factors is least likely to be associated with this tumor?

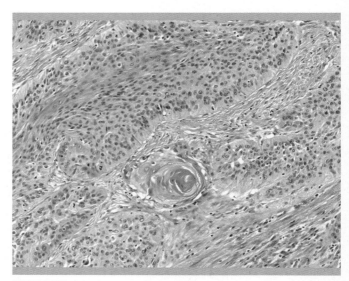

FIGURE 14-6

(A) Bladder calculi
(B) Bladder diverticulum
(C) Clonorchis sinensis infection
(D) Non-functioning bladder
(E) Renal transplantation

24. All the following criteria are helpful in classifying a tumor as urachal carcinoma, except
(A) Bulk of the tumor is located within the bladder wall rather than the luminal aspect
(B) Direct extension of another primary adenocarcinoma has been excluded
(C) Presence of an in-situ component
(D) Sharp demarcation between the tumor and normal surface epithelium
(E) Tumor is located in the dome or anterior wall of the bladder

25. Which of the following statements about inflammatory myofibroblastic tumor is incorrect?
(A) All lesions express anaplastic lymphoma kinase (ALK) by immunohistochemistry
(B) Mitotic figures may be present
(C) Neoplastic cells are composed of myofibroblastic cells resembling tissue-culture fibroblasts
(D) Some lesions may arise within months following a transurethral resection procedure
(E) The tumor cells can infiltrate the bladder wall and extend into perivesical adipose tissue

26. Which of the following tumors is the most common bladder tumor encountered in children and adolescents?
    (A) Inflammatory myofibroblastic tumor
    (B) Leiomyoma
    (C) Leiomyosarcoma
    (D) Lymphoma
    (E) Rhabdomyosarcoma

27. A 40-year-old man with history of hypertension underwent resection of a well-circumscribed 3.0 cm bladder tumor. Based on Figure 14-7, which of the following immunohistochemical markers is not expressed by this lesion?

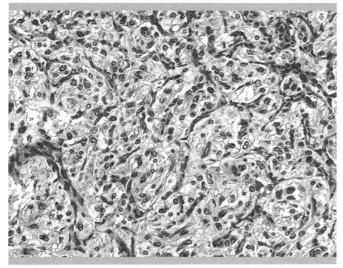

FIGURE 14-7

    (A) Chromogranin
    (B) Cytokeratin
    (C) Neuron-specific enolase
    (D) S-100
    (E) Synaptophysin

28. In what percentage of patients is metastatic disease the initial mode of presentation in patients with clear cell renal cell carcinoma?
    (A) 10%
    (B) 20%
    (C) 30%
    (D) 50%
    (E) 60%

29. Which is the most common genetic abnormality encountered in patients with sporadic clear cell renal cell carcinoma?
    (A) Deletion of chromosome Y
    (B) Deletion of 3p

    (C) Mutation of *c-met*
    (D) Trisomy 7
    (E) Trisomy 17

30. A nephrectomy specimen from a 50-year-old man with a renal mass is shown in Figure 14-8. Which of the following intracellular contents results in the typical golden-yellow appearance of this tumor?

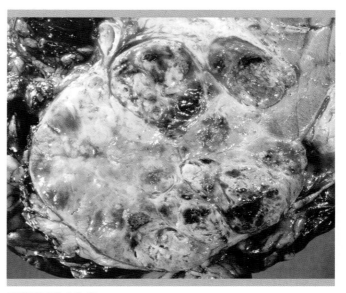

FIGURE 14-8

    (A) Glycogen
    (B) Hyaline globules
    (C) Lipid
    (D) Mitochondria
    (E) Necrosis

31. Besides stage, which of the following features is considered to be a significant prognostic factor in renal cell carcinoma?
    (A) Architectural growth pattern
    (B) Hemorrhage
    (C) Mitotic activity
    (D) Necrosis
    (E) Nuclear grade

32. From which part of the renal parenchyma does clear cell renal cell carcinoma arise?
    (A) Collecting duct
    (B) Distal convoluted tubule
    (C) Glomeruli
    (D) Loop of Henle
    (E) Proximal convoluted tubule

33. Which of the following immunohistochemical markers is least likely to be expressed by clear cell renal cell carcinoma?
    (A) CAM5.2
    (B) CD10
    (C) Epithelial membrane antigen
    (D) High molecular weight cytokeratin
    (E) Vimentin

34. Which of the following features is helpful in distinguishing multilocular cystic renal cell carcinoma from multilocular renal cyst (cystic nephroma)?
    (A) Cells lining the cysts
    (B) Cytokeratin immunostain
    (C) Gross appearance
    (D) Cyst contents
    (E) Presence of clear cells within fibrous septae

35. How large should a papillary renal tumor be in order for it to be classified as a carcinoma?
    (A) 0.1 cm
    (B) 0.2 cm
    (C) 0.4 cm
    (D) 0.5 cm
    (E) 1.0 cm

36. A 45-year-old man was found to have this single, cortical-based tumor with necrosis and hemorrhage (see Figure 14-9). Which of these genetic alterations is not typical for this entity?

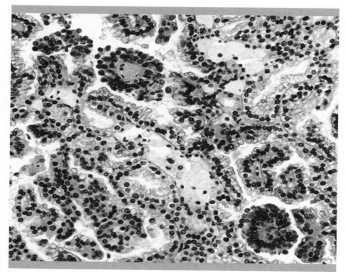

FIGURE 14-9

    (A) Deletion of chromosome 3p
    (B) Deletion of chromosome Y
    (C) Germline mutation in *c-met* gene

    (D) Trisomy 7
    (E) Trisomy 17

37. Which of the following immunohistochemical markers helps in distinguishing clear cell renal cell carcinoma with a pseudopapillary growth pattern from a papillary renal cell carcinoma?
    (A) CAM5.2
    (B) CEA
    (C) CD10
    (D) CK7
    (E) HMWCK

38. All the following features are characteristic of the tumor shown in Figure 14-10, except

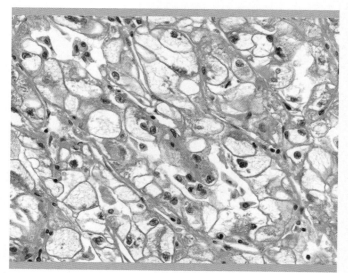

FIGURE 14-10

    (A) Composed of large pale cells with prominent cell membranes
    (B) Sarcomatoid transformation occurs in 5% of cases
    (C) Stain diffusely with Hale's colloidal iron
    (D) Ultrastructural studies show abundant rough endoplasmic reticulum
    (E) Usually located in the lower pole of the kidney

39. A 65-year-old man is noted to have a firm, tan-white kidney tumor located within the medullary pyramid (see Figure 14-11). What is the best diagnosis for this lesion?

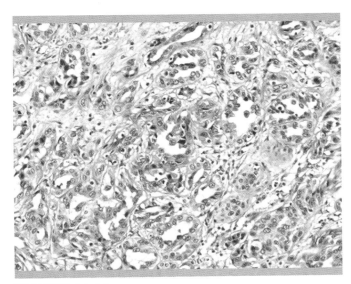

FIGURE 14-11

(A) Carcinoma of the collecting ducts of Bellini
(B) Metastatic carcinoma
(C) Papillary renal cell carcinoma
(D) Renal medullary carcinoma
(E) Urothelial carcinoma with glandular features

40. Of the tumors listed below, which of the following tumors occurs almost exclusively in patients with sickle cell hemoglobinopathy/trait?
(A) Clear cell renal cell carcinoma
(B) Chromophobe renal cell carcinoma
(C) Collecting duct carcinoma
(D) Oncocytoma
(E) Renal medullary carcinoma

41. An 11-year-old girl undergoes resection of a renal mass shown in Figure 14-12. Which of the following features is diagnostic of this entity?

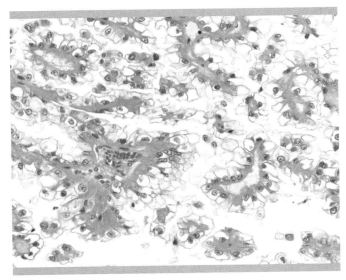

FIGURE 14-12

(A) Papillary growth pattern
(B) Solitary mass located in the cortex
(C) Tan-yellow cut-surface
(D) Nuclear labeling for TFE3 protein
(E) Young age at presentation

42. A 53-year-old asymptomatic woman is diagnosed with mucinous tubular and spindle cell carcinoma. Which of the following histologic findings is least likely to be associated with this lesion?
(A) Alcian blue reactivity
(B) Common in women
(C) Favorable prognosis
(D) High nuclear grade
(E) Vimentin and EMA positivity

43. Which of the following histologic findings would be unusual for the tumor shown in Figure 14-13?

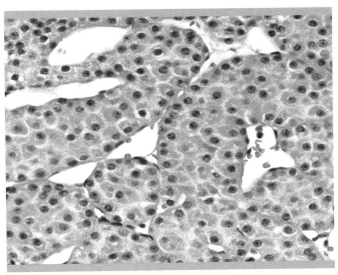

FIGURE 14-13

(A) Cystic degeneration
(B) Frequent mitotic activity
(C) Myxoid change
(D) Scattered nuclear atypia
(E) Solid nests

44. A partial nephrectomy specimen from a 21-year-old man shows a tumor composed of small, tightly packed acini and branching tubules. Which of the following features favors a diagnosis of papillary renal cell carcinoma over metanephric adenoma?
(A) Lack of encapsulation
(B) Lack of nucleoli
(C) Numerous mitotic figures
(D) Sharp interface between tumor and adjacent parenchyma
(E) WT-1 staining

45. Metanephric stromal tumor is characterized by all the following features, except
    (A) Angiodysplasia
    (B) Cartilaginous foci
    (C) Desmin immunoreactivity
    (D) Juxtaglomerular cell hyperplasia
    (E) Onion-skin arrangement of spindle cells

46. What is the peak age of incidence for the tumor shown in Figure 14-14?

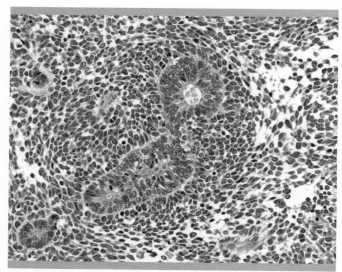

FIGURE 14-14

    (A) 3 months
    (B) 1 year
    (C) 2 years
    (D) 2–5 years
    (E) 6 years

47. Anaplasia in Wilms tumor is associated with all the following characteristics, except
    (A) Indicates aggressiveness of the tumor
    (B) It is rare in patients younger than 2 years of age
    (C) Marked nucleomegaly
    (D) Multipolar polypoid mitotic figures
    (E) Nuclear hyperchromasia

48. Perilobar nephrogenic rests are identified by all of the following features, except
    (A) Composed of blastema and tubular pattern with very little stroma
    (B) Ill-defined lesions
    (C) May remain dormant
    (D) Multiplicity
    (E) Peripheral location

49. Which of the following pediatric renal tumors typically presents at a mean age of 36 months, is composed of nests of polygonal and spindle cells with pale, vesicular nuclei, and has a propensity to metastasize to the bone?
    (A) Clear cell sarcoma
    (B) Congenital mesoblastic nephroma
    (C) Cystic nephroma
    (D) Nephroblastoma
    (E) Neuroblastoma

50. Which of the following genes is inactivated rhabdoid tumor of the kidney?
    (A) *ALK*
    (B) *c-met*
    (C) *SMARCB1*
    (D) *VHL*
    (E) *WT-1*

51. A 3-month-old infant is found to have a renal sinus mass shown in Figure 14-15. What is the best diagnosis?

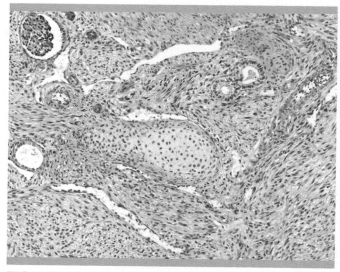

FIGURE 14-15

    (A) Clear cell sarcoma
    (B) Congenital mesoblastic nephroma
    (C) Cystic nephroma
    (D) Nephroblastoma
    (E) Rhabdoid tumor

52. Which of the following statements does not apply to the renal cortical-based lesion shown in Figure 14-16?

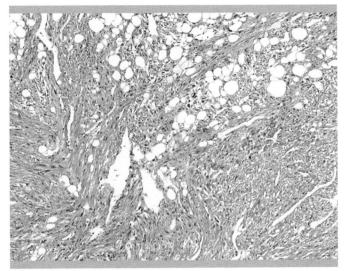

FIGURE 14-16

(A) Hemorrhage is one of the major complications
(B) Incidence is similar to renal cell carcinoma
(C) Multifocality and bilaterality are common
(D) Predominantly occurs in males
(E) Surgery is curative

53. Which of the following immunohistochemical markers is not expressed by angiomyolipoma?
(A) Actin
(B) Cytokeratin
(C) Desmin
(D) HMB-45
(E) Melan A

54. In an angiomyolipoma, which of the following features is indicative of malignant behavior?
(A) Epithelioid phenotype
(B) Inferior vena cava invasion
(C) Lymph node metastasis
(D) Pushing borders
(E) Renal vein invasion

55. Which of the following markers is least likely to be expressed by a juxtaglomerular cell tumor?
(A) Actin
(B) CD31
(C) CD34
(D) Desmin
(E) Vimentin

56. Which of the following features is least likely to be associated with this 0.8 cm renal medullary lesion shown in Figure 14-17?

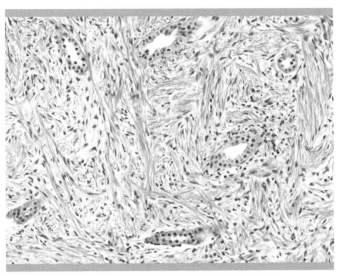

FIGURE 14-17

(A) Amyloid deposits
(B) Arises in the renal medullary pyramid
(C) Benign behavior
(D) Hypertension
(E) Incidental lesion

57. Cystic nephroma and mixed epithelial and stromal tumor of the kidney present with overlapping clinical and morphologic features listed below, except
(A) Abnormal renal architecture with remnants of nephrons in fibrous septae
(B) Cysts lined by cuboidal cells with hobnail features
(C) Expansile masses with solid and cystic areas
(D) High incidence in women
(E) Ovarian-like stroma within fibrous septae

58. Which of the following subtypes of penile squamous cell carcinoma is most likely to show evidence of human papilloma virus infection?
(A) Basaloid carcinoma
(B) Conventional keratinizing carcinoma
(C) Papillary carcinoma
(D) Pseudohyperplastic carcinoma
(E) Verrucous carcinoma

59. Penile squamous cell carcinoma most commonly arises from which of the following anatomic locations?
    (A) Mucosa of coronal sulcus
    (B) Mucosa of foreskin
    (C) Mucosa of glans
    (D) Skin of foreskin
    (E) Skin of shaft

60. The worldwide incidence of penile squamous cell carcinoma is highest in which of the following countries?
    (A) Australia
    (B) China
    (C) France
    (D) India
    (E) Uganda

61. Which of the following groups of lymph nodes is considered to be the "sentinel" drainage basin for penile squamous cell carcinoma?
    (A) Deep inguinal lymph nodes
    (B) Iliac lymph nodes
    (C) Obturator lymph nodes
    (D) Paraaortic lymph nodes
    (E) Superficial inguinal lymph nodes

62. Which of the following growth patterns of penile squamous cell carcinoma is associated with a high rate of lymph node metastasis and poor prognosis?
    (A) Condylomatous
    (B) Superficial spreading
    (C) Vertical
    (D) Verrucous
    (E) Warty

63. All the following features support a diagnosis of verrucous squamous cell carcinoma, except
    (A) Locally aggressive behavior
    (B) Prominent koilocytotic atypia
    (C) Regular, broad-based invasive front
    (D) Straight papillae with keratin cysts
    (E) Well-differentiated tumor cells

64. All the following features favor a diagnosis of Bowenoid papulosis over Bowen's disease, except
    (A) Association with HPV infection
    (B) Involvement of the penile shaft
    (C) Scaly, plaque-like appearance
    (D) Spontaneous regression
    (E) Young age of the patient

65. A 28-year-old man is found to have azoospermia, bilaterally normal testicular size, and active spermatogenesis. Which of the following condition is the most likely explanation for patient's azoospermia?
    (A) Cryptorchidism
    (B) Excurrent duct obstruction
    (C) Germinal cell aplasia
    (D) Klinefelter's syndrome
    (E) Maturation arrest

66. All the following conditions are associated with macroorchidism, except
    (A) Carney's complex
    (B) Congenital adrenal hyperplasia
    (C) Cryptorchidism
    (D) Fragile X syndrome
    (E) FSH-secreting pituitary microadenoma

67. Testicular feminization syndrome or androgen insensitivity syndrome is characterized by all the following findings, except
    (A) 46, XX karyotype
    (B) High risk for development of germ cell tumors
    (C) Lack of androgen receptor
    (D) Leydig cell hyperplasia and Sertoli cell nodules
    (E) Phenotypic female

68. A 10-year-old girl with 46, XY karyotype and ambiguous genitalia is found to have a testis on one side and a contralateral streak gonad. Which of these gonadal developmental disorders best explains these findings?
    (A) Complete androgen insensitivity syndrome
    (B) Dysgenetic male pseudohermaphroditism
    (C) Mixed gonadal dysgenesis
    (D) Persistent Müllerian duct syndrome
    (E) Pure gonadal dysgenesis

69. Which of these statements about intratubular germ cell neoplasia unspecified (ITGNU) is incorrect?
    (A) CD117 may be employed to highlight ITGNU
    (B) ITGNU is associated with testicular microlithiasis
    (C) ITGNU typically occurs in abnormal testis
    (D) 10% of adults with ITGNU will develop clinical germ cell tumor within 7 years
    (E) Tubules containing ITGNU show reduced spermatogenesis and thickened tubular membranes

70. An orchiectomy specimen from a 40-year-old man is shown in Figure 14-18. What is the most likely diagnosis?

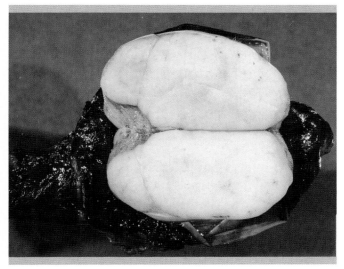

FIGURE 14-18

(A) Choriocarcinoma
(B) Embryonal carcinoma
(C) Seminoma
(D) Teratoma
(E) Yolk sac tumor

71. A 45-year-old man undergoes resection of this testicular mass (see Figure 14-19). Which of the following findings is not associated with this lesion?

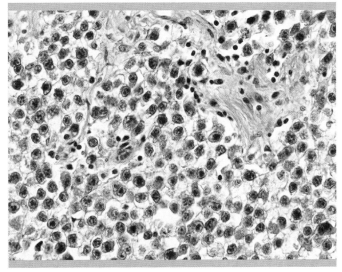

FIGURE 14-19

(A) Elevated serum LDH
(B) Immunoreactivity with inhibin
(C) Presence of glycogen within the cytoplasm
(D) Sarcoid-like granulomas
(E) Syncytiotrophoblastic giant cells

72. Spermatocytic seminoma is distinguished from classic seminoma by all the following features, except
(A) In-situ component in dilated seminiferous tubules
(B) Lack of lymphocytic tumor response
(C) More frequent unilateral involvement
(D) Older age at presentation
(E) Three distinct cell types

73. A 30-year-old man undergoes resection of a hemorrhagic and necrotic testicular mass shown in Figure 14-20. Upon immunohistochemical evaluation, the tumor cells show diffuse expression of CD30 and CK7. What is the best diagnosis for this tumor?

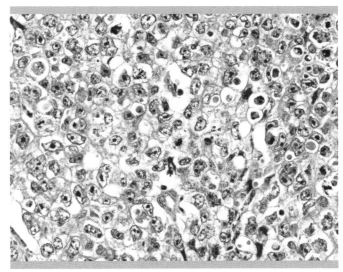

FIGURE 14-20

(A) Choriocarcinoma
(B) Embryonal carcinoma
(C) Leydig cell tumor
(D) Seminoma
(E) Yolk sac tumor

74. Which of the following histologic patterns is the most commonly encountered pattern in yolk sac tumors?
(A) Hepatoid
(B) Parietal
(C) Polyvesicular vitelline
(D) Reticular
(E) Solid

75. Which of the following findings is most helpful in distinguishing juvenile granulosa cell tumor from yolk sac tumor?
    (A) Age at diagnosis <1 year
    (B) Elevated serum AFP levels
    (C) Inhibin immunoreactivity
    (D) Solid and cystic gross appearance
    (E) Solid and microcystic pattern

76. In the pediatric population, which of the following germ cell tumors when present in its pure form, is considered to be a benign tumor?
    (A) Choriocarcinoma
    (B) Embryonal carcinoma
    (C) Seminoma
    (D) Yolk sac tumor
    (E) Teratoma

77. All the following features are characteristic of teratoma with an associated somatic malignancy, except
    (A) Malignant foci are of non-germ cell origin
    (B) Malignant foci show a non-invasive growth pattern
    (C) Malignant foci usually occur within the non-seminomatous germ cell tumor component
    (D) The most common form of somatic malignancy is sarcoma
    (E) At the primary location, malignant foci do not confer a worse prognosis than the teratoma itself

78. Which of the following features is least likely to be associated with testicular mixed germ cell tumors?
    (A) Comprise 40–60% of all testicular tumors
    (B) Higher stage is associated with poor prognosis
    (C) The finding of embryonal carcinoma and choriocarcinoma is associated with poor prognosis
    (D) They frequently affect Caucasian Americans
    (E) They usually occur in prepubertal males

79. In retroperitoneal lymph node dissection performed for treated mixed germ cell tumor of the testis, the finding of which of the following components is associated with a favorable prognosis?
    (A) Choriocarcinoma
    (B) Embryonal carcinoma
    (C) Mature teratoma
    (D) Seminoma
    (E) Yolk sac tumor

80. A 10-year-old boy presents with a history of hair loss, deepening of voice, maturation of external genitalia, and aggressive social behavior. Further examination reveals a functioning testicular tumor shown in Figure 14-21. What is the best diagnosis?

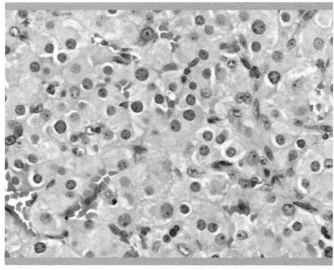

FIGURE 14-21

    (A) Gonadoblastoma
    (B) Leydig cell tumor
    (C) Seminoma
    (D) Sertoli cell tumor
    (E) Yolk sac tumor

81. Which of the following criteria is not required for a diagnosis of a malignant Leydig cell tumor?
    (A) Cellular anaplasia
    (B) Intracytoplasmic Reinke's crystals
    (C) More than 3 mitoses per high-power field
    (D) Necrosis
    (E) Vascular invasion

ANSWERS

1. **(B) Central zone.**
   The prostate gland is divided into four zones. The anterior fibromuscular stroma usually contains very few glands. The cone-shaped area that surrounds ejaculatory ducts is known as the central zone. Glands present in this region can be mistaken for high-grade prostatic intraepithelial neoplasia. Peripheral zone is located distal to the central zone, and is most commonly affected by carcinoma. Periurethral ducts and the larger transitional zone constitute the fourth zone of prostatic parenchyma.

2. **(C) They have a contractile function.**
   Basal cells are characterized by all the features listed in choices A, B, D, and E. They are not myoepithelial cells, and thus, do not have a contractile function. They do not react with muscle-specific actin or S-100 protein.

3. **(D) Sclerosing adenosis.**
   All choices listed in the question can potentially mimic prostatic adenocarcinoma. Atrophy is characterized by the presence of well-formed glands, which show

a reduction in the cytoplasmic volume of the luminal epithelial cells, acinar architectural distortion, and variable amount of stromal fibrosis. The four main subtypes of atrophy are simple, cystic, postatrophic hyperplasia, and partial atrophy. Atypical adenomatous hyperplasia is composed of benign glands lined by cells with pale, clear cytoplasm. Sclerosing adenosis is marked by the presence of thick eosinophilic basement membrane around at least some of the glands. In addition, the presence of myoepithelial cells within the basal cell lining of the glands and in the spindle cell population of the stroma.

4. **(B) Lacks AMACR expression.**
The biopsy shows nephrogenic metaplasia (or nephrogenic adenoma), which is a benign proliferation of gland-like structures that is most commonly encountered in the bladder and periurethral region. The glands may show a tubular, cystic, papillary, or solid architecture, and are composed of cells with eosinophilic cytoplasm. The individual cells often exhibit hobnailing. As AMACR immunoreactivity may be seen in up to 58% of cases, the lesion could be misdiagnosed as prostatic adenocarcinoma on TURP specimens.

5. **(A) Collagenous micronodules.**
Prostatic adenocarcinoma usually shows an infiltrative growth pattern composed of small glands with straight luminal borders. Cytologically, the cells show pale to amphophilic cytoplasm, nuclear hyperchromasia, and variably prominent nucleoli. Intraluminal crystalloids and blue mucin are a common finding. The cancer-specific features include the presence of mucinous fibroplasia or collagenous micronodules (ingrowth of fibroblasts within or around the neoplastic glands), glomeruloid formations, and perineural invasion.

6. **(D) Pattern 4.**
The figure shows neoplastic glands arranged in a cribriform architecture, with irregular and jagged contours. The intraluminal proliferation spans the entire lumen of the gland. This architecture is classified as Gleason pattern 4. The Gleason grading system for prostatic adenocarcinoma is based on the glandular architecture rather than cytologic features. Five histologic patterns are described. The primary and secondary patterns are added to generate a Gleason score. Patterns 3 and 4 can both show a cribriform architecture. However, the Gleason 3 glands have smooth and rounded contours that contrast with the irregular and jagged contours seen in the Gleason pattern 4.

7. **(E) 30 months.**
Studies have shown that on an average, it takes nearly 30 months for a complete therapeutic response following radiation therapy. Knowledge of this timeframe is important, as rebiopsy findings predict prognosis. A positive post-treatment biopsy with no radiation effect has a worse prognosis than biopsies without evidence of residual neoplasm. A repeat biopsy showing cancer glands with treatment effect carries an intermediate prognosis. Some of the post-radiation changes include decrease in the number of glands, poorly formed glands, single neoplastic cells, abundant vacuolated cytoplasm, nuclear pyknosis, and stromal fibrosis.

8. **(C) Loss of basal cells.**
Androgen deprivation by orchiectomy or pharmacologic agents is employed in patients with locally advanced or metastatic prostate cancer. All the choices, except C, describe post-hormonal therapy changes. Basal cells typically undergo hyperplasia and squamous metaplasia following therapy. The neoplastic glands show compressed or obliterated lumina. The tumor cells show pyknotic nuclei, foamy cytoplasm, or may be entirely replaced by mucin aggregates.

9. **(A) Better prognosis than acinar carcinoma.**
The figure shows a distinct subtype of prostatic adenocarcinoma known as ductal adenocarcinoma. Although the "endometrioid" pattern is more common, the tumor can exhibit papillary and cribriform areas. Ductal adenocarcinoma usually behaves more aggressively than acinar carcinoma. Although this subtype is not graded, the histology is considered to be equivalent to Gleason pattern 4.

10. **(A) Cytologic atypia and necrosis.**
Stromal proliferations of prostate are classified as prostatic stromal proliferation of uncertain malignant potential (STUMP) or prostatic stromal sarcoma. All the listed features are those of a STUMP, except choice A (cytologic atypia and necrosis), which is typically associated with prostatic stromal sarcoma.

11. **(C) Peripheral zone.**
The peripheral zone comprises 70% of the prostatic volume. Central zone and transitional zone make up 25% and 5% of the parenchyma, respectively.

12. **(B) Cystitis glandularis.**
The biopsy shows glands with columnar transformation and goblet cells, a condition referred to as cystitis glandularis of the intestinal type. Nests of urothelial cells with cystic dilatation are referred to as cystitis cystica. von Brunn's nests, cystitis cystica, cystitis glandularis, and florid proliferative cystitis are a spectrum of reactive proliferative changes that occur in the normal urothelium. At cystoscopy, the changes may appear as dome-shaped thin-walled cysts or nodular lesions. They

rarely present as a polypoid mass. Cystitis glandularis of the intestinal type may show extravasation of mucin, and thus, may be misdiagnosed as adenocarcinoma. Lack of cytologic atypia, glandular disarray, mitotic activity, desmoplasia, and necrosis is helpful in excluding an adenocarcinoma.

13. **(C) Hematuria and pyuria.**
Interstitial cystitis is associated with all the listed features, except choice C. The urine is usually sterile. A diagnosis of interstitial cystitis is based on clinical findings of urinary frequency, urgency, nocturia, and exclusion of other causes of cystitis. It has a non-ulcerative (early form) and ulcerative form (late form). Perineural inflammation is present in a majority of cases. Denuded carcinoma in -situ is an important differential diagnosis that needs to be excluded.

14. **(B) Encrusted cystitis.**
Encrusted cystitis is a form of cystitis that is common in women and occurs as a result of deposition of inorganic salts due to alkalization of urine by urea-producing bacteria. Histologically, the lesions show deposits of calcium within the lamina propria along with fibrin and necrotic debris.

15. **(B) Invasion of the renal sinus is staged as pT1.**
Invasion of renal sinus fat and renal sinus vein is staged as pT3a and pT3b, respectively. Renal sinus invasion is usually associated with renal sinus vein invasion. This phenomenon accounts for the predilection of clear cell renal cell carcinoma to metastasize to lung, liver, bone, and brain.

16. **(B) Cytoxan.**
Of the listed choices, cytoxan or cyclophosphamide is associated with hemorrhagic cystitis due to the topical effect of its active metabolites that concentrate in the urine. In addition to extensive ulceration, congestion, edema, and hemorrhage, cytoxan also produces cytologic atypia similar to radiation effect, characterized by cytoplasmic vacuolation and nuclear enlargement with degenerative changes. These changes need to be distinguished from carcinoma in-situ. BCG cystitis shows submucosal non-necrotizing granulomas, while mitomycin C and Thiotepa usually cause mucosal denudation.

17. **(E) Patent urachus/urachal cyst.**
Failure of a part or the entire urachus (regressed allantois and superior part of the bladder) to close can result in the formation of any of the following conditions: patent urachus, umbilical urachal sinus, vesicourachal diverticulum, and urachal cyst. The patient presents with leakage of urine. The urachal remnants are lined by urothelial cells admixed with inflammatory cells. Bladder exstrophy is a congenital abnormality in which the bladder mucosa is everted on the surface of the abdominal wall.

18. **(E) Trigone.**
Ectopic prostate tissue is a rare lesion that arises as a polyp/polypoid mass within the trigone. The surface epithelium is lined by urothelial cells while the submucosal tissue is composed of prostatic glands and stroma. The lesion commonly occurs in young men.

19. **(E) Urothelial dysplasia.**
All the histologic features described in the question correspond to urothelial dysplasia wherein the cytologic changes fall short of a diagnosis of urothelial carcinoma in-situ (CIS). Carcinoma in-situ is characterized by nuclear enlargement, large nucleoli, loss of nuclear polarity, mitotic activity, lack of umbrella cells, and nuclear pleomorphism. Reactive atypia usually shows nucleomegaly without any of the other cytologic features of CIS. Flat urothelial hyperplasia shows markedly thickened mucosa without cytologic atypia.

20. **(A) Arborization of papillae.**
The biopsy shows papillary urothelial hyperplasia that demonstrates all the listed histologic features, except arborization of the papillary fronds, a feature typically seen in papillary neoplasms. Per the WHO/ISUP classification, the non-invasive papillary lesions are classified as papillary hyperplasia, papilloma, papillary neoplasm of low malignant potential, and low-grade and high-grade papillary urothelial carcinoma.

21. **(A) Alcohol.**
Carcinogens present in aromatic amines, aniline dyes, cigarette smoke, and certain analgesics, such as phenacetin are associated with an increased risk for development of urothelial carcinoma. There is no such association with alcohol.

22. **(A) Invasion into adipose tissue indicates extravesical extension and constitutes pT3.**
Tumor infiltrating the adipose tissue does not always indicate the presence of extravesical extension, because fat can be present in all the layers of the bladder wall. Similarly, tumor infiltrating smooth muscle does not always constitute muscularis propria invasion, since small wispy smooth muscle bundles of muscularis mucosae are normally present within the lamina propria. Stage T1 tumors are treated with transurethral resection, with or without, adjuvant intravesical therapy. Stage T2-T4 tumors are treated with surgical resection.

23. **(C) Clonorchis sinensis infection.**
The figure shows squamous cell carcinoma of the bladder. While urothelial carcinomas can show

squamous cell differentiation, a diagnosis of squamous cell carcinoma is restricted to pure tumors. It constitutes <2% of all bladder cancers and is common in areas (Africa, Egypt) that are endemic for *Schistosoma hematobium* infection. Clonorchis sinensis or liver fluke is not associated with bladder cancers.

24. **(C) Presence of an in-situ component.**
Urachal carcinoma arises from urachal remnants. Most cases have been documented in patients who are ≥50 years of age. In general, urachal adenocarcinoma (the most common variant) is much less common that non-urachal adenocarcinoma. An in situ component is never associated with this lesion. In addition, the tumor usually does not show cystitis glandularis in the adjacent mucosa.

25. **(A) All lesions express anaplastic lymphoma kinase (ALK) by immunohistochemistry.**
Inflammatory myofibroblastic tumor of the bladder encompasses two types of spindle cells lesions: those that occur after transurethral resections (previously known as post-operative spindle cell nodule) and those that have similar morphology, but arise without a prior history of surgery (previously known as pseudosarcomatous fibromyxoid tumor). The former lesion tends to be small compared to the latter, which may reach a size of up to 10 cm. Both these lesions are composed of a myofibroblastic proliferation associated with chronic inflammatory cells and occasional mitotic figures. Atypical mitotic figures are never seen. The tumor cells express cytokeratin, vimentin, and actin, but are negative for caldesmon and EMA. Up to two-thirds of cases are positive for ALK by immunohistochemistry.

26. **(E) Rhabdomyosarcoma.**
Rhabdomyosarcoma is the most common bladder tumor in children and adolescents. Leiomyosarcoma is the most common sarcoma in adults. Most rhabdomyosarcomas are of the embryonal type. They present in two forms: polypoid or botryoid (favorable prognosis) and deeply infiltrative tumors (poor prognosis). Because of the myxoid and spindle cell areas, they need to be differentiated from inflammatory myofibroblastic tumors.

27. **(B) Cytokeratin.**
The figure shows a lesion composed of nests of round cells (*Zellballen* pattern) with amphophilic cytoplasm arranged in nests surrounded by thin-walled blood vessels, diagnostic of paraganglioma. S-100 stain usually highlights sustentacular cells located at the periphery of the tumor nests. Hypertension is found in nearly two-third of patients diagnosed with paraganglioma. Nearly 10–15% of bladder paragangliomas are malignant.

28. **(C) 30%.**
The classic clinical presentation of clear cell renal cell carcinoma is a triad that consists of hematuria, pain, and flank mass. Because of the improved imaging techniques, they are detected much earlier. In up to 30% of cases, patients present with metastatic disease.

29. **(B) Deletion of 3p.**
Majority of the renal cell carcinomas (RCCs) are sporadic tumors. In its hereditary form, the most common tumor is the von Hippel–Lindau (VHL) disease-associated clear cell RCC. This tumor suppressor gene is located on chromosome 3p25. Sporadic clear cell RCC is most commonly associated with deletion of 3p and mutations in *VHL* gene.

30. **(C) Lipid.**
The tumor shown in this specimen has the characteristic variegated gross appearance of a clear cell renal cell carcinoma. Presence of abundant intracytoplasmic lipid (and some glycogen) imparts the typical golden-yellow appearance to this tumor. Lipid does not survive tissue processing, and therefore, the cytoplasm has a clear appearance on hematoxylin–eosin stain. Higher-grade lesions usually have a more solid and tan-white appearance, as they tend to contain less lipid and glycogen.

31. **(E) Nuclear grade.**
Nuclear grade is an important indicator of prognosis in patients with renal cell carcinoma. Nuclear grade is derived using the Fuhrman grading system. This is a four-tiered system that is based on nuclear size, shape, chromatin pattern, and nucleolar prominence. At 10× magnification, grade 1 cells show small nuclei, dense chromatin, and inconspicuous nucleoli, similar to that of a small lymphocyte. Grade 2 cells show fine chromatin pattern and tiny nucleoli that are not visible at 10×. Grade 3 cells show nucleoli that are easily detected at 10×, while grade 4 cells show prominent nuclear pleomorphism, hyperchromasia, and macronucleoli.

32. **(E) Proximal convoluted tubule.**
Clear cell renal cell carcinoma arises from the proximal convoluted tubule, while papillary renal cell carcinoma arises from the distal convoluted tubule. Collecting duct carcinoma arises from the collecting duct cells in the medulla. Oncocytoma and chromophobe renal cell carcinoma arise from intercalated cells of the collecting ducts.

33. **(D) High molecular weight cytokeratin.**
Clear cell renal cell carcinoma shows immunoreactivity with antibodies against brush border antigens, such as low molecular weight cytokeratin (CAM5.2), epithelial membrane antigen, CD10, and renal cell carcinoma (RCC) marker. It is one of

the unique tumors that express both an epithelial (keratins) and a mesenchymal marker (vimentin). The tumor cells do not stain with high molecular weight cytokeratin such as 34βE12.

34. **(E) Presence of clear cells within fibrous septae.**
Both multilocular cystic renal cell carcinoma and multilocular renal cyst (cystic nephroma) can have a similar gross appearance., The finding of aggregates of neoplastic clear cells within the fibrous septae is diagnostic of multilocular cystic renal cell carcinoma. Immunohistochemical stains such as keratin and epithelial membrane antigen may be employed to highlight these cells; however, they do not help in distinguishing the two entities.

35. **(D) 0.5 cm.**
The size cut-off used to classify a papillary tumor as a carcinoma is 0.5 cm. Lesions smaller than 0.5 cm are referred to as papillary adenomas. Most papillary adenomas are found incidentally in nephrectomies performed for chronic pyelonephritis, long-term dialysis, and acquired cystic renal disease. Occasionally, the lesion may be seen in patients with VHL syndrome.

36. **(A) Deletion of chromosome 3p.**
The figure shows a papillary renal cell carcinoma (RCC) characterized by fibrovascular cores lined by cells with abundant eosinophilic cytoplasm, pseudostratified nuclei (type 2 papillary RCC) along with foamy macrophages within the fibrovascular core. In contrast, type 1 papillary RCC is composed of cells with scant, pale cytoplasm and uniform nuclei that lie against the basement membrane of the cell. Trisomy 7, 17, and deletion of chromosome Y are common genetic alterations associated with sporadic papillary RCC. Germline mutation of *c-met* gene is seen in hereditary papillary RCC.

37. **(D) CK7.**
Nearly 87% of type 1, and 20% of type 2 papillary renal cell carcinomas, express CK7. Clear cell renal cell carcinomas are usually negative for CK7. CEA and high molecular weight cytokeratin are expressed by collecting duct carcinomas.

38. **(D) Ultrastructural studies show abundant rough endoplasmic reticulum.**
The tumor shown in this figure is a chromophobe renal cell carcinoma. Chromophobe renal cell carcinomas typically show two histologic forms: classic and eosinophilic. The classic form is composed of polygonal cells with accentuated "plant-like" cell membranes (seen in this figure). Electron microscopy reveals abundant round to oval cytoplasmic microvesicles within the tumor cells. The eosinophilic variant shows abundant mitochondria, and fewer microvesicles. The tumor cells are strongly

positive for CK7. The immunoreactivity is usually prominent along the cell membranes. Genetic analysis may show loss of multiple chromosomes such as 1, 2, 6, 10, 13, 17, and 21.

39. **(A) Carcinoma of the collecting ducts of Bellini.**
The tumor is composed of complex, infiltrative cords and tubules of pleomorphic tumor cells surrounded by inflamed desmoplastic stroma. Given the location and gross description, the histologic findings are characteristic of collecting duct carcinoma. Although renal medullary carcinoma can show a similar growth pattern, this tumor usually affects young adults. Collecting duct carcinomas have a poor clinical prognosis. The tumor cells express high molecular weight cytokeratin, CK7, and CEA. Because of the overlapping morphologic and immunophenotypic features, collecting duct carcinomas are difficult to distinguish from urothelial carcinoma. The finding of an adjacent in-situ component supports the diagnosis of urothelial carcinoma.

40. **(E) Renal medullary carcinoma.**
Renal medullary carcinoma is a highly aggressive medullary tumor that almost exclusively affects patients with sickle cell hemoglobinopathy/trait. It occurs in children and young adults of African American and Mediterranean descent. The tumor is composed of nests and sheets of eosinophilic cells embedded in a desmoplastic stroma that is rich in neutrophils and lymphocytes. Sickled RBCs may be visible in adjacent blood vessels. Most patients do not survive beyond 1 year following an initial diagnosis.

41. **(D) Nuclear labeling for TFE3 protein.**
The figure shows a tumor composed of clear cells with voluminous cytoplasm and papillary growth pattern. In conjunction with the young age this morphology is consistent with an Xp11.2 translocation tumor. While all the listed features can be encountered in this tumor, positive staining with TFE3 protein is the most consistent and reliable feature that can be used to confirm the diagnosis. The most common translocations involve the *TFE3* gene on chromosome X and *PRCC* gene (chromosome 1) and *ASPL* gene (chromosome 17). *ASPL-TFE3* gene fusion is also seen in alveolar soft part sarcoma. The (X;17) tumors differ from (X;1) tumors by showing a less compact arrangement of cells, an alveolar architecture with hyaline nodules, voluminous cytoplasm with prominent cell borders, and abundant psammoma bodies. In addition, the t(X;17) tumors tend to present at an advanced stage with lymph node metastasis.

42. **(D) High nuclear grade.**
Mucinous tubular and spindle cell renal cell carcinoma is composed of tubules and spindle-shaped

epithelial cells in a background of mucinous stroma that is positive for Alcian blue. The nuclei are bland with indistinct nucleoli, and thus, choice D is incorrect. The tumor cells are usually positive for vimentin and EMA. While gains and losses of multiple chromosomes have been documented, none of them show losses of chromosome 3p or trisomy 7 and/or 17.

43. **(B) Frequent mitotic activity.**
    The figure shows a tumor composed of cells with abundant granular eosinophilic cytoplasm, characteristic of an oncocytoma. Grossly, the tumor tends to be a well-circumscribed, solid lesion with a distinct tan-brown or mahogany color. A third of the tumors show a central fibrous scar. Oncocytoma is a benign renal tumor that on ultrastructural examination shows numerous intracytoplasmic mitochondria. Nucleoli are frequently visible at 10× magnification, but mitotic activity (choice B) is either absent or very rare. Degenerative atypia is not infrequent. Invasion into the perinephric fat may be seen, but does not have any prognostic significance. The morphologic features may overlap with chromophobe renal cell carcinoma, and can be distinguished by lack of diffuse staining with Hale's colloidal iron and CK7. Oncocytoma lacks the high nuclear grade and mitotic activity that is associated with an eosinophilic variant of clear cell renal cell carcinoma.

44. **(C) Numerous mitotic figures.**
    Metanephric adenoma is a cortical-based tumor that frequently occurs in children and young adults. In addition to the listed features (choices A, B, D, and E), the tumor also shows psammoma bodies and stubby papillae. Immunohistochemically, the cells are negative for EMA and CK7, an additional feature that helps in this distinction.

45. **(C) Desmin immunoreactivity.**
    Metanephric stromal tumor is a pediatric renal tumor composed of bland spindle cells with indistinct cytoplasmic processes. Juxtaglomerular cell hyperplasia with entrapped glomeruli is a unique feature of this tumor. In addition, heterologous elements such as cartilage, glia, and fat may also be seen. The cells express CD34 and are negative for S-100, desmin, and cytokeratin.

46. **(D) 2–5 years.**
    The figure shows an example of triphasic Wilms tumor composed of undifferentiated blastema, fibroblast-like stroma, and epithelial elements in the form of abortive tubules. Undifferentiated blastema is composed of densely packed primitive small blue cells with scant cytoplasm, oval nuclei, and a fine chromatin pattern Nephroblastoma or

Wilms tumor is the most common pediatric renal tumor. The peak age of incidence is between 2 and 5 years of age. More than 90% of patients are diagnosed by age six. Clear cell sarcoma occurs around 2–3 years of age. Cystic partially differentiated nephroblastomas and rhabdoid tumors peak around 2 years of age. Congenital mesoblastic nephroma is usually occurs at 3 months of age.

47. **(A) Indicates aggressiveness of the tumor.**
    Anaplasia in Wilms tumor indicates unfavorable histology. It may be focal or diffuse in nature and is characterized by all the listed features except choice A. It predicts resistance of a tumor to adjuvant therapy and, is therefore, a predictive marker rather than a prognostic marker.

48. **(B) Ill-defined lesions.**
    Nephrogenic rests are persistent foci of embryonal renal tissue that are believed to give rise to nephroblastoma. They are divided into two types: perilobar and intralobar. All the listed features are typical of perilobar rests, except choice B. The intralobar rests tend to be solitary, ill-defined, stroma-rich, and are randomly distributed within the renal parenchyma.

49. **(A) Clear cell sarcoma.**
    Clear cell sarcoma is a rare malignant pediatric renal tumor that arises in the renal medulla and is composed of polygonal and spindle cells with pale cytoplasm and characteristic pale vesicular nuclei (classic pattern). The other patterns include myxoid, cellular, sclerosing, epithelioid, spindle cell, and palisading. The tumor cells are negative for all markers, except vimentin. Patients have a high rate of recurrent and metastatic bone disease.

50. **(C) *SMARCB1*.**
    Rhabdoid tumor is composed of sheets of large cells with vesicular nuclei, prominent nucleoli, and characteristic eosinophilic cytoplasmic inclusions. It is highly malignant tumor that occurs in children younger than 24 months of age. It is associated with hematuria and hypercalcemia. Inactivation of *SMARCB1* (*hSNF5/INI1*) gene on chromosome 22 is the hallmark genetic abnormality. Loss of INI1 protein expression by immunohistochemistry is helpful in confirming this diagnosis. The intracytoplasmic inclusions are composed of intermediate filaments and are positive for vimentin.

51. **(B) Congenital mesoblastic nephroma.**
    The tumor shown in this figure is a congenital mesoblastic nephroma composed of fascicles and whorls of bland spindled myofibroblasts and thin collagen fibers. Also seen are entrapped renal tubules and chondroid metaplasia. Grossly, these lesions show a solid, tan-white renal mass,

resembling a leiomyoma. The two histologic variants include the classic form that resembles fibromatosis and the cellular form that is identical to
infantile fibrosarcoma. The neoplastic cells express
vimentin and smooth muscle actin. The cellular
form also shares molecular features with infantile
fibrosarcoma.

52. **(D) Predominantly occurs in males.**
The lesion shown in this figure is an angiomyolipoma (AML), a neoplasm composed of three
elements: mature adipose tissue, smooth muscle,
and thick-walled hyalinized blood vessels. The
blood vessels lack tunica media and internal elastic
lamina that is normally present in arteries. The neoplastic cells appear to spin-off from the outer aspect
of these aberrant blood vessels. Occasionally, either
the fat or smooth muscle component of the neoplasm may predominate. AML commonly occurs in
women (male:female ratio of 1:3) and can arise as a
component of tuberous sclerosis.

53. **(B) Cytokeratin.**
Angiomyolipoma coexpresses smooth muscle markers (actin and desmin) and melanocytic markers
(HMB-45, Melan A, tyrosinase, and microphthalmia transcription factor). Epithelial markers are
typically negative.

54. **(A) Epithelioid phenotype.**
In contrast to an ordinary angiomyolipoma, epithelioid angiomyolipoma is capable of invasion
and metastasis, and is therefore categorized as a
malignant tumor. It often presents as a large tumor
with infiltrative borders, composed of polygonal
eosinophilic and short spindle cells with prominent nuclear atypia and mitotic activity. Ordinary
angiomyolipoma may be associated with venous or
lymph node invasion; however, none of these features have adverse prognostic significance.

55. **(D) Desmin.**
The typical clinical triad of juxtaglomerular cell
tumor is that of a renal mass, in a patient with
poorly controlled hypertension, and elevated renin
levels. Histologically, the tumor is composed of
sheets of uniform polygonal cells with eosinophilic
cytoplasm amidst scant myxoid stroma. Hemangiopericytoma-like vascular pattern is characteristic.
The tumor cells contain membrane-bound, rhomboid, renin-specific crystals. They express all the
listed markers, except desmin.

56. **(D) Hypertension.**
The figure shows a renomedullary interstitial cell
tumor composed of small fascicles of stellate to
polygonal cells embedded in a pale basophilic
stroma. The stroma can be hyalinized or amyloid-
like. Entrapped medullary tubules are often found

around the periphery of this lesion. Although the
tumor arises from interstitial cells of renal medulla,
known to regulate blood pressure, clinically, this
tumor is not associated with hypertension.

57. **(A) Abnormal renal architecture with remnants
of nephrons in fibrous septae.**
Cystic nephroma and mixed epithelial stromal tumor
are both composed of epithelial and stromal elements.
The epithelial component is in the form of cysts separated by variably cellular ovarian-like estrogen/proges-
terone receptor-positive stroma. The lesions should be
differentiated from non-neoplastic cystic conditions,
which tend to alter the native renal parenchymal
architecture, and contain remnants of glomeruli and
tubules within the fibrous septae (choice A).

58. **(A) Basaloid carcinoma.**
The risk factors for penile squamous cell carcinomas include phimosis, chronic inflammatory
conditions (balanitis xerotica obliterans), smoking,
ultraviolet irradiation, and human papilloma virus
(HPV) infection. Of the variants listed in this question, squamous cell carcinoma with basaloid and/or
warty features is associated with HPV infection.

59. **(C) Mucosa of glans.**
Nearly 75–80% of penile squamous cell carcinomas
arise from mucosa of the glans. Other less common
sites of origin include mucosa of foreskin (15%),
coronal sulcus (5%), and skin of foreskin and shaft.

60. **(E) Uganda.**
The incidence of penile squamous cell carcinoma
worldwide is highest (up to 10–12% of all malig-
nancies) in developing countries, especially in
Africa, South America, Mexico, Jamaica, and Haiti.
In western countries, the incidence is around 0.5%.

61. **(E) Superficial inguinal lymph nodes.**
The first site of metastatic disease is superficial
inguinal lymph nodes located in the upper inner
quadrant. This is generally followed by metastasis
to the deep inguinal lymph nodes, pelvic nodes,
and retroperitoneal lymph nodes.

62. **(C) Vertical.**
Histologic type, depth of invasion, and vascular
invasion are important prognostic factors of penile
squamous cell carcinoma. Vertical growth is associated with large, ulcerated, and fungating lesions,
which are deeply invasive, show high-grade morphology, and have a high rate of inguinal lymph
node metastasis. Superficial spreading carcinomas
are flat, white, plaque-like indurated tumors that
are associated with a prominent intraepithelial component. Warty or condylomatous carcinomas show
a verruciform growth pattern. Similar to verrucous
carcinoma, they have a low rate of lymph node
metastasis.

63. **(B) Prominent koilocytotic atypia.**
Verrucous carcinoma is a rare type of penile squamous cell carcinoma that is not associated with human papilloma virus infection. As a result, the tumors do no show koilocytotic atypia. Unlike giant condylomas, warty carcinomas, and papillary carcinomas, the papillae in verrucous carcinoma lack a distinct fibrovascular core. The tumors may recur if incompletely excised. Metastatic disease is almost never seen with these tumors.

64. **(C) Scaly, plaque-like appearance.**
Bowenoid papulosis and Bowen's disease are difficult to distinguish on histologic basis alone. Both are HPV-associated lesions, show high-grade squamous dysplasia, and can involve the shaft of the penis. Bowenoid papulosis usually occurs in younger patients and presents as multiple, red papules rather than the scaly, plaque-like appearance seen with Bowen's disease.

65. **(B) Excurrent duct obstruction.**
Germinal cell aplasia, Klinefelter's syndrome, and maturation arrest typically do not show active spermatogenesis. With advanced age, cryptorchid testes are usually smaller that normal descended testes. Thus, the most likely explanation for azoospermia in this case is excurrent duct obstruction, which may be congenital (cystic fibrosis, congenital bilateral absence of the vas deferens) or acquired (sterilization associated with scrotal surgery or infection).

66. **(C) Cryptorchidism.**
All the listed choices, except cryptorchidism, are associated with non-neoplastic testicular enlargement.

67. **(A) 46, XX karyotype.**
Complete androgen insensitivity syndrome (AIS) or testicular feminization syndrome is the most frequent cause of male pseudohermaphroditism. Due to lack of androgen receptors, testosterone and dihydrotestosterone are unable to stimulate the development of Wolffian duct system and male external genitalia. The syndrome is characterized by phenotypic females, 46, XY karyotype, undescended testes, female external genitalia, breast development, diminished or absent pubic and axillary hair, shallow vagina, and absence of Müllerian duct-derived organs. In addition to Leydig cell hyperplasia and Sertoli cell nodules, the tubules may contain malignant intratubular germ cells.

68. **(C) Mixed gonadal dysgenesis.**
Mixed gonadal dysgenesis is a form of gonadal dysgenesis with asymmetric gonadal morphology that includes several groups of intersex patients including (1) a testis on one side and a contralateral streak gonad, (2) a testis and contralateral gonadal agenesis, (3) hypoplastic gonads with rudimentary tubules in one, (4) a streak gonad with a contralateral tumor, and (5) a germ cell tumor with contralateral gonadal agenesis. Additionally, in mixed gonadal dysgenesis, majority of the cases show Müllerian duct-derived structures. The gonads show variable degree of development. Pure gonadal dysgenesis is a form of gonadal dysgenesis that manifests as bilateral streak gonads, internal Müllerian structures, a 46, XY karyotype, and female phenotype. Dysgenetic male pseudohermaphroditism is characterized by bilateral dysgenetic testes, persistent Müllerian duct structures, cryptorchidism, and inadequate virilization. Persistent Müllerian duct syndrome patients are phenotypically and genotypically males with persistence of Müllerian duct derivatives (uterus, cervix, fallopian tubes, and upper two-third of vagina). Please refer to Answer 67 for details of complete androgen insensitivity syndrome.

69. **(D) 10% of adults with ITGNU will develop clinical germ cell tumor within 7 years.**
Nearly 90% of adults with ITGNU eventually develop seminoma or a non-seminomatous germ cell tumor within 7 years. All other choices describe findings typically associated with ITGNU. OCT4 and PLAP are other markers that may be used to highlight ITGNU. In patients younger than 1 year of age, primordial germ cells and spermatogonia may mimic ITGNU, morphologically as well as immunohistochemically. Similarly, giant spermatogonia in adults are differentiated from ITGNU by the presence of normal spermatogenesis within the tubules and lack of CD117 staining.

70. **(C) Seminoma.**
The orchiectomy specimen shows a homogeneous, tan, multinodular mass replacing the testicular parenchyma. Given the age of this patient, the gross features are characteristic of a seminoma. Spermatocytic seminomas usually have a soft, friable, and gelatinous gross appearance. Yolk sac tumors have a tan-yellow and glistening appearance. Embryonal carcinoma and choriocarcinomas are soft and hemorrhagic tumors with foci of necrosis. Teratomas are solid and cystic tumors with or without foci of cartilage, bone and skin.

71. **(B) Immunoreactivity with inhibin.**
The figure shows sheets of round to polygonal cells with vesicular nuclei, prominent nucleoli, and distinct nuclear membranes that have "squared-off" edges. The sheets of cells are surrounded by fibrous septae and lymphocytes, findings diagnostic of a seminoma. The clear to pale eosinophilic cytoplasm is a result of abundant glycogen. The tumor cells

express CD117, PLAP, OCT4, and may show reactivity with hCG in areas with syncytiotrophoblastic differentiation. They do not express inhibin.

72. **(C) More frequent unilateral involvement.**
All the listed choices help in distinguishing spermatocytic seminoma from classic seminoma, except choice C. Unlike classic seminoma, spermatocytic seminoma frequently presents as bilateral testicular tumors. Morphologically as well as clinically (due to older age at presentation), it can be confused with lymphoma and plasmacytoma. The in-situ component of seminoma often occurs in tubules with a smaller diameter. The tumor is composed of three cell types - small lymphocyte-like cells, intermediate cells with fine chromatin and eosinophilic cytoplasm, and large cells with dense, cord-like, filamentous chromatin pattern (spireme chromatin pattern). Spermatocytic seminomas never present at extratesticular locations.

73. **(B) Embryonal carcinoma.**
The figure shows a tumor composed of cells with pleomorphic nuclei, prominent nucleoli, and indistinct cytoplasmic borders. The immunoprofile and histology of the tumor is characteristic of an embryonal carcinoma. Embryonal carcinomas typically occur in patients who are at least a decade younger than patients affected by seminoma. The cells may show a solid, tubulopapillary, or glandular architecture, with or without the formation of embryoid bodies (solid nodules of tumor surrounded by a cavity resembling amniotic cavity). In addition to CK7 and CD30, the tumor cells also express CAM5.2, cytokeratin AE1/AE3, and PLAP. They rarely express CK20 and EMA. They do not express high-molecular weight cytokeratins. Most embryonal carcinomas occur as a component of mixed germ cell tumors.

74. **(D) Reticular.**
Histologically, yolk sac tumor can show several different patterns that include reticular, macrocystic, endodermal sinus-like, papillary, solid, glandular-alveolar, myxomatous, sarcomatoid, polyvesicular vitelline, hepatoid, and parietal. The most common pattern is the reticular or the microvesicular pattern that is composed of small cysts lined by flattened cells with little cytoplasm. The characteristic Schiller-Duval bodies are found in association with the endodermal sinus pattern. These are papillary formations that contain a blood vessel within cystic structures.

75. **(C) Inhibin immunoreactivity.**
Because of the overlapping gross and microscopic appearance, distinguishing juvenile granulosa cell tumor from a yolk sac tumor can be difficult. Both

tumors present before 1 year of age and show elevated serum AFP levels. Juvenile granulosa cell tumor usually lacks the spectrum of histologic patterns seen in yolk sac tumors. Immunoreactivity with inhibin (choice C) is diagnostic of this entity, and thus helps in distinguishing the two tumors.

76. **(E) Teratoma.**
Teratomas usually occur in descended or undescended testes as well as in extratesticular tissues. When they occur in children and young adults, in their pure form, they behave as benign tumors. In contrast, in adults, metastatic disease occurs in 25% of cases.

77. **(B) Malignant foci show a non-invasive pattern.**
All the features listed in this question are associated with a teratoma with somatic malignancy, except choice B. The malignant foci usually show an invasive growth pattern, and are at least as large as one-half of a 4× microscopic field. At metastatic sites, this feature is associated with a poor prognosis.

78. **(E) They usually occur in prepubertal males.**
Mixed germ cell tumors rarely occur in prepubertal males. The average age at presentation is 30 years. In addition to higher stage, angiolymphatic space invasion, and the presence of embryonal carcinoma and choriocarcinoma, are associated with a poor prognosis.

79. **(C) Mature teratoma.**
In specimens of post-treated retroperitoneal lymph nodes, the findings of necrosis, fibrosis, and mature teratoma, are associated with a favorable prognosis. Viable foci of choriocarcinoma, embryonal carcinoma, seminoma, or yolk sac tumor, all indicate an unfavorable prognosis.

80. **(B) Leydig cell tumor.**
In the prepubertal age group, Leydig cell tumor presents with signs and symptoms of isosexual precocity. In the postpubertal age group, patients usually present with a testicular mass, although impotence and gynecomastia may be seen in some patients. Gonadoblastoma occurs in patients with mixed gonadal dysgenesis. Seminoma, Sertoli cell tumor, and yolk sac tumor, all present as testicular masses.

81. **(B) Intracytoplasmic Reinke's crystals.**
Nearly 10–15% of Leydig cell tumors are malignant. Histologic features that are suspicious for malignancy include the presence of necrosis, vascular invasion, >3 mitoses/hpf, cellular anaplasia, and tumor size >5 cm. Reinke's crystals are hexagonal or rhomboid-shaped crystals seen in about 40% of tumors. They have no prognostic significance.

SUGGESTED READING

1. Srigley JR. Benign mimickers of prostatic adenocarcinoma. *Mod Pathol.* 2004;17:328-348.
2. Luque RJ, Lopez-Beltran A, Perez-Seoane C, Suzigan S. Sclerosing adenosis of the prostate: histologic features in needle biopsy specimens. *Arch Pathol Lab Med.* 2003;127:e14-e16.
3. Skinnider BF, Oliva E, Young RH, Amin MB. Expression of alpha-methylacyl-CoA racemase (P504 S) in nephrogenic adenoma: a significant immunohistochemical pitfall compounding the differential diagnosis with prostatic adenocarcinoma. *Am J Surg Pathol.* 2004;28:701-705.
4. Epstein JI, Yang XJ. *Prostate Biopsy Interpretation.* 3rd ed. Philadelphia, PA: Lippincott Williams & Wilkins; 2002.
5. Epstein JI, Allsbrook WC, Amin MB, et al. The 2005 International Society of Urological Pathology (ISUP) consensus conference on Gleason grading of prostate carcinoma. *Am J Surg Pathol.* 2005;29:1228-1242.
6. Grignon DJ. Unusual subtypes of prostate cancer. *Mod Pathol.* 2004;17:316-327.
7. Gaudin PB, Rosai J, Epstein JI. Histopathologic effects of radiation and hormonal therapies on benign and malignant prostate tissue. *J Urol Pathol.* 1998;8:55-67.
8. Bostwick DG, Eble JN. *Prostate Urological Surgical Pathology.* St. Louis: Mosby; 1997.
9. Epstein JI, Amin MB, Reuter VR, Mostofi FK. The World Health Organization/International Society of Urological Pathology consensus classification of urothelial (transitional cell) neoplasms of the urinary bladder. Bladder Consensus Conference Committee. *Am J Surg Pathol.* 1998;22:1435-1448.
10. Taylor DC, Bhagavan BS, Larsen MP, et al. Papillary urothelial hyperplasia: a precursor to papillary neoplasms. *Am J Surg Pathol.* 1996;20:1481-1488.
11. Amin MB, McKenney JK. An approach to the diagnosis of flat intraepithelial lesions of the urinary bladder using the World Health Organization/International Society of Urological Pathology consensus classification system. *Adv Anat Pathol.* 2002;9:222-232.
12. Amin MB. Histological variants of urothelial carcinoma: diagnostic, therapeutic and prognostic implications. *Mod Pathol.* 2009;22(suppl 2):S96-S118.
13. Mostafa MH, Helmi S, Badawi AF, et al. Nitrate, nitrite and volatile N-nitroso compounds in the urine of Schistosoma haematobium and Schistosoma mansoni infected patients. *Carcinogenesis.* 1994;15:619-625.
14. Tsuzuki T, Magi-Galluzzi C, Epstein JI. ALK-1 expression in inflammatory myofibroblastic tumor of the urinary bladder. *Am J Surg Pathol.* 2004;28:1609-1614.
15. Leuschner I, Harms D, Mattke A, et al. Rhabdomyosarcoma of the urinary bladder and vagina: a clinicopathologic study with emphasis on recurrent disease. A report from the Kiel Pediatric Tumor Registry and the German CWS Study. *Am J Surg Pathol.* 2001;25:856-864.
16. Philip AT, Amin MB, Tamboli P, et al. Intravesical adipose tissue: quantitative study of its presence and location with implications for therapy and prognosis. *Am J Surg Pathol.* 2000;24:1286-1290.
17. Ro JY, Ayala AG, El-Naggar A. Muscularis mucosa of urinary bladder: importance for staging and treatment. *Am J Surg Pathol.* 1987;11:668-673.
18. Volmar KE, Chan TY, De Marzo AM, Epstein JI. Florid von Brunn nests mimicking urothelial carcinoma: a morphologic and immunohistochemical comparison to the nested variant of urothelial carcinoma. *Am J Surg Pathol.* 2003;27:1243-1252.
19. Allan CH, Epstein JI. Nephrogenic adenoma of the prostatic urethra: a mimicker of prostate adenocarcinoma. *Am J Surg Pathol.* 2001;25:802-808.
20. Gupta A, Wang HL, Policarpio-Nicolas ML, et al. Expression of alpha-methylacyl-coenzyme A racemase in nephrogenic adenoma. *Am J Surg Pathol.* 2004;28:1224-1229.
21. Long JP Jr, Althausen AF. Malakoplakia: a 25-year experience with a review of the literature. *J Urol.* 1989;141:1328-1331.
22. Warren JW, Keay SK. Interstitial cystitis. *Curr Opin Urol.* 2002;12:69-74.
23. Chan TY, Epstein JI. Radiation or chemotherapy cystitis with "pseudocarcinomatous" features. *Am J Surg Pathol.* 2004;28:909-913.
24. Bauer SB, Retik AB. Urachal anomalies and related umbilical disorders. *Urol Clin North Am.* 1978;5:195-211.
25. Dogra PN, Ansari MS, Khaitan A, et al. Ectopic prostate: an unusual bladder tumor. *Int Urol Nephrol* 2002;34:525-526.
26. Eble JN, Sauter G, Epstein JI, et al. *World Health Organization Classification of Tumors: Pathology and Genetics of Tumors of the Urinary System and Male Genital Organs.* Lyon, France: IARC Press; 2004.
27. Nassir A, Jollimore J, Gupta R, et al. Multilocular cystic renal cell carcinoma: a series of 12 cases and review of the literature [review]. *Urology.* 2002;60:421-427.
28. Tickoo SK, Reuter VE. Differential diagnosis of renal tumors with papillary architecture. *Adv Anat Pathol.* 2011;18(2):120-132.
29. Abrahams NA, Maclennan GT, Khoury JD, et al. Chromophobe renal cell carcinoma: a comparative study of histological, immunohistochemical and ultrastructural features using high throughput tissue microarray. *Histopathology.* 2004;45:593-602.
30. Srigley JR, Eble JN. Collecting duct carcinoma of kidney [review]. *Semin Diagn Pathol.* 1998;15:54-67.
31. Swartz MA, Karth J, Schneider DT, et al. Renal medullary carcinoma: clinical, pathologic, immunohistochemical, and genetic analysis with pathogenetic implications. *Urology.* 2002;60:1083-1089.
32. Bruder E, Passera O, Harms D, et al. Morphologic and molecular characterization of renal cell carcinoma in children and young adults. *Am J Surg Pathol.* 2004;28:1117-1132.
33. Kuroda N, Toi M, Hiroi M, et al. Review of mucinous tubular and spindle cell carcinoma of the kidney with a focus on clinical and pathobiological aspects. *Histol Histopathol.* 2005;20:221-224.
34. Amin MB, Crotty TB, Tickoo SK, Farrow GM. Renal oncocytoma: a reappraisal of morphologic features with clinicopathologic findings in 80 cases. *Am J Surg Pathol.* 1997;21:1-12.

35. Muir TE, Cheville JC, Lager DJ. Metanephric adenoma, nephrogenic rests, and Wilms' tumor: a histologic and immunophenotypic comparison. *Am J Surg Pathol*. 2001;25:1290-1296.
36. Hennigar RA, O'Shea PA, Grattan-Smith JD. Clinicopathologic features of nephrogenic rests and nephroblastomatosis. *Adv Anat Pathol*. 2001;8:276-289.
37. Beckwith JB. National Wilms' Tumor Study: an update for pathologists. *Pediatr Dev Pathol*. 1998;1:79-84.
38. Eble JN, Bonsib SM. Extensively cystic renal neoplasms: cystic nephroma, cystic partially differentiated nephroblastoma, multilocular cystic renal cell carcinoma, and cystic hamartoma of renal pelvis. *Semin Diagn Pathol*. 1998;15:2-20.
39. Argani P, Perlman EJ, Breslow NE, et al. Clear cell sarcoma of the kidney: a review of 351 cases from the National Wilms' Tumor Study Group Pathology Center. *Am J Surg Pathol*. 2000;24:4-18.
40. Vujanic GM, Sandstedt B, Harms D, et al. Rhabdoid tumour of the kidney: a clinicopathological study of 22 patients from the International Society of Pediatric Oncology (SIOP) nephroblastoma file. *Histopathology*. 1996;28:333-340.
41. Fitchev P, Beckwith JB, Perlman EJ. Congenital mesoblastic nephroma: prognosis and outcome. *Lab Invest*. 2003;83:2P.
42. L'Hostis H, Deminiere C, Ferriere JM, Coindre JM. Renal angiomyolipoma: a clinicopathologic, immunohistochemical, and follow-up study of 46 cases. *Am J Surg Pathol*. 1999;23:1011-1020.
43. Cibas ES, Goss GA, Kulke MH, et al. Malignant epithelioid angiomyolipoma ("sarcoma ex angiomyolipoma") of the kidney: a case report and review of the literature. *Am J Surg Pathol*. 2001;25:121-126.
44. Martin SA, Mynderse LA, Lager DJ, Cheville JC. Juxtaglomerular cell tumor: a clinicopathologic study of four cases and review of the literature. *Am J Clin Pathol*. 2001;116:854-863.
45. Tamboli P, Ro JY, Amin MB, et al. Benign tumors and tumor-like lesions of the adult kidney. Part II: benign mesenchymal and mixed neoplasms, and tumor-like lesions. *Adv Anat Pathol*. 2000;7:47-66.
46. Adsay NV, Eble JN, Srigley JR, et al. Mixed epithelial and stromal tumor of the kidney. *Am J Surg Pathol*. 2000;24:958-970.
47. Cubilla AL, Piris A, Pfannl R, et al. Anatomic levels—important landmarks in penectomy specimens: a detailed anatomic and histologic study based on examination of 44 cases. *Am J Surg Pathol*. 2001;25:1091-1094.
48. Cubilla AL, Velazques EF, Reuter VE, et al. Warty (condylomatous) squamous cell carcinoma of the penis: a report of 11 cases and proposed classification of "verruciform" penile tumors. *Am J Surg Pathol*. 2000;24:505-512.
49. Cubilla AL, Velazquez EF, Young RH. Epithelial lesions associated with invasive penile squamous cell carcinoma: a pathologic study of 288 cases. *Int J Surg Pathol*. 2004;12:351-364.
50. Cerilli LA, Kuang W, Rogers D. A practical approach to testicular biopsy interpretation for male infertility. *Arch Pathol Lab Med*. 2010 Aug;134(8):1197-1204.
51. Rutgers JL. Advances in the pathology of intersex conditions. *Hum Pathol*. 1991;22(9):884-891.
52. Ulbright TM. Germ cell tumors of the gonads. A selective review emphasizing problems in differential diagnosis, newly appreciated, and controversial issues. *Mod Pathol*. 2005;18(suppl 2):S61-S79.
53. Tumours of the urinary system and male genital organs: WHO histological classification of testis tumors. In: Eble JN, Sauter G, Epstein J, Sesterhenn I, eds. *World Health Organization Classification of Tumours: Pathology and Genetics*. Lyon, France: IARC Press; 2004:218-219.
54. Woodward P, Heidenreich A, Looijenga L, et al. Tumors of the urinary system and male genital organs: embryonal carcinoma. In: Eble J, Sauter G, Epstein J, Sesterhenn I, eds. *WHO Classification of Tumours: Pathology and Genetics*. Lyon, France: IARC Press; 2004:236-237.
55. Woodward P, Heidenreich A, Looijenga L, et al. Tumors of the urinary system and male genital organs: Tumours of more than one histological type (mixed forms). In: Eble J, Sauter G, Epstein J, Sesterhenn I, eds. *WHO Classification of Tumours: Pathology and Genetics*. Lyon, France: IARC Press; 2004:246-249.
56. Sesterhenn I, Cheville J, Woodward PJ. Tumors of the urinary system and male genital organs: Leydig cell tumour. In: Eble J, Sauter G, Epstein J, Sesterhenn I, eds. *WHO Classification of Tumours: Pathology and Genetics*. Lyon, France: IARC Press; 2004:250-251.
57. Mohanty SK, Parwani AV. Mixed epithelial and stromal tumors of the kidney: an overview. *Arch Pathol Lab Med*. 2009;133(9):1483-1486.

CHAPTER 15

GYNECOLOGIC PATHOLOGY

1. A 42-year-old woman presents with purple-colored polygonal-shaped papules on the vulva and wrist. A diagnosis of lichen planus is being entertained. All of the following findings on biopsy would support this diagnosis except
   (A) Band-like dermal chronic inflammatory infiltrate
   (B) Collections of eosinophils
   (C) Colloid bodies
   (D) Dyskeratosis of basal keratinocytes
   (E) Wedge-shaped hyperkeratosis

2. A 62-year-old woman presents with erythematous ovoid patches with associated blistering on the genitalia. She indicated that she gets a similar "rash" every time she takes antibiotics. She has been recently started on a course of tetracycline. The biopsy shows vacuolar changes and necrotic keratinocytes at the dermal–epidermal junction with subepidermal blisters and perivascular acute and chronic inflammatory cells including eosinophils. The most likely diagnosis is
   (A) Erythema multiforme
   (B) Fixed drug eruption
   (C) Lichen sclerosus
   (D) Syphilis
   (E) Vasculitis

3. A 50-year-old woman presents with white, plaque-like lesions on the vulva. A biopsy is taken and is shown in Figure 15-1. The most appropriate diagnosis is

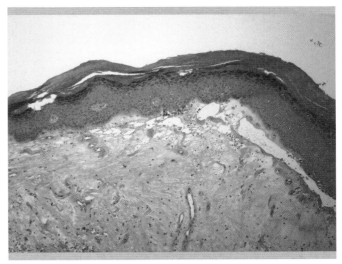

FIGURE 15-1

   (A) Lichen planus
   (B) Lichen sclerosus et atrophicus
   (C) Mycosis fungoides
   (D) Plasmacytosis mucosae
   (E) Syphilis

4. A 28-year-old woman has an indurated, painless vulvar ulcer. A biopsy is taken and is shown in Figure 15-2. Which stain would best highlight the causative organism?

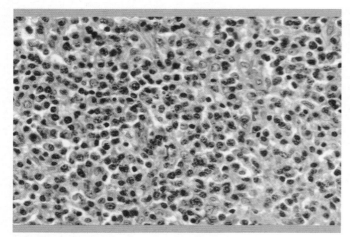

FIGURE 15-2

(A) Fite stain
(B) Gomori methenamine silver stain
(C) Gram stain
(D) Herpes virus immunostain
(E) Warthin–Starry stain

5. A 42-year-old woman has a well-established diagnosis of psoriasis. Trauma (abrasion) to the vulva region results in the development of lesions. Trauma induced lesions are referred to as
(A) Auspitz sign
(B) Inverse psoriasis
(C) Koebner phenomenon
(D) Munroe sign
(E) Spongiform pustules of Kogoj

6. A 29-year-old woman presents with elevated, flat-topped, red-brown papules on the vulva. A diagnosis of condyloma lata is made. The causative organism is
(A) *Candida albicans*
(B) *Chlamydia trachomatis*
(C) Dermatophyte
(D) Herpes simplex
(E) *Treponema pallidum*

7. A biopsy is taken (shown in Figure 15-3) from an ulcerated vulvar lesion in a previously healthy 22-year-old woman. The most likely etiology is

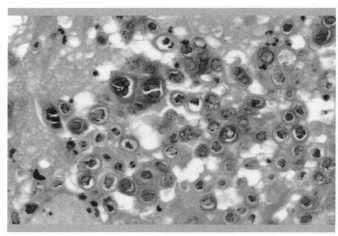

FIGURE 15-3

(A) Cytomegalovirus
(B) Epstein–Barr virus
(C) Herpes virus
(D) Rubella virus
(E) Varicella zoster virus

8. A 28-year-old pregnant woman presents with a 1 cm pedunculated mass on the vulva. A biopsy is taken and is shown in Figure 15-4. The most likely diagnosis is

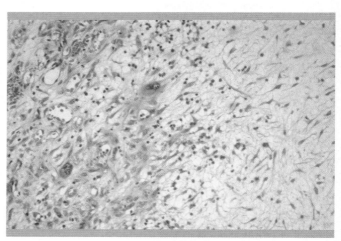

FIGURE 15-4

(A) Aggressive angiomyxoma
(B) Botryoid rhabdomyosarcoma
(C) Condyloma acuminatum
(D) Fibroepithelial stromal polyp
(E) Malignant fibrosis histiocytoma

9. The stromal cells in the lesion in Question 8 is likely to stain with all of the following immunomarkers except
   (A) CD34
   (B) Desmin
   (C) Estrogen receptor
   (D) Progesterone receptor
   (E) Vimentin

10. A 37-year-old woman presents with a perineal mass that measures 10 cm. She undergoes surgical resection of the mass, which is shown in Figure 15-5. The most likely diagnosis is

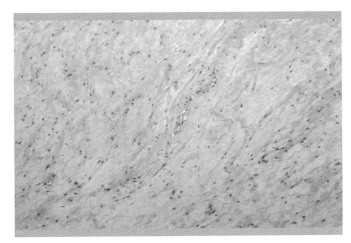

FIGURE 15-5

   (A) Aggressive angiomyxoma
   (B) Angiomyofibroblastoma
   (C) Benign fibroepithelial polyp
   (D) Cellular angiofibroma
   (E) Liposarcoma

11. The most appropriate treatment for the lesion in Question 10 is
    (A) Hormone therapy targeting estrogen/progesterone receptors
    (B) None because it will spontaneously resolve
    (C) Radiation alone
    (D) Surgical excision with 1 cm margins
    (E) Surgical excision with 1 cm margins and radiation

12. Which of the following is not true regarding cellular angiofibroma of the vulva?
    (A) Mitotic figures are commonly seen.
    (B) Most demonstrate CD34 immunoreactivity.
    (C) They have minimal cytologic atypia.
    (D) They typically arise in middle-aged women.
    (E) Usually have an infiltrative border.

13. The lesion seen (Figure 15-6) in this 65-year-old woman is best classified as

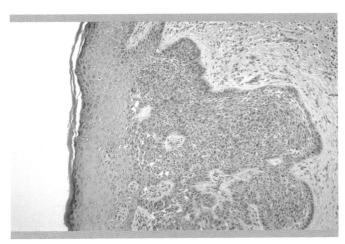

FIGURE 15-6

   (A) Basal cell carcinoma
   (B) Condyloma acuminatum
   (C) Psoriasis
   (D) Squamous cell carcinoma
   (E) Verrucous carcinoma

14. Which of the following immunomarkers would most likely be positive in this lesion from the vulva of a 41-year-old woman? (Figure 15-7)

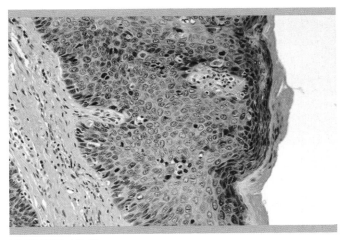

FIGURE 15-7

   (A) CD19
   (B) CD34
   (C) CEA
   (D) p16
   (E) S-100 protein

15. A 39-year-old woman's vulva lesion is stained with p53 antibody and suprabasilar staining of the surface epithelium is observed. This staining patten is seen with which pathology?
    (A) Lichen sclerosus
    (B) Lichen simplex chronicus
    (C) Normal squamous mucosa
    (D) Vulvar intraepithelial neoplasia
    (E) Yeast infections

16. A 62-year-old woman has a vulvar carcinoma that is 1.3 cm in greatest dimension, confined to the vulva, and invades the stroma to a depth of 1.2 mm. The TNM stage of this tumor would be
    (A) Tis
    (B) T1a
    (C) T1b
    (D) T2
    (E) T3

17. Which of the following is least predictive of outcome in the vulvar tumor seen (Figure 15-8) in a 75-year-old woman?

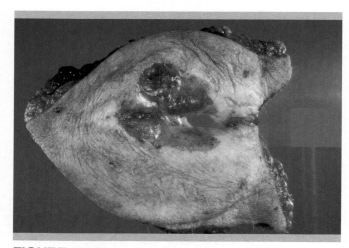

FIGURE 15-8

    (A) Host inflammatory response
    (B) Invasion depth
    (C) Lymph node involvement
    (D) Tumor stage
    (E) Tumor size

18. The lesion shown in Figure 15-9 that arises in the vulva of a 54-year-old. It is best classified as which subtype of squamous cell carcinoma?

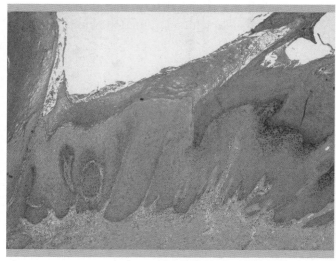

FIGURE 15-9

    (A) Basaloid carcinoma
    (B) Keratinizing squamous cell carcinoma
    (C) Keratoacanthoma-like carcinoma
    (D) Verrucous carcinoma
    (E) Warty carcinoma

19. In differentiating between Merkel cell carcinoma and a basaloid squamous cell carcinoma of the vulva, all of the following are features typical of Merkel cell carcinoma except
    (A) Cytokeratin 20 dot-like immunoreactivity
    (B) Diffuse or trabecular growth pattern
    (C) Frequent apoptosis
    (D) Low mitotic index
    (E) Tumor cells positive for neuron specific enolase

20. The least common site for the development of extramammary Paget disease is
    (A) Anogenital region
    (B) Axillae
    (C) Ears
    (D) Eyelids
    (E) Sinuses

21. This vulvar lesion is encountered in a 62-year-old woman who presented with an eczematous, pruritic plaque. The lesion demonstrates the following immunohistochemical profile: cytokeratin 7 positive, cytokeratin 20 positive, GCDFP15 negative, uroplakin III positive, MUC2 negative. The most likely site of origin for the lesion is (Figure 15-10)

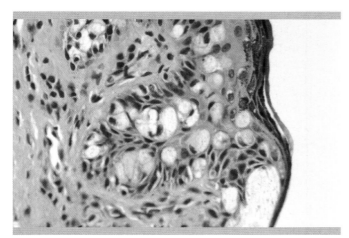

FIGURE 15-10

(A) Bladder
(B) Breast
(C) Cervix
(D) Colon
(E) Rectum

22. All of the following are true regarding this vulvar tumor except (Figure 15-11)

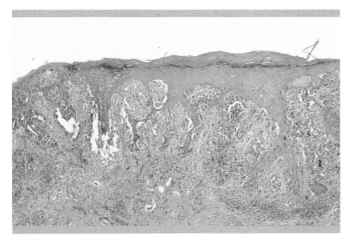

FIGURE 15-11

(A) Median survival is 3–4 years.
(B) Most commonly arises in the 3rd and 4th decades of life in this location.
(C) Second most common malignant vulvar neoplasm after squamous cell carcinoma.
(D) Stains positively with antibodies to MART1 and HMB-45.
(E) This is the most common location of this tumor in the female genital tract.

23. All of the following are common findings in the Vater syndrome except
(A) Anal atresia
(B) Deafness
(C) Renal malformations
(D) Single umbilical artery
(E) Vaginal atresia

24. A young woman presents with a thin watery vaginal discharge, a positive amine odor test, and a vaginal pH of 4.8. She is diagnosed with acute vaginitis. The most common cause of acute vaginitis is
(A) Bacterial vaginosis
(B) Candida infection
(C) Group B streptococcus
(D) Trauma
(E) *Trichomonas vaginalis*

25. A 34-year-old woman presents with pelvic pain and a malodorous vaginal discharge. She has an intrauterine device in place. Which of the following organisms is the most likely etiology of the vaginal abscess she is diagnosed with?
(A) Actinomyces
(B) Candida
(C) Group B streptococcus
(D) Herpes simplex type 2
(E) *Trichomonas vaginalis*

26. A 63-year-old woman presents with vaginal bleeding and a vaginal mass. A biopsy shows a prominent histocytic infiltrate with accompanying lymphocytes, plasma cells, and neutrophils. By electron microscopy, cytoplasmic structures are identified with an electron-lucent core, surrounded by radially oriented hydroxyapatite spicules. These findings are characteristic of which of the following?
(A) Emphysematous vaginitis
(B) Lichen planus
(C) Ligneous vaginitis
(D) Malakoplakia
(E) Toxic shock syndrome

27. A 26-year-old woman presents with a 2 cm antero-lateral wall vaginal cystic mass. The cyst is lined by cuboidal epithelium that does not stain with mucicarmine or PAS. The best diagnosis for this lesion would be which of the following?
(A) Cystic atrophy
(B) Epidermal inclusion cyst
(C) Gartner cyst
(D) Müllerian cyst
(E) Vaginal adenosis

28. All of the following are changes in the vagina associated with radiotherapy except
    (A) Atrophic squamous epithelium
    (B) Cells with cytoplasmic vacuolization
    (C) Markedly increased mitotic figures
    (D) Stromal hyalinization
    (E) Vascular hyalinization

29. The lesion shown in Figure 15-12 arose in the vagina of a 28-year-old woman, who presented with vaginal bleeding and dyspareunia. The diagnosis is which of the following?

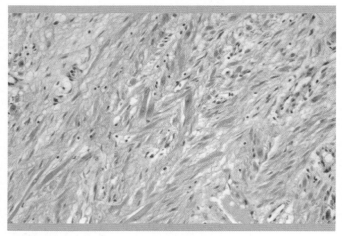

FIGURE 15-12

    (A) Leiomyoma
    (B) Müllerian papilloma
    (C) Neurofibroma
    (D) Rhabdomyoma
    (E) Spindle cell epithelioma

30. All of the following are known risk factors for the development of vaginal squamous cell carcinoma except
    (A) Alcohol
    (B) Low socioeconomic status
    (C) Pelvic radiation
    (D) Smoking
    (E) Trauma

31. A 46-year-old woman is diagnosed with vaginal squamous cell carcinoma. The tumor involves subvaginal tissue but does not extend beyond the pelvic wall. Which of the following is the correct International Federation of Gynecologists and Obstetrics (FIGO) stage?
    (A) 0
    (B) I
    (C) II
    (D) III
    (E) IV

32. Which of the following vaginal lesions is most closely associated with a history of diethylstilbestrol (DES) exposure?
    (A) Clear cell adenocarcinoma
    (B) Endometrioid adenocarcinoma
    (C) Mesonephric adenocarcinoma
    (D) Mucinous adenocarcinoma
    (E) Squamous cell carcinoma

33. This vaginal tumor shown in Figure 15-13 presented in a 4-year-old girl who presented with a mass protruding from the introitus. Which of the following immunomarkers would be expected to be positive in this lesion?
    (A) Cytokeratin 7
    (B) Cytokeratin 20
    (C) Melan-A
    (D) Myo-D1
    (E) S-100 protein

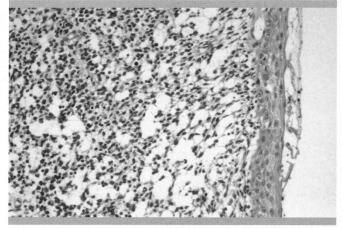

FIGURE 15-13

34. A mass was removed from the vagina of a 2-year-old girl. The lesion stains with AFP but does not stain with CD30, PLAP, or cytokeratin 7. Which of the following is the correct diagnosis of this lesion? (Figure 15-14)

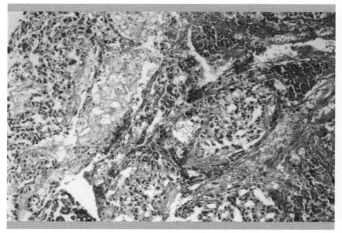

FIGURE 15-14

(A) Choriocarcinoma
(B) Embryonal carcinoma
(C) Immature teratoma
(D) Metastatic dysgerminoma
(E) Yolk sac tumor

35. Tumors from which of the following sites are most likely to metastasize to vagina?
(A) Bladder
(B) Breast
(C) Colon
(D) Kidney
(E) Stomach

36. All of the following are considered "high risk" human papilloma virus subtypes except
(A) 11
(B) 16
(C) 18
(D) 31
(E) 35

37. The best diagnosis for this lesion encountered in a 33-year-old woman on a cervical biopsy is which of the following? (Figure 15-15)

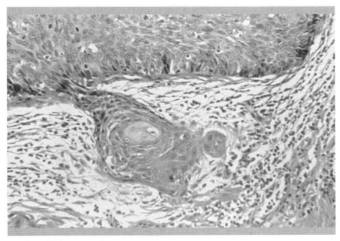

FIGURE 15-15

(A) Basal cell carcinoma
(B) Mild squamous dysplasia
(C) Reactive changes
(D) Superficially invasive squamous cell carcinoma
(E) Verrucous carcinoma

38. The cervical tumor seen in the 42-year-old woman demonstrates focal parametrial invasive but does not extend to the pelvic wall or lower third of the vagina. Using the International Federation of Gynecology and Obstetrics (FIGO) classification, what stage is this neoplasm? (Figure 15-16)

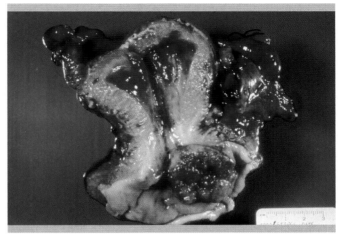

FIGURE 15-16

(A) IA
(B) IB
(C) IIA
(D) IIB
(E) IIIA

39. Squamous cell carcinoma of the cervix will most likely metastasize to which of the following sites?
(A) Bone
(B) Brain
(C) Kidney
(D) Lung
(E) Pancreas

40. A 41-year-old woman has a recent PAP smear with a diagnosis consistent with adenocarcinoma in situ. Which HPV subtype is most frequently associated with this diagnosis?
(A) 13
(B) 16
(C) 18
(D) 31
(E) 33

41. Which of the following immunostains is least likely to stain cervical adenocarcinoma in situ?
(A) Carcinoembryonic antigen
(B) Cytokeratins AE1/3
(C) p16
(D) p53
(E) Progesterone receptor

42. The changes illustrated (Figure 15-17) in this cervical biopsy from a 38-year-old woman are best classified as which of the following?

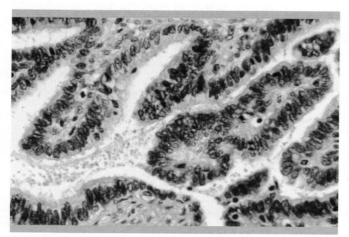

FIGURE 15-17

(A) Adenoma malignum
(B) Colonization of endocervical glands by high-grade squamous dysplasia
(C) Endometriosis
(D) Reactive atypia
(E) Tubal metaplasia

43. Which of the following cervical lesions is associated with the ovarian cord stromal tumor with annular tubules and Peutz–Jeghers syndrome?
(A) Clear cell adenocarcinoma
(B) Endocervical tunnel cluster
(C) Microglandular hyperplasia
(D) Minimal deviation mucinous adenocarcinoma
(E) Small cell carcinoma

44. The cervical lesion illustrated in Figure 15-18 is best diagnosed as which of the following?

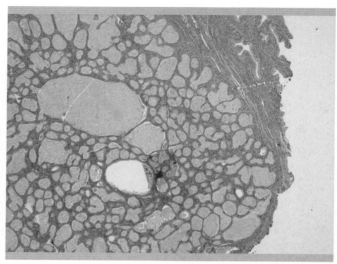

FIGURE 15-18

(A) Adenoma malignum
(B) Endocervical tunnel cluster
(C) Lobular endocervical glandular hyperplasia
(D) Nabothian cyst
(E) Normal

45. The cervical lesion illustrated in Figure 15-19 was removed. All of the following are true statements regarding this tumor except

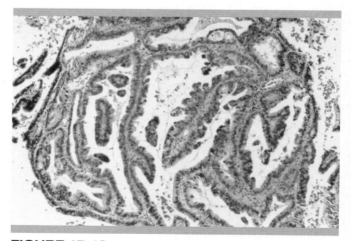

FIGURE 15-19

(A) It has a poor prognosis.
(B) It is associated with high-risk HPV.
(C) It is associated with oral contraceptive use.
(D) It is frequently associated with adenocarcinoma in situ.
(E) It is typically occurs in young women.

46. All of the following are true regarding cervical adenoid cystic carcinomas except
    (A) They are associated with a desmoplastic stromal response.
    (B) They are associated with high-risk HPV.
    (C) They commonly present with bleeding.
    (D) They do not stain with CEA antibody.
    (E) They frequently arise in elderly women.

47. The cervical lesion shown in Figure 15-20 presented with vaginal bleeding in a 40-year-old woman. The tumor is likely to stain with all of the following antibodies except

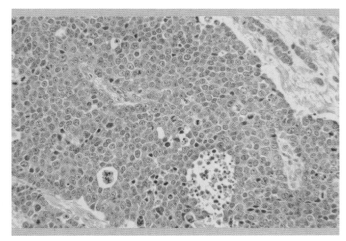

FIGURE 15-20

    (A) CEA
    (B) Chromogranin
    (C) EMA
    (D) Low molecular weight keratin
    (E) p63

48. An endometrial biopsy from a 24-year-old woman is shown in Figure 15-21. The changes are most consistent with which secretory day?

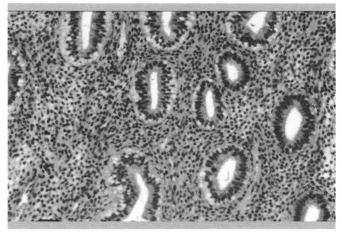

FIGURE 15-21

    (A) Day 16
    (B) Day 17
    (C) Day 19
    (D) Day 20
    (E) Day 22

49. Predecidual change in the endometrium, limited to surrounding spiral arterioles, is characteristic of which secretory day?
    (A) Day 21
    (B) Day 22
    (C) Day 23
    (D) Day 24
    (E) Day 25

50. Which of the following is the least likely cause of abnormal uterine bleeding in a 29-year-old woman?
    (A) Anovulation
    (B) Chronic endometritis
    (C) Endometrial atrophy
    (D) Endometrial polyp
    (E) Leiomyoma

51. Which of the following features is considered characteristic of chronic endometritis?
    (A) Eosinophils
    (B) Granulomas
    (C) Lymphocytes
    (D) Lymphoid aggregates
    (E) Plasma cells

52. The treatment of choice for chronic endometritis is which of the following?
    (A) Antibiotics
    (B) Curettage
    (C) Hysterectomy
    (D) No treatment required
    (E) Oral contraceptives

53. All of the following are features of anovulation on an endometrial biopsy except
    (A) Evidence of surface repair
    (B) Fibrin thrombi in spiral arterioles
    (C) Irregularly distributed and cystically dilated glands
    (D) Patchy stromal breakdown
    (E) Prominent thickened blood vessels

54. The risk of developing endometrial adenocarcinoma in the setting of isolated squamous morules is which of the following?
    (A) Never
    (B) <5%
    (C) 5–10%
    (D) 10–15%
    (E) 20–25%

55. Eosinophilic metaplasia is most likely encountered in which of the following clinical settings?
    (A) Adolescent with anovulatory cycles
    (B) Menopausal woman on hormone replacement therapy
    (C) Pregnancy
    (D) Premenopausal woman with inadequate luteal phase
    (E) Prepubertal girl with precocious puberty

56. All of the following are pregnancy-related changes of the uterus except
    (A) Arias–Stella reaction
    (B) Decidual cells
    (C) Intermediate trophoblasts
    (D) Nitabuch fibrin
    (E) Papillary syncytial metaplasia

57. A 49-year-old woman has an endometrial biopsy that shows complex atypical hyperplasia. Her approximate risk of developing carcinoma is which of the following?
    (A) <5%
    (B) 5–10%
    (C) 11–15%
    (D) 16–20%
    (E) 21–25%

58. Which of the following is not a risk factor for the development of endometrial hyperplasia?
    (A) Anovulatory cycles
    (B) Excess progesterone administration
    (C) Obesity
    (D) Polycystic ovarian syndrome
    (E) Unopposed estrogen

59. Which of the following is the most common malignant tumor of the female genital tract?
    (A) Cervical squamous cell carcinoma
    (B) Endocervical adenocarcinoma
    (C) Endometrial adenocarcinoma
    (D) Ovarian serous carcinoma
    (E) Uterine leiomyosarcoma

60. The pattern seen (Figure 15-22) in this endometrial tumor represents which variant of endometrial carcinoma?

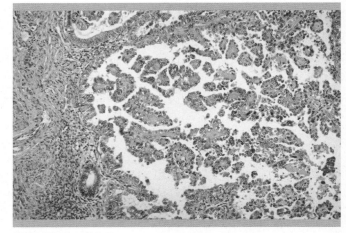

FIGURE 15-22

    (A) Clear cell
    (B) Endometrial
    (C) Mucinous
    (D) Serous
    (E) Transitional cell

61. Which of the following types of endometrial carcinoma has the worst prognosis?
    (A) Clear cell
    (B) Endometrioid
    (C) Mucinous
    (D) Squamous cell
    (E) Transitional

62. All of the following are features of typical type I endometrial carcinoma except
    (A) Hyperplasia precursor
    (B) Mucinous carcinoma
    (C) p53 alterations
    (D) Premenopausal
    (E) PTEN mutation

63. Which of the following parameters is used in grading an endometrial adenocarcinoma of the uterus?
    (A) Amount of solid growth
    (B) Depth of invasion

(C) Extent of squamous differentiation
(D) Number of mitotic figures
(E) Percent necrosis

64. All of the following features are useful in establishing the presence of squamous differentiation in an endometrial carcinoma except
(A) Discohesive cells
(B) Glassy cytoplasm
(C) Intercellular bridges
(D) Keratinization
(E) Sharp cell margins

65. A 46-year-old woman is diagnosed with a villo-glandular variant of endometrioid carcinoma of the uterus. All of the following are true regarding this variant except
(A) High-grade tumors
(B) May be associated with lymphovascular invasion
(C) Often shows areas of conventional endometrioid adenocarcinoma
(D) Second most common endometrioid carcinoma variant
(E) Villous architecture more common in superficial part of tumor

66. All of these features are characteristic of endometrioid adenocarcinoma of the uterus arising in the setting of hereditary nonpolyposis colon cancer syndrome (Lynch syndrome) except
(A) Lymphatic permeation
(B) MLH-1 positive staining
(C) Poor differentiation
(D) Prominent tumor infiltration by lymphocytes
(E) Sertoliform pattern

67. Psammoma bodies are most commonly seen in association with which of the following uterine tumors?
(A) Clear cell adenocarcinoma
(B) Mucinous adenocarcinoma
(C) Serous adenocarcinoma
(D) Small cell carcinoma
(E) Transitional cell carcinoma

68. Which of the following immunostains or special stains would be least useful in trying to differentiate endocervical versus endometrial adenocarcinoma?
(A) CEA
(B) Estrogen receptor
(C) Mucicarmine
(D) p16
(E) Vimentin

69. All of the following are features of the Arias–Stella reaction that can help in differentiating it from clear cell adenocarcinoma except
(A) Absent mitoses
(B) Hobnail cells
(C) Normal endometrial gland architecture
(D) Partial gland involvement
(E) Pseudonuclear inclusions

70. The tumor seen in this 53-year-old woman was biopsied in the uterus. The tumor stains with antibodies to cytokeratin 7, estrogen receptor, and progesterone receptor. Besides endometrioid carcinoma, what other lesion should be considered in the differential diagnosis? (Figure 15-23)

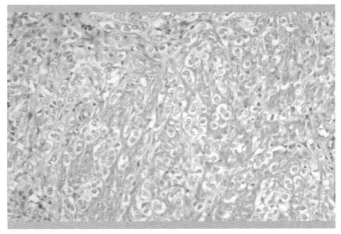

FIGURE 15-23

(A) Endometrial stromal sarcoma
(B) Leiomyosarcoma
(C) Metastatic breast carcinoma
(D) Metastatic colon cancer
(E) Placental site trophoblastic tumor

71. A 62-year-old woman is diagnosed with endometrioid adenocarcinoma of the uterus on biopsy. She undergoes a hysterectomy. Examination of the specimen shows tumor confined to the uterus and invading about 75% of the way through the myometrial wall. What stage is the tumor?
(A) Stage Ia
(B) Stage Ib
(C) Stage Ic
(D) Stage IIa
(E) Stage IIb

72. The uterine tumor shown in Figure 15-24 was resected in a 40-year-old woman. The tumor was subserosal in location and measured 3.4 cm in greatest dimension. The tumor is best classified as which of the following?

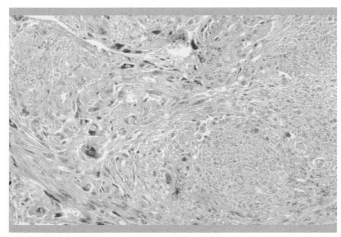

FIGURE 15-24

   (A) Apoplectic leiomyoma
   (B) Epithelioid leiomyoma
   (C) Leiomyosarcoma
   (D) Osteosarcoma
   (E) Symplastic leiomyoma

73. The uterine mass illustrated in Figure 15-25 is best classified as which of the following?

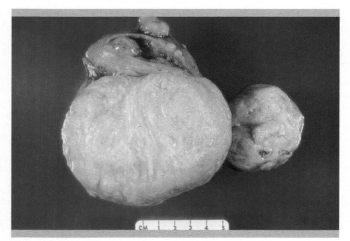

FIGURE 15-25

   (A) Apoplectic leiomyoma
   (B) Leiomyoma with diffuse perinodular hydropic change
   (C) Leiomyosarcoma
   (D) Lipoleiomyoma
   (E) Myxoid leiomyoma

74. Uterine leiomyomas are least likely to stain with which of the following antibodies?
   (A) Actin
   (B) Estrogen receptor
   (C) h-caldesmon
   (D) Oxytocin
   (E) S-100 protein

75. Which of the following morphologic features is least consistent with a diagnosis of intravenous leiomyomatosis?
   (A) Endothelium covered protrusions of smooth muscle
   (B) Intersecting fascicles of desmin positivity
   (C) Minimal cytologic atypia
   (D) Minimal p53 immunoreactivity
   (E) 6 Mitotic figures/10 high-power fields

76. The 2.6 cm uterine mass seen in this 38-year-old woman had up to 13 mitotic figures/10 high-power fields. The best diagnosis for this lesion is which of the following? (Figure 15-26)

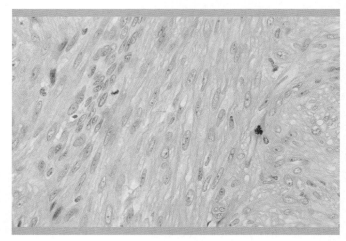

FIGURE 15-26

   (A) Cellular leiomyoma
   (B) Epithelioid leiomyoma
   (C) Gonadotropin-releasing hormone agonist treated leiomyoma
   (D) Leiomyosarcoma
   (E) Mitotically active leiomyoma

77. The most common site for benign metastasizing leiomyoma is which of the following?
   (A) Bone
   (B) Liver
   (C) Lung
   (D) Mediastinum
   (E) Retroperitoneum

78. Which of the following is not a histologic feature associated with gonadotropin-releasing hormone agonist treatment of leiomyoma?
    (A) Increased mitotic activity
    (B) Infarct-like necrosis
    (C) Lymphocyte infiltrate
    (D) Nuclear crowding
    (E) Smaller and fewer blood vessels

79. The lesion shown in Figure 15-27 was a 12 cm, partially necrotic mass arising in the uterus of a 56-year-old woman. The most likely diagnosis is which of the following?

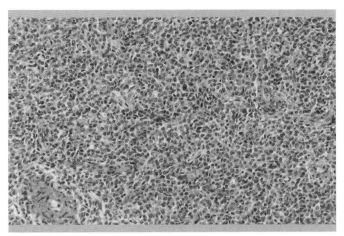

FIGURE 15-28

    (A) CD10
    (B) Desmin
    (C) CD99
    (D) Melan-A
    (E) Progesterone receptor

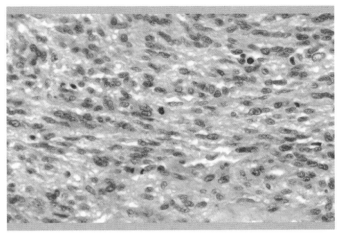

FIGURE 15-27

    (A) Bizarre leiomyoma
    (B) Cellular leiomyoma
    (C) Leiomyosarcoma
    (D) Mitotically active leiomyoma
    (E) Rhabdomyoma

80. PEComa of the uterus may stain with all of the following antibodies except
    (A) CD10
    (B) HMB-45
    (C) Inhibin
    (D) Microphthalmia transcription factor
    (E) Melan-A

81. Which of the following antibodies is most commonly positive in the uterine mass shown in Figure 15-28.

82. A 62-year-old woman presents with an enlarged uterus and pelvic pain. On hysterectomy, she is noted to have a 7 cm mass composed of a mixture of benign appearing endometrial glands and malignant stroma resembling fibrosarcoma. The best diagnosis for this lesion is which of the following?
    (A) Endometrial polyp with cellular stroma
    (B) Low-grade endometrial stromal sarcoma with sex cord-like differentiation
    (C) Malignant mixed Müllerian tumor
    (D) Müllerian adenofibroma
    (E) Müllerian adenosarcoma

83. All of the following are risk factors for the development of malignant mixed Müllerian tumor of the uterus except
    (A) Alcohol use
    (B) Nulliparity
    (C) Obesity
    (D) Previous radiation
    (E) Tamoxifen therapy

84. Median survival for malignant mixed Müllerian tumors of the uterus is best approximated by which of the following?
    (A) About 1 year
    (B) About 2 years
    (C) About 5 years
    (D) About 8–10 years
    (E) <6 months

85. Peutz–Jeghers syndrome is associated with the development of which of the following changes in the fallopian tube?
    (A) Decidual change
    (B) Mucinous metaplasia
    (C) Pseudocarcinomatosis hyperplasia
    (D) Salpingitis isthmica nodosa
    (E) Walthard cysts

86. All of the following are risk factors for the development of a tubal ectopic pregnancy except
    (A) Decidual metaplasia
    (B) Endometriosis
    (C) History of salpingitis
    (D) Pelvic inflammatory disease
    (E) Prior tubal surgery

87. Which of the following organisms is least commonly associated with pelvic inflammatory disease?
    (A) Anaerobic bacteria
    (B) *Chlamydia*
    (C) Mycoplasma
    (D) *Neisseria*
    (E) *Staphylococcus*

88. Bilateral salpingitis marked by caseating mucosal granulomas, chronic inflammation, and fibrosis in the muscularis propria and a paucity of eosinophils is most characteristic of which of the following?
    (A) Crohn disease
    (B) Parasitic infection
    (C) Reaction to lipoidal contrast agents
    (D) Sarcoidosis
    (E) Tuberculosis

89. A 1.2 cm subserosal mass is identified in the fallopian tube of a 51-year- old woman. The lesion, shown in Figure 15-29, is best classified as which of the following?

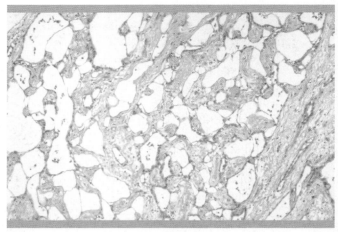

FIGURE 15-29

    (A) Adenocarcinoma
    (B) Adenomatoid tumor
    (C) Female adnexal tumor of probable Wolffian duct origin
    (D) Leiomyoma
    (E) Lymphangioma

90. The tumor shown in Figure 15-30 is the same lesion as in Question 89. The positive staining shown most likely is associated with which of the following antibodies?

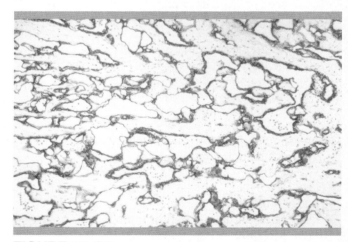

FIGURE 15-30

    (A) Calretinin
    (B) CD15
    (C) CEA
    (D) Factor VIII
    (E) TAG-72

91. Which of the following fallopian tube lesions is most frequently associated with BRCA1or BRCA2 mutations?
    (A) Adenocarcinoma
    (B) Adenomatoid tumor
    (C) Female adnexal tumor of probable Wolffian origin
    (D) Metaplastic papillary tumor
    (E) Papilloma

92. All of the following are true regarding a female adnexal tumor of probable Wolffian origin except
    (A) Commonly arise in the broad ligament
    (B) Low-grade tumor
    (C) May have tubular or sieve-like growth patterns
    (D) Stains with CEA
    (E) Stains with cytokeratins AE1/AE3

93. All of the following are features or findings commonly associated with the ovarian changes shown in Figure 15-31 except

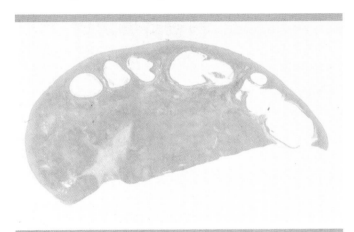

FIGURE 15-31

    (A) Anovulation
    (B) Hirsutism
    (C) Infertility
    (D) Insulin resistance
    (E) Postmenopausal peak

94. A 59-year-old woman had endometrial carcinoma diagnosed on a hysterectomy. On examination of the ovaries removed at the same time, the change shown in Figure 15-32 was noted. The best diagnosis for this lesion is which of the following?

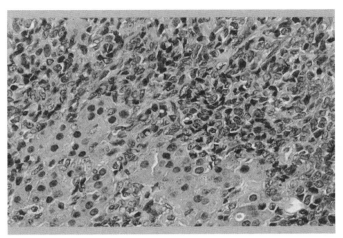

FIGURE 15-32

    (A) Decidual change
    (B) No pathologic change
    (C) Steroid cell tumor
    (D) Stromal hyperthecosis
    (E) Stromal luteoma

95. Multiple circumscribed, red-brown ovarian nodules presenting during pregnancy most likely represent which of the following?
    (A) Leydig cell hyperplasia
    (B) Leydig cell tumors
    (C) Luteinized follicular cysts
    (D) Pregnancy luteomas
    (E) Stromal hyperplasia

96. A 19-year-old woman presents with abdominal pain and a 12 cm right ovary that is excised and shown in Figure 15-33. The lesion most likely represents which of the following?

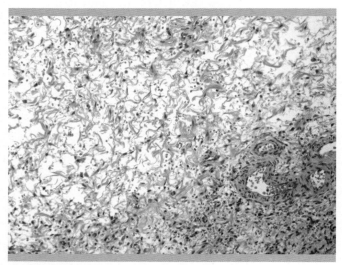

FIGURE 15-33

(A) Hyperreactio luteinalis
(B) Lymphangioma
(C) Massive ovarian edema
(D) Myxoid leiomyoma
(E) Pregnancy luteoma

97. The most common surface epithelial stromal tumor type of the ovary is which of the following?
(A) Clear cell
(B) Endometrioid
(C) Mucinous
(D) Serous
(E) Transitional

98. The overall 5-year survival for serous borderline tumor of the ovary is best approximated by which of the following
(A) 40–50%
(B) 60%
(C) 70%
(D) 80%
(E) 90%

99. Which of the following immunostains would positively stain a well-differentiated papillary mesothelioma and allow its differentiation from serous borderline tumor?
(A) CA125
(B) Calretinin
(C) BerEP4
(D) CD15
(E) Cytokeratin 7

100. The ovarian tumor shown in Figure 15-34 arose in a 46-year-old woman and is best classified as which of the following?

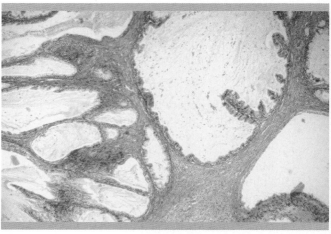

FIGURE 15-34

(A) Borderline mucinous tumor
(B) Endometrioid carcinoma
(C) Mucinous adenocarcinoma
(D) Mucinous cystadenoma
(E) Metastatic appendicial carcinoma

101. Mucinous epithelial tumors of the ovary may coexist with all of the following tumors except
(A) Brenner tumor
(B) Carcinoid tumor
(C) Granulosa cell tumor
(D) Mature cystic teratoma
(E) Sertoli–Leydig tumor

102. Primary mucinous adenocarcinomas of the ovary demonstrate positive immunostaining with all of the following antibodies except
(A) CA125
(B) CDX2
(C) CEA
(D) Cytokeratin 7
(E) Cytokeratin 20

103. All of the following are true regarding endometrioid carcinomas arising in the ovary except
(A) About 15–20% of patients have a synchronous primary endometrial adenocarcinoma.
(B) They demonstrate ER and PR immunoreactivity.
(C) Most patients present in the 5th-7th decades.
(D) Most present as bilateral ovarian masses.
(E) Serum CA125 levels are commonly elevated.

104. All of the following are true regarding clear cell carcinoma of the ovary except
    (A) It is associated with paraneoplastic hypercalcemia.
    (B) It is associated with pelvic endometriosis.
    (C) Most occur in nulliparous women.
    (D) Patients with this tumor are at risk of developing pelvic venous thromboses.
    (E) Stage for stage, clear cell carcinoma has a better prognosis than serous carcinoma.

105. The right ovarian tumor illustrated in Figure 15-35 presented in a 49-year-old woman. The best diagnosis is which of the following?

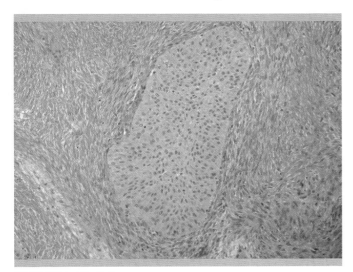

FIGURE 15-35

    (A) Benign Brenner tumor
    (B) Borderline Brenner tumor
    (C) Granulosa cell tumor
    (D) Malignant Brenner tumor
    (E) Transitional cell carcinoma

106. Which of the following ovarian tumors is associated with Gorlin syndrome?
    (A) Adult granulosa cell tumor
    (B) Fibroma
    (C) Sertoli–Leydig cell tumor
    (D) Sex cord tumor with annular tubules
    (E) Thecoma

107. A 52-year-old woman presents with a left ovarian mass and a recent history of endometrial hyperplasia. The lesion illustrated in Figure 15-36 stains with antibodies to inhibin and CD10 and shows cytoplasmic oil-red-O staining. The best diagnosis for this tumor is which of the following?

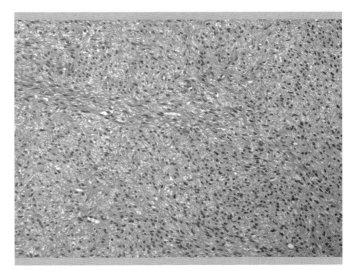

FIGURE 15-36

    (A) Fibroma
    (B) Leydig cell tumor
    (C) Granulosa cell tumor
    (D) Sclerosing stromal tumor
    (E) Thecoma

108. The lesion illustrated in Figure 15-37 presented as a 5 cm ovarian mass in a 22-year-old woman. The best diagnosis is which of the following?

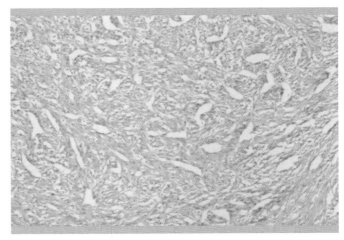

FIGURE 15-37

    (A) Fibroma
    (B) Juvenile granulosa cell tumor
    (C) Krukenberg tumor
    (D) Luteinized thecoma
    (E) Sclerosing stromal tumor

109. The ovarian tumor illustrated here is best classified as which of the following?
    (A) Adult granulosa cell tumor
    (B) Carcinoid tumor
    (C) Dysgerminoma
    (D) Endometrioid carcinoma with sex cord-like differentiation
    (E) Small cell carcinoma

110. All of the following are true regarding juvenile granulosa cell tumor of the ovary except
    (A) Has hyperchromatic nuclei with prominent grooves
    (B) Immunostaining for inhibin and calretinin is positive
    (C) May be associated with Maffucci syndrome
    (D) Mostly present in patients <30 years of age
    (E) Serum inhibin levels can be used to monitor for recurrence

111. The lesion shown in Figure 15-38 represents the retiform pattern of an ovarian mass presenting in a 23-year-old woman with a normal AFP level. The best diagnosis is which of the following?

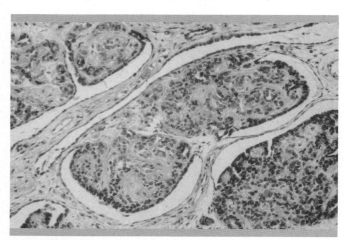

FIGURE 15-38

    (A) Endometrioid carcinoma
    (B) Immature teratoma
    (C) Krukenberg tumor
    (D) Sertoli–Leydig cell tumor
    (E) Yolk sac tumor

112. Which of the following tumors is associated with Peutz–Jeghers syndrome?
    (A) Adult granulosa cell tumor
    (B) Gonadoblastoma
    (C) Sertoli cell tumor
    (D) Sex cord tumor with annular tubules
    (E) Steroid cell tumor

113. All of the following are true regarding the ovarian tumor shown in Figure 15-39 except

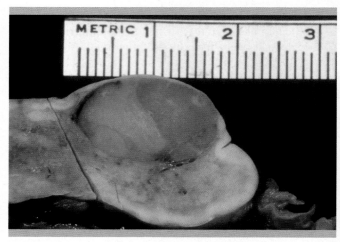

FIGURE 15-39

    (A) Cytoplasm contains Reinke crystals
    (B) May produce androgenic-related manifestations
    (C) May stain with antibodies to inhibin and calretinin
    (D) Most commonly located in the ovarian hilum
    (E) Usually bilateral

114. Which of the following represents the most common malignant ovarian germ cell tumor?
    (A) Choriocarcinoma
    (B) Dysgerminoma
    (C) Embryonal carcinoma
    (D) Mature teratoma
    (E) Yolk sac tumor

115. The most common histologic pattern observed in ovarian yolk sac tumors is which of the following?
    (A) Hepatoid
    (B) Microcystic
    (C) Pseudopapillary
    (D) Reticular
    (E) Solid

116. The most common secondary malignancy to arise in the setting of a mature cystic teratoma is which of the following?
    (A) Adenocarcinoma
    (B) Melanoma
    (C) Sarcoma
    (D) Small cell carcinoma
    (E) Squamous cell carcinoma

117. Which of the following is the most common form of a monodermal ovarian teratoma?
(A) Carcinoid tumor
(B) Ependymoma
(C) Glioblastoma
(D) Sebaceous tumor
(E) Struma ovarii

118. Which of the following parameters is used to assign a grade to immature teratomas?
(A) Amount of immature glial implants
(B) Amount of immature neuroepithelium
(C) Amount of other germ cell tumor components present
(D) Amount of vascular proliferation
(E) Degree of elevation of CA19-3

119. The tumor shown in Figure 15-40 arose in the right ovary of a 7-year-old girl. The best diagnosis is which of the following?

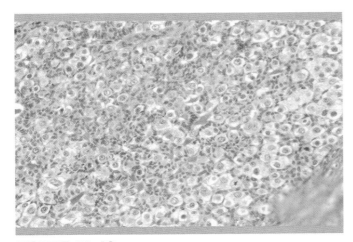

FIGURE 15-40

(A) Adult granulosa cell tumor
(B) Dysgerminoma
(C) Gonadoblastoma
(D) Polyembryoma
(E) Sertoli–Leydig all tumor

120. Which of the following features is more characteristic of a primary ovarian tumor than a metastasis?
(A) Bilateral involvement
(B) Cortical or surface involvement
(C) 15 cm size
(D) Nodular growth pattern
(E) Signet-ring cell morphology

121. The lesion illustrated in Figure 15-41 was excised from the left ovary in a 62-year-old woman. The tumor demonstrates CK20 positivity and does not stain with CK7 antibody. She has a smaller mass in the contralateral ovary. Which of the following is the best diagnosis?

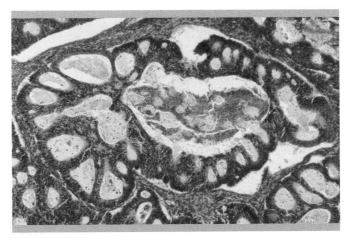

FIGURE 15-41

(A) Endometrioid carcinoma
(B) Metastatic breast carcinoma
(C) Metastatic colorectal carcinoma
(D) Metastatic gastric carcinoma
(E) Metastatic lung carcinoma

122. Involvement of the ovary by lymphoma is most likely to be of which type?
(A) Burkitt lymphoma
(B) Diffuse large B-cell lymphoma
(C) Follicular B-cell lymphoma
(D) Lymphoblastic lymphoma
(E) Peripheral T-cell lymphoma

123. A 28-year-old woman presents with a 16 cm left ovarian mass seen here in Figure 15-42 and mild hypercalcemia. All are true regarding this tumor except which of the following?
    (A) About half of patients present with advanced stage
    (B) Ki-67 labeling index is high
    (C) Necrosis and hemorrhage are common
    (D) Typically inhibin positive
    (E) Usually presents as an unilateral mass

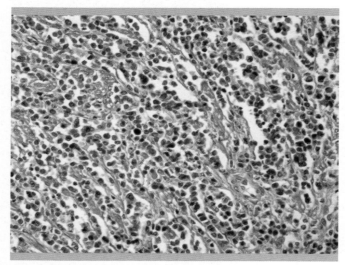

FIGURE 15-42

124. All of the following are true regarding a complete hydatidiform mole except
    (A) Absence of fetal heart sounds
    (B) Earlier onset of toxemia
    (C) Increased risk of developing choriocarcinoma
    (D) Markedly elevated beta-hCG levels
    (E) Normal or small uterus for gestational age

125. All of the following are microscopic features associated with a partial hydatidiform mole except
    (A) Focal syncytiotrophoblastic hyperplasia
    (B) Generalized hydropic villous change
    (C) Nucleated red blood cells in villous capillaries
    (D) Scalloped villous contours
    (E) Trophoblastic villous inclusions

126. An endometrial curettage reveals a focal lesion marked by nests and single cells embedded in an eosinophilic extracellular matrix. You suspect the lesion represents a placental site nodule but need to rule out an epithelioid trophoblastic tumor. Which of the following immunostains would be most useful to make this distinction?

    (A) CD146
    (B) CK18
    (C) hPL
    (D) Ki-67
    (E) p63

127. Approximately what percent of placental trophoblastic tumors are likely to metastasize?
    (A) They never do
    (B) <5%
    (C) 10–15%
    (D) 20–25%
    (E) >30%

128. Disseminated metastases from a molar pregnancy-associated choriocarcinoma are least likely to involve which of the following organs?
    (A) Brain
    (B) Liver
    (C) Lungs
    (D) Lymph nodes
    (E) Vagina

129. Excessively short umbilical cords are associated with all of the following conditions except
    (A) Fetal distress
    (B) Psychomotor abnormalities in the fetus
    (C) Twinning
    (D) Umbilical cord rupture
    (E) Uterine inversion

130. All of the following are true regarding the finding shown in Figure 15-43 except

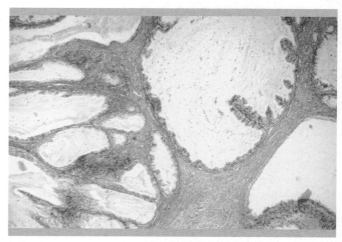

FIGURE 15-43

(A) Consists of one artery and one vein.
(B) Majority of infants with this finding have some abnormality.
(C) Occurs in approximately 1% of all placentas.
(D) Renal anomalies may be seen in this setting.
(E) The most common congenital anomaly of the cord.

131. The finding observed here in Figure 15-44 in the umbilical cord of a 36-week gestational age fetus is associated with a perinatal mortality rate of approximately
(A) <1%
(B) 1–2%
(C) 5%
(D) 10%
(E) >15%

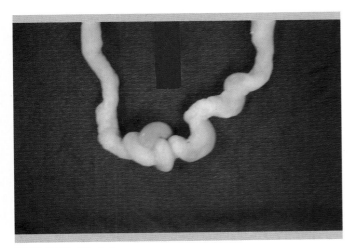

FIGURE 15-44

132. The membrane changes shown here in Figure 15-45 in a 32-week gestational age placenta are most likely associated with which of the following conditions?
(A) Amniotic band syndrome
(B) Chorangiosis
(C) Oligohydramnios
(D) Placental infarct
(E) Placenta previa

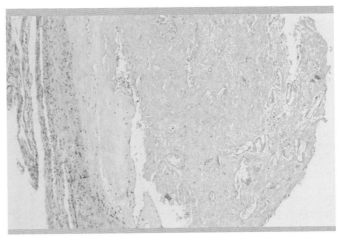

FIGURE 15-45

133. In the setting of meconium staining, meconium pigment macrophages may be observed in the amnion how many hours after discharge of the meconium?
(A) 1 hour
(B) 3 hours
(C) 5 hours
(D) 7 hours
(E) 10 hours

134. Acute villitis and intervillous abscesses are almost always due to infection by which organism?
(A) Cytomegalovirus
(B) Group B streptococci
(C) Listeria
(D) Syphilis
(E) Varicella

135. Which of the following conditions represents a placenta in which the membranes do not insert at the edge of the placenta but at some point inward toward the center?
(A) Battledore placenta
(B) Circumvallate
(C) Interpositional insertion
(D) Placenta membranacea
(E) Succenturiate

136. A placenta marked by fibrinoid necrosis of blood vessels and an accumulation of macrophages within the endothelium are showing changes consistent with which of the following processes?
(A) Accelerated maturation
(B) Immaturity
(C) Infarct
(D) Maternal underperfusion
(E) Vasculitis

137. All of the following are features associated with HELLP syndrome except
    (A) Elevated liver function tests
    (B) Hemolysis
    (C) Increased risk of placental abruption
    (D) Placenta accreta
    (E) Low platelet count

138. The lesion illustrated here in Figure 15-46 from the placenta of a 28-year-old woman at 38-week gestational age illustrates which of the following?
    (A) Chorangioma
    (B) Chorangiosis
    (C) Dysmaturity
    (D) Hemorrhagic endovasculitis
    (E) Sickle cell disease

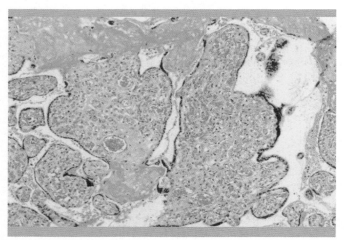

FIGURE 15-46

139. In diamniotic/dichorionic twins, approximately what fraction represents dizygotic twins?
    (A) 1/5
    (B) 1/4
    (C) 1/3
    (D) 1/2
    (E) 2/3

140. Which of the following is the most common maternal tumor to metastasize to the placenta or spread to the fetus?
    (A) Breast carcinoma
    (B) Cervical carcinoma
    (C) Lung carcinoma
    (D) Lymphoma
    (E) Melanoma

ANSWERS

1. **(B) Collections of eosinophils.**
   Lichen planus is an uncommon condition to involve the vulva; it has a predilection for the wrist, ankles, and genitalia. Patients typically present with purple polygonal papules with white lines or Wickham striae. Histologically, a biopsy would show a lichenoid pattern of inflammation, consisting primarily of lymphocytes and histiocytes, accompanied by basal keratinocyte damage. Hyperkeratosis, wedge-shaped hypergranulosis, and clefting at the dermal–epidermal junction are also frequent findings. Collections of eosinophils are typically not encountered in lichen planus.

2. **(B) Fixed drug eruption.**
   Fixed drug eruptions are associated with ingestion of an offending agent. The patients often present with erythematous ovoid patches or erythematous plaques, which may show focal blister formation. Areas of hyperpigmentation may be seen in late-stage lesions. Microscopically, vacuolar changes at the dermal–epidermal junction accompanied by necrotic keratinocytes at the dermal–epidermal junction and subepidermal blisters may be evident. Perivascular acute and chronic inflammatory cells, including eosinophils, may also be present.

3. **(B) Lichen sclerosus et atrophicus.**
   Lichen sclerosus et atrophicus typically presents as a plaque-like lesion involving the anogenital skin in women. Histologically, psoriasiform epidermal hyperplasia with a band-like lymphocytic infiltrate may be evident. Dermal homogenization with pallor and vascular dropout, as shown in this figure, is a feature of more developed lesions. These patients have a chronic waxing and waning clinical course and they are at risk of developing squamous dysplasia.

4. **(E) Warthin–Starry stain.**
   Syphilis initially presents with an indurated, painless ulcer usually 20–30 days postexposure to the *Treponema pallidum* organism. In this case, the biopsy shows a prominent band-like infiltrate of predominantly plasma cells involving the dermis with an overlying psoriasiform epidermal hyperplasia and ulceration. In a suspected case, a Warthin–Starry stain can be useful in highlighting the spiral spirochete organism that measures 6–16 μm in length.

5. **(C) Koebner phenomenon.**
   Psoriasis represents a chronic dermatitis and occasionally involves the genital area. Lesions typically appear as circumscribed patches and plaques with a "silvery" scale. Common sites include elbows, knee, sacrum, scalp, and intertriginous areas. These are sites that are often areas of persistent trauma or friction. The occurrence of lesions in response to trauma has been referred to as Koebner phenomenon. Drugs and infections may also trigger the onset. Histologic findings of psoriasis include epidermal spongiosis with perivascular

chronic inflammation and dermal vascular congestion and edema. With progression of lesions, acanthosis with increased basal mitotic activity and
neutrophil-rich parakeratosis with hypogranulosis
may be encountered. Collections of neutrophils in
areas of parakeratosis are referred to as Munroe
microabscesses or spongiform pustules of Kogoj
(if the collections are located in the spinous layer).
Auspitz sign refers to focal bleeding that occurs
when a scale of psoriasis is removed. The term
inverse psoriasis is used in reference to psoriasis
affecting intertriginous areas.

6. **(E) *Treponema pallidum.***
The presence of elevated, flat-topped, red-brown
to gray papules on the mucosal surfaces of the
labia is grossly consistent with the condyloma lata
lesion of syphilis. The causative organism is the
spirochete *Treponema pallidum.*

7. **(C) Herpes virus.**
The biopsy shows intranuclear viral inclusions in
several cells lying in an ulcer. The inclusions histologically are most consistent with those of herpes
virus infection, more commonly herpes virus type
II in this location. Infected cells may show one
or more nuclei with ground glass chromatin and
intranuclear inclusions, as seen here. Cytomegalovirus may show intranuclear inclusions as well but
are usually accompanied by nuclear enlargement
and intracytoplasmic inclusions.

8. **(D) Fibroepithelial stromal polyp.**
Fibroepithelial stromal polyps of the vulva usually
present as polypoid or pedunculated lesions.
Multiple lesions may be observed during pregnancy.
The polyp is lined by squamous epithelium. The
underlying stroma may show various degrees
of cellularity, usually with scattered stellate and
occasionally multinucleate stromal cells, as seen
here. Occasionally, scattered pleomorphic nuclei or
atypia may be observed; this appears to be of little
clinical significance. The lesion is thought to be
benign and may regress following pregnancy.

9. **(A) CD34.**
The stromal cells in the fibroepithelial stromal polyp
shown in Question 8 are known to stain with antibodies to desmin, vimentin, estrogen receptor, and
progesterone receptor. Blood vessels within the polyp
may stain with antibody to CD34, but the other components of the polyp do not stain with this antibody.

10. **(A) Aggressive angiomyxoma.**
Aggressive angiomyxoma usually presents in the
pelvic and perineal regions in women of reproductive age. As shown in this figure, the lesion is
marked by a hypocellular matrix with a myxoid
appearance. Bland spindled-shaped cells with
round-to-oval nuclei and pale cytoplasmic processes may be observed. Scattered medium to large

size, sometimes hyalinized, blood vessels associated with a surrounding condensation of collagen
may be observed. Occasional collections of smooth
muscle cells may be observed within the lesion.
Overall, the lesion is fairly poorly demarcated from
the surrounding tissue.

11. **(D) Surgical excision with 1 cm margins.**
The most appropriate treatment for aggressive
angiomyxoma is a local wide excision with 1 cm
margins. If incompletely excised, there is a 30–40%
risk of local recurrence.

12. **(E) Usually have an infiltrative border.**
Cellular angiofibromas of the vulva are benign
tumors composed of bland spindled cells mixed
with a prominent vascular component. They
typically arise in middle-aged women as small,
well-circumscribed subcutaneous masses, which
may present with pain. They usually have a well-
demarcated border (not infiltrative) and are devoid
of significant cytologic atypia. Mitotic activity may
be focally prominent in these lesions. Most lesions
demonstrate positive staining with antibody to
CD34 and about half of cases demonstrate
positive staining with antibodies to estrogen and
progesterone receptor.

13. **(A) Basal cell carcinoma.**
The lesion illustrated in the figure represents a
basal cell carcinoma marked by bland cytologic
features and peripheral palisading. Basaloid squamous cell carcinomas typically show more prominent cytologic atypia and lack peripheral palisading
of basaloid cells. p16 immunostaining is generally
not helpful in differentiating basaloid squamous
cell carcinomas from basal cell carcinoma.

14. **(D) p16.**
The lesion illustrated in the figure represents a
vulvar squamous cell carcinoma in situ, classic
or bowenoid type. p16 immunostaining is often
extensively positive in classic vulvar intraepithelial
neoplasia or carcinoma in situ. p53 overexpression
is more commonly encountered in differentiated or
simplex vulvar intraepithelial neoplasia. p16 is a surrogate marker for HPV infection. Diffuse and intense
staining correlates with HPV infection, whereas focal
or weak positivity may be nonspecific.

15. **(D) Vulvar intraepithelial neoplasia.**
p53 immunostaining can be useful in diagnosing a
differentiated or simplex vulvar intraepithelial neoplasia. In normal squamous mucosa, p53 immunostaining is generally confined to the basal keratinocytes. In differentiated vulvar intraepithelial
neoplasia, p53 staining often extends beyond the
basal layer of keratinocytes to involve suprabasilar
cells. In lichen sclerosus and lichen simplex chroni-
cus, staining would be confined to the basal layer
of keratinocytes.

16. **(C) T1b.**
Tumors confined to the vulva and peritoneum and measuring 2 cm or less in greatest dimension represent TNM T1 lesions or a FIGO grade I lesions. A T1a lesion is also marked by a stromal invasion of <1 mm in contrast to a T1b lesion that is marked by stromal invasion of 1 mm or more. T2 tumors are >2 cm in greatest dimension and confined to the vulva or peritoneum and T3 lesions show evidence of invasion of the lower urethra, vagina, or anus.

17. **(A) Host inflammatory response.**
The lesion shown in the figure most likely represents a squamous cell carcinoma, in this case arising in the background of lichen sclerosus et atrophicus. Prognostic factors for invasive squamous cell carcinoma of the vulva include the stage of tumor, tumor size, depth of invasion, the presence of lymphovascular invasion, and lymph node involvement. Host inflammatory response does not serve as an important prognostic factor in these tumors.

18. **(D) Verrucous carcinoma.**
The lesion seen in this 54-year-old woman arising in the vulva represents the verrucous carcinoma variant of squamous cell carcinoma. This lesion is marked by bulbous neoplastic cells that appear to push rather than infiltrate into the underlying stroma. The epithelial cells themselves typically show mild nuclear atypia. The lesion is often associated with prominent hyperkeratosis and parakeratosis.

19. **(D) Low mitotic index.**
Merkel cell carcinoma is composed of small blue cells with high mitotic index and frequent apoptosis. Cells are arranged in a diffuse or trabecular pattern. Squamous differentiation in Merkel cell carcinoma is a very rare finding. The tumor demonstrates positive staining with antibodies to chromogranin, neuron specific enolase, and cytokeratin 20 in a dot-like cytoplasmic pattern.

20. **(E) Sinuses.**
Extramammary Paget disease represents intraepidermal adenocarcinoma and is most commonly encountered in the anogenital region, axillae, ears, and eyelids. Sinuses, of the sites listed, are the least common site of origin for this disease.

21. **(A) Bladder.**
The lesion illustrated in the figure represents an example of Paget disease involving the vulva. The immunohistochemical profile listed for this tumor is most consistent with a lesion of urothelial or bladder origin.

22. **(B) Most commonly arises in the 3rd and 4th decades of life in this location.**
The tumor illustrated in the figure represents a melanoma arising in the vulvar region. Vulvar melanoma is the second most common malignant tumor of the vulva after squamous cell carcinoma, and the vulva is the most common location of this tumor in the female genital tract. Mean survival is typically 41 months with a 90% 5-year survival, if invasion is <1 mm in thickness. The depth of invasion is a major prognostic factor in this lesion. These tumors typically arise in postmenopausal women in the 6th and 7th decades of life, not in the 3rd and 4th decades. The tumor, as is the case with melanomas elsewhere in the body, demonstrates positive staining with antibodies to S-100 protein, HMB-45, and melan-A (MART1).

23. **(B) Deafness.**
Vaginal atresia has been seen as part of Winter syndrome (renal agenesis and deafness) and Vater syndrome, which is associated with renal and skeletal malformations, anal atresia, cardiac defects, tracheoesophageal fistula, and single umbilical artery.

24. **(A) Bacterial vaginosis.**
Bacterial vaginosis is typically characterized by a vaginal pH of >4.5, thin watery, fishy-smelling discharge, a wet mount showing >20% clue cells, and a positive amine odor test.

25. **(A) Actinomyces.**
Actinomycosis represents an infection by a gram-positive, non-acid-fast anaerobic bacterium. An association of this organism with vaginal foreign bodies, including intrauterine devices, is well established. Such infections often present with postcoital bleeding, malodorous vaginal discharge, pruritus, and abdominal or pelvic pain.

26. **(D) Malakoplakia.**
The vagina is the most frequently involved site within the female genital tract for malakoplakia. This process is the result of an acquired defect in macrophage function and is most commonly associated with *Escherichia coli*. Other organisms have been less commonly implicated in the etiology. Histologically, a biopsy would be marked by a prominent histocytic infiltrate with accompanying acute and chronic inflammatory cells. Concentrically laminated spherules, which may be seen within the cell cytoplasm of macrophages or extracellularly, are a common characteristic feature, so-called Michaelis–Gutmann bodies. Von Kossa or calcium stains may be used to highlight Michaelis–Gutmann bodies. Ultrastructurally, these bodies have electron-lucent cores surrounded by a thin layer of electron-dense hydroxyapatite spicules arranged around a core in a radial fashion.

27. **(C) Gartner cyst.**
Gartner cyst represents benign cyst arising from remnants of mesonephric or Wolffian ducts. These

cysts are typically located in the anterolateral wall of the vagina. They are lined by cuboidal or low columnar, nonmucinous epithelium (PAS negative, mucicarmine negative). Müllerian cysts are lined by mucinous epithelial cells, which demonstrate mucicarmine and PAS positivity.

28. **(C) Markedly increased mitotic figures.**
Histologic changes typically associated with radiation therapy effect include atrophic and/or reactive squamous epithelium, enlarged squamous cells with cytoplasmic vacuolization, individual cell cytologic atypia and multinucleation, rare but not increased mitotic figures, stromal hyalinization with a variable degree of inflammation, reactive stromal fibroblasts and vascular changes including sclerosis, thrombosis, and ectasia.

29. **(D) Rhabdomyoma.**
Rhabdomyomas are benign tumors of skeletal muscle that typically arise in reproductive age or perimenopausal women. The usual presentation includes vaginal bleeding or dyspareunia. The histology, as shown in the figure, is marked by spindled cells with abundance of eosinophilic cytoplasm, marked by cross striations resembling skeletal muscle tissue. A variety of muscle-related immunostains including desmin, myoglobin, myosin, and actin can be used to highlight the tumor.

30. **(A) Alcohol.**
Risk factors for the development of vaginal squamous cell carcinoma include trauma, low socioeconomic status, HPV infection, smoking, pelvic radiation, and history of cervical neoplasia, vulvar intraepithelial neoplasia, immunosuppression, or previous hysterectomy. Alcohol use is not a risk factor for the development of vaginal squamous cell carcinoma.

31. **(C) II.**
A vaginal squamous cell carcinoma that involves subvaginal tissue but does not extend beyond the pelvic wall is best classified as a FIGO stage II lesion. Stage 0 tumors correspond to carcinoma in situ. Stage I tumors are carcinomas limited to the vaginal wall. Stage III tumors are carcinomas that have extended to the pelvic sidewall. Stage IV tumors have extended beyond the true pelvis or involve the mucosa of the bladder or rectum.

32. **(A) Clear cell adenocarcinoma.**
Women with a history of intrauterine DES exposure are at risk of developing clear cell adenocarcinoma of the vagina, with a peak incidence around 20 years of age. The risk seems to be higher in patients who are exposed to the drug prior to the 18th week of gestational age. In patients without a history of DES exposure, the typical age of carcinoma presentation is 40–70 years.

33. **(D) Myo-D1.**
The lesion shown in the figure is marked by a proliferation of epithelioid, small blue cells consistent with embryonal rhabdomyosarcoma. Rhabdomyosarcomas stain with a variety of muscle-related markers including desmin, myogenin, and myo-D1; they do not generally stain with cytokeratin markers, S-100 protein, and melan-A. These tumors are the most common vaginal neoplasms of childhood, usually arising in the anterior vaginal wall. Most patients present at <5 years of age.

34. **(E) Yolk sac tumor.**
Yolk sac or endodermal sinus tumors may rarely arise in the vagina and are generally seen in children under the age of 3 years. Like their counterparts elsewhere, they stain with antibody to alpha fetoprotein (AFP). They do not generally stain with markers of other germ cell tumors including CD30, placental alkaline phosphatase (PLAP), or cytokeratin 7. PLAP typically stains germinomas and seminomas/dysgerminomas, and CD30 usually stains embryonal carcinomas.

35. **(C) Colon.**
Tumors that tend to metastasize to the vagina most commonly arise in the endometrium, cervix, colon, and ovaries. The other sites listed are less frequently the location of primary tumor resulting in a metastasis to the vagina.

36. **(A) 11.**
HPV infection is a well-known risk for the development of cervical carcinoma. Certain subtypes of HPV are considered high risk and include 16, 18, 31, 33, 35, 39, 45, 51, 52, 56, 58, 59, and 68. Low-risk HPV subtypes include 6, 11, 42, 43, 44, and 53.

37. **(D) Superficially invasive squamous cell carcinoma.**
The figure shows a nest of squamoid cells with marked cytoplasmic keratinization and extending into the submucosal space. The presence of paradoxical maturation is frequently seen at the infiltrating edge of squamous cell carcinomas of the cervix.

38. **(D) II B.**
Cervical squamous cell carcinoma, which is marked by focal parametrial invasion without extension to the pelvic wall or lower third of the vagina, is best classified as a stage IIB lesion. Stage IA lesions are carcinomas confined to the uterus and diagnosed only by microscopy, marked by a maximum stromal invasion depth of 5 mm and a horizontal spread of 7 or less millimeters. Stage IB tumors are clinically visible lesions confined to the cervix; the lesions show >5 mm of stromal invasion or >7 mm horizontal spread. Stage IIA lesions extend beyond the uterus but not the pelvic wall or

lower third of the vagina and show no evidence of parametrial invasion. Stage IIIA lesions extend to the pelvic wall and involve the lower third of the vagina. Tumors that extend to the pelvic wall or cause hydronephrosis or nonfunctioning kidney are classified as stage IIIB lesion.

39. **(D) Lung.**
The most frequent sites for metastasis of cervical squamous cell carcinomas include the lung, abdomen, liver, and gastrointestinal tract. The other sites listed as options in this question are less frequent sites of metastatic involvement.

40. **(C) 18.**
Both adenocarcinoma in situ and invasive adenocarcinoma of the cervix, like squamous cell carcinoma, are associated with HPV infection. Approximately 70% of adenocarcinoma in situ cases are associated with HPV subtype 18, with 30% related to HPV subtype 16.

41. **(E) Progesterone receptor.**
Up to two-third of adenocarcinoma in situ lesions demonstrate positive cytoplasmic staining with antibody to CEA antibody. Carcinoma in situ lesions frequently demonstrate high Ki-67 labeling indices, frequent p53 positivity, and strong p16 positivity. The epithelial cells that make up this lesion stain with cytokeratin markers. Positivity with antibodies to estrogen and progesterone receptor is less evident.

42. **(A) Adenoma malignum.**
Adenoma malignum or minimal deviation mucinous adenocarcinoma is marked by irregularly shaped glands, often with branching or papillary infoldings and angular outpouchings that deeply infiltrate the cervical wall. Cells lining the glands demonstrate nuclear enlargement and occasional mitoses. Reactive atypia is marked by nuclear enlargement, hyperchromasia, and pleomorphism, but the chromatin pattern is smudgy rather than coarse, and mitoses are rare or absent. Endometriosis is marked by the presence of the endometrial glands surrounded by endometrial-type stroma and evidence of hemorrhage. Tubal metaplasia is characterized by cells with cilia and a relatively low nuclear-to-cytoplasmic ratio. Squamous epithelial colonization of endocervical glands in the setting of high-grade squamous dysplasia is characterized by cells that tend to have more abundant cytoplasm and less evidence of pseudostratification.

43. **(D) Minimal deviation mucinous adenocarcinoma.**
Minimal deviation mucinous adenocarcinoma is well-known to be associated with mucinous or sex cord tumors such as SCTAT or Sertoli cell tumors of the ovary. The lesion is also seen in Peutz–Jeghers syndrome, which is associated with a mutation in the SKT11 gene.

44. **(B) Endocervical tunnel cluster.**
Benign endocervical tunnel clusters are marked by an arrangement of endocervical glands in a lobular configuration. The cells lining the glands are cytologically bland and the tunnel cluster should not be confused with endocervical carcinoma. The lesions do not stain with CEA antibody.

45. **(A) It has a poor prognosis.**
The lesion illustrated in the figure represents a well-differentiated villoglandular adenocarcinoma. This rare lesion typically occurs in young women and has an excellent prognosis. The tumor is associated with high-risk HPV and oral contraceptive use. Microscopically, the tumor is marked by elongated, thin papillary structures lined by cuboidal to columnar pseudostratified epithelium with mild cytologic atypia. Some of these cells lining the villi contain intracellular mucin. The tumors are frequently associated with high-grade squamous dysplasia or adenocarcinoma in situ.

46. **(D) They do not stain with CEA antibody.**
Adenoid cystic carcinomas most typically occur in elderly (postmenopausal) women in the cervix and typically present with postmenopausal bleeding. Microscopically, they resemble the adenoid cystic carcinoma pattern seen in the salivary gland and are often accompanied by a desmoplastic stromal reaction. The principal difference between the tumors in the cervix and those in the salivary gland is the absence of myoepithelial cells in the cervical tumors. Adenoid cystic carcinomas generally stain positively with epithelial markers, including low molecular weight keratins, EMA, and CEA and are associated with high-risk HPV. The tumors are fairly aggressive in terms of behavior and are often associated with local recurrences and metastases.

47. **(E) p63.**
The lesion illustrated in the figure represents a small cell neuroendocrine carcinoma arising in the cervix. These tumors generally stain with epithelial markers including low molecular weight keratin, EMA, and CEA, as well as, markers of neural differentiation including chromogranin, neuron specific enolase, synaptophysin, and Leu-7. They generally do not stain with p63.

48. **(B) Day 17.**
The changes shown in this biopsy are most consistent with an early secretory endometrium, day 17. The rows of subnuclear vacuoles are arranged in an orderly fashion. Occasional mitotic figures may still be evident. On day 16, early development of basal cytoplasmic vacuoles may be seen along with frequent mitoses in both glands and stroma

and generally tubular glands with pseudostratified nuclei. On day 19, basal nuclei, scattered subnuclear vacuoles, and increased intraluminal secretions are evident. Mitotic activity is generally not present on day 19. On day 20, rare subnuclear vacuoles may be still present. Endometrial glands are becoming increasingly complex and intraluminal secretions are most prominent. On day 22, there is maximal stromal edema with naked nuclei.

49. **(C) Day 23.**
The changes described here are most consistent with a late secretory endometrium, day 23. On day 21, there is some early stromal edema but no predecidual change is evident yet. On day 22, stromal edema is maximal, but again there is no predecidual change. On day 24, predecidual change extends from gland to gland but does not extend up to the surface of the endometrium. By day 25, there is a thin layer or patch of predecidual change just below the surface of the endometrium.

50. **(C) Endometrial atrophy.**
Endometrial atrophy is most commonly encountered in postmenopausal women. The patient's age suggests she is likely premenopausal and all of the other options listed are more common causes of abnormal uterine bleeding in a younger woman.

51. **(E) Plasma cells.**
The presence of plasma cells is considered characteristic, although not necessarily synonymous with chronic endometritis. Occasionally, one may encounter plasma cells in endometrial polyps and in late menstrual endometrium. In some cases, lymphocytes, eosinophils, and occasional lymphoid aggregates may be found but are not as specific. Granulomatous inflammation is generally not a common feature of endometritis.

52. **(A) Antibiotics.**
The treatment of choice for chronic endometritis is antibiotic therapy. Approximately 90% of women will show evidence of improvement within 2–3 days following the initiation of antibiotic therapy.

53. **(E) Prominent thickened blood vessels.**
Histologic features associated with anovulation are dependent on estrogen levels. One may encounter regularly distributed and cystically dilated endometrial glands with evidence of tubal metaplasia, patchy stromal breakdown, surface repair, and focal fibrin thrombi in spiral arterioles. The presence of prominent thickened blood vessels is more typically associated with endometrial polyps.

54. **(B) <5%.**
The risk of developing endometrial carcinoma in the setting of squamous morules or metaplasia is minimal.

55. **(B) Menopausal woman on hormone replacement therapy.**
Eosinophilic and mucinous metaplasias are most likely encountered in menopausal women undergoing hormone replacement therapy.

56. **(E) Papillary syncytial metaplasia.**
Papillary syncytial metaplasia is most frequently encountered in the setting of a menopausal woman on hormone replacement therapy. It is generally not encountered in association with pregnancy. The other features listed here are findings associated with pregnancy including decidual cells, hypersecretory endometrium, epithelial cells with Arias–Stella reaction, immature chorionic villi with trophoblastic cells, and evidence of placental implantation site with intermediate trophoblastic cells associated with a fibrin layer (Nitabuch fibrin).

57. **(E) 21–25%.**
In an endometrial biopsy that shows complex atypical hyperplasia, the approximate risk of developing carcinoma is about 25%. The risk of developing carcinoma in the setting of simple hyperplasia is about 1% and approximately 10% for complex hyperplasia without atypia.

58. **(B) Excess progesterone administration.**
There are a variety of risk factors for the development of endometrial hyperplasia. Most of these are associated with unopposed estrogen and may include conditions such as prolonged periods of anovulation, unopposed estrogen administration in the absence of progesterone, peripheral conversion of androgens to estrone, and adipose tissue in the setting of obesity or polycystic ovary disease. Excess progesterone administration is not associated with the development of endometrial hyperplasia.

59. **(C) Endometrial adenocarcinoma.**
The most common malignant tumor of the female genital tract is endometrial carcinoma, which has an incidence rate of approximately 10–20 per 1,00000 women per year in Western countries.

60. **(A) Clear cell.**
The tumor shown in the figure is marked by a papillary architectural pattern with sclerosed cores and cells lining the papillae that have a hobnail shape and sometimes clear cytoplasm. These morphologic features are most consistent with the clear cell variant of endometrial carcinoma.

61. **(A) Clear cell.**
There are a variety of indicators of poor prognosis with endometrial carcinoma. Among these is histologic type; particularly serous and clear cell carcinomas have a more aggressive behavior and poor prognosis. Additionally, histologic grade, stage, depth of myometrial invasion, serosal or adnexal

involvement, lymph node metastasis, and lympho-vascular invasion are all poor prognostic indicators with endometrial carcinoma.

62. **(C) p53 alterations.**

From a clinical perspective, endometrial carcinomas appear to be divided into two major clinico-pathologic groups. Type I cancers typically arise in premenopausal women in the presence of unopposed estrogen. The cancer is associated often with a hyperplasia precursor lesion. Most type I endometrial cancers are low-grade lesions with minimal myometrial invasion and most commonly are endometrioid or mucinous-type carcinomas. Molecular alterations that are common in this setting include microsatellite instability and PTEN and K-ras mutations. Type II endometrial cancers are more commonly seen in postmenopausal women. An unopposed estrogen state is not present and hyperplasia is not frequently observed. These typically are high-grade lesions that are deeply invasive and most commonly are serous, clear cell, squamous cell, and undifferentiated carcinomas. These tumors are frequently associated with p53 alterations.

63. **(A) Amount of solid growth.**

The grading of endometrioid adenocarcinoma of the uterus is based on the amount of solid growth of the glandular component of the tumor and not the squamous component. Grade I tumors typically have <5% solid growth pattern. Grade II tumors have 5–50% solid growth pattern areas, and grade III tumors have over 50% solid growth pattern.

64. **(A) Discohesive cells.**

A number of features can be looked for in order to establish the presence of squamous differentiation in an endometrioid adenocarcinoma. Characterization of an increased eosinophilic cytoplasm is one such feature. Other features include the presence of identifiable intercellular bridges, sheet-like growth with glandular formation or palisading, sharp cell margins, eosinophilic and thicker glassy cytoplasm, and decreased nuclear-to-cytoplasmic ratio as compared with foci elsewhere in the same tumor. The presence of discohesive cells is generally not a feature particularly suggestive of squamous differentiation.

65. **(A) High-grade tumors.**

The villoglandular variant of endometrioid carcinoma is the second most common variant. These are usually low-grade tumors marked by long papillae with delicate fibrovascular cores lined by pseudostratified columnar epithelium. These tumors are frequently admixed with areas resembling conventional endometrioid carcinoma. The villous architectural patten is more commonly seen in the superficial portion of the tumor. Lymphovas-

cular invasion with lymph node metastasis may be encountered.

66. **(E) Sertoliform pattern.**

Endometrioid carcinomas are known to be associated with hereditary nonpolyposis colon cancer syndrome (Lynch syndrome). These usually arise in young premenopausal women. The syndrome is associated with a defect in DNA mismatch repair genes, MLH-1 or MSH-2. Features characteristic of the endometrioid adenocarcinomas arising in this setting include poor differentiation, a Crohn-like lymphoid reaction, the presence of tumor infiltrating lymphocytes, and lymphatic permeation. Staining with antibodies to MLH-1, MSH-2, or MSH-6 may be helpful identifying such cases. The Sertoliform pattern of endometrioid carcinoma is not particularly associated with this syndrome.

67. **(C) Serous adenocarcinoma.**

Psammoma bodies are present in up to 30% of serous adenocarcinomas of the uterus. They may also be encountered occasionally (but less frequently) in other types such as clear cell carcinoma.

68. **(C) Mucicarmine.**

Distinguishing endocervical from endometrial adenocarcinoma may be difficult, particularly in limited biopsy specimens. Features that may be helpful in sorting these two lesions out include coexpression of vimentin and cytokeratin, which is more characteristic of endometrial carcinomas. Strong nuclear immunoreactivity with antibody estrogen receptor is also more frequently encountered with endometrial carcinomas. CEA immunoactivity is more commonly encountered with endocervical adenocarcinomas. Evidence of HPV infection, including p16 immunostaining, is more commonly encountered with endocervical adenocarcinomas. Mucicarmine positivity may be seen in either tumor type.

69. **(B) Hobnail cells.**

Arias–Stella reaction can sometimes resemble clear cell adenocarcinoma of endometrium. Characteristic features of the Arias–Stella reaction that can help in differentiating it from clear cell adenocarcinoma include preserved nuclear-to-cytoplasmic ratio, smudged appearance of the nuclei without prominent nucleoli or mitotic activity. The normal architecture of the endometrial gland is preserved with the Arias–Stella reaction in contrast to the disorganized architecture of carcinoma. Partial gland involvement by Arias–Stella and evidence of nuclei showing degenerative changes with pseudo-nuclear inclusions also are features more common of Arias–Stella reaction. Mitotic activity is more prominently observed with clear cell carcinoma.

70. **(C) Metastatic breast carcinoma.**
Metastatic carcinomas to the endometrium can occasionally mimic primary endometrial cancers. Breast carcinoma typically expresses cytokeratin 7, estrogen receptor, and progesterone receptor immunoactivity. GCDFP15 immunoreactivity is more frequently observed with metastatic breast carcinomas. Endometrioid adenocarcinomas may also express cytokeratin 7, ER and PR immunoreactivity. Metastatic colon adenocarcinomas demonstrate positive staining with antibody to cytokeratin 20 but are negative for cytokeratin 7 and typically demonstrate a garland architectural pattern with central dirty necrosis.

71. **(C) Stage Ic.**
The FIGO staging of endometrial carcinoma indicates that tumors confined to the uterus are stage I lesions, as described in this case. Stage Ia lesions are confined to the endometrium. Stage Ib tumors invade to a depth of <50% of the myometrial wall. Stage Ic tumors invade through 50% or more of the myometrial wall. Stage II tumors involve the uterine cervix, either extending to the endocervical epithelial surface or glands (stage IIa) or infiltrating the cervical stroma (stage IIb).

72. **(E) Symplastic leiomyoma.**
The lesion illustrated in the figure represents a smooth muscle tumor with large atypical "bizarre" nuclei. This feature is characteristic of the leiomyoma with bizarre nuclei or bizarre leiomyomas.

73. **(D) Lipoleiomyoma.**
The figure represents a smooth muscle tumor with an associated adipose tissue component, most consistent with a lipoleiomyoma. Occasionally, leiomyomas may contain heterologous elements that may include adipose tissue, skeletal muscle, osseous tissue, or cartilaginous tissue. Prognosis is not adversely impacted by the presence of any of these elements.

74. **(E) S-100 protein.**
Uterine leiomyomas may stain with a variety of antibodies including actin, smooth muscle myosin, desmin, h-caldesmon, and oxytocin. They frequently demonstrate evidence of estrogen or progesterone immunoreactivity and may also on occasion stain with antibodies to cytokeratins and EMA. S-100 protein immunoreactivity is not a salient feature of uterine leiomyomas.

75. **(E) 6 Mitotic figures/10 high-power fields.**
Intravenous leiomyomatosis is marked by endothelium-covered protrusions of smooth muscle. Plugs of tumor involve vascular, usually venous, spaces. There is usually minimal cytologic atypia associated with these tumors and one may see intersecting fascicles of muscle that stain with antibodies, which usually target this tissue type including des-

min. p53 immunoactivity is generally not a feature of these tumors. Mitotic activity is typically low, usually <5 mitotic figures/10 high-power fields.

76. **(E) Mitotically active leiomyoma.**
The lesion shown in the figure represents a smooth muscle tumor of the uterus marked by minimal cytologic atypia but readily identifiable mitotic figures. The high mitotic count in this lesion, coupled with relatively small size of the mass and lack of appreciable cytologic atypia, is most consistent with a mitotically active leiomyoma.

77. **(C) Lung.**
A common site for involvement by benign metastasizing leiomyoma is the lung in women who have uterine leiomyomas, leiomyomas with vascular invasion or intravenous leiomyomatosis. Other less commonly involved sites include the retroperitoneum, mediastinal lymph nodes, bone, and soft tissues.

78. **(A) Increased mitotic activity.**
Histologic alterations associated with gonadotropin-releasing hormone agonist treatment of leiomyoma are variable. The most common alterations that have been described in the literature include nuclear crowding; decreased tumor size; lymphocytic infiltrate; areas of infarct-like necrosis; small cell size; increased hyalinization; increased apoptotic bodies; and a variety of vascular wall alterations including thickening, myxoid change, fibrinoid change, thrombosis, or fibrosis.

79. **(C) Leiomyosarcoma.**
The smooth muscle tumor illustrated in the figure is characterized by prominent cellularity, nuclear atypia, and mitotic activity that are readily identifiable. Given the large size of the tumor and the presence of necrosis, these features are most consistent with a diagnosis of leiomyosarcoma.

80. **(C) Inhibin.**
PEComa of the uterus is a rare lesion marked by perivascular epithelioid cells with abundant clear to eosinophilic cytoplasm. These lesions generally demonstrate HMB-45 immunoreactivity in addition to melan-A and MiTF staining. They can variably stain with antibody to CD10. They generally do not stain with cytokeratin markers, inhibin, and S-100 protein.

81. **(A) CD10.**
The lesion shown in the figure represents an endometrial stromal sarcoma marked by a proliferation of relatively small cells with scant cytoplasm, oval-to-round nuclei, and inconspicuous nucleoli. This lesion typically stains with antibodies to CD10 and vimentin. Keratin and smooth muscle actin immunoreactivity are also frequently noted. Occasionally, ER/PR positive staining may be observed. In tumors with evidence of sex cord-like differentiation, melan-A and CD99 positivity may also be

encountered. Of the antibodies listed as options, CD10 is the most likely to be positive in a diffuse fashion in this tumor.

82. **(E) Müllerian adenosarcoma.**
Müllerian adenosarcoma is a low-grade tumor marked by a biphasic pattern composed of a benign or atypical epithelial component and a low-grade malignant stromal component. Findings described in the patient histologically appear to be most consistent with that diagnosis. These patients typically present with abnormal vaginal bleeding and pelvic pain. On examination, they have an enlarged uterus. Müllerian adenofibromas are extremely rare lesions that have benign epithelial and stromal components. Mixed Müllerian tumors have malignant epithelial and stromal components. The stromal component in an endometrial polyp, although it may demonstrate some focal atypia, generally does not show features of a malignancy such as fibrosarcoma.

83. **(A) Alcohol use.**
Risk factors for the development of a malignant mixed Müllerian tumor are similar to those of endometrial carcinoma and include estrogen, obesity, tamoxifen therapy, and nulliparity. A history of prior radiation may also place patient at risk. Alcohol use is not a known risk factor for the development of malignant mixed Müllerian tumors of the uterus.

84. **(B) About 2 years.**
Median survival for all stages of malignant mixed Müllerian tumors is around 2 years. Five-year survival rates have ranged from 5% to 35% for patients with tumor of all stages with a better than 5-year survival (40–60%) for stage I and II tumors.

85. **(B) Mucinous metaplasia.**
Mucinous metaplasia may be associated with Peutz–Jeghers syndrome. Mucinous metaplasia of the fallopian tube typically appears as a single layer of mucinous epithelium replacing the usual ciliated-type epithelium of the fallopian tube. The overall architecture of the tube is maintained.

86. **(A) Decidual metaplasia.**
Risk factors for the development of a tubal ectopic pregnancy include any condition that potentially interferes with passage of the fertilized egg into the uterus. These conditions may include a history of salpingitis, pelvic inflammatory disease, endometriosis, tubal surgery, or structural defects of the fallopian tube. Decidual metaplasia is usually not thought of as a risk factor for the development of a tubal ectopic pregnancy.

87. **(E) *Staphylococcus*.**
A variety of organisms are known to be associated with pelvic inflammatory disease. Among the more common organisms are *Neisseria*, *Chlamydia*, Mycoplasma, and anaerobic bacteria. Of the organisms listed, *Staphylococcus* is the least likely to be the etiologic agent for pelvic inflammatory disease.

88. **(E) Tuberculosis.**
The presence of caseating mucosal granulomas with chronic inflammation and fibrosis and a paucity of eosinophils are most consistent with a diagnosis of tuberculous salpingitis. Sarcoidosis may result in granulomas, although typically nonnecrotizing. Parasitic infections are often associated with eosinophils and the organism may be evident. Lipoidal salpingitis is a granulomatous reaction secondary to lipoidal contrast agent; the lipid droplets are usually surrounded by histocytes and foreign body giant cells.

89. **(B) Adenomatoid tumor.**
The lesion illustrated in the figure best represents an adenomatoid tumor arising in the fallopian tube. These lesions are typically encountered in middle-aged or elderly women, usually as an incidental finding. It presents as well circumscribed but nonencapsulated lesion with gland-like and slit-like spaces. In between these spaces, single signet-ring-like cells may be evident. Another population of cuboidal flat cells with bland cytologic features can be seen. Variable numbers of lymphocytes may be intermixed in the tumor.

90. **(A) Calretinin.**
The tumor shown in Question 89 represents an adenomatoid tumor. Immunohistochemistry wise, these tumors will stain with antibodies to calretinin, WT1, and low molecular weight cytokeratin markers. They typically do not show staining with antibodies to CEA, CD15, factor VIII, or TAG-72.

91. **(A) Adenocarcinoma.**
Adenocarcinoma of the fallopian tube is known to be associated with BRCA1/BRCA2 germline mutations. These mutations are also known to be associated with an increased risk of breast carcinoma.

92. **(D) Stains with CEA.**
Female adnexal tumors of probable Wolffian origin commonly arise in the fallopian tube, broad ligament, and ovarian hilar region. These are low-grade lesions, which usually present with abdominal pain or palpable mass. Histologically, the tumor may be marked by a diffuse, cystic or sieve-like, or tubular growth pattern. The tumors generally stain with keratin markers, CD10, calretinin, and vimentin. CEA immunoactivity is not a feature of this neoplasm.

93. **(E) Postmenopausal peak.**
The lesion shown in the figure is most consistent with polycystic ovarian disease. This condition is associated with a variety of other things that can contribute to increased morbidity including infertility and insulin resistance. Association of this entity

with hirsutism, acne, and male-pattern baldness may be evident. Most patients present early in life in the perimenarchal, not in the postmenopausal, period.

94. **(D) Stromal hyperthecosis.**
The figure shows ovarian stroma with intermixed single and small collections of cells with large rounded contour and abundant eosinophilic cytoplasm. Findings here are most consistent with stromal luteinization or stromal hyperthecosis. This condition may be associated with increased androgen production and evidence of virilization, obesity, hypertension, and glucose intolerance.

95. **(D) Pregnancy luteomas.**
Multiple circumscribed, red-brown ovarian nodules presenting during pregnancy are most consistent with a diagnosis of pregnancy luteomas. The entity is usually encountered in the second half of pregnancy and is considered benign, regressing after delivery. Histologically, the nodules are well circumscribed and composed of luteinized cells with abundant eosinophilic cytoplasm, prominent nucleoli, and centrally placed round and regular nuclei. Mitotic activity may be readily identified. Some lesions may demonstrate evidence of necrosis.

96. **(C) Massive ovarian edema.**
The figure shown here is marked by prominent stromal edema. This morphology is most consistent with a massive ovarian edema. Patients often present with an enlarged ovary. Enlargement is almost always unilateral and more frequently involves the right versus left ovary. There is a well-known increased risk of torsion associated with this lesion. Typical age of presentation is in the first 3 decades of life. In a subset of cases, aggregates of luteinized cells may be observed in the stroma.

97. **(D) Serous.**
The most common epithelial stroma tumors of the ovary are the serous types, comprising nearly half of this group. Mucinous and endometrioid tumors are the next most common epithelial stromal tumors of the ovary.

98. **(E) 90%.**
The overall survival for a serous borderline tumor or serous tumor of low malignant potential is approximately 90–95% at 5 years and 80% at 20 years. The presence of invasive implants is associated with a poor prognosis. The transformation to a low-grade serous carcinoma is also associated with a poor prognosis.

99. **(B) Calretinin.**
Serous borderline tumors generally stain with antibodies to cytokeratin 7, WT1, BerEP4, and CD15. While they typically do not stain with antibody to cytokeratin 20, staining with antibody CA125 may be evident. Calretinin positivity is more commonly seen with mesotheliomas and not serous borderline tumors.

100. **(A) Borderline mucinous tumor.**
The lesion illustrated in the figure is best classified as a borderline mucinous tumor. These lesions microscopically are marked by a stratification of intestinal-type epithelium demonstrating mild-to-moderate cytologic atypia. Goblet cells may be frequently seen. Occasionally, Paneth cells and endocrine cells may be present. There is minimal stromal invasion evident in these tumors.

101. **(C) Granulosa cell tumor.**
Mucinous epithelial tumors of the ovary are known to coexist with Brenner tumors, carcinoid tumors, Sertoli–Leydig cell tumors, and mature cystic teratomas. Granulosa cell tumors are not known to be associated with mucinous epithelial tumors of the ovary.

102. **(A) CA125.**
Mucinous adenocarcinomas or cystadenocarcinomas of the ovary generally will stain with antibodies to cytokeratins 7 and 20, CEA, and CDX2. These tumors generally do not stain with antibody to CA125. Many of these tumors demonstrate K-ras mutations and are generally not associated with BRCA1/BRCA2 mutations.

103. **(D) Most present as bilateral ovarian masses.**
Endometrioid carcinomas of the ovary are typically unilateral, not bilateral masses, in the majority of patients (70%). Significant subsets of patients, approximately 15–20%, have a synchronous primary endometrial adenocarcinoma. Most patients present during the 5th-7th decades of life. Tumors may demonstrate estrogen and progesterone receptor immunoactivity and CA125 levels are commonly elevated.

104. **(E) Stage for stage, clear cell carcinoma has a better prognosis than serous carcinoma.**
Clear cell carcinomas of the ovary are typically unilateral masses that most commonly present between the 5th and 7th decades of life. These tumors are more prevalent in the Japanese population versus Western countries. Most patients are nulliparous and the tumor is known to be associated with pelvic endometriosis. The patients are at increased risk of developing pelvic venous thromboses and the tumor is known to be associated with paraneoplastic hypercalcemia. Stage clear cell carcinoma of the ovary has a worse prognosis than other surface epithelial carcinomas, including serous carcinoma.

105. **(A) Benign Brenner tumor.**
The lesion shown in the figure is marked by a nest of uniform transitional-type epithelium embedded in a fibromatous stroma. The cells are generally ovoid with small nuclei and indistinct nucleoli. The

morphologic features shown here are most consistent with that of a benign Brenner tumor. Borderline Brenner tumors typically exhibit papillary architectural pattern. Malignant tumors are marked by evidence of stromal invasion, often accompanied by a more appreciable cytologic atypia.

106. **(B) Fibroma.**
Fibromas can arise at any age but are most commonly seen in middle-aged women. Earlier age of presentation for fibromas may be associated with Gorlin syndrome (nevoid basal cell carcinoma syndrome); this is an autosomal-dominant condition marked by a variety of defects of the skeletal muscle system, multiple basal cell carcinomas and ovarian fibromas, which are frequently multinodular and bilateral. Fibromas are also associated with Meigs syndrome, which is marked by ascites and pleural effusion.

107. **(E) Thecoma.**
The lesion illustrated in the figure is marked by cells with abundant pale vacuolated cytoplasm with generally round-to-oval nuclei. These morphologic features are consistent with that of a thecoma. These tumors demonstrate evidence of lipid within the cytoplasm (oil-red-O positive). Thecomas typically are positive for inhibin, calretinin, CD10, and vimentin.

108. **(E) Sclerosing stromal tumor.**
Sclerosing stromal tumors are generally marked by a pseudolobular architecture. The more cellular nodules alternate with hypocellular edematous or collagenized appearing areas. The tumor is composed of a prominent number of thin-walled blood vessels intermixed with spindled and rounded cells. There is minimal cytologic atypia or evidence of mitotic activity in these low-grade tumors. The vast majority of the patients with this lesion present before the age of 30 years.

109. **(A) Adult granulosa cell tumor.**
Adult granulosa cell tumors are generally marked by a proliferation of granulosa cells in a fibrothecomatous background. Occasional microfollicular structures, referred to as Call–Exner bodies, may be observed in these lesions. The tumor may have diffuse, trabecular, follicular, insular, gyriform, or watered-silk growth patterns. Individual cell nuclei are generally round-to-oval with a characteristic longitudinal groove. Features illustrated in the tumor are most consistent with that of the adult granulosa cell tumor.

110. **(A) Has hyperchromatic nuclei with prominent grooves.**
Hyperchromatic nuclei with prominent grooves are generally not a feature of the juvenile granulosa cell tumor. Grooved nuclei are more commonly encoun-

tered with the adult-type granulosa cell tumor. Juvenile granulosa cell tumor is a unilateral mass that typically presents in the first 3 decades of life. The lesion is known to be associated with Maffucci syndrome and Ollier disease. Serum inhibin levels can be used to monitor for evidence of tumor recurrence. These tumors demonstrate immunoreactivity with antibodies to inhibin and calretinin.

111. **(D) Sertoli–Leydig cell tumor.**
The lesion illustrated in the figure represents the retiform pattern of a Sertoli–Leydig cell tumor. This pattern is marked by the presents of cyst-like tubules and cysts with short and rounded papillae. The papillary cores are often hyalinized. Mitotic activity may be variably seen. Alpha-fetoprotein (AFP) levels are usually normal, which allow distinction of this lesion from a yolk sac tumor.

112. **(D) Sex cord tumor with annular tubules.**
The sex cord tumor with annular tubules is well-known to be associated with Peutz–Jeghers syndrome. In this setting, the majority of tumors are bilateral. Approximately one-third of patients with sex cord tumors with annular tubules have Peutz–Jeghers syndrome.

113. **(E) Usually bilateral.**
The tumor illustrated in the figure represents a Leydig cell tumor and is marked by cells with abundant eosinophilic cytoplasm. These tumors most commonly arise in the ovarian hilum and typically present as a unilateral mass in a peri- or postmenopausal woman. Many of these tumors produce androgens. A characteristic microscopic finding is the presence of Reinke crystals in the cytoplasm of the tumor cells. These neoplasms will stain with antibodies to vimentin, CD56, inhibin, and calretinin.

114. **(B) Dysgerminoma.**
Dysgerminoma of the ovary represents the most common malignant ovarian germ cell tumor (approximately 50% of them). It most commonly arises in the 2nd–3rd decades of life. The tumors, like seminomas of the testis, are marked by a proliferation of large polygonal cells with clear or light eosinophilic cytoplasm, prominent nuclei with nucleoli, and brisk mitotic activity. Intermixed lymphocytes and occasional granulomas may be observed in these neoplasms.

115. **(D) Reticular.**
There are a variety of different microscopic growth patterns for yolk sac tumor that makes their diagnosis a challenge. The most common pattern is the reticular pattern. The less common architectural patterns include microcytic, pseudopapillary, solid, polyvesicular vitelline, hepatoid, glandular, and parietal patterns. The presence of Schiller–Duval bodies, albeit pathognomonic, is seen in only

about a third of cases. Eosinophilic hyaline glob-ules are a common and useful diagnostic feature of yolk sac tumors.

116. **(E) Squamous cell carcinoma.**
The most common secondary malignancy to arise in the setting of a mature cystic teratoma is squamous cell carcinoma. Less commonly, adeno-carcinoma, small cell carcinoma, sarcoma, and malignant melanoma have been described arising in teratomas.

117. **(E) Struma ovarii.**
The most common form of a monodermal ovarian teratoma is a struma ovarii. These lesions consist of thyroid follicles and may resemble a normal thy-roid gland, thyroid adenoma, or goiter. Rarely, the lesion may show features of papillary carcinoma. Other forms of monodermal teratoma include car-cinoid tumors, neuroectodermal tumors, sebaceous tumors, and endodermal lesions.

118. **(B) Amount of immature neuroepithelium.**
The grading of immature teratomas is based on the amount of immature neuroepithelium present in the lesion. Grade I lesions are marked by 1 low-power field of immature neuroepithelium on any 1 slide. Grade II lesions are marked by 1 to 3 low-power fields of immature neuroepithelium on any 1 slide. Grade III tumors exceed 3 low-power fields on any 1 slide.

119. **(C) Gonadoblastoma.**
The lesion illustrated in the figure represents a gonadoblastoma. These tumors are marked by large germ cells surrounded by smaller sex cord-type cells. About a third of patients have bilateral tumors. These tumors do show an increased risk of evolving into a dysgerminoma.

120. **(C) 15 cm size.**
Typical features suggestive of a metastasis to the ovary versus a primary ovarian neoplasm include the presence of bilateral ovarian involvement, tumor size <10 cm, surface and superficial cortical involvement, nodular growth pattern, signet-ring cell component, hilar involvement or lympho-vascular invasion, and an infiltrative growth pat-tern with stromal desmoplasia. The presence of a very large mass is more commonly indicative of a primary ovarian tumor.

121. **(C) Metastatic colorectal carcinoma.**
The lesion shown in the figure is marked by a cribriform pattern with central dirty necrosis. This morphology is suggestive of metastatic colorec-tal carcinoma. The morphologic impression is confirmed by the immunohistochemical profile that supports this diagnosis. Many primary ovar-ian tumors demonstrate cytokeratin 7 immuno-reactivity.

122. **(B) Diffuse large B-cell lymphoma.**
Diffuse large B-cell lymphoma is the most common non-Hodgkin lymphoma to involve the ovary. The other lymphoma types listed as options for this question have been described less frequently to arise in the ovary.

123. **(D) Typically inhibin positive.**
The lesion illustrated in the figure is marked by a proliferation of small cells with minimal cytoplasm consistent with a small carcinoma. These tumors typically present in younger women with abdomi-nal distention or pain and frequently with hyper-calcemia (approximately two-thirds of patients). About half of the patients present with advanced disease, with a spread beyond the ovary at the time of presentation. Favorable prognostic factors include older age (>30 years), normal preopera-tive calcium level, smaller size (<10 cm), and an absence of large atypical cells. Ki-67 labeling indi-ces are typically high. These tumors will stain with low molecular weight cytokeratin markers such as cytokeratins 8 or 18. They generally do not stain with inhibin antibody. Necrosis and hemorrhage are frequent gross features of these lesions.

124. **(E) Normal or small uterus for gestational age.**
A complete hydatidiform mole is androgenetic diploid. There is an increased prevalence of com-plete moles in lower socioeconomic status women and at the extremes of reproductive age. Com-plete moles are characterized by excessive uterine enlargement for gestational age, an absence of fetal heart sounds, earlier onset of toxemia, and markedly elevated serum beta-hCG levels. Approxi-mately 2–5% of complete moles may go on to develop choriocarcinoma.

125. **(B) Generalized hydropic villous change.**
Generalized hydropic villous change is a feature more characteristic of a complete rather than par-tial mole. The other features listed here are typical of a partial mole including scalloped villous con-tours, a mixture of small and normal sized villi, trophoblastic inclusions or invaginations, focal syncytiotrophoblastic proliferation or hyperplasia, and nucleated red cells within villous capillaries or other evidence of fetal development.

126. **(D) Ki-67.**
Placental site nodules represent benign lesions of intermediate trophoblast. The epithelioid tropho-blastic tumor represents the malignant counterpart of the placental site nodule. A Ki-67 labeling index in excessive of 10% is more suggestive of the epi-thelioid trophoblastic tumor rather that a placental site nodule. Both lesions may stain with antibodies to cytokeratin 18, p63, and variably with CD 146 and hPL.

127. **(C) 10–15%.**

Approximately 10–15% of patients with placental site trophoblastic tumor will demonstrate evidence of metastasis. The most common site of metastasis is the lung. In general, predictive prognostic factors in patients with placental site trophoblastic tumor include stage, older age (>35 years), depth of myometrial invasion, mitotic activity in excess of five mitoses per high-power fields, tumor size, clear cytoplasm, necrosis, elevated hCG levels, previous term pregnancy, and increased interval from previous pregnancy of >2 years.

128. **(D) Lymph nodes.**

Metastases from choriocarcinoma are more likely to be hematogenous and most frequently involve the lungs followed by the vagina, liver, and brain. Of the sites listed, lymph nodes are the least likely site of metastatic disease in this clinical setting.

129. **(C) Twinning.**

An umbilical cord <35 cm is considered excessively short. An excessively short umbilical cord may be associated with a variety of other findings including fetal distress, failure to descend during labor, umbilical cord rupture, umbilical cord hematoma, fetal anomalies, uterine inversion, poor outcome, and psychomotor abnormalities in the newborn. Twinning is generally not considered to be associated with excessively short umbilical cords. Long cords (>70 cm) have been associated with entanglement, cord prolapse, fetal distress, fetal growth restrictions and demise, and poor neurologic outcome.

130. **(B) Majority of infants with this finding have some abnormality.**

The lesion shown in the figure represents a two-vessel umbilical cord or a single umbilical artery cord. This is one of the most common congenital anomalies of the placenta and occurs in approximately 1% of births. The cord consists of one artery and one vein. Renal and cardiac anomalies have been described in association with this lesion. Although the majority of infants born with a single umbilical artery cord are normal, there is an increased incidence of placental abnormalities, prematurity, multiple gestations, intrauterine growth restriction, and increased perinatal morbidity and mortality.

131. **(D) 10%.**

The lesion illustrated in the figure represents a true knot of the umbilical cord. True knots are found in approximately 0.5% of all umbilical cords and more commonly in male fetuses and the setting of a long umbilical cord. False knots are more common and represent focal twisting or varicosities of the umbilical vessels and are generally thought to be of no clinical significance.

132. **(C) Oligohydramnios.**

The lesion illustrated in the figure represents amnion nodosum. In this setting, one often sees multiple small nodules on the surface of the amnion. The nodules represent amniotic fluid debris and vernix that become attached to the surface. This condition is associated with oligohydramnios and conditions resulting in decreased amount of amniotic fluid including certain malformative lesions involving the urinary tract.

133. **(A) 1 hour.**

In the setting of meconium staining, meconium pigment macrophages may be observed in the amnion within 1 hour after discharge. After 3 hours, macrophages may be observed within the chorion.

134. **(C) Listeria.**

An acute villitis or acute inflammation within the placental villi and the presence of intervillous abscesses are suggestive of an infection by *Listeria monocytogenes*. Cytomegalovirus is more commonly marked by a plasmacytic villitis with hemosiderin deposition and villous capillary thrombosis; typical cytoplasmic or intranuclear inclusions may be evident. In varicella infection, chronic villitis characterized by multinucleated giant cells may be evident. Syphilis infection in the placenta is associated with a large, heavy pale placenta and microscopically demonstrates evidence of chronic villitis with prominent numbers of plasma cells and obliterative endarteritis. Group B streptococcal infection is more commonly associated with chorioamnionitis.

135. **(B) Circumvallate.**

The findings described here are characteristic of a circumvallate placenta. Circummarginate insertion of the fetal membranes is similar to circumvallation, in that the membranes do not insert at the margin. In circummargination, there is no folding back of the membranes at the margin; this finding does not appear to be associated with the same adverse perinatal outcomes that circumvallation is (premature delivery, bleeding, intrauterine growth restriction, abruption, and premature rupture of membranes). Placenta membranacea is characterized by the presence of chorionic villi around all or nearly the entire circumference of the amniotic sac. Succenturiate lobes represent placental tissue separated from the major placental disk by membranes and/or connecting vessels. Interpositional insertion and battledore placenta represent conditions in which there is an abnormal attachment of the umbilical cord to the placental disk.

136. **(D) Maternal underperfusion.**

The changes described in the placenta represent a vascular condition associated with maternal underperfusion known as acute atherosis. In atherosis, there is necrosis of blood vessel walls, usually a fibrinoid necrosis, accompanied by an accumulation of foamy macrophages within the endothelium.

137. **(D) Placenta accreta.**
The HELLP syndrome is marked by hemolysis, elevated liver enzymes, and low platelets. The syndrome is associated with placental abruption. Placenta accreta or deficiency of the decidual, resulting in a deep invasion of trophoblastic cells and villi into the myometrium, is not a feature associated with HELLP syndrome.

138. **(B) Chorangiosis.**
The lesion shown in the figure is marked by placental villi that contain increased numbers of blood vessels. This finding is consistent with a diagnosis of chorangiosis. Chorangiosis is more precisely defined as 10 or more villi containing 10 or more capillaries each in 10 microscopic fields at a magnification of 100× in 3 areas of the placenta. This condition has been associated with poor perinatal outcome and associated more commonly with placentas from women living at high altitude. Chorangioma represents a benign vascular tumor or hemangioma of the placenta.

139. **(E) 2/3.**
Two-thirds of diamniotic/dichorionic twins represent dizygotic twins.

140. **(E) Melanoma.**
The most common tumors in pregnant women include cervical and breast carcinomas. The most common maternal tumor to metastasize to the placenta or spread to the fetus is melanoma.

SUGGESTED READING

1. Aguirre P, Thor AD, Scully RE. Ovarian small cell carcinoma histogenetic considerations based on immunohistochemical and other findings. *Am J Clin Pathol.* 1989;92:140-149.

2. Altshuler G. A conceptual approach to placental pathology and pregnancy outcome. *Semin Diagn Pathol.* 1993;10:204-221.

3. Alvarado-Cabrero I, Young RH, Vamvakas EC, et al. Carcinoma of the fallopian tube: a clinicopathological study of 105 cases with observations on staging and prognosis factors. *Gynecol Oncol.* 1999;72:367-379.

4. Ayhan A, Tuncer ZS, Tuncer R, et al. Granulosa cell tumor of the ovary: a clinicopathological evaluation of 60 cases. *Eur J Gynecol Oncol.* 1994;108:786-791.

5. Brainard JA, Hart WR. Proliferative epidermal lesions associated with anogenital Paget's disease. *Am J Surg Pathol.* 2000;24:543-552.

6. Calaminus G, Wessalowski R, Harms D, et al. Juvenile granulosa cell tumors of the ovary in children and adolescents: results from 33 patients registered in a prospective cooperative study. *Gynecol Oncol.* 1997;65:447-452.

7. Clement PB. Pathology endometriosis. *Pathol Ann.* 1990;25:245-295.

8. Clement PG, Young RH. Endometrioid carcinoma of the uterine corpus: a review of its pathology with emphasis on recent advances and problematic aspects. *Adv Anat Pathol.* 2002;9:145-184.

9. Comerci JT Jr., Licciardi F, Bergh PA, et al. Mature cystic teratoma: a clinicopathologic evaluation of 517 cases and review of the literature. *Obstetr Gynecol.* 1994;84:22-28.

10. Deavers MT, Malpica A, Ordonez NG, et al. Ovarian steroid cell tumors: an immunohistochemical study including a comparison of calretinin with inhibin. *Int J Gynecol Pathol.* 2003;22:162-167.

11. DeBrito PA, Silverberg SG, Orenstein JM. Carcinosarcoma (malignant mixed müllerian [mesodermal] tumor) of the female genital tract: immunohistochemical and ultrastructural analysis of 28 cases. *Hum Pathol.* 1993;24:132-142.

12. Deligdisch L. Hormonal pathology of the endometrium. *Mod Pathol.* 2000;13:285-294.

13. Devouassoux-Shisheboran M, Silver SA, Tavassoli FA. Wolffian adnexal tumor, so-called female adnexal tumor of probable Wolffian origin (FATWO): immunohistochemical evidence in support of a Wolffian origin. *Hum Pathol.* 1999;26:69-74.

14. Downes KA, Hart WR. Bizarre leiomyomas of the uterus: a comprehensive pathologic study of 24 cases with long-term follow-up. *Am J Surg Pathol.* 1997;21:1261-1270.

15. Duggan MA, Brashert P, Östör A, et al. The accuracy and interobserver reproducibility of endometrial dating. *Pathology.* 2001;33:292-297.

16. Eichhorn JH, Young RH. Neuroendocrine tumors of the genital tract. *Am J Clin Pathol.* 2001;115:S94-S112.

17. Feakins RM, Lowe DG. Basal cell carcinoma of the vulva: a clinicopathologic study of 45 cases. *Int J Gynecol Pathol.* 1997;16:319-324.

18. Ferry JA, Scully RE. 'Adenoid cystic' carcinoma and adenoid basal carcinoma of the uterine cervix. A study of 28 cases. *Am J Surg Pathol.* 1998;12:134-144.

19. Ferry JA, Young RH. Malignant lymphoma, pseudolymphoma and hematopoietic disorders of the female genital tract. *Pathol Ann.* 1991;26:227-263.

20. Franks S. Medical progress—polycystic ovary syndrome. *N Engl J Med.* 1995;33:853-861.

21. Gagnon Y, Tëtu B. Ovarian metastases of breast carcinoma: a clinicopathologic study of 59 cases. *Cancer.* 1989;64:892-898.

22. Genest DR. Partial hydatidiform mole: clinicopathological features, differential diagnosis, ploidy and molecular studies, and gold standards for diagnosis. *Int J Gynecol Pathol.* 2001;20:315-322.

23. Gopalan R, Simsir A. Metaplasias of the endometrium. *Pathol Case Rev.* 2000;5:153-157.

24. Guerrieri C, Högberg T, Wingren S, et al. Mucinous borderline and malignant tumors of the ovary: a clinicopathologic and DNA ploidy study of 92 cases. *Cancer.* 1994;74:2329-2340.

25. Heller DS, Moomjy M, Koulos J, et al. Vulvar and vaginal melanoma. A clinicopathologic study. *J Reprod Med.* 1994;39:945-948.

26. Hellstrom AC, Tegerstedt G, Silfversward C, et al. Malignant mixed müllerian tumors of the ovary: histopathologic

and clinical review of 36 cases. *Int J Gynecol Cancer.* 1999; 9:312-316.

27. Hirai Y, Takeshima N, Haga A, et al. A clinicocytopathologic study of adenoma malignum of the uterine cervix. *Gynecol Oncol.* 1998;70:219-223.

28. Jordan LB, Abdul-Kader M, Al-Nafussi A. Uterine serous papillary carcinoma. Histopathologic changes within the female genital tract. *Int J Gynecol Cancer.* 2001;11:283-289.

29. Kumar NB, Hart WR. Metastases to the uterine corpus from extragenital cancers. A clinicopathologic study of 63 cases. *Cancer.* 1982;50:2163-2169.

30. Kurman RJ, Norris HJ. Malignant germ cell tumors of the ovary. *Hum Pathol.* 1997;8:551-564.

31. Lage JM, Mark SD, Roberts DJ, et al. A flow cytometric study of 137 fresh hydropic placentas: correlation between types of hydatidiform moles and nuclear DNA ploidy. *Obstet Gynecol.* 1992;79:403-410.

32. Lee KR, Young RH. The distinction between primary and metastatic mucinous carcinomas of the ovary: gross and histologic findings in 50 cases. *Am J Surg Pathol.* 2003;27: 281-292.

33. Leung AKC, Robson WLM. Single umbilical artery: a report of 159 cases. *Amer J Dis Child.* 1989;143:108-111.

34. Matias-Guiu X, Catasus L, Bussaglia E, et al. Molecular pathology of endometrial hyperplasia and carcinoma. *Hum Pathol.* 2001;32:569-577.

35. McCluggage WG, Sumathi VO, McBride HA, et al. A panel of immunohistochemical stains, including carcinoembryonic antigen, vimentin, and estrogen receptor, aids the distinction between primary endometrial and endocervical adenocarcinomas. *Int J Gynecol Pathol.* 2001;21:11-15.

36. McCormack WM. Pelvic inflammatory disease. *N Engl J Med.* 1994;30:115-119.

37. McLennan H, Price E, Urbanska M, et al. Umbilical cord knots and encirclements. *Aust NZ J Obstet Gynecol.* 1988; 28:116-119.

38. Merino MJ, Edmonds P, LiVolsi V. Appendiceal carcinoma metastatic to the ovaries and mimicking primary ovarian tumors. *Int J Gynecol Pathol.* 1985;4:110-120.

39. Miller PW, Coen RW, Benirschke K. Dating the time interval from meconium passage to birth. *Obstet Gynecol.* 1985;66: 459-462.

40. Negri G, Egarter-Vigl E, Kasal A, et al. p16INK4 a is a useful marker for the diagnosis of adenocarcinoma of the cervix uteri and its precursors: an immunohistochemical study with immunocytochemical correlations. *Am J Surg Pathol.* 2003;27:187-193.

41. Nogales FF, Isaac MA, Hardisson D, et al. Adenomatoid tumors of the uterus: an analysis of 60 cases. *Int J Gynecol Pathol.* 2002;21:34-40.

42. Nucci MR, Oliva E (eds.). *Gynecologic Pathology.* Philadelphia, PA: Churchill Livingstone Elsevier; 2009.

43. Oliva E, Young RH, Amin MB, et al. An immunohistochemical analysis of endometrial stromal and smooth muscle tumors of the uterus: a study of 54 cases emphasizing the importance of using a panel because of overlap in immunoreactivity for individual antibodies. *Am J Surg Pathol.* 2002; 26:403-412.

44. Östör AG, Rome RM. Micro-invasive squamous cell carcinoma of the cervix: a clinico-pathologic study of 200 cases with long-term follow-up. *Int J Gynecol Cancer.* 1994;4:257-264.

45. Paradinas FJ, Fisher RA, Browne P, et al. Diploid hydatidiform moles with fetal red blood cells in molar villi. 1—pathology, incidence, and prognosis. *J Pathol.* 1997;181:183-188.

46. Pelkey TJ, Frierson HF Jr, Mills SE, et al. The diagnostic utility of inhibin staining in ovarian neoplasms. *Int J Gynecol Pathol.* 1998;17:97-105.

47. Prat J. Ovarian tumors of borderline malignancy (tumors of low malignant potential): a critical appraisal. *Adv Anat Pathol.* 1999;6:247-274.

48. Prayson RA, Goldblum JR, Hart WR. Epithelioid smooth-muscle tumors of the uterus. A clinicopathologic study of 18 patients. *Am J Surg Pathol.* 1997;21:383-391.

49. Prayson RA, Hart WR. Mitotically active leiomyomas of the uterus. *Am J Clin Pathol.* 1992;97:14-20.

50. Redline RW, Abramowsky CR, Clinical and pathologic aspects of recurrent placental villitis. *Hum Pathol.* 1985;16: 727-731.

51. Robboy SJ, Kaufman RH, Prat J, et al. Pathologic findings in young women enrolled in the National Cooperative Diethylstilbestrol Adenosis (DESAD) project. *Obstet Gynecol.* 1979;53:309-317.

52. Robboy SJ, Scully RE. Strumal carcinoid of the ovary: an analysis of 50 cases of a distinctive tumor composed of thyroid tissue and carcinoid. *Cancer.* 1980;46:2019-2034.

53. Robert ME, Fu YS. Squamous cell carcinoma of the uterine cervix—a review with emphasis on prognostic factors and unusual variants. *Semin Diagn Pathol.* 1990;7:173-189.

54. Rodriguez IM, Prat J. Mucinous tumors of the ovary: a clinicopathologic analysis of 75 borderline tumors of intestinal type) and carcinomas. *Am J Surg Pathol.* 2002;26: 139-152

55. Ross JC, Eifel PH, Cox RS, et al. Primary mucinous adenocarcinoma of the endometrium: a clinicopathologic and histochemical study. *Am J Surg Pathol.* 1983;7:715-729.

56. Saito J, Fukuda T, Hoshiai H, et al. High-risk types of human papillomavirus associated with the progression of cervical dysplasia to carcinoma. *J Obstet Gynaecol Res.* 1999;25: 281-286.

57. Saitoh A, Tsutsumi Y, Osamura RY, et al. Sclerosing stromal tumor of the ovary. Immunohistochemical and electron microscopic demonstration of smooth-muscle differentiation. *Arch Pathol Lab Med.* 1989;113:372-376.

58. Scurry J, Whitehead J. Healey M. Histology of lichen sclerosus varies according to site and proximity to carcinoma. *Am J Dermatopathol.* 2001;23:413-418.

59. Seidman JD, Kurman RJ. Subclassification of serous borderline tumors of the ovary into benign and malignant types—a clinicopathologic study of 65 advanced stage cases. *Am J Surg Pathol.* 1996;20:1331-1345.

60. Shen K, Wu P-C, Lang J-H, et al. Ovarian sex cord tumor with annular tubules: a report of six cases. *Gynecol Oncol.* 1993;48:180-184.

61. Shih IM, Kurman RJ. The pathology of intermediate trophoblastic tumors and tumor-like lesions. *Int J Gynecol Pathol.* 2001;20:31-47.

62. Silverberg SG. Problems in the differential diagnosis of endometrial hyperplasia and carcinoma. *Mod Pathol*. 2000; 13:309-327.

63. Steeper TA, Rosai J. Aggressive angiomyxoma of the female pelvis and perineum. Report of nine cases of a distinctive type of gynecologic soft-tissue neoplasm. *Am J Surg Pathol*. 1983;7:463-475.

64. Stoler MH, Mills SE, Gersell DH, et al. Small-cell neuroendocrine carcinoma of the cervix. A human papillomavirus type 18-associated cancer. *Am J Surg Pathol*. 1991;15: 28-32.

65. Stoler MH. Human papillomaviruses and cervical neoplasia: a model for carcinogenesis. *Int J Gynecol Pathol*. 2000; 19:16-28.

66. Szulman AE. Examination of the early conceptus. *Arch Pathol Lab Med*. 1991;115:696-700.

67. Tanaka Y, Sasaki Y, Nishihira H, et al. Ovarian juvenile granulosa cell tumor associated with Maffucci's syndrome. *Am J Clin Pathol*. 1992;97:523-527.

68. Trebeck CE, Friedlander ML, Russell P, et al. Brenner tumours of the ovary: a study of the histology, immunohistochemistry and cellular DNA content in benign, borderline and malignant ovarian tumors. *Pathology*. 1987;19:241-246.

69. van Bogaert L-J. Clinicopathologic findings in endometrial polyps. *Obstet Gynecol*. 1988;71:771-773.

70. Vang R, Whitaker BP, Farhood A, et al. Immunohistochemical analysis of clear cell carcinoma of the gynecologic tract. *Int J Gynecol Pathol*. 2001;20:252-259.

71. Wong PC, Ferenczy A, Fan LD, et al. Krukenberg tumors of the ovary. Ultrastructural, histochemical an immunohistochemical studies of 15 cases. *Cancer*. 1986;57:751-760.

72. Young RH, Hart WR. Metastases from carcinomas of the pancreas simulating primary mucinous tumors of the ovary: a report of seven cases. *Am J Surg Pathol*. 1989;13: 748-756.

73. Young RH, Kurman RJ, Scully RE. Placental site nodules and plaques: a clinicopathologic analysis of 20 cases. *Am J Surg Pathol*. 1990;14:1001-1009.

74. Young RH, Scully RE. Fibromatosis and massive edema of the ovary, possibly related entities: a report or 14 cases of fibromatosis and 11 cases of massive edema. *Int J Gynecol Pathol*. 1984;3:153-178.

75. Young RH, Scully RE. Metastatic tumors in the ovary: a problem-oriented approach and review of the recent literature. *Semin Diagn Pathol*. 1991;8:250-276.

76. Young RH, Scully RE. Ovarian Sertoli-Leydig cell tumors a clinicopathological analysis of 207 cases. *Am J Surg Pathol*. 1985;9:543-569.

77. Young RH, Scully RE. Invasive adenocarcinoma and related tumors of the uterine cervix. *Semin Diagn Pathol*. 1990;7: 205-227.

78. Young RH, Welch WR, Dickersin GR, et al. Ovarian sex cord tumor with annular tubules: review of 74 cases including 27 with Peutz-Jeghers syndrome and four with adenoma malignum of the cervix. *Cancer*. 1982;50:1384-1402.

79. Zaloudek CJ, Norris HJ. Adenofibroma and adenosarcoma of the uterus. A clinicopathologic study of 35 cases. *Cancer*. 1981;48:354-366.

CHAPTER 16

HEAD AND NECK PATHOLOGY

1. A 61-year-old man presents with a parotid mass, and an excision is performed (see Figure 16-1). All of the following are true regarding this lesion except

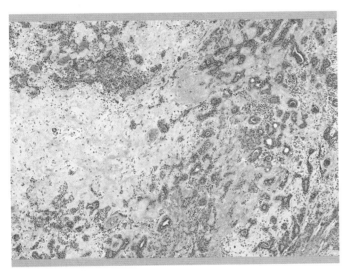

FIGURE 16-1

(A) Enucleation of the nodule is the treatment of choice
(B) Immunohistochemical staining for S-100 and p63 will be positive in a subset of cells
(C) Most common salivary gland neoplasm
(D) Recurrence generally results in multiple discontinuous nodules in the operative site
(E) The presence of necrosis and hyalinization is concerning for transformation to malignancy

2. A patient presents with a parotid mass, which is excised (see Figure 16-2). What is the most likely clinical history associated with this lesion?

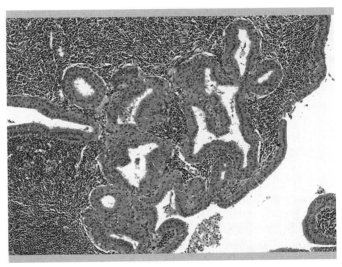

FIGURE 16-2

(A) A 12-year-old girl with slow growing mass associated with facial nerve paralysis
(B) A 47-year-old woman with dry mouth and dry eyes
(C) A 48-year-old man with a tonsil mass
(D) A 50-year-old man with human immunodeficiency virus (HIV) infection
(E) A 60-year-old man with heavy smoking history

3. A 46-year-old woman presents with a parotid mass, and a superficial parotidectomy is performed (see Figure 16-3). What genetic abnormality is commonly present in these tumors?

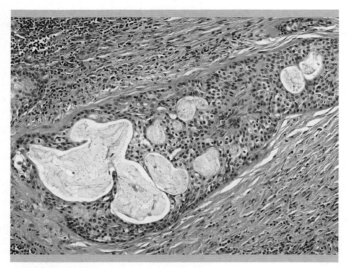

FIGURE 16-3

(A) t(2;13)(q35;q14) PAX3–FOXO1 fusion
(B) t(11;19)(q21;p13) MECT1–MAML2 fusion
(C) t(12;15) (p13;q25) ETV6–NTRK3 fusion
(D) t(12;22)(q13;q12) ATF1–EWSR1 fusion
(E) t(15;19) (q13;p13) NUT–BRD4 fusion

4. A 32-year-old woman has a radiolucent well-circumscribed unilocular cyst of the posterior mandible associated with an unerupted wisdom tooth on x-ray films. Curettage is performed (see Figure 16-4). What genetic syndrome is this lesion associated with?

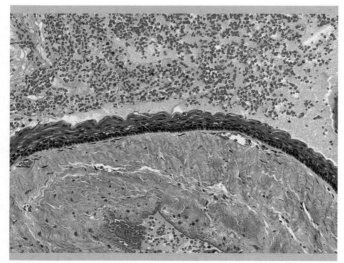

FIGURE 16-4

(A) Cowden's syndrome
(B) Hereditary breast and ovarian carcinoma syndrome (*BRCA1*)
(C) Hereditary nonpolyposis colorectal carcinoma syndrome (Lynch syndrome)
(D) Nevoid basal cell carcinoma syndrome (Gorlin syndrome)
(E) von Hippel–Lindau syndrome (*VHL*)

5. A 36-year-old woman presents with a mass in the posterior jaw. Imaging shows a multiloculated cyst with a "soap-bubble" appearance in the posterior mandible, which is associated with an impacted tooth. A biopsy is performed (see Figure 16-5). Which of the following statements is true regarding this lesion?

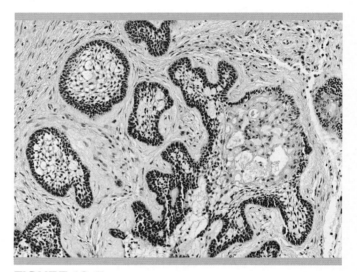

FIGURE 16-5

(A) Curettage is the treatment of choice to prevent fractures
(B) Recurrence rate is <10% for conventional-type tumors
(C) The presence of severe cytologic atypia does not affect prognosis
(D) The unicystic type has a worse prognosis
(E) Tumors are considered "malignant" only with documented metastasis

6. A 52-year-old man has the following process on a sinonasal biopsy (see Figure 16-6). What is the most likely clinical history associated with this process?

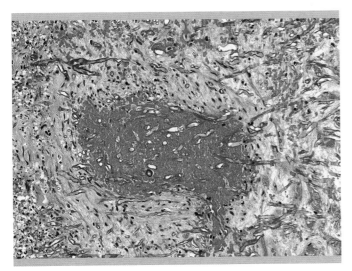

FIGURE 16-6

(A) Chronic sinusitis refractory to medical therapy and increased peripheral blood IgE
(B) Diabetic who presented with headache and vision changes
(C) Epistaxis, hemoptysis, and destructive septal lesion
(D) Nasal obstruction with large polyp arising from the nasopharynx
(E) Woodworker with large destructive mass of the nasal cavity

7. A 68-year-old man with no significant past medical history presents with facial pain and a parotid mass. An excision is performed (see Figure 16-7). Which of the following statements is true regarding this lesion?

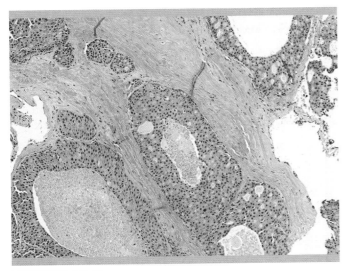

FIGURE 16-7

(A) Gross cystic disease fluid protein 15 (GCDFP-15) staining is positive in most tumors
(B) Immunohistochemical staining with HER-2 will be negative in most tumors
(C) Likely represents metastasis from an occult breast primary
(D) Most tumors are estrogen receptor and progesterone receptor positive
(E) Overall prognosis is good, with >80% 5-year survival

8. A 15-year-old girl presents with visual disturbance, and imaging shows an area of maxillary bone expansion causing nerve compression. A biopsy of the abnormal bone is performed (see Figure 16-8). Which of the following statements regarding this lesion is true?

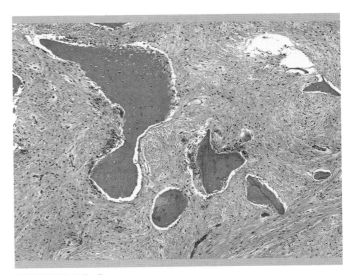

FIGURE 16-8

(A) High risk of transformation to osteosarcoma requires complete surgical excision
(B) Monostotic type may be associated with endocrinopathies (e.g., growth hormone excess)
(C) Mutations in cAMP G-protein are present in most polyostotic cases
(D) Osteoblastic rimming of the bone trabeculae is characteristic
(E) Radiologic imaging typically shows an area of sharply demarcated radiolucency

9. A 63-year-old woman presents with a submandibular gland mass, which is excised (see Figure 16-9). Which of the following stains/markers will be positive in the clear cell population of tumor cells?

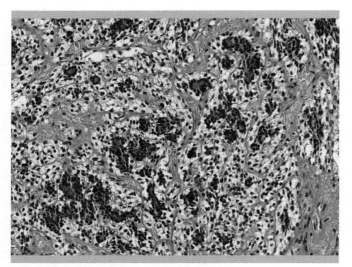

FIGURE 16-9

   (A) Calponin
   (B) Epithelial membrane antigen (EMA)
   (C) P53
   (D) Periodic acid Schiff with diastase (PASD)
   (E) Renal cell carcinoma (RCC) antigen

10. A 47-year-old man presents with chronic sinusitis. Endoscopic sinus surgery is performed, and the following material is removed from the maxillary sinus (see Figure 16-10). Which of the following statements is incorrect regarding this process?

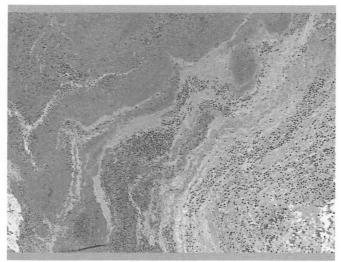

FIGURE 16-10

   (A) Aggressive therapy is warranted due to high mortality from this process
   (B) Charcot-Leyden crystals are almost always seen
   (C) Grossly, the material is thick and putty-like
   (D) Most commonly associated with *Aspergillus*
   (E) Peripheral blood eosinophilia may be present

11. A 42-year-old man presents with a palate mass, and undergoes excisional biopsy. The lesion is largely cystic, and shows the following morphologic appearance (see Figure 16-11). What is the most likely diagnosis?

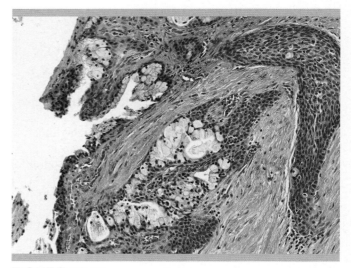

FIGURE 16-11

   (A) High-grade mucoepidermoid carcinoma
   (B) Low-grade mucoepidermoid carcinoma
   (C) Necrotizing sialometaplasia
   (D) Pleomorphic adenoma with squamous metaplasia
   (E) Squamous cell carcinoma

12. A 23-year-old man presents with sinusitis, chest pain, cough, bloody urine, and epistaxis. An ulcerated lesion of the nasal septum is biopsied (see Figure 16-12). All of the following statements are true regarding this process except

FIGURE 16-12

(A) Elevated serum antineutrophil cytoplasmic antibody (ANCA) is characteristic
(B) Nasal cavity is the most frequently involved site of the upper aerodigestive tract
(C) Pathologic triad of vasculitis, granulomatous inflammation, and necrosis is seen in a minority of cases
(D) Septal perforation may result in a "saddle nose" deformity
(E) The target antigen of the ANCA antibody is myeloperoxidase (MPO)

13. A 62-year-old man presents with nasal obstruction; a biopsy is performed (see Figure 16-13). All of the following statements are correct about this process except

(A) High-grade adenocarcinoma is the most common form of malignant transformation
(B) Local invasion can result in bony destruction
(C) Most common location is along the lateral nasal wall
(D) Over 80% are unilateral
(E) Up to 40% have been associated with low-risk human papilloma virus (lr-HPV) infection

14. A 70-year-old woman presents with hoarseness, and a mass in the supraglottic larynx is identified and biopsied (see Figure 16-14). Over 4 mitotic figures are identified in 10 high-power fields. All of the following immunohistochemical stains are likely to be positive in this tumor except

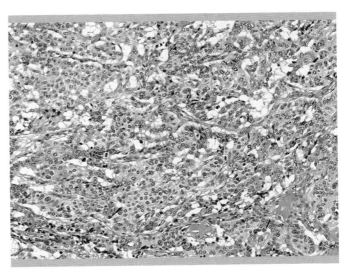

FIGURE 16-14

(A) Calcitonin
(B) CD56
(C) Cytokeratin
(D) S-100
(E) Synaptophysin

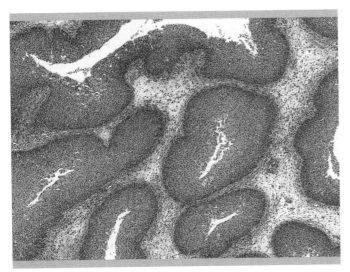

FIGURE 16-13

15. A 42-year-old woman presents with an upper lip mass that is mobile, slowly enlarging, and submucosal. An excision is performed (see Figure 16-15). Which immunohistochemical stain is most likely to be positive in the majority of tumor cells?

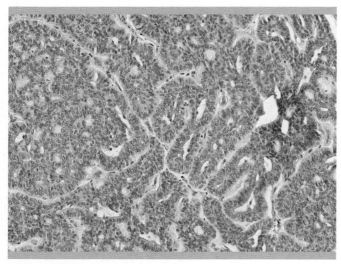

FIGURE 16-15

(A) Calponin
(B) p16
(C) S-100
(D) Smooth muscle actin (SMA)
(E) Thyroid transcription factor 1 (TTF-1)

16. A 38-year-old woman presents with a 0.5 cm polypoid anterior maxillary gingival mass, and a biopsy is performed (see Figure 16-16). What other condition does this woman most likely have?

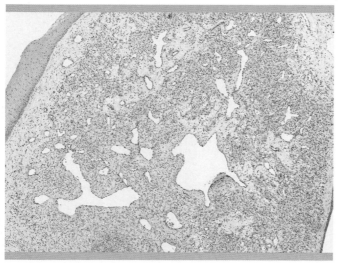

FIGURE 16-16

(A) Dentures causing trauma to the area
(B) Gorlin syndrome
(C) Heavy smoking history
(D) Human immunodeficiency virus (HIV) infection
(E) Pregnancy

17. An 11-year-old boy presents with hoarseness and stridor. Direct laryngoscopy shows multiple papillary frond-like lesions involving the vocal cord and trachea. A biopsy is performed (see Figure 16-17). What virus is this process most commonly associated with?

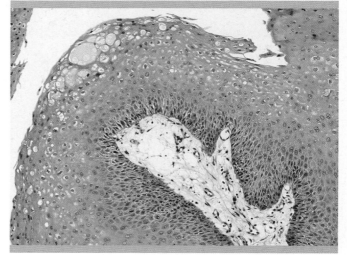

FIGURE 16-17

(A) Epstein–Barr virus (EBV)
(B) High-risk human papilloma virus (hr-HPV)
(C) Human herpesvirus 8 (HHV-8)
(D) Human immunodeficiency virus (HIV)
(E) Low risk human papilloma virus (lr-HPV)

18. A 42-year-old man presents with a dorsal tongue mass. An incisional biopsy is performed (see Figure 16-18). All of the following stains will be positive in the neoplastic cells except

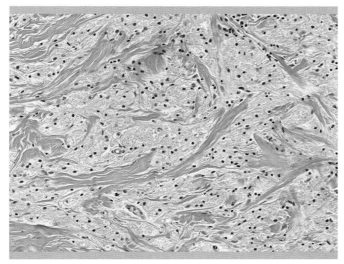

FIGURE 16-18

(A) CD68
(B) Desmin
(C) Periodic acid Schiff with diastase (PASD)
(D) S-100
(E) Vimentin

19. A 42-year-old woman presents with an asymptomatic, slowly enlarging neck mass. Imaging shows a mass at the level of the carotid artery bifurcation. An excision is performed (see Figure 16-19). All of the following are true regarding this lesion except

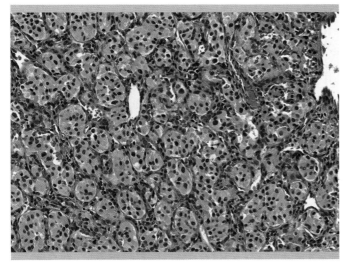

FIGURE 16-19

(A) Associated with multiple endocrine neoplasia 2 (MEN 2)
(B) Associated with mutations in succinate dehydrogenase
(C) Biopsy is recommended prior to excision to plan extent of resection
(D) S-100 staining will highlight sustentacular cells
(E) The only criteria for malignancy is metastasis

20. A 68-year-old man presents with hoarseness, and a mass is identified in the vocal cord. A biopsy is performed (see Figure 16-20). All of the following statements are true regarding this lesion except

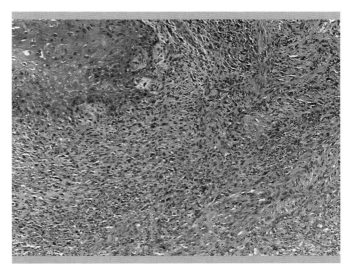

FIGURE 16-20

(A) Areas of classical squamous cell carcinoma can be identified in most cases
(B) Epithelial markers are negative within the spindle cells in up to 30% of cases
(C) Not associated with tobacco smoking
(D) Prognosis is good, with over 80% 5-year survival
(E) Vast majority are polypoid and/or pedunculated

21. A 38-year-old man presents with a neck mass located in the lateral neck, which on imaging is cystic. The lesion is excised and is composed of a unilocular cyst with the following appearance (see Figure 16-21). What is the most likely origin of this cyst?

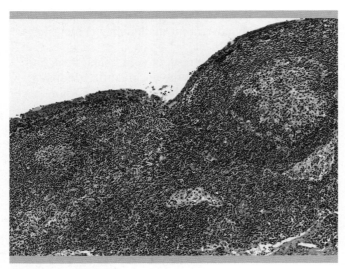

FIGURE 16-21

(A) Acquired inclusion cyst
(B) Cystic lymph node metastasis
(C) First branchial apparatus
(D) Second branchial apparatus
(E) Thyroglossal duct remnant

22. A 32-year-old man with a recent diagnosis of human immunodeficiency (HIV) syndrome presents with leukoplakia along the lateral borders of his tongue. A biopsy is performed (see Figure 16-22). What other virus is this process associated with?

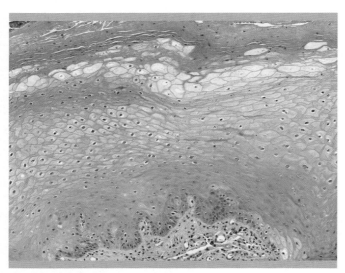

FIGURE 16-22

(A) Epstein–Barr virus (EBV)
(B) Human herpesvirus 8 (HHV-8)
(C) High risk human papilloma virus (hr-HPV)
(D) Human T-cell leukemia virus 1 (HTLV-1)
(E) Low risk human papilloma virus (lr-HPV)

23. A 58-year-old woman presents with facial pain and a mass in the parotid gland, which is excised (see Figure 16-23). All of the following statements are true regarding this lesion except

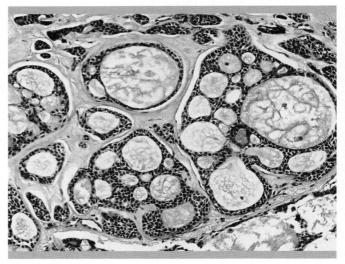

FIGURE 16-23

(A) More than 30% solid component is associated with a worse prognosis
(B) The 5-year overall survival is good (>70%)
(C) The amorphous pink material is a product of luminal secretions
(D) The most common site of distant metastasis is lung
(E) Two distinct cell types (ductal and myoepithelial) are present

24. A 62-year-old man presents with a neck mass, and excisional biopsy is performed (see Figure 16-24). All of the following statements are true regarding this lesion except

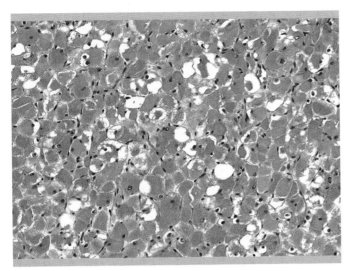

FIGURE 16-24

(A) Associated with tuberous sclerosis
(B) Cytoplasmic cross striations are characteristic
(C) Immunohistochemistry for myoglobin and desmin are positive
(D) Over 70% of the adult type occur in the head and neck
(E) Positive cytoplasmic staining with periodic acid Schiff (PAS) stain is seen, which is lost with diastase

25. A 46-year-old woman presents with a parotid mass. An excisional biopsy is performed (see Figure 16-25). Which of the following ancillary tests would be most helpful in confirming the diagnosis?

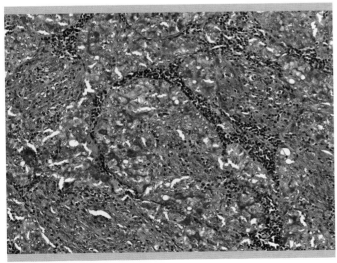

FIGURE 16-25

(A) Calponin
(B) CD117 (c-kit)
(C) Fontana–Masson
(D) Mucicarmine
(E) Periodic acid Schiff with diastase (PASD)

26. A 55-year-old man presents with a mass in the posterior neck. A biopsy is performed (see Figure 16-26). Which of the following immunohistochemical stains will be strongly positive in the spindle cells?

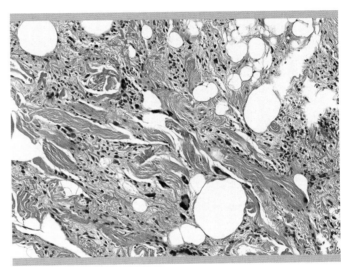

FIGURE 16-26

(A) CD31
(B) CD34
(C) Epithelial membrane antigen
(D) S-100
(E) Smooth muscle actin

27. A 50-year-old man from China presents with nasal septal destruction and palate perforation. A biopsy is performed, which shows an angiocentric and angiodestructive pattern of atypical cells (see Figure 16-27). Immunohistochemical stains for CD56 and granzyme B are positive within the atypical cells. What infectious agent is this process highly associated with?

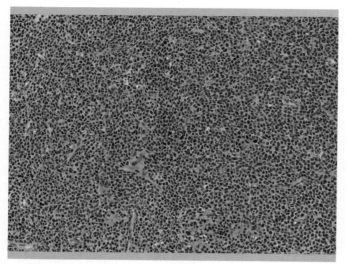

FIGURE 16-27

(A) Epstein–Barr virus (EBV)
(B) Human herpesvirus 8 (HHV-8)
(C) Human immunodeficiency virus (HIV)
(D) Human papilloma virus (HPV)
(E) Human T-cell leukemia virus 1 (HTLV-1)

28. A 32-year-old woman presents with a cystic neck mass, which is excised (see Figure 16-28). What clinical history did she most likely present with?

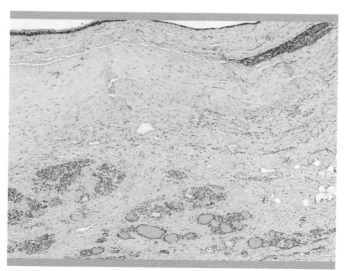

FIGURE 16-28

(A) Lateral neck mass along anterior border of the sternocleidomastoid muscle
(B) Lateral neck mass and simultaneous large exophytic tonsillar mass
(C) Lateral neck mass that is pulsatile and causes fainting when manipulated
(D) Midline neck mass that arises from the thyroid cartilage
(E) Midline neck mass that moves with swallowing

29. A 72-year-old woman presents with nasal obstruction and headache, and a 3 cm nasal mass is excised (see Figure 16-29). The majority of the tumor cells (small bland spindle cells) will be positive for which immunohistochemical stain?

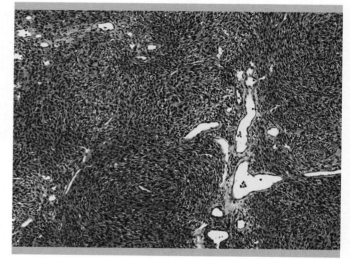

FIGURE 16-29

(A) Androgen receptor (AR)
(B) CD34
(C) Desmin
(D) Epithelial membrane antigen (EMA)
(E) Smooth muscle actin (SMA)

30. A 45-year-old man presents with unilateral hearing loss, and a mass is seen on imaging in the middle ear. Excisional biopsy is performed (see Figure 16-30). All of the following statements are true regarding this lesion except

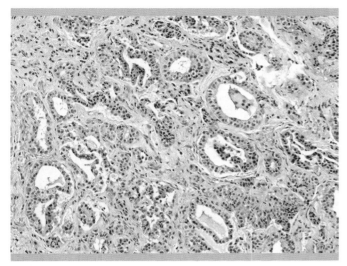

FIGURE 16-30

(A) Complete excision is the treatment of choice
(B) Good prognosis, with infrequent local recurrences and no metastatic potential
(C) Immunohistochemical staining for cytokeratin 7 and synaptophysin will be positive in most cases
(D) Mastoid bone and ossicle destruction on imaging is characteristic
(E) Tumor nests can have a pseudoinfiltrative appearance

31. A 45-year-old man with no past medical problems presents with nasal obstruction and epistaxis. A nasal mass arising in the ethmoid sinus is biopsied (see Figure 16-31). All of the following are true regarding this neoplasm except

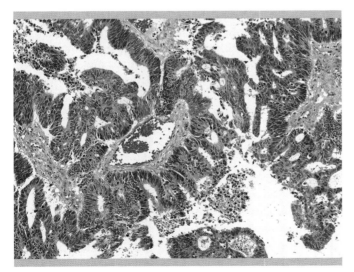

FIGURE 16-31

(A) An occult colorectal carcinoma metastasis should be excluded clinically
(B) Associated with woodworking and leather working professions
(C) Immunohistochemical staining for cytokeratin 20 and CDX2 is negative in the majority of cases
(D) Prognosis is poor, with <50% 5-year survival
(E) The papillary subtype has a better prognosis than other morphologic patterns

32. A 52-year-old woman presents to her physician complaining of hearing a clicking in her ear that is in time with her heartbeat. A computed tomography (CT) scan shows a mass in the middle ear. An excision is performed (see Figure 16-32). What immunohistochemical stain will be positive within the neoplastic cells?

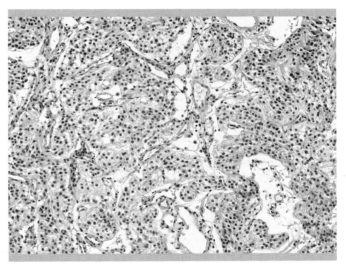

FIGURE 16-32

(A) Calponin
(B) CD34
(C) Cytokeratin
(D) Epithelial membrane antigen
(E) Synaptophysin

33. A 37-year-old man presents with vertigo, tinnitus, and hearing loss. Imaging demonstrates a destructive mass within the inner ear, middle ear, and cerebellopontine angle. A biopsy is performed (see Figure 16-33). What genetic syndrome is this lesion associated with?

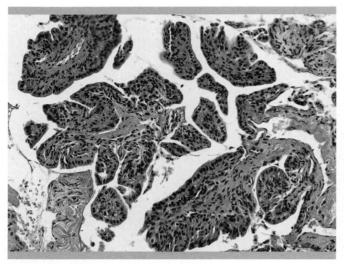

FIGURE 16-33

   (A) Cowden's syndrome
   (B) Familial adenomatosis polyposis (FAP) syndrome
   (C) Multiple endocrine neoplasia 2a (MEN 2a)
   (D) Neurofibromatosis 1 (NF-1)
   (E) von Hippel–Lindau syndrome (VHL)

34. A 44-year-old woman presents with dysphasia, and exam shows a nodular red mass in the base of tongue. A biopsy is performed (see Figure 16-34). What other clinically important finding is this woman likely to have?

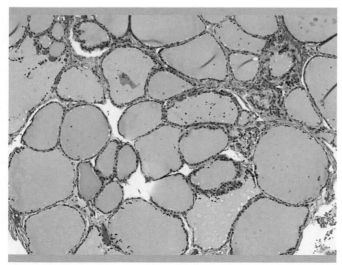

FIGURE 16-34

   (A) Absent thyroid gland
   (B) Branchial cleft cyst
   (C) DiGeorge syndrome
   (D) Elevated peripheral blood calcitonin level
   (E) Malignant tumor in the thyroid gland

35. A recent immigrant from Taiwan presents with a neck mass, and a nasopharyngeal lesion is biopsied (see Figure 16-35). What infectious agent is this process highly associated with?

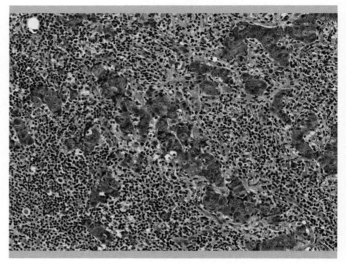

FIGURE 16-35

   (A) Epstein–Barr virus (EBV)
   (B) Human herpesvirus 8 (HHV-8)
   (C) Human immunodeficiency virus (HIV)
   (D) Human papilloma virus (HPV)
   (E) Human T-cell leukemia virus 1 (HTLV-1)

36. A 61-year-old woman presents with nasal obstruction, and a polypoid mass arising from the anterior nasal septum is found. A biopsy is performed and is consistent with sinonasal malignant melanoma (see Figure 16-36). No skin lesions are identified. Which of the following statements is true regarding this lesion?

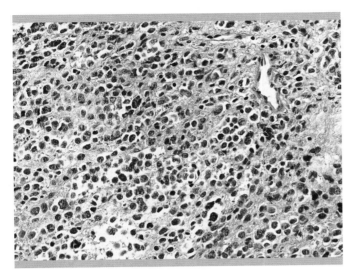

FIGURE 16-36

(A) Clark's level and Breslow thickness are important to report
(B) Fontana–Masson staining will be positive
(C) Immunohistochemical staining for S-100 will highlight sustentacular cells
(D) More common in Caucasian patients with heavy sun exposure
(E) Pagetoid spread along mucosal epithelium is helpful in confirming metastasis

37. A 58-year-old man presents with anosmia and nasal obstruction. A dumbbell-shaped mass involving the nasal cavity and intracranial fossa is found, and a biopsy is performed (see Figure 16-37). Which of the following statements is correct regarding this process?

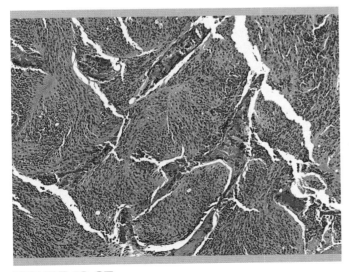

FIGURE 16-37

(A) Almost all tumors involve the maxillary sinus
(B) Believed to arise from specialized sensory neuroepithelium
(C) Flexner–Wintersteiner rosettes are seen in grade 1 and 2 tumors only
(D) Immunohistochemical staining for S-100 is diffusely positive in the neoplastic cells.
(E) *MYC* amplification is seen in almost all cases

38. A 41-year-old woman presents with nasal obstruction. Biopsy of a nasopharyngeal mass is performed, and is diagnosed as a nasopharyngeal papillary adenocarcinoma. There is no radiologic evidence of another site of origin (lung or thyroid). Which of the following statements is true regarding this neoplasm?
(A) Associated with Epstein-Barr virus (EBV)
(B) Metastasis occurs in over 40% of cases
(C) Nuclear pseudoinclusions are easily identified
(D) Positive for thyroid transcription factor 1 (TTF-1)
(E) Positive for thyroglobulin (TG)

39. A recent immigrant from central Africa has had chronic sinus drainage and a mass causing nasal obstruction. A biopsy is diagnosed as rhinoscleroma. What is the causative agent for this process?
(A) *Aspergillus fumigatus*
(B) Epstein–Barr virus
(C) Human papilloma virus
(D) *Klebsiella rhinoscleromatis*
(E) *Rhinosporidium seeberi*

40. A 38-year-old woman presents with several yellow, 2 mm papules on her buccal mucosa that were noticed by her dentist. A biopsy is performed and demonstrates nests of sebaceous glands in the submucosa. What is the best diagnosis for this lesion?
(A) Fordyce granules
(B) Juxtaoral organ of Chievitz
(C) Lingual thyroid
(D) Oral hairy leukoplakia
(E) Ranula

41. A 45-year-old woman presents with dry mouth and dry eyes. A lower lip minor salivary gland biopsy is performed and shows several lymphoid aggregates in each lobule. What serologic test is the most specific for this disease?
(A) Elevated erythrocyte sedimentation rate (ESR)
(B) Positive antineutrophil cytoplasmic antibody (ANCA)
(C) Positive antinuclear antibody (ANA)
(D) Positive anti-SSB (anti-La)
(E) Positive double-stranded DNA antibody (anti-dsDNA)

42. A 74-year-old man presents with a parotid mass that recently rapidly increased in size. A total parotidectomy is performed and demonstrates a carcinoma ex pleomorphic adenoma. All of the following statements are true regarding this lesion except
    (A) Any malignant salivary gland tumor type can be seen as part of this tumor
    (B) Lung metastases may have the appearance of a benign pleomorphic adenoma
    (C) Minimally invasive and noninvasive (encapsulated) tumors are associated with a better prognosis
    (D) Minimally invasive tumors must show <1.5 mm of invasion beyond the tumor capsule
    (E) The histologic subtype of malignant tumor present is important for prognosis

43. A 14-year-old girl is diagnosed with dysgenetic polycystic disease of the parotid gland. Which of the following is true regarding this lesion?
    (A) Associated with adult polycystic kidney disease
    (B) Complete resection is required to prevent malignant transformation
    (C) Occurs almost exclusively in women
    (D) Secondary to large duct obstruction by a sialolith
    (E) Swelling worsens with eating

44. All of the following immunohistochemical stains will be positive in myoepithelial cells of salivary gland origin except
    (A) Calponin
    (B) Carcinoembryonic antigen (CEA)
    (C) Pancytokeratin
    (D) S-100
    (E) Smooth muscle actin (SMA)

45. A 43-year-old woman presents with a mass in the tongue, and biopsy demonstrates a malignant neoplasm composed of infiltrating nests of cells with abundant clear cytoplasm in a dense hyalinized stroma. All of the following salivary gland tumors can have prominent clear cell change except
    (A) Adenoid cystic carcinoma
    (B) Clear cell carcinoma of salivary gland origin
    (C) Epithelial–myoepithelial carcinoma
    (D) Mucoepidermoid carcinoma
    (E) Myoepithelioma

46. A 6-year-old boy presents with a radiodense irregular lesion in the maxilla on routine dental x-ray. Biopsy shows an admixture of dentin, enamel matrix, and cementum, forming small irregular toothlike structures. All of the following statements are true regarding this lesion except
    (A) Complex lesions are characterized by recognizable tooth formation
    (B) Compound lesions most often occur in the anterior maxilla
    (C) Considered a hamartoma of odontogenic origin
    (D) Most common odontogenic lesion
    (E) Simple excision is the treatment of choice given the absence of local recurrence in these lesions

47. A 25-year-old man presents with a rapidly enlarging mass in the neck. What histologic findings would be diagnostic of nodular fasciitis?
    (A) Epithelioid and spindled cells with marked nuclear pleomorphism and atypical mitotic figures
    (B) Highly cellular spindle cell proliferation with a herringbone appearance
    (C) Rhabdoid cells with atypical mitotic figures
    (D) Tissue culture-like plump myofibroblasts in a background of inflammation and extravasated erythrocytes
    (E) Wavy spindle cells with varying hypocellular and hypercellular areas and palisaded nuclei

48. A man presents with recurrent epistaxis, and is found to have a large nasopharyngeal mass. Excisional biopsy shows large- to medium-sized disorganized vessels within a fibrous stroma; the vessels have variably thickened walls with a smooth muscle component. Which of the following statements is accurate regarding this lesion?
    (A) Biopsy is recommended prior to complete excision
    (B) Estrogen receptor is positive in the stromal cells
    (C) Metastasis occurs in over 25% of patients
    (D) Most commonly occurs in males under 20 years of age
    (E) Radiation is the treatment of choice

49. A 48-year-old man presents with multiple enlarged neck lymph nodes, and a fine needle aspiration biopsy is consistent with metastatic nonkeratinizing squamous cell carcinoma. Immunohistochemical staining with p16 is positive in the tumor cells. What is the most likely site of the primary squamous cell carcinoma?
    (A) Base of tongue
    (B) Esophagus
    (C) Floor of mouth
    (D) Nasopharynx
    (E) True vocal cord

50. A 12-year-old boy presents with a large mass in the nasal cavity, which on biopsy is composed of an undifferentiated carcinoma with focal areas of squamous differentiation. No mucocytes are identified. Immunohistochemical staining for cytokeratin 7 and p63 is positive, and negative for smooth muscle actin and S-100. What molecular alteration is most likely present in this tumor?
    (A) t(11;19)(q21;p13) MECT1–MAML2 fusion
    (B) t(11;22)(p13:q12) EWS–WT1 fusion
    (C) t(11;22)(q24;q12) EWS–FLI1 fusion
    (D) t(15;19) (q13;p13.1) NUT–BRD4 fusion
    (E) t(2;13)(q35;q14) PAX3–FOXO1 fusion

51. Which of these environmental exposures is not associated with the development of squamous cell carcinoma of the upper aerodigestive tract?
    (A) Alcohol use
    (B) Betel quid (betel leaf) use
    (C) High-fat diet
    (D) Radiation exposure
    (E) Tobacco use

52. A 50-year-old man presents with an orbital mass, causing headaches and diplopia. A biopsy is interpreted as extrapulmonary solitary fibrous tumor. All of the following are features of solitary fibrous tumor except
    (A) Bland spindle cells with hypocellular and hypercellular areas
    (B) Immunohistochemical staining for CD99
    (C) Palisading of spindle cell nuclei
    (D) Thick bands of keloid-like hyalinized collagen
    (E) Thin-walled staghorn-shaped vessels

53. A 51-year-old man presents with a squamous cell carcinoma of the tonsil that is positive for high-risk human papilloma virus (hr-HPV). All of the following statements regarding this process are true except
    (A) Immunohistochemical staining for p16 will be strong and diffuse
    (B) Lymph node metastases are frequently cystic
    (C) Prognosis is better than non-HPV-associated squamous cell carcinoma
    (D) The majority of patients present with high-stage disease (lymph node metastasis)
    (E) The most common high-risk HPV subtype in these tumors is HPV-18

54. An 82-year-old man with a scalp lesion is diagnosed with an atypical fibroxanthoma. All of the following are true regarding this lesion except
    (A) Atypical mitotic figures can be seen
    (B) Depth of invasion does not affect prognosis
    (C) Exclusion of melanoma and spindle cell carcinoma by immunohistochemistry is required for diagnosis
    (D) Good prognosis, with very low rate of local recurrence and metastasis
    (E) Morphologically is a poorly differentiated neoplasm with marked pleomorphism and atypia

55. A 34-year-old man presents with a unilocular radiolucent cyst in the posterior mandible, which is associated with a tooth. Which of the following findings would favor a dentigerous cyst over a periapical (radicular) cyst?
    (A) Abundant acute and chronic inflammation is present
    (B) Associated with a nonvital tooth
    (C) Cyst surrounds the crown of an impacted wisdom tooth
    (D) Radiologic evidence of tooth root absorption is present
    (E) Squamous epithelium lining the cyst wall

56. A 54-year-old woman presents with leukoplakia of her tongue. All of the following can clinically appear as leukoplakia on the tongue except
    (A) Amalgam tattoo
    (B) Frictional hyperkeratosis
    (C) Keratinizing squamous dysplasia
    (D) Lichen planus
    (E) Mucosal candidiasis

57. A 61-year-old man presents with bilateral ears that are red-purple, swollen, and tender. His nose is also red and tender. A biopsy demonstrates necrotic cartilage in association with a mixed inflammatory infiltrate composed of neutrophils, lymphocytes, plasma cells, and eosinophils. Which of the following statements is true regarding this disorder?
    (A) Immunofluorescence will be negative for immunoglobulin deposition around cartilage
    (B) Leading cause of death is airway compromise due to laryngotracheal collapse
    (C) Mutually exclusive with other autoimmune disorders, such as rheumatoid arthritis
    (D) Postulated etiology is autoimmune antibodies to type IV collagen
    (E) The acute phase is characterized by floppy ears and saddle nose deformity

58. A 64-year-old man presents with stridor, and a 5 cm mass is found in the posterior larynx, arising from the cricoid cartilage. A biopsy demonstrates cartilage with increased cellularity and mild nuclear atypia. What is the most likely diagnosis?
    (A) Chondrometaplasia
    (B) Extraskeletal mesenchymal chondrosarcoma
    (C) Laryngeal chondroma
    (D) Pleomorphic adenoma
    (E) Low-grade chondrosarcoma

59. A 34-year-old opera singer presents with hoarseness. Clinical exam shows a lesion along the anterior one-third of the true vocal cord, and he is clinically diagnosed with a vocal cord nodule. What histologic findings would you expect to see with this lesion?
    (A) Abundant granulation tissue with surface ulceration and fibrinoid necrosis
    (B) Infiltrative squamous nests with marked nuclear pleomorphism
    (C) Plump polygonal cells with abundant granular eosinophilic cytoplasm
    (D) Submucosal amorphous eosinophilic material that is positive on Congo red stain
    (E) Submucosal edematous, myxoid stroma with dilated vessels and hemorrhage

60. A 53-year-old man presents with an ulcer on the hard palate. The biopsy demonstrates numerous squamous nests within the submucosa, admixed with minor salivary gland acini. All of the following features would favor a diagnosis of necrotizing sialometaplasia over invasive squamous cell carcinoma except
    (A) Acinar coagulative necrosis
    (B) Lack of nuclear atypia
    (C) Lobular architecture
    (D) Smooth borders to the squamous nests
    (E) Surface keratinizing squamous dysplasia

61. A 55-year-old man presents with an ear mass. A biopsy is performed, which shows a proliferation of small glands with apocrine change, yellow-brown pigment in the cytoplasm, and eosinophilic secretions in the lumens. Immunohistochemical stains demonstrate a dual cell population with well-developed ductal and myoepithelial cells. What is the most likely site of this tumor?
    (A) Cerebellopontine angle
    (B) External ear canal
    (C) Inner ear/temporal bone
    (D) Middle ear
    (E) Parotid tail

62. A 74-year-old man is diagnosed with a verrucous carcinoma. Which of the following statements is true regarding this lesion?
    (A) Any component of conventional squamous cell carcinoma invasion alters prognosis
    (B) Characteristic findings are typically found on superficial biopsies
    (C) Associated with low risk human papilloma virus (lrPHV) infection.
    (D) Lymph node metastases are found in over 30% of patients
    (E) These lesions can show focal significant atypia and atypical mitotic figures

63. A 37-year-old woman presents with a mass on the anterior dorsal tongue, and is diagnosed with an ectomesenchymal chondromyxoid tumor. All of the following are pathologic features of this tumor except
    (A) Background myxoid to chondromyxoid stroma
    (B) Proliferation of uniform spindle and stellate cells
    (C) Strong staining for glial fibrillary acidic protein and cytokeratin
    (D) Strong staining for p63 and calponin
    (E) Well-circumscribed nodular growth pattern

64. An 11-year-old boy presents with a history of chronic otitis media and unilateral hearing loss. At surgery, his middle ear is filled with flaky keratin debris, and biopsy shows bland keratinizing squamous epithelium with a granular cell layer. All of the following statements are true regarding this process except
    (A) Congenital lesions are caused by a neoplastic proliferation of squamous epithelium
    (B) Destruction of the ossicular chain can occur, leading to hearing loss
    (C) Early treatment of otitis media in children can reduce the chance of developing this lesion
    (D) Local recurrence can occur in up to 20% of patients if incompletely excised
    (E) Tympanic membrane perforation is important in acquired lesions

65. A 45-year-old man is found to have an incidental polypoid mass in the superior nasal cavity; a biopsy is performed and shows brain tissue (see Figure 16-38). A connection with the intracranial cavity is not found on imaging or at the time of biopsy. What is the most likely explanation of these findings?

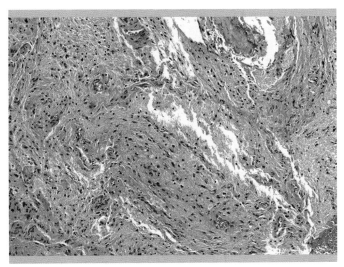

FIGURE 16-38

(A) Accidental intracranial biopsy
(B) Encephalocele
(C) Extension of intracranial glioma into the nasal cavity
(D) Metastatic glioblastoma
(E) Nasal glial heterotopia

66. A 7-year-old girl presents with a rapidly growing orbital mass, which is biopsied (see Figure 16-39). Which of the following statements is true regarding this lesion?

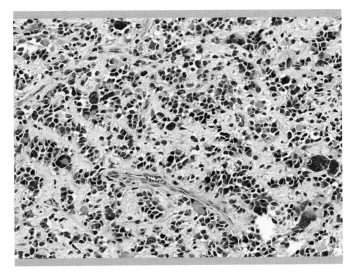

FIGURE 16-39

(A) A cambium layer is seen in the spindle cell variant
(B) Immunohistochemical staining for myogenin is positive in the tumor cytoplasm
(C) The alveolar subtype is associated with translocations involving the *FKHR* gene
(D) The embryonal subtype is associated with *PAX3* gene mutations
(E) Tumors with a t(1;13)(p36;q14) are more aggressive and have worse overall survival

67. A 50-year-old woman presents with headaches, and magnetic resonance imaging (MRI) demonstrates a mass within the sphenoid sinus. A biopsy was performed (see Figure 16-40). She also has symptoms of Cushing disease, but the MRI shows a normal pituitary. What immunohistochemical stain is most likely to be positive in this biopsy?

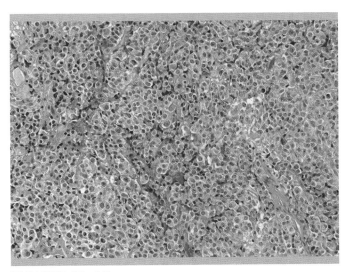

FIGURE 16-40

(A) Adrenocorticotropic hormone (ACTH)
(B) CD45
(C) Growth hormone (GH)
(D) HMB-45
(E) S-100

68. A 34-year-old man presents with hearing loss, and imaging shows a mass in the skull base. An excision is performed (see Figure 16-41). Which of the following statements is true regarding this lesion?

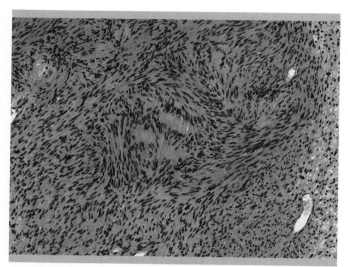

FIGURE 16-41

(A) Bilateral tumors are associated with neurofibromatosis 1
(B) Commonly arise from cranial nerve VIII
(C) Mass effect causes conductive hearing loss
(D) Neoplasm derived from neurons
(E) Strong and diffuse staining for synaptophysin

69. A 38-year-old man presents with headaches and a skull base mass is found and biopsied (see Figure 16-42). The cells are positive for epithelial membrane antigen (EMA) and S-100. What is the best diagnosis for this tumor?

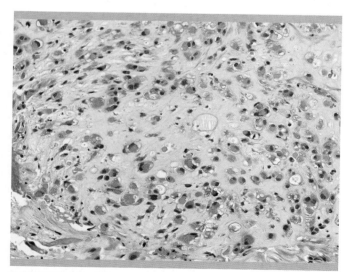

FIGURE 16-42

(A) Chordoma
(B) Chondrosarcoma
(C) Glioma, chordoid type
(D) Metastatic adenocarcinoma
(E) Rhabdomyosarcoma

70. A 44-year-old woman presents with a mass of the posterior neck, which has the following appearance (see Figure 16-43). Which of the following statements is true regarding this lesion?

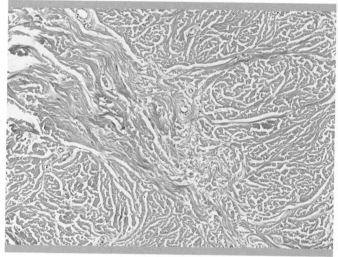

FIGURE 16-43

(A) Elastic fibers are a major component of this lesion
(B) Highly associated with Lynch syndrome
(C) Nuclear staining for β-catenin is positive in most cases
(D) Present as rapidly growing mass of short duration
(E) Spindle cells are positive for CD34 and pancytokeratin

71. A 32-year-old asymptomatic woman at routine dental x-rays is found to have a well-circumscribed radiolucent expansile lesion in the posterior mandible. Biopsy demonstrates spicules of bone with prominent osteoblastic rimming admixed with a cellular, fibrous stroma. Based on the imaging and microscopic appearance, what is the most likely diagnosis?
(A) Fibrous dysplasia
(B) Keratocystic odontogenic tumor
(C) Ossifying fibroma
(D) Osteoma
(E) Osteosarcoma

72. A 50-year-old man presents with bilateral cystic lesions of the parotid glands. An excisional biopsy is performed, and demonstrates multilocular lymphoepithelial cysts lined by squamous epithelium, associated with lymphoid hyperplasia and irregularly shaped germinal centers. What additional clinical history or clinical finding is most likely present?
    (A) Heavy smoking history
    (B) Human immunodeficiency virus (HIV) infection
    (C) Lung non-small cell carcinoma and enhancing nodules in the neck
    (D) Recent tuberculosis exposure and cough
    (E) Right tonsil enlargement due to an exophytic mass

73. A 2-month-old child has a large mass in the parotid gland, which on biopsy is diagnosed as a sialoblastoma. All of the following statements are true regarding this lesion except
    (A) Can be detected prenatally by ultrasound in many patients
    (B) Contains a mixture of ductal and myoepithelial cells
    (C) Distant metastases are common at presentation
    (D) Occurs exclusively in children under 2 years of age
    (E) The presence of anaplasia is a poor prognostic risk factor

74. A 3-month-old girl presents with a rapidly growing mass of the anterior maxillary alveolar ridge, which has a blue discoloration. A biopsy is performed, and is diagnosed as a melanotic neuroectodermal tumor of infancy (MNTI). All of the statements regarding this lesion are true except
    (A) Good prognosis, despite rapid growth and local destruction
    (B) Immunohistochemical staining is positive for multiple lineage markers (epithelial, melanocytic, and neural)
    (C) More than 90% of cases are diagnosed before 1 year of age
    (D) Necrosis and increased mitotic activity are associated with an increased risk of malignancy
    (E) Urinary vanilmandelic acid (VMA) is elevated in some cases

75. A 2-week-old baby girl has feeding difficulties, and her mother notices a mass on the anterior maxillary gingiva. Biopsy demonstrates a submucosal tumor composed of polygonal cells with abundant eosinophilic granular cytoplasm, which is CD68 positive, but negative for S-100 immunohistochemical staining. What is the best diagnosis for this tumor?
    (A) Alveolar rhabdomyosarcoma
    (B) Congenital epulis of the newborn
    (C) Granular cell tumor
    (D) Hemangioma of infancy
    (E) Melanocytic neuroectodermal tumor of infancy

76. A 33-year-old woman is found to have antrochoanal polyp causing nasal obstruction. All of the following statements are correct regarding this lesion except
    (A) Atypical stromal cells are an indication of malignancy
    (B) Infarction, fibrosis and vascular compromise is common
    (C) Occurs in younger patients than usual type sinonasal polyps
    (D) Originates in the maxillary sinus and extends out the ostium into the nasal cavity
    (E) Removal of the stalk is required to prevent recurrence

77. What is the most common salivary gland neoplasm?
    (A) Acinic cell carcinoma
    (B) Adenoid cystic carcinoma
    (C) Epithelial–myoepithelial carcinoma
    (D) Mucoepidermoid carcinoma
    (E) Pleomorphic adenoma (benign mixed tumor)

78. A 59-year-old man is diagnosed with a conventional squamous cell carcinoma of the anterior tongue, which is 2 cm in greatest dimension. His neck examination is negative. At what tumor thickness does the risk of occult lymph node metastasis significantly increase?
    (A) >1 mm
    (B) >5 mm
    (C) >7 mm
    (D) >10 mm
    (E) >15 mm

79. What is the most common malignant salivary gland tumor in children?
    (A) Acinic cell carcinoma
    (B) Adenoid cystic carcinoma
    (C) Mucoepidermoid carcinoma
    (D) Pleomorphic adenoma
    (E) Salivary duct carcinoma

ANSWERS

1. **(A) Enucleation of the nodule is the treatment of choice.**

   The photomicrograph shows an example of a pleomorphic adenoma (benign mixed tumor) of the parotid, characterized by epithelial, myoepithelial, and mesenchymal differentiation. The most common mesenchymal change is chondromyxoid stroma that is admixed with plasmacytoid myoepithelial cells. Pleomorphic adenomas are the most common salivary gland neoplasm, and are generally regarded as benign tumors, although a small subset (<10%) will undergo transformation to malignancy (carcinoma ex pleomorphic adenoma). Features in a pleomorphic adenoma that are concerning for malignant transformation include hyalinization, necrosis, high mitotic activity, perineural or vascular invasion, and marked pleomorphism. The myoepithelial cell component will be positive for S-100, p63, smooth muscle actin, vimentin, and cytokeratin 7. The treatment of choice is superficial or total parotidectomy, to ensure the lesion is completely excised. Enucleation is not recommended, as this can result in recurrence in up to 50% of patients. Recurrent pleomorphic adenoma most commonly presents as multiple discrete nodules of benign-appearing pleomorphic adenoma within the original operative field, and it can be difficult to achieve surgical control subsequently.

2. **(E) A 60-year-old man with heavy smoking history.**

   The photomicrograph demonstrates a cystic and papillary proliferation of oncocytic cells that have a classic bilayered appearance with underlying lymphoid stroma, consistent with a Warthin tumor (papillary cystadenoma lymphomatosum). Warthin tumors are highly associated with cigarette smoking, and are most common in older men. About 10% of Warthin tumors will be bilateral. This lesion is seen almost exclusively in the parotid gland, and is believed to arise from entrapped salivary duct epithelium within intraparotid lymph nodes. Warthin tumors are benign, and malignant transformation is exceedingly rare. Similar neoplasms, lacking the lymphoid stroma, can be seen, and are called oncocytic papillary cystadenomas. A teenager with a slow growing mass of the parotid and worrisome nerve symptoms most likely has a mucoepidermoid carcinoma (the most common malignant salivary gland tumor in children). A parotid mass in a 47-year-old man with a tonsil mass most likely represents metastasis to a periparotid lymph node from a human papilloma virus-associated squamous cell carcinoma. A middle-aged man with

   human immunodeficiency virus (HIV) infection is likely to have HIV-associated salivary gland disease, which causes lymphoepithelial cysts with abnormal germinal centers. A middle-aged woman with dry mouth, dry eyes, and parotid enlargement may have Sjögren disease, which can cause firm, diffuse enlargement of the gland in severe disease.

3. **(B) t(11;19)(q21;p13) MECT1–MAML2 fusion.**

   The photomicrograph demonstrates a neoplasm composed of mucinous goblet cells, epidermoid cells, and intermediate cells, consistent with a mucoepidermoid carcinoma. Mucoepidermoid carcinoma is the most common malignant salivary gland tumor in adults and children, and more commonly occurs in the major salivary glands. Frequently a tumor-associated lymphoid proliferation is present. Several different grading schemes exist that stratify prognosis. Recently, a recurring translocation involving chromosome 11q21 [mucoepidermoid carcinoma translocated gene 1 (*MECT1*) gene] and chromosome 19p13 [mastermind-like 2 gene (*MAML2*) gene] has been described in the majority of tumors, particularly low-grade and intermediate-grade tumors. The PAX3–FOXO1 translocation is seen in alveolar rhabdomyosarcoma; the ETV6–NTRK3 translocation is seen in mammary analogue secretory carcinoma (MASC) of the salivary gland; the ATF1–EWSR1 translocation is seen in clear cell carcinoma of salivary gland origin (formerly hyalinizing clear cell carcinoma); and the NUT–BRD4 translocation is seen in NUT midline carcinomas of the head and neck.

4. **(D) Nevoid basal cell carcinoma syndrome (Gorlin syndrome).**

   The photomicrograph demonstrates a cyst lined by squamous epithelium that has a corrugated (wavy) surface with parakeratosis and a basal layer with nuclear palisading, consistent with a keratocystic odontogenic tumor (also known as odontogenic keratocyst). Keratocystic odontogenic tumors are most commonly found in the posterior portion of the mandible, and are associated with an unerupted tooth in over 50% of cases. Radiologically, the lesion is radiolucent, well circumscribed, and unilocular. While most keratocystic odontogenic tumors are sporadic, they are seen with a high frequency in patients with the nevoid basal cell carcinoma syndrome (Gorlin syndrome) that is caused by mutation of the *PTCH* gene on chromosome 9. Gorlin syndrome is characterized by early and multifocal development of basal cell carcinomas in young patients, along with skeletal abnormalities and rarely medulloblastoma of the central nervous system. Keratocystic odontogenic tumors are considered a benign neoplasm, but may recur unless completely excised. Malignant transformation is extremely rare. Cowden's syndrome (*PTEN* mutation) is associated with benign hamartomatous growths and uterine, breast, and thyroid cancers. Hereditary breast and ovarian carcinoma syndrome (*BRCA1*) is associated with breast and ovarian cancer development. Lynch syndrome (*MLH1*, *MSH2*, *MSH6* or *PMS2*) is associated with colorectal and endometrial carcinomas, while von Hippel–Lindau syndrome (*VHL* mutation) is associated with hemangioblastomas (particularly of the central nervous system) and kidney carcinomas.

5. **(E) Tumors are considered "malignant" only with documented metastasis.**

The photomicrograph demonstrates an infiltrative tumor composed of islands of epithelial cells that have central, loosely arranged angular cells (stellate reticulum) surrounded by a single layer of basal cells with palisading and reverse polarity, consistent with an ameloblastoma. Ameloblastoma is the second most common odontogenic tumor (after odontoma), and is a locally aggressive neoplasm that most commonly affects the posterior portion of the jaw. Radiologically, these tumors classically have a multiloculated "soap-bubble" appearance with thin walls, and are often associated with an impacted tooth. Recurrence is common, and occurs in approximately 35% of conventional ameloblastomas, so en bloc excision with a 1 cm margin is the treatment of choice. Unicystic tumors have a better prognosis, with <10% recurrence rate, and can be treated with local enucleation. Severe cytologic atypia, high mitotic rate, or necrosis typically occur in ameloblastic carcinomas, which appear as an undifferentiated carcinoma arising from an otherwise conventional ameloblastoma. Ameloblastic carcinomas have a significantly higher recurrence rate and overall poor prognosis. Only tumors with documented metastasis are diagnosed as "malignant ameloblastomas" and the most common site of metastasis is lung.

6. **(B) Diabetic who presented with headache and vision changes.**

The photomicrograph demonstrates sinonasal tissue with fungal hyphae invading into vascular spaces, consistent with invasive fungal sinusitis. When the fungal organism is a Zygomycetes, this process is called mucormycosis. The most common fungal organism to cause invasive fungal sinusitis is *Aspergillus*. Fulminant invasive fungal sinusitis is classically described as occurring in immunocompromised patients, including bone marrow transplant patients, and patients with malignancy

(e.g., lymphoma). Mucormycosis was described in diabetic patients who present with sinus pain and swelling, which can progress to blindness from invasion of the orbit. Aggressive surgical therapy to debride necrotic tissue and antifungal therapy is necessary, due to the high mortality rates associated with this disease. Allergic fungal sinusitis is associated with refractory sinusitis and increased peripheral blood IgE. A patient with epistaxis, hemoptysis, and a destructive septal lesion likely has Wegener's granulomatous. A woodworker with a destructive nasal mass likely has an intestinal-type sinonasal adenocarcinoma. A young man with nasal obstruction and a large polyp arising from the nasopharynx likely has a juvenile angiofibroma.

7. **(A) Gross cystic disease fluid protein 15 (GCDFP-15) staining is positive in most tumors.**

The photomicrograph demonstrates a high-grade adenocarcinoma that has cribriform and "Roman bridge" architecture associated with comedonecrosis, consistent with a salivary duct carcinoma. Salivary duct carcinoma is an uncommon malignant salivary gland tumor that can occur de novo or arise as part of a carcinoma ex pleomorphic adenoma. These tumors occur almost exclusively in older adults (>50 years of age) and more commonly in men. The classic morphologic appearance often mimics high-grade ductal carcinoma of the breast, with comedonecrosis, "Roman bridges," cribriform, and solid growth. Along with the morphologic similarities, these tumors are also positive for several breast markers, including gross cystic disease fluid protein (GCDFP-15), and may be focally positive for estrogen receptor. However, almost no tumors are positive for progesterone receptor, and instead, these tumors are positive for androgen receptor (AR) in over 90% of cases. In addition, these tumors typically have a 3+ pattern of immunohistochemical staining for HER-2, although *HER-2* gene amplification is not always present. Metastasis from a breast primary to the parotid region can occur; however, it is very rare, and the breast carcinomas are almost always known and have had multiple metastases already. Salivary duct carcinoma is a very aggressive tumor with a poor prognosis, and the 5-year overall survival is <35%.

8. **(C) Mutations in cAMP G-protein are present in most polyostotic cases.**

The photomicrograph demonstrates a proliferation of fibrous tissue containing spindled cells along with fine, branching, curvilinear trabeculae of woven bone that are irregular in shape (Chinese characters) and have a nearly complete lack of osteoblastic rimming, consistent with fibrous dysplasia. Fibrous dysplasia is an uncommon disease of bone that occurs most commonly in children and young adults, and results in bony expansion and distortion due to replacement of the bone by a fibrous stroma containing irregular woven bony trabeculae. This disease can involve only one bone (monostotic type) or multiple bones (polyostotic type). The polyostotic type involves craniofacial bones in nearly 100% of cases. The polyostotic type is also rarely associated with multiple endocrinopathies, which is called McCune–Albright syndrome. Most cases (both sporadic and inherited) are associated with mutations of the GNSA1 gene, which encodes a G-protein involved in cAMP cell signaling. The characteristic radiologic appearance is bone expanded by an ill-defined ground-glass (or cotton wool) appearance that merges imperceptibly with normal nearby bone. The characteristic microscopic appearance is a fibrous stroma with irregularly shaped (Chinese character or alphabet soup) woven bony trabeculae that lack osteoblastic rimming. The risk of transformation to malignancy is extremely low, and surgery is typically used for cosmesis and to alleviate symptoms from nerve entrapment. In contrast, ossifying fibroma is a clearly demarcated radiolucency that on biopsy demonstrates bony trabeculae with prominent osteoblastic rimming and a highly cellular fibrous stroma.

9. **(A) Calponin.**
    The photomicrograph shows a malignant salivary gland tumor that is composed of tubules formed by an inner cuboidal cell layer and an outer layer of large polygonal cells with clear cytoplasm, consistent with an epithelial–myoepithelial carcinoma. Epithelial–myoepithelial carcinoma is a rare malignant salivary gland tumor that predominantly occurs in adults, and is characterized by a distinct biphasic pattern of inner ductal type cells and outer myoepithelial cells with abundant clear cytoplasm. The clear myoepithelial cells contain abundant glycogen, which is positive on periodic acid Schiff stain, but is lost when digested by diastase. The clear myoepithelial cells are also positive for p63, calponin, S-100, smooth muscle actin, and other myoepithelial markers. The ductal cells are highlighted by epithelial membrane antigen and low molecular weight cytokeratins. Epithelial–myoepithelial carcinoma is not positive for p53 unless the tumor has undergone high-grade transformation/ dedifferentiation. Renal cell carcinoma (RCC) antigen is negative in these tumors.

10. **(A) Aggressive therapy is warranted due to high mortality from this process.**
    The photomicrograph demonstrates thick mucin with abundant inflammatory debris, eosinophils, and Charcot-Leyden crystals in alternating layers forming "tree ring" or "tide lines" of pink and blue material from low power, consistent with allergic-type mucin due to allergic fungal sinusitis. Allergic fungal sinusitis is caused by an allergic reaction to inhaled fungal elements, most commonly *Aspergillus* species. This process should not be confused with invasive fungal sinusitis, which is characterized by fungal hyphae invading into necrotic and viable sinonasal tissue with a marked host inflammatory reaction that does not typically include eosinophils. Invasive fungal sinusitis has a high mortality, and requires aggressive surgical and medical management. In contrast, allergic fungal sinusitis may be present for years without serious consequences, and has a good prognosis with an integrated medical and surgical approach to remove the fungal elements causing the allergic response. Allergic-type mucin has been grossly described as "peanut butter-like" or "putty-like" due to its thick consistency. The allergic response includes recruitment of numerous eosinophils that degranulate, resulting in Charcot-Leyden crystals, which are needle or bipyramidal shaped deeply eosinophilic crystals that are refractile. The allergic response can also result in a peripheral blood eosinophilia. Gomori methenamine silver (GMS) staining may highlight the fungal elements, but demonstration of the fungal hyphae is not required to make this diagnosis.

11. **(B) Low-grade mucoepidermoid carcinoma.**
    The photomicrograph demonstrates a lesion containing a proliferation of mucus-containing goblet cells, epidermoid (squamous) cells, and intermediate cells, consistent with a mucoepidermoid carcinoma. The gross description of a largely cystic lesion, along with these features, favors a low-grade tumor. Mucoepidermoid carcinoma is graded as low grade, intermediate grade, or high grade based on a variety of morphologic features. Two competing grading schemes are available, but several features are common to both systems. Features of low-grade tumors include >25% cystic component, a pushing (rather than infiltrative) invasive edge, and the absence of perineural invasion. In contrast, high-grade mucoepidermoid carcinomas have <25% cystic component, have an infiltrative border with small nests, show perineural invasion, and have a predominance of squamous-type epithelium. This case has features most consistent with a low-grade

tumor. High-grade mucoepidermoid carcinomas can be confused with squamous cell carcinoma; features that favor squamous cell carcinoma include surface mucosal dysplasia, marked keratinization, and the absence of goblet cells. Necrotizing sialo-metaplasia occurs when minor salivary gland tissue infarcts and squamous metaplasia extends into the residual salivary ducts. Necrotizing sialometaplasia will have a lobular architecture, recapitulating the original salivary gland structure, and will be surrounded by necrotic acini. Other salivary gland tumors can have squamous metaplasia, such as pleomorphic adenomas, but will also show the other components of these tumors, such as chondromyxoid stroma, myoepithelial cells, and ducts.

12. **(E) The target antigen of the ANCA antibody is myeloperoxidase (MPO).**
The clinical presentation of nasal cavity, lung, and kidney involvement, along with a biopsy demonstrating granulomatous inflammation and necrosis, is highly suggestive of Wegener's granulomatosis. Unfortunately, the classic triad of vasculitis, granulomatous inflammation, and geographic necrosis is present in <20% of patients, and requiring all 3 features in a single biopsy will result in underdiagnosis of this process. Serologic testing is extremely important in the diagnosis of this disease. Almost all patients with systemic Wegener's granulomatosis will have elevated levels of antineutrophil cytoplasmic antibody (ANCA) in the peripheral blood. In fact, it is almost always a positive c-ANCA, which specifically targets the proteinase 3 (PR3) antigen in the cytoplasm of neutrophils. A p-ANCA targets the myeloperoxidase (MPO) antigen in neutrophils, and is elevated in patients with primary sclerosing cholangitis and ulcerative colitis. The most commonly involved site in the upper aerodigestive tract is the nasal cavity (causing chronic, refractory sinusitis), and when severe and untreated can lead to nasal septal perforation and the classic "saddle nose" deformity.

13. **(A) High-grade adenocarcinoma is the most common form of malignant transformation.**
The photomicrograph shows epithelium with an endophytic (or inverting) growth pattern composed of columnar to transitional cells admixed with mucocytes (goblet cells) and intraepithelial mucous cysts containing acute and chronic inflammation, consistent with an sinonasal schneiderian papilloma, inverting type. Schneiderian papillomas are most commonly unilateral (90%), and the inverting and oncocytic types most commonly occur along the lateral nasal wall. The exophytic (or fungiform) type most commonly occurs on the nasal septum. These tumors are generally regarded as benign, although unchecked growth can result in local invasion into bone and nearby structures. Rarely, malignant transformation can occur, and is most commonly a keratinizing squamous cell carcinoma. The etiology of these tumors remains uncertain; however, up to 40% of inverting and 50% of exophytic schneiderian papillomas have been associated with low risk human papilloma virus (lr-HPV), usually types 6 and 11.

14. **(D) S-100.**
The photomicrograph demonstrates a carcinoid tumor of the larynx, characterized by an organoid or nested growth pattern of cells with salt and pepper nuclei, and the report of over 4 mitotic figures in 10 high-power fields is diagnostic of an atypical carcinoid. Atypical carcinoid tumors are the most common neuroendocrine tumor of the larynx, and most often are found in the supraglottis. Like other neuroendocrine neoplasms, atypical carcinoid tumors of the larynx are positive for cytokeratin, synaptophysin, chromogranin, CD56, and other neuroendocrine markers. However, over 80% of atypical carcinoid tumors of the larynx are notable for immunohistochemical staining with calcitonin, unlike atypical carcinoid tumors at other sites. This can make differentiation from metastatic medullary thyroid carcinoma challenging, although patients with laryngeal atypical carcinoid tumors do not have elevated calcitonin peripheral blood levels. S-100 will highlight the sustentacular cells in laryngeal paragangliomas, a major differential diagnostic consideration for laryngeal carcinoid tumors, but S-100 is negative in carcinoid tumors.

15. **(C) S-100.**
The photomicrograph shows a neoplastic proliferation of columnar cells forming cords and ribbons in a canalicular pattern with occasional beading (cords of cells fusing together at intervals), consistent with a canalicular adenoma. Canalicular adenomas are a type of monomorphic adenoma, and have a unique clinical presentation, with the majority of tumors occurring in the upper lip, and are well circumscribed, mobile, and submucosal. Women are more commonly affected than men, and these lesions can occur over a wide age range. Only a single cell type is seen on hematoxylin and eosin sections, which often is described as having oval uniform nuclei with pale, fine chromatin. On immunohistochemistry, the tumor cells are positive for cytokeratins, S-100, and CD117, but negative for other myoepithelial markers, such as smooth muscle actin and calponin. These tumors are not associated with human papilloma virus, and do not show

increased p16 staining. Although some tumors can show nuclear features similar to papillary thyroid carcinoma, thyroid transcription factor 1 staining is negative.

16. **(E) Pregnancy.**
The photomicrograph shows a vascular proliferation characterized by central large arborizing vessels surrounded by small capillary-like vessels in a lobular growth pattern with surface ulceration, consistent with a lobular capillary hemangioma. Lobular capillary hemangiomas classically occur on the gingiva of pregnant women, and are thought to be due to an excessive vascular proliferative response to the hormonal changes in pregnancy (but can be seen in women taking oral contraceptives). Lobular capillary hemangiomas can also occur in other locations, including the nasal cavity where they can cause epistaxis and other sites in the oral cavity. Chronic trauma can result in a fibroma or a peripheral giant cell granuloma of the gingiva. Human immunodeficiency virus (HIV) infection is associated with the vascular proliferation Kaposi sarcoma, which is caused by human herpesvirus 8 (HHV-8). Gorlin syndrome (nevoid basal cell carcinoma syndrome) is associated with keratocystic odontogenic tumor of the jaw. A heavy smoking history would most likely be associated with a dysplastic or malignant squamous proliferation.

17. **(E) Low-risk human papilloma virus (lr-HPV).**
The photomicrograph demonstrates a squamous papilloma, characterized by branching projections of bland-appearing squamous epithelium over a fibrovascular stroma. Focal koilocytic change can be seen in the epithelium. The presence of multiple squamous papillomas in the larynx and trachea of a child is consistent with a diagnosis of respiratory papillomatosis (laryngeal papillomatosis). Respiratory papillomatosis is seen in children and young adults, and is believed to be primarily due to low-risk human papilloma virus (lr-HPV) infection of the upper aerodigestive tract, which in children is likely to be acquired perinatally, and in adults is likely due to sexual transmission. The most common HPV subtypes involved are HPV-6 and HPV-11, although rarely high-risk HPV subtypes can be present. Respiratory papillomatosis in children can cause significant airway obstruction; therefore, surgical excision (including laser debridement) is the treatment of choice, but recurrence rates are high. Malignant transformation can rarely occur, usually in patients with a significant smoking history, so the presence of high-grade dysplasia, when present, should be documented in the pathology report.

18. **(B) Desmin.**
The photomicrograph demonstrates an example of a granular cell tumor of the tongue, which is characterized by plump polygonal to spindled cells with abundant eosinophilic granular cytoplasm. Granular cell tumors can occur at any site, but over half occur in the head and neck, particularly the oral cavity and tongue. These tumors are believed to be derived from Schwann cells, with abundant lysozymes resulting in the characteristic granular cytoplasm. Granular cell tumors are typically nonencapsulated and often have an infiltrative edge involving adjacent skeletal muscle. When involving a mucosal site, marked reactive change of the overlying squamous epithelium frequently occurs, called pseudoepitheliomatous hyperplasia. Pseudoepitheliomatous hyperplasia is characterized by squamous rete extending deep into the lamina propria, which often have keratin pearl formation, mimicking squamous cell carcinoma. Granular cell tumors are strongly and diffusely positive for S-100, vimentin, and CD68. A periodic acid Schiff with diastase stain (PASD) will be positive in the lysozyme granules. Desmin is negative in these tumors, in contrast to adult rhabdomyomas, which can have similar plump eosinophilic polygonal cells.

19. **(C) Biopsy is recommended prior to excision to plan extent of resection.**
The photomicrograph demonstrates a proliferation of cells in rounded nests and balls (zellballen) within a highly vascular stroma. The cells have abundant cytoplasm and round bland nuclei. These features, along with the history, are consistent with a carotid body paraganglioma (carotid body tumor). Carotid body paragangliomas are the most common extraadrenal paraganglioma of the head and neck, and are more common in women. The classic imaging appearance is a mass at the level of the carotid artery bifurcation that appears to sit between the two artery branches. These tumors are highly vascular, and biopsy is contraindicated as life-threatening hemorrhage can occur. Instead, preoperative embolization is commonly used, along with en bloc excision, for treatment. The chief cells are easily recognized on hematoxylin and eosin stain, and are positive for synaptophysin and chromogranin. Each nest is surrounded by delicate sustentacular cells that are best seen on S-100 stain. Paragangliomas have been associated with several inherited syndromes, including multiple endocrine neoplasia 2 (MEN 2) and mutations in several subunits of the succinate dehydrogenase enzyme (*SDHB*, *SDHC*, and *SDHD*). Most tumors are benign, but rarely paragangliomas can behave

in a malignant fashion. Unfortunately, no histologic features within the primary tumor are predictive of malignancy; therefore, metastasis is the only criterion for a diagnosis of malignant paraganglioma.

20. **(C) Not associated with tobacco smoking.**
The photomicrograph shows an example of spindle cell (sarcomatoid) squamous cell carcinoma, which is characterized by a markedly atypical spindle cell proliferation that blends into areas of conventional squamous cell carcinoma. Spindle cell squamous cell carcinomas of the larynx are almost always polypoid or exophytic tumors, and many are pedunculated. Differentiating spindle cell squamous cell carcinoma from a true sarcoma can be difficult, but in most cases an area of conventional squamous cell carcinoma can be found at least focally. Immunohistochemical staining for epithelial markers is helpful when positive, but up to 30% of spindle cell squamous cell carcinomas are negative for these stains. Despite the poorly differentiated appearance, patients with these tumors do very well, with a 5-year survival of over 80%. This is most likely due to the polypoid nature of these tumors, which often present at low stage and can be cured by polypectomy in many cases. Like other forms of squamous cell carcinoma, these tumors are highly associated with significant tobacco smoke exposure, as well as alcohol intake.

21. **(D) Second branchial apparatus.**
The photomicrograph demonstrates a cyst lined by thin bland squamous epithelium showing no atypia or mitotic activity, with an underlying lymphoid proliferation with germinal center formation, consistent with a branchial cleft cyst. The clinical location in the lateral neck is consistent with a second branchial cleft abnormality, as first branchial cleft abnormalities are usually found in and around the ear. Second branchial cleft cysts are most commonly located along the anterior border of the sternocleidomastoid muscle, and are most commonly found in patients between 20 and 40 years of age, although they are frequently seen in young children. Clinically, these lesions may wax and wane in size over time. A thyroglossal duct cyst would be located in the midline, and frequently have thyroid tissue in the wall of the cyst. An acquired inclusion cyst (or epidermal inclusion cyst) may be caused by prior trauma or surgery, would be lined by squamous epithelium with abundant keratin debris, and would lack a well-developed lymphoid stroma. The most important differential diagnosis to consider, particularly in patients over 35, is cystic metastatic squamous cell carcinoma to a cervical lymph node. Metastatic cystic squamous cell carcinomas typi-

cally show band or ribbon-like uniformly thick epithelium that lacks maturation, shows atypia and increased mitotic activity, and proliferation into the underlying lymphoid tissue. The underlying lymphoid tissue shows true lymph node architecture (subcapsular sinus, interfollicular zones, and a capsule).

22. **(A) Epstein–Barr virus (EBV).**
The photomicrograph shows an example of oral hairy leukoplakia, which is characterized by squamous hyperkeratosis and parakeratosis, epithelial hyperplasia, and "balloon cells" in the spinous layer, which show ballooning degeneration and nuclear viral cytopathic effect. Oral hairy leukoplakia occurs almost exclusively in human immunodeficiency virus (HIV)-infected patients, and correlates with low CD4 counts. It classically presents as white patches (leukoplakia) along the lateral border of the tongue, which may change in appearance over time, resolving and then reappearing. Oral hairy leukoplakia is caused by Epstein–Barr virus, and Epstein–Barr virus-encoded RNA (EBER) will be positive within the balloon cells of the squamous epithelium. Superficial candida infection is also commonly seen in the superficial layers of oral hairy leukoplakia.

23. **(C) The amorphous pink material is a luminal secretion.**
The photomicrograph demonstrates a salivary gland neoplasm characterized by cribriform and tubular architecture with abundant pink amorphous material forming ribbons and Swiss cheese-like holes, and cells with dark and angulated nuclei with scant cytoplasm. These features are consistent with an adenoid cystic carcinoma. Adenoid cystic carcinoma is the fourth most common malignant salivary gland neoplasm, and occurs in major and minor salivary glands. These tumors are composed of two cell populations: (1) a myoepithelial population (the predominant cell type in most tumors) characterized by small dark and angulated nuclei with scant cytoplasm and (2) ductal cells that form small inconspicuous lumens and may have small nucleoli. Immunohistochemical staining with p63, S-100, and calponin will highlight the myoepithelial cells, while CD117 will highlight the ductal population. The amorphous material present is basement membrane proteins deposited by the myoepithelial tumor cells, not luminal secretions. The 5-year survival for patients with adenoid cystic carcinoma is good, with >75% survival. However, these tumors tend to recur in an aggressive fashion, and have a propensity for nerve invasion, leading to a late poor survival (<35% at 15 years). Adenoid cystic

carcinoma can metastasize to regional lymph nodes, but more commonly hematogenously disseminate, and the most common site for distant metastasis is lung, followed by bone.

24. **(A) Associated with tuberous sclerosis.**
The photomicrograph demonstrates an example of adult rhabdomyoma, which is characterized by large polygonal cells with abundant eosinophilic cytoplasm that often is vacuolated, imparting a "spider web-like" appearance of radially oriented strands of cytoplasm. Rhabdomyomas are divided into cardiac and extracardiac types, and extracardiac types are divided into adult, fetal, and genital types. Over 70% of adult rhabdomyomas occur in the head and neck, and can involve the larynx or soft tissues of the neck. Rhabdomyomas have skeletal muscle differentiation, and cytoplasmic cross striations are characteristic; immunohistochemistry for myoglobin and desmin will be positive. The vacuolated cells contain glycogen, which is positive on periodic acid Schiff (PAS) stain, but negative after diastase digestion (PASD). Tuberous sclerosis is highly associated with cardiac rhabdomyomas, but is not associated with extracardiac types of rhabdomyoma.

25. **(E) Periodic acid Schiff with diastase (PASD).**
The photomicrograph shows sheets of cells with abundant, granular, lightly basophilic cytoplasm, and round vesicular nuclei, consistent with acinic cell carcinoma. Acinic cell carcinoma is the second most common malignant salivary gland tumor, and the majority of these tumors occur in the parotid. Acinic cell carcinoma is characterized by serous type cells (large polygonal cells with abundant basophilic, granular cytoplasm containing dense purple granules), intercalated duct type cells (smaller, eosinophilic and cuboidal, lacking granules), vacuolated cells (clear cytoplasmic vacuoles lacking granules), and nonspecific glandular cells (also lacking granules). The serous type cells are often the main cell type, but may be in the minority in some tumors. A prominent lymphoid infiltrate is typically present at the periphery of the tumor, which can have germinal center formation, and should not be interpreted as lymph node involvement. A variety of growth patterns can also be seen, including solid sheets, microcystic pattern, papillary cystic, or follicular. The most helpful ancillary test is periodic acid Schiff with diastase (PASD), which will highlight the zymogen granules in the serous cells. Acinic cell carcinoma will be positive for cytokeratin 7, alpha-1-antitrypsin, amylase, and PAS. Mucicarmine, all myoepithelial cell markers (such as calponin), and CD117 are negative

in acinic cell carcinoma. A Fontana–Masson stain is used to highlight melanin pigment, and is negative in this tumor.

26. **(B) CD34.**
The photomicrograph shows an example of spindle cell lipoma, which is characterized by mature adipose tissue interspersed with fibroblast-like spindle cells and collagen. Scattered multinucleated giant cells with hyperchromatic nuclei arranged in a floret pattern can be seen. Spindle cell lipomas occur almost exclusively in men, usually in the posterior neck or upper back. The adipocytes will be focally positive for S-100, but the spindle cells are very strongly positive for CD34, and negative for S-100, epithelial membrane antigen, and smooth muscle actin. Spindle cell lipomas should not contain lipoblasts, which are indicative of a well-differentiated liposarcoma.

27. **(A) Epstein–Barr virus (EBV).**
The photomicrograph demonstrates an atypical lymphoid proliferation that according to the history is positive for natural killer (NK) cell and T-cell antigens, consistent with an extranodal, nasal-type NK/T-cell lymphoma. These tumors are highly destructive, usually causing septal perforation and in some cases palate destruction and perforation. Angioinvasion, angiodestruction, and necrosis are often identified. The typical immunophenotype these cells show is a combination of NK markers (CD56) and T-cell markers (CD2, cytoplasmic CD3, TIA, granzyme B, perforin, and CD45RB). Epstein–Barr virus (EBV) infection can be demonstrated in nearly all cases, and peripheral blood EBV viral load can be used to monitor therapy and for relapse. This lymphoma is unusual in Western countries, and is more frequent in areas with endemic EBV infection, including Asia and South America. HHV-8 is associated with Kaposi sarcoma, primary effusion lymphoma, and Castleman's disease; HPV is associated with cervical cancer and some squamous cell carcinomas of the head and neck; HTLV-1 infection is associated with adult T-cell leukemia/lymphoma. Human immunodeficiency virus causes acquired immunodeficiency syndrome (AIDS), but does not directly cause any known human cancers.

28. **(E) Midline neck mass that moves with swallowing.**
The photomicrograph shows a cyst lined by respiratory mucosa with benign thyroid tissue in the wall, consistent with a thyroglossal duct cyst. Thyroglossal duct cysts classically present as midline neck masses that move upward on swallowing, since they usually are connected to the hyoid bone. Therefore, removal of the middle one-third of the

hyoid bone is required to ensure complete excision (Sistrunk procedure). A lateral neck mass along the anterior border of the sternocleidomastoid muscle might be a branchial cleft cyst. A lateral neck mass that is pulsatile and causes fainting is most likely a carotid body tumor. A lateral neck mass in association with an exophytic tonsillar mass most likely is metastatic squamous cell carcinoma to a cervical lymph node. A midline neck mass arising from the thyroid cartilage may be a chondroma or chondrosarcoma.

29. **(E) Smooth muscle actin (SMA).**
The photomicrograph shows an example of sinonasal-type hemangiopericytoma (glomangiopericytoma), which is characterized by a proliferation of bland small spindle cells that have a "patternless" growth pattern (lack fascicles or whorls) along with staghorn vessels, which often have a prominent perivascular hyalinization. These tumors also classically have an overlying intact respiratory mucosa, and the subepithelial stroma is uninvolved (Grenz zone). Sinonasal-type hemangiopericytomas most commonly occur in older women, and form a polypoid mass that may cause bony erosion due to compression, but do not show direct invasion. The differential diagnosis includes solitary fibrous tumor (ropy dense collagen and thin-walled vessels), nasopharyngeal angiofibroma (dense stromal hyalinization and large vessels with a smooth muscle wall and location in the nasopharynx of young men), and meningioma (whorled pattern of spindled to epithelioid cells with intracytoplasmic inclusions). Sinonasal-type hemangiopericytomas are believed to arise from pericytic cells; this is supported by the immunohistochemical staining pattern of the spindle cells, which are positive for vimentin and smooth muscle actin, and negative for vascular markers (CD34, CD1), bcl-2, desmin, cytokeratins and epithelial membrane antigen (EMA). CD34 and bcl-2 would be positive in a solitary fibrous tumor; desmin would be positive in a rhabdomyosarcoma; and EMA would be positive in a meningioma. The spindle cells of nasopharyngeal angiofibromas typically lack staining for actins, and are positive for androgen receptor.

30. **(D) Mastoid bone and ossicle destruction on imaging is characteristic.**
The photomicrograph demonstrates proliferation of bland, cuboidal to columnar cells that form nests, trabeculae, cords, and glands with a back-to-back configuration. The cells have salt and pepper chromatin, and there is no pleomorphism, necrosis, or mitotic activity. These features are consistent with a middle ear adenoma. Middle ear adenomas are a

rare benign primary tumor of the middle ear that most commonly presents as unilateral hearing loss in adults. While the glands and nests often have an "infiltrative" appearance, true invasion into nearby structures is not seen, and this pseudoinfiltration is a product of the fibrous stroma and lack of encapsulation. Middle ear adenomas often fill cavities (such as the middle ear or mastoid air spaces) without bony destruction, although long-standing tumors can cause pressure erosion. The ossicles are typically encased by tumor but not destroyed, although complete excision (the treatment of choice) usually requires removal of the ossicles as well. Middle ear adenomas are positive for epithelial and neuroendocrine markers, such as cytokeratin 7, CAM5.2, synaptophysin, chromogranin, and human pancreatic polypeptide. These tumors are considered benign, and have a good prognosis, with rare recurrence only in patients with incomplete excision, and no risk of metastasis.

31. **(C) Immunohistochemical staining for cytokeratin 20 and CDX2 is negative in the majority of cases.**
The photomicrograph shows an invasive carcinoma composed of tall columnar cells and goblet cells with moderate-to-severe nuclear atypia and brisk mitotic activity, consistent with a sinonasal intestinal-type adenocarcinoma (ITAC). ITACs are morphologically identical to colorectal adenocarcinomas, and metastasis from an occult primary should be excluded clinically. In addition, the immunohistochemical staining pattern of ITAC is identical to colorectal carcinomas; both are positive for cytokeratin 20, CDX2, villin, and MUC2. These tumors have been associated with occupational exposure to hardwood dust, leather working chemicals, and softwood dust, although cases not associated with these exposures do occur. Five morphologic subtypes have been described (papillary, solid, colonic, mucinous, and mixed), of which the papillary type has been associated with a better prognosis. However, these tumors are typically locally aggressive and are associated with a poor prognosis, with only 40% 5-year survival.

32. **(E) Synaptophysin.**
The photomicrograph demonstrates a proliferation of cells in rounded nests and balls (zellballen) within a highly vascular stroma. The cells have abundant cytoplasm and round bland nuclei, and these features are consistent with a jugulotympanic paraganglioma. Jugulotympanic paragangliomas are the most common middle ear tumor, and arise from paraganglia along the tympanic nerve, jugular foramen, or cranial nerve X. Jugulotympanic

paragangliomas are most common in adults, and sporadic tumors are more common in women, while inherited/familial tumors are more common in men. The most common presenting complaint is pulsatile tinnitus, which is the perception of noise that accompanies the patient's heartbeat. About 50% of patients also present with hearing loss. The chief cells form rounded nests (zellballen) within a rich capillary network, and are bland, with no significant atypia or mitotic activity. Immunohistochemical staining for synaptophysin and chromogranin will be positive within the chief cells, and the surrounding sustentacular cells are highlighted on S-100 stain. Although this is a benign neoplasm, there is a 15% mortality due to the proximity of these tumors to vital anatomic structures, and surgical excision and radiation therapy are options for treatment.

33. **(E) von Hippel–Lindau syndrome (VHL).**
The photomicrograph demonstrates a papillary proliferation of cuboidal to low columnar cells lining broad papillary projections within a cystic space, consistent with an endolymphatic sac tumor (aggressive papillary tumor of endolymphatic sac origin). Endolymphatic sac tumors are extremely rare tumors of the inner ear, which are believed to arise from the endolymphatic sac/duct. These tumors are highly associated with von Hippel-Lindau syndrome (VHL); nearly 10% of patients with VHL will develop this lesion, and almost all patients with bilateral endolymphatic sac tumors have VHL. The tumor is typically centered in the inner ear region, but can involve the middle ear, cranial fossa, and cerebellopontine angle. Bony destruction is characteristic of these tumors, which often have a multiloculated lytic appearance. Despite the locally aggressive nature of these tumors, there is no metastatic potential, and the prognosis is good if completely excised.

34. **(A) Absent thyroid gland.**
The photomicrograph demonstrates an example of lingual thyroid, which is characterized by normal-appearing thyroid follicles underlying the tongue mucosa. Lingual thyroid is a rare developmental anomaly, which results from failure of the thyroid gland to descend from the foramen cecum of the tongue. Therefore, over 75% of patients with lingual thyroid will lack a normal thyroid gland. DiGeorge syndrome is characterized by congenital heart disease and abnormalities of branchial cleft development, with resulting hypocalcemia and an absent thymus. Metastasis of papillary thyroid carcinoma to the tongue is vanishingly rare, and would show nuclear and architectural features of

malignancy. Branchial cleft cysts occur in the lateral neck, and are developmentally unrelated to the thyroglossal duct. An elevated peripheral blood calcitonin level is seen in patients with medullary thyroid carcinoma.

35. **(A) Epstein–Barr virus (EBV).**
The photomicrograph shows a malignant undifferentiated carcinoma infiltrated by lymphocytes, and when found in the nasopharynx is diagnostic of an undifferentiated nasopharyngeal carcinoma. The nonkeratinizing and undifferentiated types of nasopharyngeal carcinoma are highly associated with Epstein–Barr virus; in almost 100% of cases, in situ hybridization and/or polymerase chain reaction (PCR) techniques can demonstrate EBV DNA within the tumor. In addition, peripheral blood quantitative PCR for EBV DNA can be used in both initial diagnosis and monitoring for recurrence. Nasopharyngeal carcinoma occurs with the highest frequency in China (particularly Kwangtung Province) and surrounding areas, including Taiwan. High dietary levels of nitrosamines have also been implicated in the development of this disease. The keratinizing type of nasopharyngeal carcinoma has only a weak association with EBV, and has a worse prognosis. Occasionally, high-risk human papilloma virus (HPV)-related squamous cell carcinomas can have a similar lymphoepithelial appearance, but these tumors typically arise in the oropharynx.

36. **(B) Fontana–Masson staining will be positive.**
The photomicrograph demonstrates a malignant neoplasm characterized by large pleomorphic epithelioid cells with abundant cytoplasmic brown-black pigment, consistent with a sinonasal mucosal malignant melanoma (MMM). Sinonasal MMM most commonly occurs in the anterior nasal septum or maxillary sinus in older patients, presenting as a polypoid mass that can cause nasal obstruction and epistaxis. There is no association with sun exposure or lighter-skin ethnic types. Pagetoid spread along overlying mucosa is helpful in confirming the primary site of origin, and is not typically seen in metastatic disease. Immunohistochemical staining for S-100 is usually positive in all tumor cells, not in a sustentacular cell pattern as seen in olfactory neuroblastoma. Other markers that are typically positive are HMB-45, MelanA, tyrosinase, and vimentin. Fontana–Masson stain is a histochemical stain that is specific for melanin pigment, and is positive in pigmented MMMs. Unlike cutaneous malignant melanomas, there is no role for Clark level and Breslow thickness in sinonasal MMM.

37. **(B) Believed to arise from specialized sensory neuroepithelium.**

The photomicrograph shows a neoplasm characterized by a lobular growth pattern of primitive neuroblastoma cells present in a neurofibrillary matrix, consistent with olfactory neuroblastoma (esthesioneuroblastoma). These tumors almost always involve the cribriform plate, and frequently will have intranasal and intracranial extension, resulting in a "dumbbell-shaped" appearance on imaging. Involvement of the maxillary sinus is very rare, and only seen in high-stage tumors. These tumors are believed to arise from the specialized olfactory sensory neuroepithelium present in the cribriform plate. Pseudorosettes (Homer–Wright type: neoplastic cells palisading around neural matrix) are seen in up to 30% of cases; true rosettes (Flexner–Wintersteiner type: gland-like tight groups of neoplastic cells around a central lumen) are rarely seen, and only in high-grade (3 and 4) tumors. The majority of the tumor cells will be positive for neuroendocrine markers (synaptophysin, chromogranin, etc.), but only the supporting sustentacular cells are positive for S-100. Although morphologically very similar to pediatric neuroblastomas, *MYC* amplification is not seen in these tumors.

38. **(D) Positive for thyroid transcription factor 1 (TTF-1).**

Nasopharyngeal papillary adenocarcinoma is a rare primary neoplasm of the posterior/lateral nasopharynx, which has many morphologic features similar to papillary thyroid carcinoma. The tumor has an infiltrative appearance and is composed of papillary structures lined by columnar to cuboidal cells with vesicular to clear chromatin and nuclear crowding and overlap. Similar to papillary thyroid carcinoma, psammoma bodies can be present, and immunohistochemical staining for TTF-1 is positive in the tumor cells. However, unlike papillary thyroid carcinoma, nuclear pseudoinclusions are not typically seen, and immunohistochemical staining for thyroglobulin is negative. Nasopharyngeal papillary adenocarcinoma is an indolent tumor, with no reported cases of metastasis, and complete surgical excision is curative. No association with infectious agents (such as Epstein–Barr virus) has been described, and the etiology of this tumor remains unknown.

39. **(D) *Klebsiella rhinoscleromatis*.**

Rhinoscleroma is an infectious disease secondary to *Klebsiella rhinoscleromatis* that is endemic in Central America, tropical Africa, Indonesia, and Eastern Europe. Patients with rhinoscleroma are immunocompetent, but are unable to properly phagocytize and kill the bacteria, leading to a granulomatous

and chronic inflammatory infection of the upper airway. If untreated, the inflammatory process can lead to significant disfigurement due to destruction of the nasal cavity and nose. Biopsies of rhinoscleroma show sheets of lymphocytes, plasma cells, and scattered foamy histiocytes. A Warthin–Starry stain would highlight rod-shaped organisms within the foamy histiocytes. Treatment includes long-term antibiotics and debridement. *Rhinosporidium seeberi* is the causative agent of rhinosporidiosis, which is characterized by mucosal and submucosal cysts filled with endospores. Epstein–Barr virus is the causative agent of nasopharyngeal carcinoma, along with other lymphoid neoplasms. *Aspergillus fumigatus* is the most common infectious mold in humans, and can cause allergic fungal sinusitis and invasive fungal sinusitis. Human papilloma virus is associated with oropharyngeal squamous cell carcinomas and respiratory papillomatosis.

40. **(A) Fordyce granules.**

Fordyce granules are a normal variant found in the oral cavity, composed of ectopic sebaceous glands that arise from ectodermal inclusions left behind during embryogenesis. Fordyce granules are most commonly found on the lateral upper and lower inner lips and buccal mucosa. Often multiple sebaceous glands occur in a group, forming yellow-appearing papules and plaques on the oral mucosa. The juxtaoral organ of Chievitz is a normal anatomic structure within the deep buccal fascia that is composed of benign-appearing squamous nests within stromal tissue. Lingual thyroid is a remnant of the thyroglossal duct, which leaves residual normal-appearing thyroid tissue within the posterior one-third of the tongue, usually near the foramen cecum. Ranula is the clinical term for mucoceles of minor salivary glands involving the floor of mouth, which often have a bluish discoloration clinically. Oral hairy leukoplakia occurs on the lateral tongue of HIV-infected patients, and appears as squamous hyperplasia, parakeratosis, and balloon cell change with viral cytopathic changes, and is due to Epstein–Barr virus infection of the oral mucosa.

41. **(D) Positive anti-SSB (anti-La).**

The clinical presentation is suggestive of Sjögren's syndrome. The diagnosis of Sjögren's syndrome requires the presence of at least 4 of 6 clinical and pathologic criteria, which include ocular symptoms, oral symptoms, a positive Schirmer test, a positive lip biopsy, positive parotid gland sialography, and a positive anti-SSA or anti-SSB serology. Therefore, in most patients with suspected Sjögren's syndrome, a lower lip (labial) biopsy is performed to assess the minor salivary glands. In Sjögren's syndrome, minor salivary glands will typically show patchy lymphoid aggregates composed of lymphocytes and plasma cells, in the absence of atrophy, fibrosis, duct ectasia, or acute inflammation. A focus score is calculated; a single focus is considered a lymphoid aggregate of >50 lymphocytes within salivary tissue, and the number of "foci" are counted in a 4 mm^2 area. A focus score of ≥1 is supportive of Sjögren's syndrome. Patients with Sjögren's syndrome will often have positive serology for antinuclear antibody (ANA), rheumatoid factor (RF), an elevated erythrocyte sedimentation rate (ESR), and anti-SSA, but anti-SSB is the most specific serologic test for Sjögren's syndrome.

42. **(B) Lung metastases may have the appearance of a benign pleomorphic adenoma.**
The clinical history and microscopic description are highly suggestive of a carcinoma ex pleomorphic adenoma. Carcinoma ex pleomorphic adenoma is a heterogeneous group of malignant salivary gland tumors that by definition must arise from a previous pleomorphic adenoma (benign mixed tumor). Therefore, identification of residual pleomorphic adenoma or prior documentation of a pleomorphic adenoma at the site of the tumor is required for this diagnosis. The malignant tumor may result in substantial destruction of the underlying pleomorphic adenoma, and extensive sections may be required for this diagnosis. Almost any malignant salivary gland tumor can be seen in a carcinoma ex pleomorphic adenoma, but the most common tumors are adenocarcinoma not otherwise specified, salivary duct carcinoma, myoepithelial carcinoma, and adenoid cystic carcinoma. The histologic subtype present affects the overall prognosis; tumors with a polymorphous low-grade adenocarcinoma component have a 95% 5-year overall survival rate; while tumors with a salivary duct carcinoma component have a 62% 5-year overall survival rate; and tumors with a myoepithelial carcinoma component have a 50% 5-year overall survival rate. The malignant component may be confined to the area of the original pleomorphic adenoma (so-called noninvasive, or encapsulated), which is associated with an extremely good prognosis. Minimally invasive tumors are defined as having 1.5 mm or less of invasion beyond the capsule of the tumor, and are associated with a better prognosis than widely invasive tumors. Metastases are invariably of the malignant tumor component. The presence of lung nodules with the appearance of a benign pleomorphic adenoma is most likely due to a benign metastasizing pleomorphic adenoma, which is

believed to be caused by an iatrogenic tumor embolus of benign pleomorphic adenoma during surgery for pleomorphic adenoma.

43. **(C) Occurs almost exclusively in women.**
Dysgenetic polycystic disease of the parotid is characterized by a parotid gland with multiple cysts caused by dilations of the intercalated ducts and an uninvolved main parotid duct. Key features are retained normal lobular architecture, lack of inflammatory reaction, and retained interspersed acinar cells and striated ducts. The cysts are thin walled, irregularly sized, and lined by epithelium that may be flattened, cuboidal, apocrine, or vacuolated. Occasional cysts may contain proteinaceous eosinophilic material. The overwhelming majority of patients with this disease are women, and a sex-linked inheritance to this disease has been postulated. There is no association with other inherited polycystic disorders. These patients typically present with bilateral swelling of the parotid glands that fluctuates over time, but is not associated with eating or painful. Malignant transformation has never been reported in these patients, and surgery is typically only performed for diagnosis and cosmesis. In contrast, cystic dilation of the parotid secondary to a sialolith would be associated with a significant inflammatory reaction, dilation of the main parotid duct, and the swelling would worsen with eating.

44. **(B) Carcinoembryonic antigen (CEA).**
Immunohistochemical markers are increasingly used in the diagnosis of salivary gland neoplasms. Many salivary gland tumors contain a neoplastic population of myoepithelial cells, identification of which can be helpful for definitive diagnosis. The most commonly used markers for myoepithelial cells include calponin, p63, S-100, and smooth muscle actin. Myoepithelial cells can also be positive for GFAP, pancytokeratins, and other smooth muscle markers such as smooth muscle myosin and muscle specific actin. In contrast, the ductal component of salivary gland tumors will be positive for CEA and low molecular weight cytokeratins, and lack expression of smooth muscle markers, p63, and S-100.

45. **(A) Adenoid cystic carcinoma.**
The clinical history and microscopic description in the case presentation are highly suggestive of clear cell carcinoma of salivary gland origin (previously called hyalinizing clear cell carcinoma). Clear cell carcinoma of salivary gland origin most commonly occurs in women at minor salivary gland sites, with tongue and palate most frequent. This tumor is characterized by infiltrative nests of clear epithelial

cells embedded within a hyalinized, dense, sclerotic stroma. Recently, a recurring genetic abnormality has been described in these tumors, t(12;22) (q13;q12) ATF1–EWSR1 fusion. The presence of clear cells is not specific to this tumor, however, and can be seen in a significant number of other salivary gland tumors, benign and malignant. Myoepithelial cells with prominent clear cell change are characteristic of epithelial–myoepithelial carcinoma, and can been seen in myoepitheliomas. A clear cell variant of mucoepidermoid carcinoma can be particularly difficult to distinguish from clear cell carcinoma. Other tumors that can have a clear cell change include pleomorphic adenomas, oncocytomas, acinic cell carcinomas, and sebaceous tumors. Adenoid cystic carcinoma, on the other hand, is characterized by cells with scant cytoplasm and small dark and angulated nuclei, and almost never shows clear cell change.

46. **(A) Complex lesions are characterized by recognizable tooth formation.**
Odontomas are hamartomatous lesions of odontogenic origin, and are characterized by an abnormal production of dentin, enamel matrix, cementum, and pulp tissue. Odontomas are the most common lesion of odontogenic origin, and are subclassified as compound and complex odontomas. Compound odontomas are most commonly found in the anterior maxilla, and show formation of tooth-shaped structures that are often smaller than normal teeth. Complex odontomas contain a haphazard arrangement of the same material, but lack recognizable toothlike structures, and are more common in the posterior mandible. Since these are benign tumors, there is no risk of recurrence, so simple excision is the treatment of choice.

47. **(D) Tissue culture-like plump myofibroblasts in a background of inflammation and extravasated erythrocytes.**
Nodular fasciitis is a rare mass-forming reactive proliferation of myofibroblastic cells that most commonly occurs in the head and neck and upper extremities. Nodular fasciitis most commonly occurs in young patients, and may be associated with a recent trauma. Classically, it presents as a rapidly enlarging mass of short duration. Microscopically, it is characterized by plump myofibroblasts arranged in a tissue culture-like pattern with short storiform and interlacing fascicles. The background usually contains inflammation and extravasated erythrocytes. Mitotic figures may be frequent, but atypical mitotic figures should not be seen. Over time, these lesions will spontaneously involute. A tumor composed of a highly cellular

spindle cell proliferation with a herringbone appearance would favor a fibrosarcoma. A tumor with epithelioid and spindled cells with marked nuclear pleomorphism and atypical mitotic figures would favor a malignant high-grade sarcoma. A tumor with rhabdoid cells and atypical mitotic figures would favor a rhabdomyosarcoma. A tumor with wavy spindle cells with varying hypocellular and hypercellular areas and palisaded nuclei would favor a schwannoma.

48. **(D) Most commonly occurs in males under 20 years of age.**
The histologic description is of a nasopharyngeal angiofibroma (juvenile angiofibroma), which occurs almost exclusively in young males under 20 years of age, and arises from the nasopharynx, although large lesions may obscure this clinical clue. These tumors are highly vascular, and are composed of disorganized, variably sized vessels, which often show irregular smooth muscle thickening of the vascular walls and staghorn configuration. The vessels are embedded within a cellular fibrotic stroma. Nasopharyngeal angiofibromas express androgen receptor in the stromal and endothelial cells, leading to growth during puberty due to increases in testosterone. The stromal cells are negative for estrogen receptor and progesterone receptor. These tumors are considered benign, although they can have aggressive local growth with bony destruction. The treatment of choice is complete surgical excision, usually with preoperative embolization to control bleeding, and radiation is only used to manage large inoperative tumors. Biopsy is not recommended, as fatal exsanguination can occur.

49. **(A) Base of tongue.**
Immunohistochemical staining for p16 in a squamous cell carcinoma is a surrogate marker for high risk human papilloma virus (hr-HPV). HPV-related squamous cell carcinomas of the head and neck most commonly occur in the oropharynx, which includes the palatine tonsils and base of tongue. Approximately 60% of oropharyngeal squamous cell carcinomas will be HPV associated, and more commonly occur in younger patients without a history of tobacco use. The squamous cell carcinoma is most commonly nonkeratinizing, and has been associated with the papillary subtype of squamous cell carcinoma. The most common initial presentation of HPV-associated squamous cell carcinoma is neck lymph node metastasis, and the primary tumor can be occult, even on direct laryngoscopy evaluation. Rarely, HPV-associated squamous cell carcinomas can occur at nonoropharyngeal sites.

50. **(D) t(15;19) (q13;p13.1) NUT–BRD4 fusion.**
    The clinical history of a child or adolescent with a midline (nasal cavity, mediastinum, and larynx) undifferentiated carcinoma that shows squamous differentiation is highly suggestive of a NUT midline carcinoma. NUT midline carcinomas were first described in the mediastinum, although almost as many have been described in the head and neck, particularly the nasal cavity and nasopharynx. These tumors occur in adolescents and young adults, although some have been reported in patients as old as 78 years. The defining feature of this neoplasm is the presence of a unique translocation involving the nuclear protein of the testis (NUT) gene on chromosome 15 and the BRD4 gene on chromosome 19. The t(11;19)(q21;p13) translocation fuses the MECT1 and MAML2 genes in mucoepidermoid carcinoma of salivary gland origin. The t(2;13)(q35;q14) translocation fuses the PAX3 and FOXO1 genes in alveolar rhabdomyosarcoma. The t(11;22)(q24;q12) translocation fuses the EWS and FLI1 genes in Ewing sarcoma. The t(11;22)(p13;q12) translocation fuses the EWS and WT1 genes in desmoplastic small round cell tumors.

51. **(C) High-fat diet.**
    Squamous cell carcinoma is the most common malignancy of the upper aerodigestive tract. Many different environmental exposures can increase the risk of developing this tumor. The most important cause of squamous cell carcinoma is tobacco use, either smoking or smokeless, followed by alcohol use. In Asia, the use of betel quid, which is a combination of palm nut, betel leaf, and lime, has also been associated with the development of squamous cell carcinoma. Patients with a prior history of radiation exposure are also at increased risk of developing squamous cell carcinoma. While a high-fat diet has been associated with the development of colorectal carcinoma, it has not been shown to affect the rate of upper aerodigestive tract squamous cell carcinoma.

52. **(C) Palisading of spindle cell nuclei.**
    Extrapulmonary solitary fibrous tumors have been reported in almost every site in the body. In the head and neck, the most common site is orbit and maxillary sinus. Solitary fibrous tumors are in many ways a diagnosis of exclusion, as the diagnosis rests of a combination of cytologic, architectural, and immunohistochemical findings. Solitary fibrous tumors are composed of bland, blunt, spindle-shaped cells that often appear to have a "patternless" growth pattern. The tumor often has areas of high cellularity and low cellularity that alternate. Thin-walled vessels with a hemangiopericytoma-like (or staghorn) shape are frequently seen, although this finding is nonspecific. One of the most helpful morphologic features is the presence of thick, ropy, or keloid-like collagen fibers that are interspersed between tumor cells. Nuclear palisading is almost never seen, and should suggest an alternative diagnosis, such as schwannoma. Solitary fibrous tumors show immunohistochemical staining for CD34, bcl-2, and CD99, and are negative for cytokeratins and S-100.

53. **(E) The most common high-risk HPV subtype in these tumors is HPV-18.**
    Human papilloma virus (HPV)-associated squamous cell carcinomas of the head and neck most commonly occur in the oropharynx (palatine tonsil, base of tongue, etc.). Immunohistochemical staining for p16 will be strong and diffuse in HPV-associated tumors, while only patchy and weak in non-HPV-associated tumors. HPV-associated squamous cell carcinoma has a better prognosis than non-HPV-associated squamous cell carcinoma, despite the fact that these tumors most commonly present at high stage with unilateral or bilateral lymph node metastasis. Lymph node metastases are frequently cystic, and can be confused with branchial cleft cysts on radiologic imaging, particularly due to the younger age and absence of tobacco use seen in HPV-associated squamous cell carcinoma patients. The most common HPV subtype associated with head and neck squamous cell carcinoma is HPV-16, although rarely other high-risk types, including HPV-18, have been found.

54. **(B) Depth of invasion does not affect prognosis.**
    Atypical fibroxanthoma is a rare skin tumor that most commonly occurs in the scalp of elderly men. Histologically, atypical fibroxanthoma is characterized by a poorly differentiated neoplasm that has marked pleomorphism and atypia, including bizarre cells. The atypical cells can be spindled, epithelioid, or giant multinucleated cells. High mitotic activity, as well as atypical mitotic figures, is frequently seen. Exclusion of melanoma and spindle cell carcinoma is required for this diagnosis; atypical fibroxanthomas are negative for cytokeratins, p63, S-100, and melanocytic markers, and will be positive for vimentin, CD68, and CD10. Atypical fibroxanthomas occur in the dermis of the skin, and are not associated with an overlying epithelial dysplasia. The depth of invasion of these tumors is critical, as lesions that are confined to the dermis have a good prognosis, with a very low rate of local

recurrence (<10%) and only case reports of metastasis. Involvement of the subcutaneous soft tissues implies a more aggressive behavior and increased risk of metastasis, and many pathologists diagnose lesions with features of atypical fibroxanthoma that extend into the subcutaneous fat as malignant fibrous histiocytoma.

55. **(C) Cyst surrounds the crown of an impacted wisdom tooth.**

The two most common cysts of the jaw are dentigerous cysts and periapical (radicular) cysts. Dentigerous cysts are the most common developmental cyst, and typically are found in asymptomatic young patients at routine dental imaging. Dentigerous cysts most commonly occur in association with an
impacted mandibular molar (wisdom) tooth, although other teeth can be involved. The classic appearance is a cyst that surrounds the crown of an impacted tooth, and is attached to the tooth at the enamel–cementum junction. Dentigerous cysts are lined by two to three layers of squamous to cuboidal epithelium with occasional mucus cells or ciliated cells. Periapical cysts almost exclusively occur in association with carious teeth that are frequently nonvital. The cavity and bacteria result in infection and inflammation of the tooth root, leading to cystic change of odontogenic rests around the tooth root. Periapical cysts are lined by squamous epithelium and are associated with a marked acute and chronic inflammatory reaction. The cyst is always associated with the root of the tooth, and root absorption of the affected tooth can be seen in many cases.

56. **(A) Amalgam tattoo.**

Leukoplakia is a clinical diagnosis of an area of white discoloration on a mucosal surface, most commonly in the oral cavity. Most causes of leukoplakia histologically show hyperkeratosis of the squamous epithelium, which results in the thickened, white clinical appearance. The most common causes of leukoplakia include frictional hyperkeratosis, lichen planus, mucosal candidiasis, and keratinizing squamous dysplasia. In contrast, amalgam tattoos are areas of blue-black discoloration, caused by spread of amalgam material used in tooth fillings (silver, tin, mercury, and other materials) underneath nearby mucosal surfaces. Amalgam tattoos often are clinically concerning for mucosal malignant melanoma, due to the dark discoloration.

57. **(B) Leading cause of death is airway compromise due to laryngotracheal collapse.**

The description of bilateral ear and nose involvement by a process resulting in necrotic cartilage, associated with a mixed inflammatory infiltrate,
is highly suggestive of relapsing polychondritis. Relapsing polychondritis is an autoimmune disorder that selectively destroys cartilage and proteoglycan-rich tissues. It is believed to be due to antibodies against type II collagen, the primary component of cartilage. Type IV collagen is the primary component of basement membranes. In the acute phase, involved structures are red, swollen, and tender, which is indicative of ongoing cartilage destruction. In the chronic phase, patients have lost most cartilage in the involved structures, which results in floppy ears and saddle nose deformity of the nasal bridge. Over 30% of patients with relapsing polychondritis have another autoimmune disease, most commonly rheumatoid arthritis. Immunofluorescence on an acute phase biopsy will show deposition of immunoglobulins and C3 at the periphery of cartilage and in perichondral vessels. This disease can involve cartilage at other sites, including the larynx, trachea, and joints. The leading cause of death is airway compromise due to tracheobronchial and laryngeal damage and collapse. Treatment with steroids can be helpful, as well as immunomodulatory therapy.

58. **(E) Low-grade chondrosarcoma.**

Cartilaginous neoplasms rarely occur in the larynx. Chondrosarcoma of the larynx occurs in older patients, arises from the posterior cricoid cartilage in over 80% of patients, and typically presents with stridor or hoarseness, due to airway obstruction. Chondrosarcomas of the larynx occur >15 times more frequently than chondromas of the larynx. Therefore, even when there is minimal atypia, any cartilaginous neoplasm of the larynx is concerning for malignancy, and caution should be used when making the diagnosis of chondroma. Chondromas of the larynx also most commonly arise in the posterior cricoid cartilage, but by definition are never >2 cm in greatest dimension, and should have an appearance very similar to normal hyaline cartilage, with minimal increased cellularity and no atypia. At least 10% of chondromas of the larynx will recur, and these most likely represent underdiagnosed well-differentiated chondrosarcomas. Complete surgical excision that is larynx-preserving, if possible, is the treatment of choice for laryngeal chondrosarcomas, with a very good overall survival (>95% at 10 years). Laryngeal chondrometaplasia occurs in the vocal cord, and forms submucosal, elastic-rich cartilaginous nodules that do not connect with the underlying thyroid cartilage. Pleomorphic adenomas rarely arise from minor salivary glands in the larynx, and will show intermixed ductal and myoepithelial cells. Extraskeletal mesenchymal chondrosarcomas have not been reported in the larynx, and do not show well-differentiated cartilaginous differentiation.

59. **(E) Submucosal edematous, myxoid stroma with dilated vessels and hemorrhage.**
Vocal cord nodules and vocal cord polyps are reactive changes caused by laryngeal mucosal trauma, which result in a polypoid or nodular growth. Vocal cord nodules are more common on the anterior third of the true vocal cord and are almost always bilateral, while vocal cord polyps occur at any site and are usually unilateral. Histologically, nodules and polyps are indistinguishable. Both show a submucosal expansion by edema, myxoid stroma, fibrous connective tissue, and ectatic vessels with associated hemorrhage and fibrin. The overlying squamous mucosa often shows reactive changes. Vocal cord amyloidosis can mimic a vocal cord polyp, but would have a more uniform appearance of acellular amorphous eosinophilic material that is positive for Congo red. A contact ulcer occurs on the posterior vocal cord, and is composed of granulation tissue with surface ulceration, fibrinoid necrosis, and inflammation. Granular cell tumors rarely can occur in the larynx, and show large polygonal cells with abundant eosinophilic granular cytoplasm. Older patients with a significant smoking history are most likely to have a squamous cell carcinoma of the vocal cord and larynx, which would show infiltrative squamous nests with marked nuclear pleomorphism.

60. **(E) Surface keratinizing squamous dysplasia.**
Necrotizing sialometaplasia occurs in older men, most commonly on the hard palate. It is believed to arise in areas of ischemic injury to minor salivary glands or trauma, resulting in squamous metaplasia of the minor salivary gland ducts. Important histopathologic features of necrotizing sialometaplasia include the presence of surrounding necrotic minor salivary gland acini, retained lobular architecture in the squamous nests, smooth rounded contours to the squamous nests, and absence of atypia. In contrast, features that would favor invasive squamous cell carcinoma include marked atypia, dyskeratosis, abnormal mitotic figures, irregular squamous nest contours, haphazard arrangement of squamous nests, and normal-appearing surrounding minor salivary gland. In addition, the presence of keratinizing squamous dysplasia of the surface mucosa is highly concerning for an invasive squamous cell carcinoma.

61. **(B) External ear canal.**
The lesion described is classic for a ceruminous adenoma of the ear. Ceruminous adenomas are characterized by a proliferation of well-formed small glands that have two cell populations—an inner ductal layer and an outer myoepithelial cell layer. The ductal cell layer in ceruminous adenomas typically has apocrine snouts (decapitation or surface blebbing), and the cytoplasm contains yellow-brown lipofuscin-like pigment that is cerumen. The gland lumens typically contain eosinophilic secretory material. Ceruminous adenomas arise exclusively in the outer one-third to outer half of the external ear canal, which recapitulates the normal distribution of ceruminous glands of the ear. Rarely, ceruminous adenomas can undergo malignant transformation, in which case an infiltrative destructive growth pattern is seen, with pleomorphism, increased mitotic activity, and necrosis. Although many salivary gland neoplasms also show a biphasic ductal/myoepithelial cell pattern, the location in the external ear canal, abundant luminal secretory products, and cerumen pigment are clues to the correct diagnosis. Middle ear adenomas are distinguished from ceruminous adenomas by their location in the middle ear, lack of cerumen pigment, and lack of a well-developed myoepithelial cell layer.

62. **(A) Any component of conventional squamous cell carcinoma invasion alters prognosis.**
Verrucous carcinoma is a variant of squamous cell carcinoma that is characterized by very well-differentiated squamous carcinoma with minimal to absent atypia and full maturation with abundant hyperkeratosis forming filiform (finger-like) projections. The keratinized surface can be orthokeratotic or parakeratotic, which has a characteristic "church-spire" appearance. Unlike conventional squamous cell carcinoma, verrucous carcinoma invades with a broad pushing front, usually associated with a marked inflammatory infiltrate in the underlying stroma. Verrucous carcinoma can be very difficult to diagnose, due to the lack of atypia and surface hyperplasia, which is very similar to verrucous hyperplasia. Definitive diagnosis requires well-oriented samples with sufficient stroma to identify the broad pushing invasive front; therefore, this diagnosis is almost never made on superficial biopsies. Clinically, these lesions can appear as a squamous papilloma, but the large size and destructive growth pattern are clinical signs of malignancy. Recognition of this variant is very important, as these patients essentially never develop metastasis to lymph nodes or distant sites, and have an extremely good prognosis. However, any component of conventional-type squamous cell carcinoma mitigates the difference

in prognosis, and these patients have a significant risk of metastasis and reduced overall survival. The presence of significant atypia and/or atypical mitotic figures in an otherwise verrucous carcinoma is almost unheard of, and should prompt a search for a conventional squamous cell carcinoma component. Verrucous carcinomas are not associated with HPV infection.

63. **(D) Strong staining for p63 and calponin.**
Ectomesenchymal chondromyxoid tumors are rare tumors of the anterior dorsal tongue, which predominantly occur in adults. These tumors are believed to be derived from undifferentiated neural crest cells, and not from minor salivary glands, which do not usually occur in the anterior dorsal tongue. These tumors are characterized by uniform-appearing small round to oval spindle and stellate cells arranged in cords, strands, and sheets, which form well-circumscribed nodules. A background chondromyxoid to myxoid stroma is typically present. The tumor cells are always positive for glial fibrillary acidic protein (GFAP) and almost always positive for cytokeratin. However, unlike myoepithelial cells, the tumor is negative for p63 and calponin. Hence the designation as "ectomesenchymal." These tumors are benign, and rarely recur after complete excision.

64. **(A) Congenital lesions are caused by a neoplastic proliferation of squamous epithelium.**
The description is classic for a case of cholesteatoma. Cholesteatoma is caused by the proliferation of non-neoplastic keratinizing squamous epithelium within the middle ear, which results in abundant keratin debris, and leads to ossicular bone destruction and hearing loss. Cholesteatomas are divided into congenital and acquired types. Congenital cholesteatomas arise from fetal epidermoid formations within the middle ear, which usually are resorbed in infancy. Patients with congenital cholesteatomas usually lack a history of chronic otitis media, and have an intact tympanic membrane. Acquired cholesteatomas are believed to largely arise in the setting of chronic otitis media that has caused tympanic membrane perforation. The tympanic membrane perforation allows keratinizing squamous epithelium entrance into the middle ear; then the chronic inflammation stimulates epithelial proliferation and growth. Early and aggressive treatment of otitis media with antibiotics can decrease the chance of developing acquired cholesteatoma in children. Although this process is non-neoplastic (and nonclonal), it can be locally aggressive and recur in up to 20% of patients, especially if incompletely excised.

Complete surgical excision is the treatment of choice.

65. **(E) Nasal glial heterotopia.**
The photomicrograph shows nests and sheets of glial tissue intermixed with fibrosis, which lacks neurons. No meninges or dura are seen. In the correct clinical setting, these findings are consistent with nasal glial heterotopia, a form of choristoma. Nasal glial heterotopia most commonly is found on the bridge of the nose underneath intact skin (second most common site is superior nasal cavity) and by definition does not have a connection with the intracranial fossa. It is composed most commonly of normal, mature glial tissue that often has an appearance similar to gliosis, with rare or absent neurons. An encephalocele is defined as herniation of brain and leptomeninges through a bony defect of the skull, and requires continuity with the cranial cavity. Indeed, after biopsy of an encephalocele, almost all patients develop a cerebrospinal fluid (CSF) leak. Accidental intracranial biopsy rarely occurs, and typically results in a CSF leak and imaging findings postoperatively of intracranial injury. Extension of an intracranial glioma into the nasal cavity is also rare, and imaging would show a destructive process with extension from the cranial cavity. Metastatic glioblastoma is very rare, and on biopsy would show marked pleomorphism and necrosis, not seen in this biopsy.

66. **(C) The alveolar subtype is associated with translocations involving the *FKHR* gene.**
The photomicrograph shows an example of rhabdomyosarcoma, which is characterized by primitive mesenchymal cells, some of which have rhabdoid morphology (eccentric eosinophilic cytoplasm) and cytoplasmic extensions, often in a myxoid or edematous stroma. Rhabdomyosarcoma is the most common soft tissue of the head and neck, and occurs primarily in children and adolescents. It is divided into two major subtypes: embryonal and alveolar. Embryonal rhabdomyosarcomas lack a translocation involving *FKHR*, and some show abnormalities of chromosome 11. Alveolar rhabdomyosarcomas characteristically have an alveolar growth pattern (nests of cells that are dyshesive and have the appearance of cells lining alveolar septae of the lung), and are unified by the presence of a translocation involving the Forkhead homolog 1 (*FKHR*) gene on chromosome 13. The most common translocations involve *PAX3* resulting in a t(2;13)(q35;q14) or *PAX7* resulting in a t(1;13)(p36;q14). Tumors with the *PAX3* translocation are more aggressive and have a worse overall survival compared to tumors with the *PAX7* translocation.

The botyroid variant is unique in that it occurs at mucosal sites (nasal cavity and ear in the head and neck), and classically appears polypoid (bunch of grapes) and has a cambium layer. A cambium layer is an area of increased tumor cellularity immediately under an intact, otherwise normal mucosal surface. All rhabdomyosarcomas demonstrate skeletal muscle differentiation both histologically (rhabdoid cells) and immunohistochemically (positive for myogenin, desmin, MyoD1, etc.). Myogenin is a nuclear stain.

67. **(A) Adrenocorticotropic hormone (ACTH).**
The photomicrograph demonstrates an ectopic pituitary adenoma, characterized by a proliferation of monotonous cells with an organoid, solid, and trabecular growth pattern and round to oval nuclei with salt and pepper chromatin and eosinophilic cytoplasm. The most common location for ectopic pituitary adenomas is the sphenoid sinus, followed by the nasopharynx. The pituitary may be normal, as these adenomas are most likely derived from embryologic remnants of the migration path of Rathke's pouch that ultimately forms the anterior pituitary. This patient also has symptoms of Cushing disease so the most likely hormonal peptide the cells will stain with is ACTH. Regardless of functional type, ectopic pituitary adenomas are also positive for cytokeratin and neuroendocrine markers, including synaptophysin and chromogranin. CD45 would be positive in a hematolymphoid proliferation; S-100 would be positive in an olfactory neuroblastoma; and S-100 and HMB-45 would be positive in sinonasal mucosal melanoma. Growth hormone would most likely be positive in a pituitary adenoma that was associated with acromegaly or gigantism.

68. **(B) Commonly arise from cranial nerve VIII.**
The photomicrograph demonstrates a schwannoma, characterized by wavy spindle cells that have densely cellular areas (Antoni A) and hypocellular areas (Antoni B), with areas of palisaded nuclei (Verocay body). Schwannomas in the head and neck are most commonly derived from cranial nerve VIII, so-called acoustic neuromas. Another common site is the sympathetic chain in the neck. Bilateral acoustic neuromas are nearly always associated with neurofibromatosis 2. Neurofibromatosis-1 is associated with neurofibromas, cafe au lait spots, and Lisch nodules. Acoustic neuromas cause hearing loss by damaging the vestibular nerve (sensorineural hearing loss), not by a mass effect damaging the ossicles of the ear (conductive hearing loss). Schwannomas are a neoplasm derived from Schwann cells (which support neurons and produce myelin), and therefore are positive for S-100 staining, but negative for neuronal markers such as synaptophysin and chromogranin.

69. **(A) Chordoma.**
The photomicrograph shows an example of chordoma, characterized by large epithelioid physaliphorous cells with vacuolated cytoplasm arranged in cords, clusters, and nests within a mucinous/myxoid matrix. Chordomas are rare tumors believed to arise from notochord remnants, and therefore are found in the midline, most commonly in the sacrococcygeal region, followed by sphenoid/occipital and vertebral sites. Immunohistochemically, chordomas are positive for epithelial markers (pancytokeratin, epithelial membrane antigen, etc.), S-100 and vimentin, but are negative for glial fibrillary acidic protein (GFAP). This profile distinguishes chordomas from chondrosarcomas, which are positive for S-100 but negative for epithelial markers and GFAP, and from chordoid gliomas, which are positive for GFAP.

70. **(C) Nuclear staining for β-catenin is positive in most cases.**
The photomicrograph demonstrates a nuchal-type fibroma, which is characterized by a mass composed of thick, haphazardly arranged collagen fibers and an overall low cellularity. Nuchal-type fibromas generally present as an asymptomatic, slow growing mass that has been present for years, which occur in the posterior neck. Nuchal-type fibromas are highly associated with Gardner syndrome (familial adenomatosis polyposis with fibromatosis) and diabetes mellitus. Rarely, nuchal-type fibromas may be the sentinel presentation of Gardner syndrome. Immunohistochemical cytoplasmic staining for CD34 and vimentin, and nuclear staining for β-catenin, is seen in the spindle cell population, but the spindle cells are negative for cytokeratin. Elastic fibers may focally be entrapped by this process, but are not a major component of this lesion, such as seen in elastofibroma.

71. **(C) Ossifying fibroma.**
The microscopic description of admixed cellular fibrous stroma and spicules of bone with osteoblastic rimming, in conjunction with radiologic imaging showing a well-circumscribed and radiolucent lesion, is consistent with an ossifying fibroma. Ossifying fibroma is considered to be a benign neoplasm of bone, and most commonly involves the posterior mandible. It is much more common in women, and usually only involves a single bone. The classic microscopic appearance is of a bland

cellular fibrous stroma at the center of the lesion, with evenly distributed bony spicules that show prominent osteoblastic rimming. Near the periphery of the lesion, the bony spicules transform to lamellar bone. Although this location and radiologic appearance would be good for a keratocystic odontogenic tumor, microscopically a cyst lined by squamous epithelium with parakeratosis and a palisading basal layer would be seen. Fibrous dysplasia would more commonly have an ill-defined ground-glass appearance on imaging, and have bony trabeculae that lack osteoblastic rimming. An osteoma would be radio-opaque on imaging, and be composed of mature cortical bone. Osteosarcomas of the craniofacial bones are very rare, and would show an infiltrative appearance on imaging and markedly atypical cells within the fibrous stroma and bony trabeculae on pathologic examination.

72. **(B) Human immunodeficiency virus (HIV) infection.**
The presence of bilateral cysts, combined with the pathologic description, is classic for human immunodeficiency virus (HIV) salivary gland disease. HIV salivary gland disease is seen in approximately 5% of patients with HIV infection, and often occurs early in the disease course, prior to the development of acquired immunodeficiency syndrome (AIDS). This disease should be differentiated from sporadic lymphoepithelial cysts, which are typically unilateral, unilocular, and lack the altered germinal centers seen in HIV salivary gland disease. A heavy smoking history in a patient with bilateral cystic parotid lesions is suggestive of Warthin's tumor. Tonsil enlargement due to an exophytic mass is suggestive of cystic metastatic human papilloma virus (HPV)-associated squamous cell carcinoma. Recent tuberculosis exposure and cough is suggestive of a granulomatous inflammatory process. A history of lung non-small cell carcinoma and enhancing nodules in the neck is suggestive of metastatic carcinoma, possibly squamous, with cystic necrosis.

73. **(C) Distant metastases are common at presentation.**
Sialoblastoma is a rare malignant tumor of infancy, which is believed to recapitulate the primitive salivary gland anlage. Histopathologically, it appears as solid nests and trabeculae composed of a mixture of ductal and basal/myoepithelial cells. The basal cells have scant cytoplasm, large nuclei with open chromatin and a single large nucleolus and may show peripheral palisading. The ductal cells are cuboidal and may form small lumens, but often represent only a small component of the tumor. These

tumors occur almost exclusively in children under 2 years of age, and can be detected prenatally in many cases on prenatal ultrasounds. The presence of nuclear anaplasia, necrosis, vascular invasion, and perineural invasion are adverse prognostic risk factors. These tumors are considered to be low grade, and surgical resection is curative in most patients. Only a minority of patients (<30%) will develop recurrence, and distant metastasis is very uncommon.

74. **(D) Necrosis and increased mitotic activity are associated with an increased risk of malignancy.**
Melanotic neuroectodermal tumor of infancy (MNTI) is a rare tumor which is clinically and pathologically distinctive, due to its classic presentation and unique microscopic appearance. Patients with MNTI are almost always under 1 year of age (80% younger than 6 months of age), and present with a rapidly growing, destructive mass of the anterior maxilla along the alveolar ridge (gingiva). Microscopically, these tumors show a distinctive biphasic appearance of large epithelioid cells with vesicular nuclei that are heavily pigmented (due to melanin), interlaced with nests of small, dark, crowded cells with scant cytoplasm that have a similar appearance to neuroblastoma cells. A dense sclerotic stroma is usually present. Interestingly, these tumors will show immunohistochemical staining for epithelial (cytokeratin), melanocytic (HMB-45), and neural (synaptophysin, neuron specific enolase) markers. These tumors are postulated to arise from neural crest cells, and the presence of elevated vanilmandelic acid (VMA) levels in some patients supports the neuroectodermal derivation of these tumors. Despite the rapid growth and local destruction, these tumors are largely considered benign with a good prognosis. Less than 2% of tumors will behave in a malignant fashion. However, no pathologic features have been shown to be predictive of malignancy in these tumors.

75. **(B) Congenital epulis of the newborn.**
Congenital epulis of the newborn is a rare benign tumor of newborns, which occurs exclusively on the gingiva, most commonly on the anterior maxillary gingiva. These tumors present at birth or within a few weeks, and can cause feeding difficulties and respiratory obstruction. Microscopically, these tumors appear nearly identical to granular cell tumors, with polygonal cells containing abundant eosinophilic granular cytoplasm. The tumors are positive for CD68 and vimentin, and negative for desmin, cytokeratin, and smooth muscle actin. However, unlike granular cell tumors, congenital

epulis of the newborn is negative for S-100 staining. These tumors will naturally regress after birth, but may require surgery if causing significant obstruction.

76. **(A) Atypical stromal cells are an indication of malignancy.**

Antrochoanal polyps are a clinically distinct type of sinonasal polyps, which occur in younger patients and are characterized by origin from the maxillary sinus with extension through the maxillary sinus ostium and into the nasal cavity. This results in a long stalk, with resulting vascular compromise and injury commonly causing infarction, fibrosis, and reactive atypia. Because of the vascular injury, atypical stromal cells are commonly seen, and are not a sign of malignancy. These atypical stromal cells are of myofibroblastic origin and typically are enlarged with pleomorphic and hyperchromatic nuclei. Distinction from a rhabdomyosarcoma is based on the limited number of atypical cells that are usually clustered in areas of injury, and the absence of staining for myogenin, desmin, or myoglobin. Complete excision, with removal of the stalk, is required to prevent recurrence.

77. **(E) Pleomorphic adenoma (benign mixed tumor).**

By far the most common salivary gland neoplasm is pleomorphic adenoma (benign mixed tumor), which represents over 75% of all salivary gland tumors (benign and malignant combined). It occurs in both major and minor salivary gland sites. The most common malignant salivary gland tumor is mucoepidermoid carcinoma, followed by adenoid cystic carcinoma and adenocarcinoma not otherwise specified.

78. **(B) >5 mm.**

Several studies have shown that in patients with oral squamous cell carcinoma of low stage (pT1 or pT2), tumor thickness is an important prognostic factor for the development of lymph node metastasis. Most studies have shown a significant increase in risk in patients with tumors 5 mm in thickness or greater, although some studies have used a cutoff of 3 mm and shown a similar result. Therefore, patients with a clinically negative neck (cN0) and a small oral cavity squamous cell carcinoma, which has a thickness over 5 mm will often undergo elective neck dissection to detect occult metastasis. It is important to report this clinically significant information in any primary resection of an oral squamous cell carcinoma.

79. **(C) Mucoepidermoid carcinoma.**

The most common malignant salivary gland tumor for all adults and children is mucoepidermoid carcinoma. Pleomorphic adenoma is the most common benign salivary gland tumor in both adults and children. Acinic cell carcinoma is the second most common malignant salivary gland tumor and is seen in adults and children. Adenoid cystic carcinoma is the fourth most common malignant salivary gland tumor and is seen almost exclusively in adults. Salivary duct carcinoma is a rare, high-grade malignant salivary gland tumor that is seen almost exclusively in adults, typically over the age of 50.

SUGGESTED READING

1. Ang KK, Harris J, Wheeler R, et al. Human papillomavirus and survival of patients with oropharyngeal cancer. *N Engl J Med.* 2010;363(1):24-35.
2. Angiero F. Ectomesenchymal chondromyxoid tumour of the tongue. A review of histological and immunohistochemical features. *Anticancer Res.* 2010;30(11):4685-4689.
3. Antonescu CR, Katabi N, Zhang L, et al. EWSR1-ATF1 fusion is a novel and consistent finding in hyalinizing clear-cell carcinoma of salivary gland. *Genes Chromosomes Cancer.* 2011;50(7):559-570.
4. Auclair PL, Ellis GL. Atypical features in salivary gland mixed tumors: their relationship to malignant transformation. *Mod Pathol.* 1996;9(6):652-657.
5. Berns S, Pearl G. Middle ear adenoma. *Arch Pathol Lab Med.* 2006;130(7):1067-1069.
6. Cheuk W, Chan JK. Advances in salivary gland pathology. *Histopathology.* 2007;51(1):1-20.
7. deShazo RD, O'Brien M, Chapin K, Soto-Aguilar M, Gardner L, Swain R. A new classification and diagnostic criteria for invasive fungal sinusitis. *Arch Otolaryngol Head Neck Surg.* 1997;123(11):1181-1188.
8. Ferlito A, Silver CE, Bradford CR, Rinaldo A. Neuroendocrine neoplasms of the larynx: an overview. *Head Neck.* 2009;31(12):1634-1646.
9. Gonzalez-Alva P, Tanaka A, Oku Y, et al. Keratocystic odontogenic tumor: a retrospective study of 183 cases. *J Oral Sci.* 2008;50(2):205-212.
10. Goode RK, Auclair PL, Ellis GL. Mucoepidermoid carcinoma of the major salivary glands: clinical and histopathologic analysis of 234 cases with evaluation of grading criteria. *Cancer.* 1998;82(7):1217-1224.
11. Kapadia SB, Frisman DM, Hitchcock CL, Ellis GL, Popek EJ. Melanotic neuroectodermal tumor of infancy. Clinicopathological, immunohistochemical, and flow cytometric study. *Am J Surg Pathol.* 1993;17(6):566-573.
12. Katabi N, Gomez D, Klimstra DS, Carlson DL, Lee N, Ghossein R. Prognostic factors of recurrence in salivary carcinoma ex pleomorphic adenoma, with emphasis on the carcinoma histologic subtype: a clinicopathologic study of 43 cases. *Hum Pathol.* 2010;41(7):927-934.
13. Kempermann G, Neumann HP, Volk B. Endolymphatic sac tumours. *Histopathology.* 1998;33(1):2-10.
14. Khan AJ, DiGiovanna MP, Ross DA, et al. Adenoid cystic carcinoma: a retrospective clinical review. *Int J Cancer.* 2001;96(3):149-158.

15. Lawson W, Schlecht NF, Brandwein-Gensler M. The role of the human papillomavirus in the pathogenesis of Schneiderian inverted papillomas: an analytic overview of the evidence. *Head Neck Pathol.* 2008;2(2):49-59.

16. Machado de Sousa, SO, Soares de Araujo N, Correa L, Pires Soubhia AM, Cavalcanti de Araujo V. Immunohistochemical aspects of basal cell adenoma and canalicular adenoma of salivary glands. *Oral Oncol.* 2001;37(4):365-368.

17. Maiorano E, Favia G, Viale G. Lymphoepithelial cysts of salivary glands: an immunohistochemical study of HIV-related and HIV-unrelated lesions. *Hum Pathol.* 1998;29(3):260-265.

18. Marie PJ. Cellular and molecular basis of fibrous dysplasia. *Histol Histopathol.* 2001;16(3):981-988.

19. Mendenhall WM, Amdur RJ, Vaysberg M, Mendenhall CM, Werning JW. Head and neck paragangliomas. *Head Neck.* 2011;33(10):1530-1534.

20. Nava VE, Jaffe ES. The pathology of NK-cell lymphomas and leukemias. *Adv Anat Pathol.* 2005;12(1):27-34.

21. O'Devaney K, Ferlito A, Hunter BC, Devaney SL, Rinaldo A. Wegener's granulomatosis of the head and neck. *Ann Otol Rhinol Laryngol.* 1998;107(5 Pt 1):439-445.

22. Pentenero M, Gandolfo S, Carrozzo M. Importance of tumor thickness and depth of invasion in nodal involvement and prognosis of oral squamous cell carcinoma: a review of the literature. *Head Neck.* 2005;27(12):1080-1091.

23. Seethala RR, Dacic S, Cieply K, Kelly LM, Nikiforova MN). A reappraisal of the MECT1/MAML2 translocation in salivary mucoepidermoid carcinomas. *Am J Surg Pathol.* 2010;34(8):1106-1121.

24. Skalova A, Starek I, Vanecek T, et al. Expression of HER-2/neu gene and protein in salivary duct carcinomas of parotid gland as revealed by fluorescence in-situ hybridization and immunohistochemistry. *Histopathology.* 2003;42(4):348-356.

25. Skalova A, Vanecek T, Sima R, et al. Mammary analogue secretory carcinoma of salivary glands, containing the ETV6-NTRK3 fusion gene: a hitherto undescribed salivary gland tumor entity. *Am J Surg Pathol.* 2010;34(5):599-608.

26. Stelow EB, French CA. Carcinomas of the upper aerodigestive tract with rearrangement of the nuclear protein of the testis (NUT) gene (NUT midline carcinomas). *Adv Anat Pathol.* 2009;16(2):92-96.

27. Stelow EB, Mills SE, Jo VY, Carlson DL. Adenocarcinoma of the upper aerodigestive tract. *Adv Anat Pathol.* 2010;17(4):262-269.

28. Thompson LD. Diagnostically challenging lesions in head and neck pathology. *Eur Arch Otorhinolaryngol.* 1997;254(8):357-366.

29. Thompson LD. Olfactory neuroblastoma. *Head Neck Pathol.* 2009;3(3):252-259.

30. Thompson LD, Gannon FH. Chondrosarcoma of the larynx: a clinicopathologic study of 111 cases with a review of the literature. *Am J Surg Pathol.* 2002;26(7):836-851.

31. Thompson LD, Miettinen M, Wenig BM. Sinonasal-type hemangiopericytoma: a clinicopathologic and immunophenotypic analysis of 104 cases showing perivascular myoid differentiation. *Am J Surg Pathol.* 2003;27(6):737-749.

32. Vered M, Dobriyan A, Buchner A. Congenital granular cell epulis presents an immunohistochemical profile that distinguishes it from the granular cell tumor of the adult. *Virchows Arch.* 2009;454(3):303-310.

33. Vitali C, Bombardieri S, Jonsson R, et al. Classification criteria for Sjogren's syndrome: a revised version of the European criteria proposed by the American-European Consensus Group. *Ann Rheum Dis.* 2002;61(6):554-558.

34. Williams SB, Ellis GL, Warnock GR. Sialoblastoma: a clinicopathologic and immunohistochemical study of 7 cases. *Ann Diagn Pathol.* 2006;10(6):320-326.

CHAPTER 17

HEMATOPATHOLOGY: LYMPH NODE AND SPLEEN

1. Which of the following markers is exclusively expressed by centrocytes and centroblasts located within the germinal center?
   (A) CD3
   (B) CD10
   (C) CD20
   (D) CD45
   (E) CD68

2. In addition to T-lymphocytes, which of the following cells populate the paracortical region of the lymph node?
   (A) B-lymphocytes
   (B) Dendritic reticulum cells
   (C) Interdigitating cells
   (D) Mast cells
   (E) Plasma cells

3. Which of the following conditions is not a cause of generalized lymphadenopathy?
   (A) Autoimmune hemolytic anemia
   (B) Hyperthyroidism
   (C) Metastatic carcinoma
   (D) Lymphoma
   (E) Sarcoidosis

4. Which of the following cytochemical stains is most helpful in diagnosing hairy cell leukemia?
   (A) Methyl green pyronine
   (B) Nonspecific esterase
   (C) Periodic acid-Schiff
   (D) Sudan Black B
   (E) Tartrate-resistant acid phosphatase

5. A 15-year-old girl presents with fever, pharyngitis, and lymphadenopathy. The paracortical region of an enlarged cervical lymph node shows a polymorphic population of lymphoid cells, including Reed-Sternberg-like cells. These large cells are positive for CD45 and CD30, and lack CD15 expression. Based on these findings, what is the best diagnosis?
   (A) Classical Hodgkin lymphoma
   (B) Cytomegalovirus lymphadenitis
   (C) Diffuse large B-cell lymphoma
   (D) Infectious mononucleosis lymphadenitis
   (E) Toxoplasma lymphadenitis

6. All the following lymphadenitides are associated with lymph node necrosis, except
   (A) Cat-scratch lymphadenitis
   (B) Kikuchi-Fujimoto lymphadenitis
   (C) Herpes simplex virus lymphadenitis
   (D) Mycobacterial tuberculosis lymphadenitis
   (E) Toxoplasma lymphadenitis

7. Warthin-Finkeldey type of giant cells are least likely to be associated with which of the following conditions?
   (A) Follicular lymphoma
   (B) Gonococcal lymphadenitis
   (C) HIV lymphadenitis
   (D) Lymphocyte-predominant Hodgkin lymphoma
   (E) Measles lymphadenitis

8. All the following features can be seen in the acute phase of HIV lymphadenitis, except:
   (A) Aggregates of monocytoid cells along blood vessels
   (B) Atrophic follicles
   (C) Diminished mantle zone
   (D) Numerous tingible body macrophages
   (E) Scattered multinucleate giant cells

9. An axillary lymph node excision with the corresponding Warthin-Starry stain is shown in Figure 17-1. These findings are diagnostic of

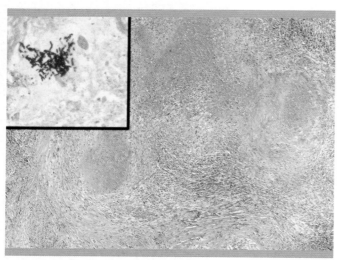

FIGURE 17-1

(A) Cat-scratch lymphadenitis
(B) Fungal lymphadenitis
(C) HIV lymphadenitis
(D) Kikuchi lymphadenitis
(E) Tuberculous lymphadenitis

10. A 42-year-old man with a history of fever, diarrhea, and weight loss is found to have widespread lymphadenopathy. An image from his cervical lymph node excision is shown in Figure 17-2. Stains for acid-fast bacilli and fungal organisms were negative. A PAS-diastase stain was positive. These findings are diagnostic of

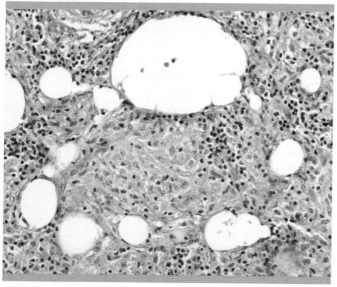

FIGURE 17-2

(A) Fungal lymphadenitis
(B) Hodgkin lymphoma
(C) Niemann-Pick disease
(D) Tuberculous lymphadenitis
(E) Whipple disease

11. All the following features are associated with toxoplasma lymphadenitis, except
(A) Aggregates of epithelioid histiocytes
(B) Aggregates of monocytoid cells surrounding blood vessels
(C) Follicular hyperplasia
(D) Necrosis
(E) Posterior cervical lymph node involvement

12. Which of the following carcinomas is least likely to metastasize to the supraclavicular lymph nodes?
(A) Colon
(B) Esophagus
(C) Lung
(D) Pancreas
(E) Stomach

13. All the following diseases cause matted lymphadenopathy, except
(A) Cat-scratch disease
(B) Cancer
(C) Lymphogranuloma venereum
(D) Measles
(E) Tuberculosis

14. All the following findings support a diagnosis of reactive lymphoid hyperplasia, except
(A) Distended germinal centers
(B) Enlarged, oddly shaped follicles
(C) Frequent mitoses
(D) Germinal centers are bcl-2 positive
(E) Peripheral rim of inactivated lymphocytes

15. Progressive transformation of germinal centers is associated with all the following findings, except
(A) Occurs in young adults
(B) Occasional Reed-Sternberg cells are present in the interfollicular space
(C) Presence of a large lymphoid nodule that is 3–5 times the diameter of an adjacent follicle
(D) Small lymphocytes infiltrate the germinal centers
(E) Usually presents as a single, enlarged lymph node

16. A 35-year-old man presents with a nodular lesion in the infraauricular region and an enlarged cervical lymph node. Lymph node examination shows diffuse eosinophilia with eosinophilic microabscesses and infiltration of the germinal centers. In addition, there is prominent vascular hyperplasia of postcapillary venules. Based on these findings, what is the best diagnosis?
    (A) Angiolymphoid hyperplasia with eosinophilia
    (B) Castleman's disease
    (C) Hodgkin lymphoma
    (D) Kikuchi disease
    (E) Kimura's disease

17. A 14-year-old teenager with a history of massive lymphadenopathy and polyclonal hypergammaglobulinemia undergoes lymph node excision that shows marked sinusoidal dilatation with effacement of follicles. Emperipolesis is conspicuous. Which of following immunohistochemical stains is least likely to be expressed by the cells of interest?
    (A) CD1a
    (B) CD4
    (C) CD30
    (D) CD68
    (E) S-100

18. A young woman of Japanese descent complains of mild fever and painless lymphadenopathy. An image from her cervical lymph node excision is shown in Figure 17-3. What is the most likely diagnosis?

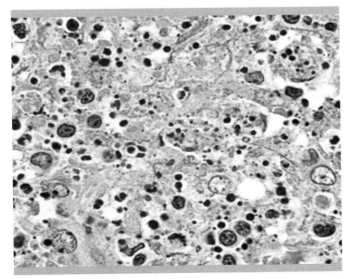

FIGURE 17-3

(A) Bacterial lymphadenitis
(B) Cat-scratch disease
(C) Kikuchi disease
(D) Lupus lymphadenitis
(E) Tuberculous lymphadenitis

19. A 25-year-old woman with a history of fever, weight loss, and a butterfly-patterned malar rash is noted to have generalized lymphadenopathy. The clinician is concerned about an infectious process and performs a lymph node excision that is shown in Figure 17-4. Based on these clinicopathologic findings, what is the most likely cause of patient's lymphadenopathy?

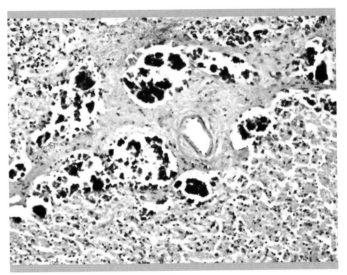

FIGURE 17-4

(A) Cat-scratch disease
(B) Kikuchi lymphadenitis
(C) Lupus lymphadenitis
(D) Luetic lymphadenitis
(E) Toxoplasma lymphadenitis

20. An axillary lymph node biopsy from a patient with a history of psoriasis is shown in Figure 17-5. The findings depicted in this figure are diagnostic of

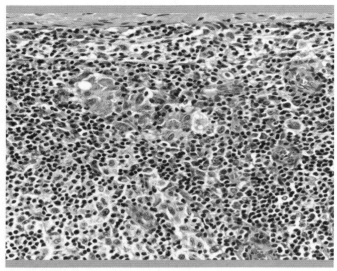

FIGURE 17-5

(A) Dermatopathic lymphadenitis
(B) Hodgkin lymphoma
(C) Metastatic melanoma
(D) Mycosis fungoides
(E) Toxoplasma lymphadenitis

21. All the following features are typically associated with the entity depicted in Figure 17-6, except

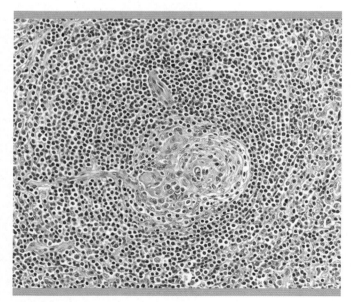

FIGURE 17-6

(A) Follicles with two or more small germinal centers
(B) Lymphocyte-depleted germinal centers
(C) PAS-positive hyaline deposits within germinal centers
(D) Sclerotic blood vessels radially penetrating the follicles
(E) Sheets of plasma cells

22. Which of the following neoplasms is not associated with Castleman's disease?
(A) Classic Hodgkin lymphoma
(B) Diffuse large B-cell lymphoma
(C) Follicular dendritic cell sarcoma
(D) Kaposi's sarcoma
(E) Multiple myeloma

23. Regional lymph nodes that drain tumors can be associated with all the following findings, except
(A) Desmoplastic reaction
(B) Granulomas
(C) Lymphocyte depletion
(D) Sinus histiocytosis
(E) Vascular transformation of sinuses

24. A 29-year-old patient with a history of convulsive disorder is noted to have atypical lymphocytosis in peripheral blood. A lymph node excision specimen shows relative preservation of nodal architecture and paracortical expansion by a mixed cellular infiltrate, including numerous immunoblasts. Occasional CD30-positive large cells are also present. What is the best diagnosis?
(A) Anaplastic large cell lymphoma
(B) Angioimmunoblastic T-cell lymphoma
(C) Hodgkin lymphoma
(D) Phenytoin lymphadenitis
(E) Viral lymphadenitis

25. In which group of lymph nodes are you most likely to find lipogranulomas?
(A) Celiac
(B) Cervical
(C) Iliac
(D) Inguinal
(E) Mediastinal

26. A lymph node shows dilated sinusoids with sheets of polyethylene-containing foamy macrophages containing needle-like flakes of black material. Which of the following clinical situations can result in this finding?
(A) A patient with a history of breast implant
(B) A patient with a history of smoking
(C) A patient with a large joint prosthesis

(D) A patient with a history of intravenous drug abuse

(E) A patient with a history of rheumatoid arthritis

27. All the following features are helpful in differentiating benign glandular inclusions from metastatic adenocarcinoma, except
    (A) Capsular/subcapsular location
    (B) Cytokeratin CAM5.2 stain
    (C) Lack of mitotic activity
    (D) Lack of nuclear pleomorphism
    (E) Lack of vascular/sinus invasion

28. All subtypes of Hodgkin lymphoma share the following features, except
    (A) Majority of the patients are young adults
    (B) Preferential involvement of cervical lymph node
    (C) Presence of extensive parenchymal fibrosis
    (D) Tumor cells surrounded by T cells
    (E) Scattered mononuclear and multinuclear tumor cells

29. A mediastinal lymph node excision from a 40-year-old man is shown in Figure 17-7. The overall lymph node had a nodular architecture and these large cells were seen in the interfollicular region. The cells shown in this figure would express all the following immunohistochemical markers, except

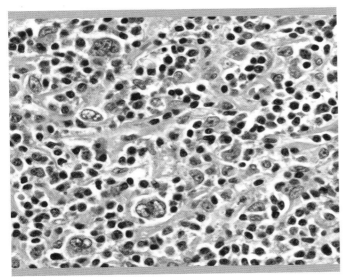

FIGURE 17-7

(A) BCL6
(B) CD15
(C) CD20
(D) CD45
(E) CD79a

30. Based on Figure 17-8, how is this variant of Hodgkin lymphoma best classified?

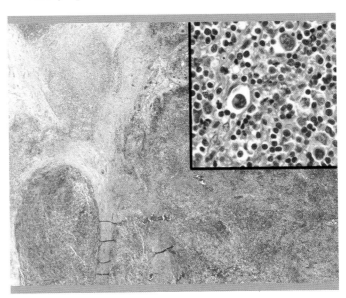

FIGURE 17-8

(A) Lymphocyte-depleted Hodgkin lymphoma
(B) Lymphocyte-predominant Hodgkin lymphoma
(C) Mixed cellularity Hodgkin lymphoma
(D) Nodular lymphocyte-predominant Hodgkin lymphoma
(E) Nodular sclerosis Hodgkin lymphoma

31. With respect to classical Hodgkin lymphoma, what is the frequency of OCT-2 and BOB.1 expression in Hodgkin Reed-Sternberg cells?
    (A) 5%
    (B) 10%
    (C) 50%
    (D) 90%
    (E) 100%

32. Within lymphoblastic lymphomas, what percentage of cases are of the B-cell phenotype?
    (A) 5%
    (B) 10%
    (C) 50%
    (D) 90%
    (E) 100%

33. Which of the following molecular alterations is associated with the worst clinical prognosis in patients with B-cell acute lymphoblastic leukemia?
    (A) t(4;11)
    (B) t(9;22)
    (C) t(12;21)
    (D) Hyperdiploidy
    (E) Hypodiploidy

34. What is the most common type of leukemia encountered in infants less than 1 year of age?
    (A) ALL with hyperdiploidy
    (B) ALL with hypodiploidy
    (C) ALL with *MLL* gene rearrangement
    (D) AML with monoblastic and monocytic features
    (E) Myeloid leukemia associated with Down syndrome

35. Hyperdiploid B-cell acute lymphoblastic leukemia is most commonly associated with extra copies of the following chromosomes, except
    (A) 3
    (B) 4
    (C) 14
    (D) 21
    (E) X

36. Which of the following genetic alterations in B-cell acute lymphoblastic leukemia is associated with a favorable prognosis?
    (A) Hyperdiploidy
    (B) Hypodiploidy
    (C) t(1;19)
    (D) t(4;11)
    (E) t(5;14)

37. A lymph node excision from a 70-year-old patient with chronic lymphocytic leukemia/small lymphocytic lymphoma is shown in Figure 17-9. The larger cells present within this proliferation center are referred to as

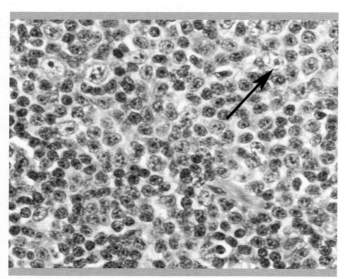

FIGURE 17-9

(A) Centroblasts
(B) Centrocytes
(C) Paraimmunoblasts
(D) Plasma cells
(E) Tingible body macrophages

38. In chronic lymphocytic leukemia, all the following factors are associated with a poor prognosis, except
    (A) Deletion 11q
    (B) Expression of ZAP-70
    (C) Expression of CD38
    (D) *IgHV* gene mutation
    (E) Rapid lymphocyte doubling time in peripheral blood

39. What percentage of peripheral blood prolymphocytes is required for a diagnosis of B-cell prolymphocytic leukemia?
    (A) 5%
    (B) 10%
    (C) 50%
    (D) 55%
    (E) 90%

40. Splenic B-cell marginal zone lymphoma is associated with all of the following features, except
    (A) Bone marrow may show intrasinusoidal lymphoma cells
    (B) Most patients are >50 years old
    (C) Peripheral blood shows presence of villous lymphocytes
    (D) Tumor cells express CD5 and annexin-1
    (E) Tumor involves spleen and splenic hilar lymph node

41. A splenectomy specimen from 60-year-old woman with splenomegaly, weakness, fatigue, monocytopenia, and a red pulp predominant infiltrate is shown in Figure 17-10. The cells express CD20, CD11c, CD103, CD25, and annexin-1. What is the best diagnosis?

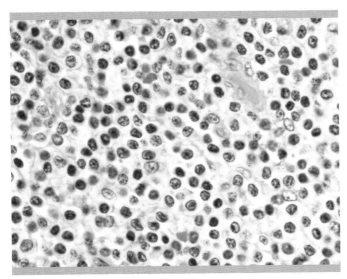

FIGURE 17-10

(A) Chronic lymphocytic leukemia/small lympho-
cytic lymphoma
(B) Chronic myeloid leukemia
(C) Diffuse large B-cell lymphoma
(D) Hairy cell leukemia
(E) Splenic lymphoma with villous lymphocytes

42. Which hematolymphoid malignancy is most likely
to be associated with IgM paraproteinemia and PAS-
positive material within the lymph node sinuses?
(A) Chronic lymphocytic leukemia/small lympho-
cytic lymphoma
(B) Lymphoplasmacytic lymphoma
(C) Mantle cell lymphoma
(D) Marginal zone lymphoma
(E) Multiple myeloma

43. A 70-year-old woman with a history of anemia is
found to have a clonal plasma cell disorder with
lytic bone lesions, hypercalcemia, and renal insufficiency. The finding of elevated M-protein in this
patient is due to overproduction of which of the
following serum proteins?
(A) IgA
(B) IgD
(C) IgE
(D) IgG
(E) Light chain kappa

44. In addition to the lack of surface immunoglobu-
lin expression, plasma cell myeloma cells lack
expression of which of the following markers?
(A) CD19
(B) CD38
(C) CD56
(D) CD79a
(E) CD138

45. Antibiotic therapy for *Helicobacter pylori* (*H. pylori*)
infection usually induces protracted remission in all
cases of *H. pylori*-associated marginal zone lympho-
mas, except in those that demonstrate the following
translocation
(A) t(1;14)
(B) t(3;14)
(C) t(11;18)
(D) t(14;18)
(E) +3

46. Which of the following oncogenes is most
frequently rearranged in follicular lymphoma?
(A) *bcl-2*
(B) *bcl-6*
(C) *myc*
(D) *p16*
(E) *p53*

47. A 60-year-old man with a history of numerous gastrointestinal polyps was found to have a lymphoid
neoplasm composed of CD20-positive, small-to
medium-sized lymphocytes with irregular nuclear
contours, and *CCDN1* translocation. Which of the
following choices is the most reproducible adverse
prognostic parameter associated with this neoplasm?
(A) Blastoid morphology
(B) Bone marrow involvement
(C) Increased mitotic rate
(D) Increased plasma cells
(E) Peripheral blood involvement

48. What is the most common extranodal site of
involvement by diffuse large B-cell lymphoma,
not otherwise specified?
(A) Bone
(B) Gastrointestinal tract
(C) Skin
(D) Spleen
(E) Testis

49. A 35-year-old woman with superior vena cava syndrome is found to have an anterosuperior mediastinal mass shown in Figure 17-11. She does not have involvement of the lymph nodes or bone marrow. The tumor cells express CD20, CD30, and CD23. These findings are diagnostic of

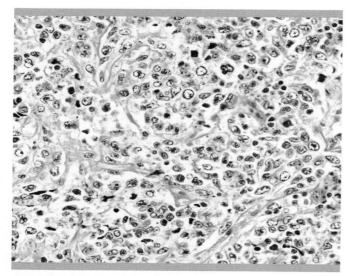

FIGURE 17-11

    (A) Diffuse large B-cell lymphoma
    (B) Hodgkin lymphoma
    (C) Primary mediastinal (thymic) large B-cell lymphoma
    (D) T-cell acute lymphoblastic leukemia
    (E) Thymoma

50. Which of the following finding is unusual for nevus cell inclusions found within a lymph node?
    (A) Capsular aggregates
    (B) HMB-45 immunoreactivity
    (C) Lack of marginal sinus involvement
    (D) Lack of nuclear pleomorphism
    (E) Monomorphic cell population

51. Autoinfarction of the spleen occurs in which of the following conditions?
    (A) Amyloidosis
    (B) Gaucher's disease
    (C) Rheumatoid arthritis
    (D) Sickle cell anemia
    (E) Systemic lupus erythematosus

52. A 4-year-old boy of African descent born in a malaria-endemic region presents with a large jaw tumor composed of medium-sized lymphoid cells with cytoplasmic lipid vacuoles. Which immunohistochemical stain is least likely to be expressed by these cells?
    (A) CD10
    (B) CD20
    (C) CD38
    (D) Ki-67
    (E) TdT

53. A 25-year-old man with cervical lymphadenopathy undergoes an excisional biopsy shown in Figure 17-12. The lesional cells show ALK protein immunoreactivity and membranous and Golgi pattern of staining with CD30. These findings are diagnostic of

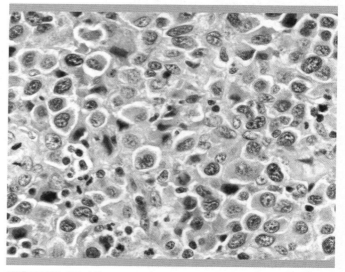

FIGURE 17-12

    (A) Anaplastic large cell lymphoma, ALK-positive
    (B) Burkitt lymphoma
    (C) B-lymphoblastic lymphoma
    (D) Diffuse large B-cell lymphoma
    (E) Hodgkin lymphoma

54. A 55-year-old man from Caribbean islands presents with widespread lymphadenopathy and peripheral blood lymphocytosis. The peripheral blood shows large lymphoid cells with basophilic cytoplasm and irregular convoluted/lobulated nuclei. Which of the following statements does not apply to the entity described here?
    (A) Associated with EBV infection
    (B) Associated with frequent opportunistic infections
    (C) Hepatosplenomegaly
    (D) Hypercalcemia
    (E) Skin rash

ANSWERS

1. **(B) CD10.**
   The secondary or reactive lymphoid follicles are composed of a peripheral mantle of small lymphocytes and a central germinal center that contains centroblasts, centrocytes, small lymphocytes, tingible body macrophages, and dendritic reticulum cells. Centrocytes and centroblasts specifically express CD10 (common acute lymphoblastic leukemia antigen, CALLA). CD3 is a pan T-cell marker, while CD20 is a pan B-cell marker. CD45 or leukocyte common antigen (LCA) is expressed by all hematopoietic cells, except erythrocytes and platelets. CD68 is expressed by histiocytes.

2. **(C) Interdigitating cells.**
   Paracortical region (deep cortex) is the region of the lymph node present between the follicles. It is the thymus-dependent area of a lymph node and contains T-lymphocytes that have undergone differentiation within the thymic cortex and medulla. Interdigitating cells (IDCs) are antigen-presenting cells located in the paracortical region that play an important role in initiating an immune response. Similar to Langerhans cells, they contain Birbeck granules, and express CD1a and S-100 protein.

3. **(C) Metastatic carcinoma.**
   All the listed conditions can present with generalized lymphadenopathy, except metastatic carcinoma, which usually presents with localized or regional lymphadenopathy.

4. **(E) Tartrate-resistant acid phosphatase.**
   Tartrate-resistant acid phosphatase is an isoenzyme, which is almost exclusively expressed by hairy cell leukemia cells. This property can be useful in differentiating it from other lymphocytic lymphomas and leukemias. Methyl green pyronine-positive material is present in immunoglobulin-secreting plasma cells and immunoblasts. Nonspecific esterases are enzymes located within the cytoplasm of monocytes/histiocytes. Periodic acid-Schiff stains glycogen in the form of block-like intracytoplasmic aggregates in acute lymphoblastic leukemia, or as chunk-like regular aggregates in erythroblastic leukemia. Sudan Black B is strongly positive in myeloid cells and eosinophils, faintly positive in monocytes, and negative in lymphocytes and erythroid cells.

5. **(D) Infectious mononucleosis lymphadenitis.**
   Although the findings are very suggestive of Hodgkin lymphoma, the immunoprofile does not support this diagnosis (large cells in Hodgkin lymphoma are usually CD30 and CD15 positive, and lack CD45 expression). In conjunction with the history, the changes are diagnostic of infectious mononucleosis

lymphadenitis. The lymph nodes often show marked follicular hyperplasia along with dilated sinuses. Large B-cell lymphoma is associated with a monotonous proliferation of lymphoid cells.

6. **(E) Toxoplasma lymphadenitis.**
   All the choices listed here show foci of lymph node necrosis, except toxoplasma lymphadenitis.

7. **(B) Gonococcal lymphadenitis.**
   Warthin-Finkeldey type of giant cells or polykaryocytes are multinucleated giant cells that are frequently associated with viral infections and low-grade lymphomas. They are most commonly observed in the prodromal phase of measles infection and in the acute phase of HIV lymphadenitis.

8. **(B) Atrophic follicles.**
   Acute HIV lymphadenitis is marked by the presence of follicular hyperplasia with serpiginous or hourglass-shaped lymphoid follicles (pattern A). The germinal centers show widespread apoptosis and numerous tingible body macrophages. As the disease progresses, there is effacement of the lymphoid follicles with involution of germinal centers (pattern B). Pattern C is characterized by atrophic or burned out follicles with diffuse and extensive vascular proliferation. Hyalinized follicles with arterioles surrounded by collagen ("lollipop" follicle) are often present in the chronic stage of HIV lymphadenitis.

9. **(A) Cat-scratch lymphadenitis.**
   The figure demonstrates necrotizing granulomas with central microabscess formation and clumps of bacteria highlighted by the Warthin-Starry stain (inset), findings diagnostic of cat-scratch lymphadenitis. Cat-scratch lymphadenitis is caused due to a cat scratch, lick, or bite, which results in cutaneous inoculation of the organism *Bartonella henselae*. Fungal and tuberculous lymphadenitis can be differentiated by the use of special stains. The latter infection usually shows caseous necrosis without nuclear debris or neutrophils. Lymph nodes affected by Kikuchi lymphadenitis do not show neutrophils or granulomas. Cat-scratch lymphadenitis can be difficult to distinguish from lymphogranuloma venereum lymphadenitis and this distinction requires the use of additional techniques such as serology.

10. **(E) Whipple disease.**
    The figure shows numerous histiocytes within the lymph node sinuses along with large cystic spaces representing fat vacuoles. In combination with the PAS-diastase positivity, these changes are diagnostic of Whipple disease. Whipple disease often presents with multisystem illness including lymphadenopathy. Niemann-Pick macrophages show clear intracytoplasmic vacuoles that do not stain with

PAS-diastase. Hodgkin lymphoma may be associated with epithelioid granulomas; however, prominent sinusoidal histiocytosis is not a common finding.

11. **(D) Necrosis.**
The triad of toxoplasma lymphadenitis includes findings described in choices A, B, and C. Posterior cervical lymph nodes are most commonly involved. In less than 1% of cases, macrophages may show trophozoite forms of the organism.

12. **(A) Colon.**
Right supraclavicular lymph node involvement is seen in carcinomas originating from esophagus and lung. Left supraclavicular lymph node (Virchow sign) enlargement may be seen in metastatic carcinoma from the stomach, pancreas, or gallbladder. Colon usually does not metastasize to this group of lymph nodes.

13. **(D) Measles.**
Viral diseases usually cause "shotty" lymphadenopathy. These lymph nodes are small in size. All the other conditions listed here cause matted lymphadenopathy, which occurs due to fibrous adhesions between the lymph node capsule and adjacent soft tissues.

14. **(D) Germinal centers are bcl-2 positive.**
Both reactive lymphoid hyperplasia and follicular lymphoma are associated with enlarged follicles distributed within the cortex and medulla. Features that favor reactive lymphoid hyperplasia include the presence of a mantle zone, tingible body macrophages within the germinal centers, and bcl-2-negative germinal centers. Follicular lymphoma shows numerous follicles with a back-to-back arrangement, with variable infiltration into the perinodal fat. The characteristic t(14;18) translocation found in >90% cases of follicular lymphoma leads to overexpression of bcl-2 in the germinal center cells.

15. **(B) Occasional Reed-Sternberg cells are present in the interfollicular space.**
Progressive transformation of germinal centers (PTGC) is a benign reactive condition that causes partial effacement of lymph node architecture. It is associated with reactive follicular hyperplasia. PTGC is characterized by the presence of large nodules of lymphocytes that are 3–5 times the size of adjacent reactive follicles. In these nodules, small lymphocytes migrate into the germinal center in multiple areas and disrupt the germinal center. The interfollicular region is typically uninvolved, and Reed-Sternberg cells are never present in this entity. In contrast to PTGC, nodular lymphocyte-predominant Hodgkin lymphoma and lymphocyte-rich Hodgkin lymphoma show neoplastic "popcorn" cells and Reed-Sternberg cells, respectively and cause diffuse effacement of nodal architecture.

16. **(E) Kimura's disease.**
Kimura's disease is a chronic inflammatory disorder characterized by angiolymphoid hyperplasia and eosinophilia. It is most prevalent in the Asian male population and has features that overlap with the entity angiolymphoid hyperplasia with eosinophilia (ALHE). Kimura's disease affects the deep subcutaneous tissue and regional lymph nodes. In contrast, ALHE involves the dermis, and often presents in Caucasian female population, without evidence of lymphadenopathy. Kimura's disease is usually associated with peripheral blood eosinophilia and elevated IgE levels. Other conditions that can cause lymph node eosinophilia include Hodgkin disease, drug reaction, and parasitic infection. Because of the pronounced vascular proliferation, Castleman's disease is also in the differential.

17. **(A) CD1a.**
The condition described here is Rosai-Dorfman disease or sinus histiocytosis with massive lymphadenopathy, a benign disorder of histiocytes that typically demonstrates intracellular engulfment of lymphocytes. The cells within the histiocytes are present inside a vacuole and, are therefore, protected from cytolysis. These lymphocytes are viable and seem to traffic in and out of these histiocytes (emperipolesis means wandering in and around). The histiocytes express CD68, CD4, CD30 (activated macrophage marker), and S-100 (stain of choice). They are usually negative for CD1a. The disease usually affects cervical lymph nodes in children and adolescents. The differential diagnosis includes non-specific sinus histiocytosis (histiocytes do not stain with S-100), malignant histiocytosis, granulomatous reaction, Langerhans cell histiocytosis (CD1a positive), and Hodgkin lymphoma.

18. **(C) Kikuchi disease.**
The figure shows irregular areas of necrosis with numerous apoptotic cells and aggregates of histiocytes with typical crescent-shaped nuclei. Note the absence of neutrophils or eosinophils. These changes in a young Asian woman are diagnostic of Kikuchi-Fujimoto lymphadenitis, a form of subacute necrotizing lymphadenitis. Cervical lymph nodes are affected in nearly 8% of patients. Fibrinoid necrosis with apoptosis, and a mixture of predominantly CD8-positive T-lymphocytes, plasmacytoid monocytes, and immunoblasts, is characteristic. Depending on the cell population, four different forms have been described: lymphohistiocytic (most common), necrotic, foamy cell type, and phagocytic type. Electron microscopy shows tubuloreticular structures (TRS) within histiocytes. TRS

have also been described in HIV infection, autoimmune diseases, and with alpha interferon therapy.

19. **(C) Lupus lymphadenitis.**
The figure shows necrotic lymph node parenchyma with basophilic hematoxylin bodies. These changes in conjunction with the clinical findings are typical of lupus lymphadenitis. Hematoxylin bodies are composed of aggregates of nuclear DNA, polysaccharides, and immunoglobulins. The lymph nodes show numerous plasma cells, while neutrophils and eosinophils are absent. Blood vessels often show Azzopardi phenomenon, which results from the deposition of hematoxylin-staining nuclear material within the vessels walls that demonstrate fibrinoid necrosis. Kikuchi lymphadenitis is a close differential, and is distinguished by the absence of hematoxylin bodies and antinuclear antibodies.

20. **(A) Dermatopathic lymphadenitis.**
The findings in this figure are those of dermatopathic lymphadenitis, a reactive paracortical hyperplasia of lymph nodes that is associated with increased numbers of interdigitating dendritic cells, Langerhans cells, and histiocytes, with cytoplasmic melanin and lipid vacuoles. These findings are typically associated with skin diseases such as psoriasis and mycosis fungoides. Pruritus is a common symptom.

21. **(E) Sheets of plasma cells.**
The figure shows the characteristic hyaline vascular lesion of Castleman's disease. Two forms of Castleman's disease have been recognized: localized and multicentric. The localized form shows two histologic variants: hyaline-vascular and plasma cell. All the features listed here are typical of the hyaline vascular variant, except for the presence of sheets of plasma cells. Most lymphoid follicles often contain more than one germinal center (twinning) and a broad mantle zone composed of small lymphocytes arranged in a concentric fashion (onion-skinning). Choice D describes the hyaline vascular or "lollipop" lesion found in the classic hyaline-vascular type of Castleman's disease.

22. **(E) Multiple myeloma.**
Due to the causal association with HHV-8 infection, patients with Castleman's disease may develop several other neoplasms such as primary effusion lymphoma, plasmablastic lymphoma, mantle cell lymphoma, and peripheral T-cell lymphoma.

23. **(A) Desmoplastic reaction.**
Lymph nodes draining tumors show many nonspecific changes such as granulomas, lymphocyte depletion, lymphocyte predominance, sinus histiocytosis, and vascular transformation of sinuses. Desmoplastic reaction represents stromal response

to tumor cells, and is usually absent in lymph nodes draining tumors.

24. **(D) Phenytoin lymphadenitis.**
Many drugs can induce hypersensitivity-related lymphadenopathy. Phenytoin and carbamazepine are the best-known examples of this condition. The histologic findings include paracortical, mixed cellular infiltrate composed of immunoblasts, eosinophils, and plasma cells. The findings typically regress following withdrawal of the drug.

25. **(A) Celiac.**
Lipogranulomas may be seen in lymph nodes draining the biliary system, especially in the setting of hyperlipidemia and diabetes mellitus. Histologic findings include the presence of microcysts and lipid droplets within multinucleated foreign-body type giant cells.

26. **(C) A patient with a large joint prosthesis.**
Lymph nodes draining joints with prosthesis are often enlarged and show a black or dark brown cut surface. They are associated with sinus histiocytosis and needle-like flakes of black polyethylene material that is strongly birefringent under polarized light. Patients with a history of breast implant show silicone-filled, vacuolated histiocytes. Rheumatoid arthritis patients may show methotrexate-related lymphoproliferative disorders that range from polymorphous to monomorphous lesions, and Hodgkin lymphoma. Those with a history of smoking may show refractile, brown-black pigment within lymph node histiocytes.

27. **(B) Cytokeratin CAM5.2 stain.**
Epithelial cell inclusions are incidental findings that may mimic metastatic carcinoma. The common types of inclusions include salivary gland inclusions in upper cervical lymph nodes, thyroid follicles (devoid of papillae) in central neck lymph node, mammary ducts and cysts in axillary lymph nodes, mesothelial inclusions in mediastinal lymph nodes, and Müllerian epithelium in pelvic nodes. Cytologic and architectural features are most helpful in distinguishing benign inclusions from metastatic carcinoma.

28. **(C) Presence of extensive parenchymal fibrosis.**
Hodgkin lymphoma is composed of two entities: nodular lymphocyte predominant Hodgkin lymphoma (NLPHL) and classical Hodgkin lymphoma. Both entities differ in morphology and immunophenotype. Classical Hodgkin lymphoma is classified into four subtypes: nodular sclerosis, mixed cellularity, lymphocyte-rich, and lymphocyte-depleted. NLPHL and classical Hodgkin lymphoma share some features (choices A, B, D, and E), except for the presence of parenchymal fibrosis, a

feature typically associated with nodular sclerosis-type of classical Hodgkin lymphoma.

29. **(B) CD15.**
The figure shows the characteristic lymphocyte predominant (LP) cells or "popcorn" cells found in nodular lymphocyte predominant Hodgkin lymphoma. The disease is characterized by a nodular, or nodular and diffuse architecture, with scattered neoplastic cells exhibiting folded or multilobated nuclei and multiple basophilic nucleoli. LP cells are positive for CD20, CD79a, BCL6, and CD45, Nearly 50% of cases also express EMA. In contrast to classical Hodgkin lymphoma, OCT-2 and BOB.1 are co-expressed in NLPHL. LP cells typically lack CD15 and CD30 expression.

30. **(E) Nodular sclerosis Hodgkin lymphoma.**
The low magnification figure shows nodular lymph node architecture with bands of fibrosis. The inset shows "lacunar" cells that are diagnostic of nodular sclerosis subtype of classical Hodgkin lymphoma. The "lacunae" are a manifestation of cytoplasmic retraction caused due to formalin-fixation.

31. **(B) 10%.**
Hodgkin Reed-Sternberg cells lack expression of transcription factor OCT-2 and its co-activator, BOB.1, in nearly 90% of cases. The background non-neoplastic B cells serve as a good internal control for both these markers.

32. **(B) 10%.**
Most cases of lymphoblastic lymphomas are of T-cell lineage. The B-cell phenotype accounts for nearly 10% of all cases of lymphoblastic lymphoma.

33. **(B) t(9;22).**
B-lymphoblastic leukemia/lymphomas are associated with recurrent genetic abnormalities that have variable clinical prognosis. Of the choices listed, t(9;22) is associated with the worst prognosis among patients with ALL.

34. **(C) ALL with *MLL* gene rearrangement.**
MLL gene located on chromosome 11q23 is involved in translocation with a variety of fusion partners. This type of leukemia occurs in infants <1 year of age, presents with a very high white blood cell count (usually >1,00000/µl), and is associated with a high frequency of CNS involvement at diagnosis.

35. **(A) 3.**
B-lymphoblastic leukemia/lymphoma with hyperploidy is characterized by lymphoblasts that contain >50 and usually <66 chromosomes, typically without any translocations or structural alterations. Extra copies of chromosomes 21, X, 14, and 4, are more commonly found, compared to chromosomes 1, 2, and 3.

36. **(A) Hyperdiploidy.**
Among the B-lymphoblastic leukemia/lymphomas with recurrent translocations, t(1;19) and t(5;14) are associated with a good prognosis. Hypodiploidy, t(4;11), and t(9;22) are associated with a poor prognosis, while patients with hyperdiploidy and t(12;21) have a favorable clinical prognosis.

37. **(C) Paraimmunoblasts.**
Lymph nodes involved by chronic lymphocytic leukemia/small lymphocytic lymphoma (CLL/SLL) show a pseudofollicular architecture (they are not surrounded by a mantle zone) consisting of regularly distributed pale areas known as proliferation centers. Proliferation centers are composed of small, medium, and large cells. Prolymphocytes are small-to-medium-sized lymphocytes with clumped chromatin and small nucleoli, while paraimmunoblasts (shown in this figure) are large cells with open chromatin and central eosinophilic nucleoli. The predominant cell population in CLL/SLL is a small lymphocyte with clumped chromatin pattern and a small nucleolus.

38. **(D) *IgHV* gene mutation.**
Rai and Binet clinical staging system is used to define the extent of CLL and clinical prognosis. In addition, newer parameters are now used to evaluate disease prognosis, especially in the early stages. In general, patients with mutated CLL (choice D) have a better prognosis than unmutated CLL.

39. **(D) 55%.**
In order to diagnose prolymphocytic leukemia, the number of prolymphocytes in the peripheral blood must exceed 55%. Prolymphocytes are medium-sized cells that are at least twice the size of a small lymphocyte. They show a round nucleus and prominent central nucleolus. Most patients are >60 years old.

40. **(D) Tumor cells express CD5 and annexin-1.**
Splenic B-cell marginal zone lymphoma or splenic lymphoma with circulating villous lymphocytes is a tumor that involves white pulp of spleen and splenic hilar lymph nodes. Peripheral blood villous lymphocytes (short polar villi) may be variably present. The individual cells resemble marginal zone cells with abundant pale cytoplasm. The tumor cells are CD20+, CD79 a+, and usually express surface IgM. They are typically negative for CD5, CD10, CD23, CD43, annexin-1, and CD103. Lack of annexin-1 is helpful in distinguishing this entity from hairy cell leukemia. Even with bone marrow involvement, the clinical course is indolent.

41. **(D) Hairy cell leukemia.**
All of the listed choices can result in splenomegaly. However, only hairy cell leukemia involves the red

pulp. The clinical presentation as well as the immunoprofile of neoplastic cells is diagnostic of hairy cell leukemia. In solid organs such as spleen or bone marrow, the abundant cytoplasm and prominent cell borders impart a characteristic "fried-egg" appearance to the infiltrate (shown in this figure). Circulating hairy cells are small-to-medium- sized cells, with oval-to-indented nuclei, and homogeneous nuclear chromatin. Nucleoli are usually inconspicuous. The cell derives it name from the circumferential "hairy" cytoplasmic projections.

42. **(B) Lymphoplasmacytic lymphoma.**
While any lymphoproliferative disorder can present with IgM paraproteinemia, lymphoplasmacytic lymphoma is more frequently associated with this phenomenon. It is an indolent neoplasm composed of small lymphocytes, plasmacytoid lymphocytes, and plasma cells. IgM deposits may be found within lymph nodes, skin, or gastrointestinal tract. Dutcher bodies (intranuclear cytoplasmic inclusions), increased mast cells, and hemosiderin, are other findings typically associated with this entity. A subset of these patients has Waldenstrom's macroglobulinemia defined by presence of lymphoplasmacytic lymphoma with bone marrow involvement, and IgM monoclonal gammopathy of any concentration. Multiple myeloma mostly presents with increased IgG or IgA.

43. **(D) IgG.**
The clinical findings presented in this case are those of symptomatic plasma cell myeloma defined by end-organ damage (CRAB: hypercalcemia, renal insufficiency, anemia, and bone lesions). The most common cause of elevated M-protein in serum or urine is overproduction of IgG (50%), followed by IgA (20%), and light chains (20%). IgD, IgM, and IgE immunoglobulins are found in <10% cases. Less than 3% of cases are classified as non-secretory myelomas.

44. **(A) CD19.**
Plasma cell myelomas demonstrate monotypic cytoplasmic Ig and lack surface Ig. Similar to normal plasma cells, they express CD38, CD138, and CD79a. However, in contrast to normal plasma cells, they lack expression of CD19 and show aberrant expression of CD56 in up to 79% cases.

45. **(C) t(11;18).**
MALT lymphomas show several cytogenetic abnormalities that include translocations t(11;18), t(14;18), t(1;14), and t(3;14). These translocations result in the formation of a chimeric protein API2-MALT1, or cause transcriptional deregulation of bcl-10, MALT1, or FOXP1. Trisomy 3 and 18 are less commonly encountered. t(11;18) is mainly found in

pulmonary and gastric tumors, t(14;18) is found in ocular adnexal/orbital and salivary gland tumors, while t(3;14) is found in MALT lymphomas arising in the thyroid, ocular adnexal/orbit, and skin. t(11;18) tumors are resistant to *H. pylori* eradication therapy.

46. **(A) bcl-2.**
Majority of follicular lymphomas are characterized by t(14;18) and *bcl-2* gene rearrangements. As a result of this molecular alteration, bcl-2 protein is expressed in 85–90% of cases of grade 1 and 2 follicular lymphomas, and up to 50% of grade 3 follicular lymphomas. Bcl-2 protein overexpression is useful in distinguishing neoplastic from reactive lymphoid follicles, although its absence does not exclude a diagnosis of follicular lymphoma.

47. **(C) Increased mitotic rate.**
The morphologic features and immunophenotype of the neoplasm described in this question are those of a mantle cell lymphoma. Lymph nodes are the most common site of involvement. In addition, extranodal locations that are frequently affected include gastrointestinal tract and Waldeyer's ring. Most cases of lymphomatous polyposis of the gastrointestinal tract represent mantle cell lymphomas. Patients usually present at an advanced stage of disease with lymphadenopathy, hepatosplenomegaly, and bone marrow involvement. The characteristic translocation t(11;14) occurs between immunoglobulin heavy chain and *cyclin D1* genes. The median survival for patients diagnosed with mantle cell lymphoma is 3–5 years, and increased mitotic rate appears to be the most consistently reported pathologic indicator of adverse prognosis.

48. **(B) Gastrointestinal tract.**
Diffuse large B-cell lymphoma constitutes 25–30% of adult non-Hodgkin lymphomas. The most common extranodal site of involvement is the gastrointestinal tract, especially stomach and ileocecal valve.

49. **(C) Primary mediastinal (thymic) large B-cell lymphoma.**
The differential diagnosis of an anterior/anterosuperior mediastinal mass includes teratoma, T-cell lymphoma, and thymoma. In this case, the figure shows a neoplasm composed of medium-to-large cells with abundant pale cytoplasm and round-to-oval nuclei separated by collagenous fibrous bands (often referred to as compartmentalizing alveolar fibrosis). Based on the immunoprofile, these findings are diagnostic of primary mediastinal (thymic) large B-cell lymphoma. Superior vena cava syndrome is a frequent clinical presentation. Diffuse large B-cell lymphomas are usually negative for

CD30. The uniform cell population present in this lesion would be unusual for Hodgkin lymphoma.

50. **(B) HMB-45 immunoreactivity.**

    Aggregates of nevus cells may be seen within the lymph node hilum, capsule, or trabeculae. In addition to cytologic features, lack of HMB-45 immunoreactivity in nevus cells is helpful in distinguishing them from metastatic melanoma.

51. **(D) Sickle cell anemia.**

    All the listed choices can lead to splenomegaly. However, sickle cell anemia specifically results in splenic insufficiency from autoinfarction. The importance of monitoring this complication is that patients with splenic insufficiency are prone to sepsis caused by encapsulated bacteria such as pneumococcus, meningococcus, and *Haemophilus influenzae*. All asplenic individuals, therefore, need to be vaccinated against these agents to prevent this serious complication.

52. **(E) TdT.**

    The neoplasm described in this patient is Burkitt lymphoma, a highly aggressive mature B-cell neoplasm that occurs in children and young adults. In Africa, endemic form is the most common form of the disease, and jaw, abdomen, orbit, and paraspinal region, are the most common sites of involvement. Histologically, the tumor shows "starry-sky" appearance characterized by tingible body macrophages distributed throughout the atypical lymphoid infiltrate. The tumor cells express B-cell markers, but are negative for TdT (expressed by lymphoblastic lymphoma). Ki-67 index is nearly 100%. Molecular alterations typically involve the *MYC* gene and include t(8;14), t(2;8), and t(8;22).

53. **(A) Anaplastic large cell lymphoma, ALK-positive.**

    The figure shows large lymphoid cells with abundant cytoplasm and pleomorphic or horseshoe-shaped nuclei, which often show a paranuclear eosinophilic region (hallmark cells). In combination with the immunohistochemical stains, the findings are diagnostic of anaplastic large cell lymphoma, ALK-positive (ALCL, ALK-positive). The neoplastic cells tend to cluster around blood vessels. The tumor is characterized by translocation involving the *ALK* gene, expression of ALK protein, and CD30 positivity. A majority of ALCL ALK-positive cases also express EMA and, therefore, can be confused with metastatic carcinoma.

54. **(A) Associated with EBV infection.**

    The clinicopathologic findings described here are those of adult T-cell leukemia/lymphoma (ATLL), a peripheral T-cell neoplasm caused by human T-cell leukemia virus type 1 (HTLV-1). The neoplasm is indolent in Southwestern Japan, Caribbean islands,

and parts of central Africa. All the listed choices are associated with ATLL. Lytic bone lesions result in hypercalcemia. The neoplastic cells are positive for T-cell associated antigens CD2, CD3, CD5, and typically do not express CD7.

SUGGESTED READING

1. Childs CC, Parham DM, Berard CW. Infectious mononucleosis. The spectrum of morphologic changes simulating lymphoma in lymph nodes and tonsils. *Am J Surg Pathol.* 1987;11:122-132.

2. Said JW. AIDS-related lymphadenopathies. *Semin Diagn Pathol.* 1988;5:365-375.

3. Lamps LW, Scott MA. Cat-scratch disease: historic, clinical, and pathologic perspectives. *Am J Clin Pathol.* 2004; 121(suppl):S71-S80

4. Alkan S, Beals T, Schnitzer B. Primary diagnosis of Whipple disease manifesting as lymphadenopathy: use of polymerase chain reaction for detection of Tropheryma whippelii. *Am J Clin Pathol.* 2001;116:898-904.

5. Lin M, Kuo T. Specificity of the histopathological triad for the diagnosis of toxoplasmic lymphadenitis: polymerase chain reaction study. *Pathol Int.* 2001;51:619-623.

6. Shapira Y, Weinberger A, Wysenbeek A. Lymphadenopathy in systemic lupus erythematosus. Prevalence and relation to disease manifestations. *Clin Rheumatol.* 1996;15: 335-338.

7. Bosch X, Guilabert A, Miquel R, et al. Enigmatic Kikuchi-Fujimoto disease: a comprehensive review. *Am J Clin Pathol.* 2004;122:141-152.

8. Chen H, Thompson LD, Aguilera NS, et al. Kimura disease: a clinicopathologic study of 21 cases. *Am J Surg Pathol.* 2004; 28:505-513.

9. Abbondanzo SL, Irey NS, Frizzera G. Dilantin-associated lymphadenopathy. Spectrum of histopathologic patterns. *Am J Surg Pathol.* 1995;19:675-686.

10. Burke J, Khalil S, Rappaport H. Dermatopathic lymphadenopathy. An immunophenotypic comparison of cases associated and unassociated with mycosis fungoides. *Am J Pathol.* 1986;123:256-263.

11. Albores-Saavedra J, Vuitch F, Delgado R, et al. Sinus histiocytosis of pelvic lymph nodes after hip replacement. A histiocytic proliferation induced by cobalt-chromium and titanium. *Am J Surg Pathol.* 1994;18:83-90

12. Cronin DM, Warnke RA. Castleman disease: an update on classification and the spectrum of associated lesions. *Adv Anat Pathol.* 2009;16(4):236-246.

13. Muller-Hermelink HK, Montserrat E, Catovsky D, Campo E, Harris NL, Stein H. Chronic lymphocytic leukaemia/ small lymphocytic lymphoma. In: Swerdlow SH, Campo E, Harris NL, et al., eds. *WHO Classification of Tumours of Haematopoietic and Lymphoid Tissue.* 4th ed. Lyon, France: IARC; 2008:180-182.

14. Hoster E, Dreyling M, Klapper W, et al. A new prognostic index (MIPI) for patients with advanced-stage mantle cell lymphoma. *Blood.* 2008;111(2):558-565.

15. Swerdlow SH, Campo E, Seto M, Muller-Hermelink HK. Mantle cell lymphoma. In: Swerdlow SH, Campo E, Harris NL, et al., eds. *WHO Classification of Tumours of Haematopoietic and Lymphoid Tissue*. 4th ed. Lyon, France: IARC; 2008:229-232.

16. Harris NL, Swerdlow SH, Jaffe ES, et al. Follicular lymphoma. In: Swerdlow SH, Campo E, Harris NL, et al., eds. *WHO Classification of Tumours of Haematopoietic and Lymphoid Tissue*. 4th ed. Lyon, France: IARC; 2008:220-226.

17. Isaacson PG, Chott A, Nakamura S, Muller-Hermelink HK, Harris NL, Swerdlow SH. Extranodal marginal zone lymphoma of mucosa-associated lymphoid tissue (MALT lymphoma. In: Swerdlow SH, Campo E, Harris NL, et al., eds. *WHO Classification of Tumours of Haematopoietic and Lymphoid Tissue*. 4th ed. Lyon, France: IARC; 2008:214-217.

18. Liu H, Ye H, Ruskone-Fourmestraux A, et al. t(11;18) is a marker for all stage gastric MALT lymphomas that will not respond to H. pylori eradication. *Gastroenterology*. 2002; 122(5):1286-1294.

19. Isaacson PG, Piris MA, Berger F, et al. Splenic marginal zone lymphoma. In: Swerdlow SH, Campo E, Harris NL, et al., eds. *WHO Classification of Tumours of Haematopoietic and Lymphoid Tissue*. 4th ed. Lyon, France: IARC; 2008:185-187.

20. Swerdlow S, Berger F, Pileri SA, Harris NL, Jaffe E, Stein H: Lymphoplasmacytic lymphoma. In: Swerdlow SH, Campo E, Harris NL, et al., eds. *WHO Classification of Tumours of Haematopoietic and Lymphoid Tissue*. 4th ed. Lyon, France: IARC; 2008:194-195.

21. Alizadeh AA, Eisen MB, Davis RE, et al. Distinct types of diffuse large B-cell lymphoma identified by gene expression profiling. *Nature*. 2000;403:503-511.

22. Pileri SA, Zinzani PL, Gaidano G, et al. Pathobiology of primary mediastinal B-cell lymphoma. *Leuk Lymphoma*. 2003;44(suppl 3):S21-S26.

23. Kinney MC, Higgins RA, Medina EA. Anaplastic large cell lymphoma. Twenty-five years of discovery. *Arch Pathol Lab Med*. 2011;135:19-43.

24. Borowitz MJ, Chan JKC. B lymphoblastic leukemia/lymphoma with recurrent genetic abnormalities. In: Swerdlow SH, Campo E, Harris NL, et al. eds. *WHO Classification of Tumours of Haematopoietic and Lymphoid Tissue*. 4th ed. Lyon, France: IARC; 2008:171-175.

25. McKenna RW, Kyle RA, Kuehl WM, Grogan TM, Haris NL, Coupland RW: Plasma cell neoplasms. In: Swerdlow SH, Campo E, Harris NL, et al. eds. *WHO Classification of Tumours of Haematopoietic and Lymphoid Tissue*. 4th ed. Lyon, France: IARC; 2008:200-213.

26. Ohshima K, Jaffe ES, Kikuchi M. Adult T-cell leukemia/lymphoma. In: Swerdlow SH, Campo E, Harris NL, et al., eds. *WHO Classification of Tumours of Haematopoietic and Lymphoid Tissue*. 4th ed. Lyon, France: IARC; 2008: 281-284.

27. Popperna S, Delsol G, Pileri SA, et al. Nodular lymphocyte predominant Hodgkin lymphoma. In: Swerdlow SH, Campo E, Harris NL, et al. eds. *WHO Classification of Tumours of Haematopoietic and Lymphoid Tissue*. 4th ed. Lyon, France: IARC; 2008:323-325.

28. Stein H, Delsol G, Pileri SA, Weiss LM, Popperna S, Jaffe ES: Classical Hodgkin lymphoma. In: Swerdlow SH, Campo E, Harris NL, et al., eds. *WHO Classification of Tumours of Haematopoietic and Lymphoid Tissue*. 4th ed. Lyon, France: IARC;2008:326-330.

CHAPTER 18

LABORATORY MANAGEMENT

1. All of the following types of certificates are issued by Clinical Laboratory Improvement Amendments (CLIA), except
   (A) Compliance
   (B) Mild complexity
   (C) Physician-performed microscopy procedures
   (D) Registration
   (E) Waiver

2. Which of the tests listed below does not qualify as a waived or physician-performed microscopic test?
   (A) Dipstick urinanalysis for bilirubin
   (B) Fecal occult blood test
   (C) HER2 test
   (D) Pinworm preparation
   (E) Spun hematocrit

3. Each lab performing any tests (except certain waived tests) is required by CLIA to participate in the following number of proficiency testing events per year
   (A) 1
   (B) 2
   (C) 3
   (D) 4
   (E) 5

4. All of the following measures need to be followed for proficiency testing samples, except
   (A) Evaluation scores should be reviewed by laboratory staff and director
   (B) Processed as a patient sample using the existing methodology
   (C) Processed in a timely manner
   (D) Processed in the lab for which the CLIA certificate is obtained
   (E) Split and sent to a reference lab for confirmation of results

5. The maximum number of laboratories that a director can direct is
   (A) 1
   (B) 2
   (C) 3
   (D) 4
   (E) 5

6. The workload limit for non-automated microscopic examination of gynecologic or non-gynecologic slides per 24-hour period is
   (A) 40
   (B) 60
   (C) 80
   (D) 100
   (E) 120

7. All of the following theories are well-known examples of motivational theories, except
   (A) Fulfillment theory
   (B) Need-hierarchy theory
   (C) Preference-expectation theory
   (D) Theories X and Y
   (E) Two-factor theory

8. According to Maslow's hierarchy of needs, the highest order need is
   (A) Esteem
   (B) Physiologic
   (C) Safety
   (D) Self-actualization
   (E) Social

9. According to McGregor's theory of management attitudes, a manager who creates an environment that allows employees to achieve their goals would be classified as
(A) Theory A manager
(B) Theory B manager
(C) Theory X manager
(D) Theory Y manager
(E) Theory Z manager

10. The right to organize unions and represent employees equally is a provision under which of the following Acts?
(A) Civil Rights Act
(B) Equal Opportunity Employment Act
(C) Fair Labor Standards Act
(D) National Labor Relations Act
(E) Labor-Management Relations Act

11. As a part of process control program for any given test, the minimum number of controls that must be run at least once a day is
(A) 1
(B) 2
(C) 3
(D) 4
(E) 5

12. Which of the following is a measure of accuracy or systematic error?
(A) Coefficient of variance
(B) Mean
(C) Median
(D) Mode
(E) Standard deviation

13. An imprecise test/method is most likely to demonstrate which of the following result?
(A) Higher median
(B) Higher mode
(C) Narrower standard deviation
(D) Smaller random error
(E) Wider distribution about the expected mean

14. In a gaussian distribution, what percentage of test results is expected to fall within ±2 standard deviations?
(A) 50%
(B) 63.8%
(C) 68.2%
(D) 95.5%
(E) 99.7%

15. Increased dispersion or contraction of data plots in a Levey-Jennings chart is caused by all of the following, except
(A) Deterioration of reagents
(B) Inattention to critical steps in the procedure
(C) New individuals performing the test
(D) Stable line voltage
(E) Variability in pipetting

16. Which of the following observations on a Levey-Jennings chart is a signal for remedial action, and is generally apparent when at least 10 consecutive data points are above or below the mean?
(A) Contraction
(B) Dispersion
(C) Outlier
(D) Shift
(E) Trend

17. The results of a control recorded on a Levey-Jennings chart are shown in Figure 18-1. Which of the following Westgard rules is violated by this run?

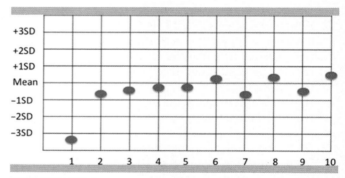

FIGURE 18-1

(A) 1_{2s}
(B) 1_{3s}
(C) 2_{2s}
(D) 4_{1s}
(E) R_{4s}

18. When comparing two methods, which of the following statistical tests is a measure of proportional bias?
(A) Correlation coefficient
(B) Coefficient of variance
(C) Slope of line
(D) Standard error
(E) Y intercept of line

19. All the following are examples of personal protective equipment (PPE), except
    (A) Cardiopulmonary resuscitation masks
    (B) Face shields
    (C) Gloves
    (D) Laboratory coats
    (E) Prescription eyeglasses

20. In the system for identifying hazardous chemical materials in a lab, which color on the diamond-shaped label indicates that the material may be susceptible to explosion?
    (A) Black
    (B) Blue
    (C) Red
    (D) White
    (E) Yellow

21. Which of the following examples is not considered to be a safe work practice?
    (A) Applying lip balm when working in a hood where chemicals are stored
    (B) Appropriate labeling of chemical reagents
    (C) Disposing chemicals in sealed containers
    (D) Storing flammable reagents in specially designated storage cabinets
    (E) Washing hands before eating

22. In case of an unknown chemical spill in the lab, you must take which of the following steps?
    (A) Attempt to clean up the spill immediately
    (B) Leave the lab premises immediately
    (C) Notify your supervisor
    (D) Open all the doors and windows to allow the vapors to escape
    (E) Try to breathe the vapors to identify the reagent

23. What does the acronym RACE stand for?
    (A) Reach, alarm, confine, escape
    (B) Rescue, alarm, confine, evacuate
    (C) Rescue, avoid, confine, escape
    (D) Run, alert, confine, evacuate
    (E) Run, avoid, confine, escape

24. Which of the following choices is an example of fixed cost?
    (A) Controls
    (B) Disposable supplies
    (C) Reagents
    (D) Supervisor wages
    (E) Technologist wages

25. All the following examples are categorized as indirect costs, except
    (A) Billing services
    (B) Building maintenance
    (C) Depreciation
    (D) Reagents
    (E) Utilities

26. What non-profit organization is responsible for developing standards for evaluating hospitals, assisted living facilities, outpatient services, and clinical laboratories?
    (A) College of American Pathologists
    (B) Council for Accreditation of Allied Health Education Programs
    (C) Food and Drug Administration
    (D) Joint Commission
    (E) Occupational Safety and Health Administration

27. How often are College of American Pathologists surveys for laboratory certification performed?
    (A) Every year
    (B) Every 2 years
    (C) Every 3 years
    (D) Every 5 years
    (E) Every 10 years

28. Which of the following organization/Act protects privacy of medical information and health coverage for those who change jobs?
    (A) American Society for Clinical Pathology
    (B) Civil Rights Act
    (C) Food and Drug Administration
    (D) Health Insurance Portability and Accountability Act
    (E) Occupational Safety and Health Administration

29. Per Federal regulations, Pap smear slides must be retained for a period of
    (A) 2 years
    (B) 3 years
    (C) 5 years
    (D) 10 years
    (E) 15 years

30. The data analysis method that calculates the difference between present value of cash flow and initial investment is referred to as
    (A) Average rate of return (ARR)
    (B) Net present value (NPV)
    (C) Payback method
    (D) Systems analysis
    (E) Time-adjusted return (TAR)

31. Which of these statements does not apply to Class I analyte-specific reagents (ASR)?
    (A) Per federal regulations, an ASR disclaimer should accompany any test result issued by a lab using ASR reagents
    (B) They are active ingredients of a laboratory-developed test system
    (C) They are subject to preclearance by U.S. Food and Drug Administration
    (D) They can be purchased from an outside vendor
    (E) They include antibodies used for immunohisto-chemistry

32. Surgical pathology glass slides must be retained for a period of
    (A) 1 year
    (B) 2 years
    (C) 5 years
    (D) 10 years
    (E) Forever

33. When used as a negative control, which of the following tissues may show non-specific staining with a biotin-based detection system?
    (A) Liver
    (B) Lung
    (C) Muscle
    (D) Pancreas
    (E) Small bowel

34. For a lab assessing HER2 protein overexpression by immunohistochemistry or HER2 gene amplification by in-situ hybridization, breast specimens should be fixed in 10% neutral buffered formalin for a minimum and maximum period of
    (A) 2 hours and 36 hours
    (B) 4 hours and 72 hours
    (C) 4 hours and 48 hours
    (D) 6 hours and 48 hours
    (E) 6 hours and 72 hours

35. Which of the following choices is an example of a critical diagnosis in anatomic pathology?
    (A) *Actinomyces* in tonsil resections
    (B) Leiomyoma
    (C) Pleomorphic adenoma
    (D) Transplant rejection
    (E) Tubular adenoma

36. Which of the following statements is not applicable to Medicare?
    (A) A laboratory must hold a CLIA certificate to qualify for Medicare reimbursement
    (B) It is administered by Centers for Medicare and Medicaid Services (CMS)
    (C) It is applicable to individuals 65 years and older
    (D) It is a state health insurance
    (E) It is for individuals with end-stage renal disease

37. The parameter that describes the ability of a test to detect disease, and is expressed as the proportion of persons with disease in whom the test is positive, is called?
    (A) Efficiency
    (B) Negative predictive value
    (C) Positive predictive value
    (D) Sensitivity
    (E) Specificity

ANSWERS

1. **(B) Mild complexity.**
   The Clinical Laboratory Improvement Amendments of 1988 (CLIA'88) Act requires each lab to operate under a correct active certificate with documentation of employee qualification, training, and competency. Tests that are simple to perform, without the need for on-site surveys, are categorized as waived tests. The other levels of test complexity are moderate and high. In addition to the certificates listed above, CLIA also issues a certificate of accreditation through a non-profit accreditation organization that is deemed by Centers for Medicare and Medicaid services (CMS), as able to act in place of CMS to provide laboratory evaluation.

2. **(C) HER2 test.**
   Waived tests are defined as simple laboratory examinations and procedures that are cleared by Food and Drug Administration (FDA) for home use. They employ simple and accurate methodologies with a negligible likelihood of erroneous results, and pose no reasonable risk of harm to the patient if the test is performed incorrectly. HER2 qualifies as a high complexity test.

3. **(C) 3.**
   Proficiency testing involves testing of unknown samples sent to a laboratory by a CMS-approved proficiency testing program. Most sets of proficiency testing samples are sent to participating laboratories 3 times per year.

4. **(E) Split and sent to a reference lab for confirmation of results.**
   The proficiency testing samples should never be split or sent to another lab for confirmation of results. Similarly, the test results should never be discussed with another lab. These activities may cause a lab to lose their CLIA certification. A test score of >80% is required in order to maintain the CLIA certificate.

5. **(E) 5.**
A physician can be listed as a director on no more than 5 laboratory certificates.

6. **(D) 100.**
The maximum number of slides that may be screened is 100 per 24-hour period. This applies to anyone who does primary screening. The minimum amount of time spent for screening 100 slides should be 8 hours (average of 12.5 slides per hour). If a cytotechnologist spends less than 8 hours screening, the maximum number of slides that can be screened is prorated using this formula: number of hours examining slides $\times$ 100/8.

7. **(A) Fulfillment theory.**
All the options, except choice A, are examples of theories that were developed to understand the process of motivation and associated behaviors.

8. **(D) Self-actualization.**
Maslow described hierarchy of needs as a predictor and descriptor of human motivation. According to this system, the five categories, from the lowest to the highest order, are physiologic, safety, social, esteem, and self-actualization.

9. **(D) Theory Y manager.**
McGregor described two basic management attitudes: theory X and Y. Theory X managers assume that employees are lazy and closely supervise their personnel. In contrast, theory Y managers help their employees grow, by allowing them to direct and control themselves. They create an environment that facilitates achievement of personal and organizational goals.

10. **(D) National Labor Relations Act.**
The Labor Management Relations Act outlaws unfair labor practices by unions. The Fair Labor Standards Act provides for minimum wage, overtime, and limits working hours for children. Civil Rights Act and Equal Opportunity Employment Act prevent discrimination based on color, race, religion, gender, or national origin.

11. **(B) 2.**
Per CLIA regulations, each lab must design, document, and implement a process control program. At least two controls, at different concentrations, must be analyzed at least once a day when a test is performed.

12. **(B) Mean.**
Mean is an indicator of central tendency and is therefore related to accuracy or systematic error.

13. **(E) Wider distribution about the expected mean.**
Standard deviation is related to the spread or distribution of control results around the expected mean. It is a measure of the width of the distribution, and is related to imprecision or random error. The

bigger the standard deviation, the wider the distribution, the greater the random error, and poorer the precision of the method.

14. **(D) 95.5%.**
For control results that fit a gaussian distribution, 68.2% of the observed results would be expected to be within $\pm$ 1SD of the mean, 95.5% would be within $\pm$ 2 SD of the mean, and 99.7% of results would be within $\pm$ 3SD of the mean.

15. **(D) Stable line voltage.**
A change in precision causes increased dispersion or contraction of the data plots on Levey-Jennings chart. Unstable line voltage is among several factors that can contribute to imprecise results.

16. **(E) Trend.**
Trend is usually caused by a gradual deterioration in standards, reagents, and instrument condition. Levey-Jennings charts are an excellent way to record these changes.

17. **(B) 1_{3s}.**
The first reading falls beyond $\pm$ 3SD of the mean, and thus, violates the 1_{3s} rule. Violation of this rule indicates either a random or a large systemic error. 1_{2s} rule is violated when either of the two control results are outside the $\pm$ 2SD limits from the mean value, and therefore, the run is rejected. A run is also rejected when the 2_{2s} rule is violated, wherein both the controls exceed their mean value beyond $\pm$ 2SD limits. R_{4s} rule is violated when one control exceeds a mean value of +2SD limit, and the other exceeds the mean –2SD limit, or when the range of a group of controls exceeds 4SD. A run is rejected per the 4_{1s} rule when four consecutive control results exceed the mean beyond $\pm$ 1SD limits. The 10_x rule is violated when 10 consecutive control results fall on the same side of the mean. A violation of 1_{3s} or R_{4s} control rules generally indicates a random error, while violation of 2_{2s}, 4_{1s}, or 10_x rules indicates a systemic error.

18. **(C) Slope of line.**
In a regression plot, the slope of a line is a measure of proportional bias. A slope of 1.12 means that the y-axis values are 12% higher than the values on the x-axis. Intercept of the line indicates that the method has a constant bias. In the formula $y = mx + b$, "b" is a measure of constant bias. This means that all y-axis values are higher than x-axis values by "b" units. Standard error and correlation coefficient R are measures of random error.

19. **(E) Prescription eyeglasses.**
Occupational Safety and Health Administration (OSHA) mandates the use of Personal Protective Equipment (PPE) to protect the employee's skin, clothing, and mucous membranes against contact

with all body fluids. Prescription eyeglasses are not considered PPE and workers are required to wear separate eye protection gear over the glasses.

20. **(E) Yellow.**
The U.S.-based National Fire Protection Association (NFPA) has a standard system for identification of hazardous agents known as NFPA 704. The code consists of a diamond with four colored sections. Each section contains a number between 0 and 4 (0 for no hazard, 4 indicates a severe hazard). Yellow color stands for reactivity, and advises the firefighter or responder that the material may be susceptible to explosion, either through self-reaction, polymerization, or by exposure to certain conditions or substances. Blue color stands for health, and indicates that the material may directly or indirectly cause injury due to acute exposure by physical contact, ingestion, or inhalation. Red color indicates flammability, and assesses the relative susceptibility of materials to catch fire. White color indicates a specific hazard, for example, oxidize, corrosive, and radiation.

21. **(A) Applying lip balm when working in a hood where chemicals are stored.**
Eating, drinking, smoking, chewing gum, or applying cosmetics or lip balm in areas where lab chemicals are present, is not considered safe work practice.

22. **(C) Notify your supervisor.**
Only trained personnel should be allowed to handle an unknown chemical spill. Always ensure your safety and safety of your coworkers. The area of spill must be secured according to laboratory safety plan and the immediate supervisor must be notified of the event.

23. **(B) Rescue, alarm, confine, evacuate.**
When a fire is discovered, the first step is to rescue any personnel or patients. Alert the authorities and call out to other staff so they can sound the alarm. Close all doors and windows to confine the fire. If fire is out of control, you must evacuate the area.

24. **(D) Supervisor wages.**
Operating laboratory expenditures are categorized into fixed costs and variable costs, depending on the sensitivity of the costs to increase or decrease in response to change in the volume of clinical tests. If a cost remains unchanged with fluctuations in volume, it is considered to be a fixed cost.

25. **(D) Reagents.**
Any costs that can be linked to a test are called direct costs. Other examples of direct costs include technicians, clerical and supervisory personnel, overtime, and on-call payments. Indirect or overhead costs are those that are not directly related to a test, but are included in the total lab expenditure.

26. **(D) Joint Commission.**
The Joint Commission (Joint Commission on Accreditation of Healthcare Organizations) also provides accreditation to hospitals. Laboratories surveyed by the Joint Commission are deemed certifiable under Clinical Laboratory Improvement Amendments of 1988 (CLIA '88) requirements. To earn an accreditation, a hospital or laboratory undergoes an on-site survey. To maintain accreditation, hospitals are surveyed (unannounced) every 3 years and laboratories every 2 years.

27. **(B) 2 years.**
College of American Pathologists (CAP) performs peer-reviewed laboratory inspections every 2 years, and similar to Joint Commission-inspected laboratories, CAP-inspected laboratories are eligible for CLIA certifications. In few states, such as, Washington and New York, a laboratory may obtain a state license in lieu of a CLIA certificate.

28. **(D) Health Insurance Portability and Accountability Act.**
Health Insurance Portability and Accountability Act (HIPAA) of 1996 regulates the use of "patient identifiers" and ensures that the information is used only for health purposes unless permission is obtained for other purposes.

29. **(C) 5 years.**
The test requisition forms must be retained for 2 years. The final reports (electronic or hard copy) must be retained for a period of 10 years. Pap smears are typically retained for a period of 5 years, while fine-needle aspiration (FNA) cytology slides are retained for 10 years.

30. **(B) Net present value (NPV).**
NPV accounts for time value of money and a positive NPV is considered to be financially acceptable. Payback method calculates the years until original investment is recovered from cash flows. Time-adjusted return method calculates the rate of return at which NPV equals zero. This rate is termed as the internal rate of return (IRR). The average rate of return (ARR) method calculates the average of the initial investment over the useful life of an instrument or project, and compares this value with the average investment return over the same time period. Thus, ARR is average annual investment return divided by average annual investment. Systems analysis is a process of evaluating a problem or a requirement, and offering a solution using a combination of software, hardware, or an operational process.

31. **(C) They are subject to preclearance by US Food and Drug Administration.**
Class I Analyte Specific Reagents (ASRs) are not subject to preclearance by the US Food and Drug

Administration or to special controls by FDA. The disclaimer is not required when using reagents that are sold in the form of a kit, with other materials and/or an instrument, and/or with instructions for use, and/or when labeled by the manufacturer as Class I for in vitro diagnostic use (IVD), Class II IVD, or Class III IVD.

32. **(D) 10 years.**
Glass slides, paraffin blocks, and reports should be retained for a minimum period of 10 years. Wet tissue (surgical specimens) should be stored for a minimum period of 2 weeks after the final report has been issued.

33. **(A) Liver.**
Liver and renal tubules have high endogenous biotin activity that leads to non-specific immunohistochemical staining using streptavidin-horse radish peroxidase system. This problem can be overcome by using a biotin-blocking step. A negative control is processed by replacing the primary antibody by any of the following reagent: an unrelated antibody of same isotype as the primary antibody, a negative control reagent, or a diluent/buffer solution.

34. **(D) 6 hours and 48 hours.**
Proper fixation of tissue is a requirement for labs performing HER2 analysis. The volume of formalin used for fixation should be 10 times the volume of the specimen. If a fixative other than 10% neutral buffered formalin is used, a validation study must be performed to ensure that the results are concordant with the standard procedure.

35. **(D) Transplant rejection.**
Abnormalities or findings that may be life threatening, or require a rapid corrective action for better patient outcomes, are referred to as critical diagnoses. Some examples include kidney biopsy finding of crescents in >50% of the glomeruli, uterine contents without villi or trophoblastic tissue, leukocytoclastic vasculitis, fat in endoscopic mucosal biopsies of the colon, mesothelial cells in cardiac biopsy, malignancies in superior vena cava syndrome, neoplasms causing paralysis, infections, unexpected malignancy, and unexpected or discrepant findings.

36. **(D) It is a state health insurance.**
Medicare is a federal health insurance that is provided under three sections, part A, B, and C. Part A covers inpatient hospitalization, hospice care,

skilled nursing care, and home health care. Part B covers outpatient lab tests, physician professional services, and other medical services and devices. Part C is an alternative to the traditional part B fee-for-service program. It provides services through health maintenance organizations and is designed to reduce patient "out of pocket" costs.

37. **(D) Sensitivity.**
Sensitivity also refers to the true-positive rate [true positive/(true positive + false negative) × 100]. Specificity is the ability of a test to detect absence of a disease, and is also referred to as the true-negative rate. The positive predictive value of a test is the probability that a positive test correlates with the presence of a disease. Thus, it is the proportion of individuals with a positive test who have the disease. Negative predictive value is the proportion of individuals with a negative test who do not have the disease.

SUGGESTED READING

1. Clark GB. *Laboratory Regulation, Certification, and Accreditation.* Philadelphia, PA: Lippincott; 1998.
2. Fine DJ, Salmon BC, Butterfield RJ, Doheny JE. *Budgeting Laboratory Resources.* Philadelphia, PA: Lippincott; 1998.
3. Fine DJ, Salmon BC, Butterfield RJ, Doheny JE. *Introduction to Laboratory Financial Management.* Philadelphia, PA: Lippincott; 1998.
4. Jaros ML, Lifshitz MS, De Cresce RP. *Financial Management.* Philadelphia, PA: Saunders Elsevier; 2007.
5. John R, Lifshitz MS, Jhang J, Fink D. *Post-Analysis: Medical Decision-Making.* Philadelphia, PA: Saunders Elsevier; 2007.
6. Kurec AS. *Staffing and Scheduling of Laboratory Personnel.* Philadelphia, PA: Lippincott; 1998.
7. Lott JA. *Process Control and method Evaluation.* Philadelphia, PA: Lippincott; 1998.
8. Luebbert PP. *Clinical Laboratory Safety and OSHA.* Philadelphia, PA: Lippincott; 1998.
9. Mass D. *Motivation-Managerial Assumptions and Effects.* Philadelphia, PA: Lippincott; 1998.
10. Passey RB. *The Clinical Laboratory Improvement Amendments (CLIA).* Philadelphia, PA: Lippincott; 1998.
11. Renshaw AA, Gould EW. Measuring errors in surgical pathology in real-life practice: defining what does and does not matter. *Am J Clin Pathol.* 2007;127:144-152.
12. Silverman JF. Critical diagnoses (critical values) in anatomic pathology. *Am J Clin Pathol.* 2006;125:815-817.

CHAPTER 19

MEDICAL RENAL PATHOLOGY

1. The glomerular filter is composed of all the following structures, except
   (A) Fenestrated endothelial cells
   (B) Lamina densa
   (C) Lamina rara externa
   (D) Lamina rara interna
   (E) Mesangial matrix

2. Which of the following statements regarding the normal glomerular filtration/barrier function is incorrect?
   (A) High permeability to cationic molecules
   (B) High permeability to molecules larger than the size of albumin
   (C) High permeability to small solutes
   (D) High permeability to water
   (E) Mutation in genes encoding proteins such as nephrin leads to loss of barrier function

3. A nephrectomy specimen from a 15-year-old patient with a unilateral renal mass shows multiple cysts ranging in size from 0.5 to 1.0 cm, distributed throughout the cortex and medulla. Based on Figure 19-1, what is the best diagnosis?

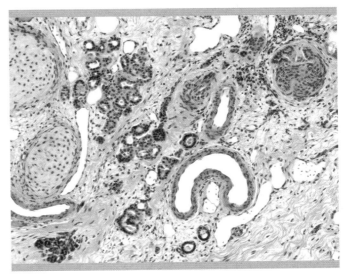

FIGURE 19-1

   (A) Autosomal-dominant polycystic kidney disease
   (B) Autosomal-recessive polycystic kidney disease
   (C) Cystic renal dysplasia
   (D) Medullary sponge kidney
   (E) Simple renal cysts

4. A nephrectomy specimen from a 40-year-old man is shown in Figure 19-2. Both the kidneys have a similar appearance. Which of the following statements does not apply to this condition?

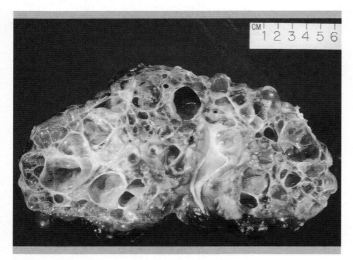

FIGURE 19-2

(A) Adult form shows an autosomal-recessive pattern of inheritance
(B) Cysts initially involve only portion of a nephron
(C) 40% patients have polycystic liver disease
(D) Mutations in *PKD1* occur in 85% of patients
(E) Renal function is maintained until 4th or 5th decade of life

5. Which of the following mechanisms of glomerular injury causes a diffuse linear pattern of staining by immunofluorescence?
(A) Antibodies against antigen complex located on the basal surface of visceral epithelial cells
(B) Antibodies against exogenous/endogenous antigens not present in the glomerulus ("planted antigens")
(C) Antibodies directed against circulating tumor antigens
(D) Antibodies directed against circulating Hepatitis C virus antigen
(E) Antibodies against NC1 domain of collagen type IV in glomerular basement membrane

6. A 10-year-old boy with history of fever and impetigo presents with abrupt onset oliguria and hematuria. A renal biopsy and the corresponding electron microscopic findings are shown in Figure 19-3. What is the best diagnosis?

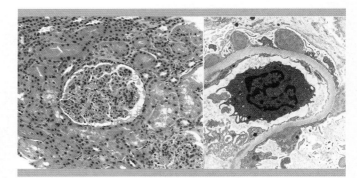

FIGURE 19-3

(A) Acute poststreptococcal glomerulonephritis
(B) Goodpasture syndrome
(C) Idiopathic rapidly progressing glomerulonephritis
(D) Membranous glomerulopathy
(E) Minimal change disease

7. A 45-year-old man presents with rapid and progressive deterioration of renal function and severe oliguria. His renal biopsy shows this finding in most of the glomeruli (see Figure 19-4). All the following statements are associated with this condition, except

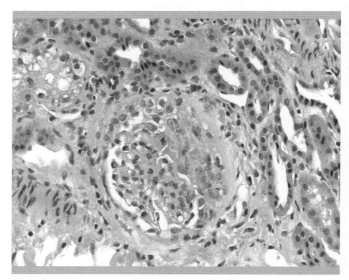

FIGURE 19-4

(A) Electron microscopy shows no changes
(B) Fatal, if the condition is left untreated
(C) Greater than 90% of patients with type III disease have circulating antineutrophil cytoplasmic antibodies

(D) Type I form of this disease is associated with anti-glomerular basement membrane antibodies

(E) Type II form of this disease is associated with immune complex deposits

8. Which of the following glomerular diseases is the most common cause of nephrotic syndrome in children?
   (A) Focal segmental glomerulosclerosis
   (B) IgA nephropathy
   (C) Membranoproliferative glomerulonephritis
   (D) Membranous glomerulopathy
   (E) Minimal change disease

9. A renal biopsy and electron microscopic findings from a 53-year-old man with history of nephrotic syndrome is shown in Figure 19-5. Which of the following conditions is the most common cause of this pattern of renal injury?

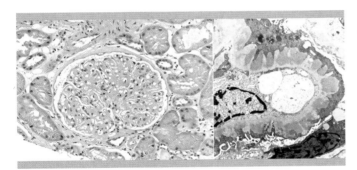

FIGURE 19-5

   (A) Drugs
   (B) Idiopathic
   (C) Infections
   (D) Malignancy
   (E) Systemic lupus erythematosus

10. A 2-year-old boy following routine prophylactic immunization is found to have highly selective proteinuria. Based on the clinical suspicion of minimal change disease, steroid therapy is instituted, and his condition rapidly returns to normal. Which of the following statements is least likely to be associated with this condition?
    (A) Excellent long-term prognosis
    (B) Hypercellular glomeruli
    (C) Intracytoplasmic lipid and protein droplets in proximal tubules
    (D) Normal blood pressure
    (E) Uniform and diffuse effacement of foot processes on electron microscopy

11. Which of the following patterns of glomerular injury is common to patients with HIV infection, heroin addicts, and sickle cell disease?
    (A) Focal segmental glomerulosclerosis
    (B) Membranoproliferative glomerulonephritis
    (C) Membranous glomerulopathy
    (D) Minimal change disease
    (E) Rapidly progressive glomerulonephritis

12. Which of the following forms of glomerular diseases is the most common cause of nephrotic syndrome in adults in United States?
    (A) Focal segmental glomerulosclerosis
    (B) Membranoproliferative glomerulonephritis
    (C) Membranous glomerulopathy
    (D) Minimal change disease
    (E) Rapidly progressive glomerulonephritis

13. IgA nephropathy is characterized by all of the following features, except
    (A) Frequent recurrence in transplanted kidneys
    (B) Increased association with celiac disease and liver disease
    (C) Most common cause of glomerulonephritis worldwide
    (D) Monoclonal deposits of IgA in mesangial region
    (E) Recurrent gross and/or microscopic hematuria

14. A 15-year-old teenager with history of gross hematuria and vision problems is found to have nerve deafness and dislocation of the left ocular lens. Electron microscopy study shows irregular foci of thickening and thinning of the glomerular basement membrane with a "basket-weave" appearance of the lamina densa. Which of the following choices best describes this renal condition?
    (A) Alport syndrome
    (B) IgA nephropathy
    (C) Minimal change disease
    (D) Poststreptococcal glomerulonephritis
    (E) Thin basement membrane disease

15. Which of the following conditions is least likely to progress towards chronic glomerulonephritis?
    (A) Focal segmental glomerulosclerosis
    (B) Membranoproliferative glomerulonephritis
    (C) Membranous glomerulopathy
    (D) Poststreptococcal glomerulonephritis
    (E) Rapidly progressive glomerulonephritis

16. A biopsy from a patient with active lupus nephritis is shown in Figure 19-6. Based on the pattern of disease shown here, in which of the following portions of the nephron are the immune complexes typically deposited?

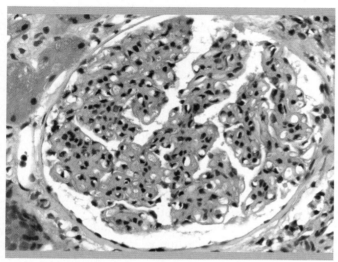

FIGURE 19-6

(A) Intramembranous
(B) Mesangial
(C) Subendothelial
(D) Subepithelial
(E) Tubular

17. A renal biopsy obtained from a patient with history of microalbuminuria is shown in Figure 19-7. What is the best diagnosis?

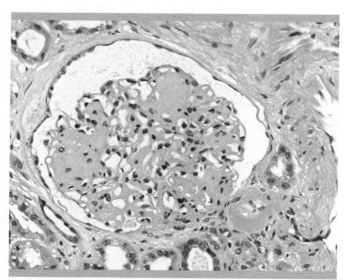

FIGURE 19-7

(A) Diabetic glomerulosclerosis
(B) Henoch-Schönlein purpura
(C) HIV nephropathy
(D) IgA nephropathy
(E) Lupus nephritis

18. Which of the following conditions is associated with deposition of IgG-IgM cryoglobulin complexes and membranoproliferative glomerulonephritis pattern of injury?
(A) Henoch-Schönlein purpura
(B) Hepatitis C infection
(C) HIV infection
(D) Lupus nephritis
(E) Sickle cell disease

19. Which of the following agents is not associated with nephrotoxic type of acute tubular necrosis?
(A) Antibiotics
(B) Heavy metals
(C) Mismatched blood transfusion
(D) Organic solvents
(E) Radiographic contrast agents

20. Autopsy examination of a 55-year-old man with history of multisystem organ failure reveals bilateral, asymmetric, shrunken kidneys with irregular coarse scarring. Upon bivalving the kidneys, the scars appear to be localized to the upper and lower poles, and are associated with dilated and blunted calyces. What is the most common cause for this pattern of injury?
(A) Acute pyelonephritis
(B) Benign nephrosclerosis
(C) Chronic glomerulonephritis
(D) Chronic pyelonephritis
(E) Malignant hypertension

21. Renal papillary necrosis can result from all the following conditions, except
(A) Analgesics
(B) Antibiotics
(C) Diabetes mellitus
(D) Sickle cell disease
(E) Urolithiasis-related obstruction

ANSWERS

1. **(E) Mesangial matrix.**
   Glomerular capillary wall is the filtering membrane, and is composed of vascular endothelial cells and glomerular basement membrane (consists of thick electron-dense central layer of lamina densa and peripheral thin layers composed of lamina rara externa and lamina rara interna). Mesangial matrix

forms a supporting framework for the mesangial cells. Mesangial cells are located between the capillaries and support the entire glomerular tuft.

2. (B) High permeability to molecules larger than the size of albumin.

The glomerular filtration is a based on a highly selective process of filtering substances across the glomerular barrier. Due to it's fenestrated nature, it is highly permeable to water and small solutes. However, larger molecules, including proteins larger than or equal to the size of albumin, are impermeable. Thus, presence of albumin in urine indicates loss of this barrier function. The glomerular barrier is highly permeable to cationic molecules. Because of the acidic glycoproteins present within its structure, the glomerular basement membrane is anionic in nature, and thus repels anionic proteins, such as albumin. Nephrin and other proteins, such as, CD2AP extend between the podocyte foot processes, dimerize across the slit diaphragm, and help in maintaining the glomerular permeability.

3. (C) Cystic renal dysplasia.

The figure shows abnormal structures including cartilage, undifferentiated mesenchyme, and immature collecting ductules, characteristic of cystic renal dysplasia. It is caused by an abnormality in metanephric differentiation and may affect one or both kidneys. The parenchyma is replaced by multiple irregular cysts. The differential diagnosis of renal cysts includes cystic renal dysplasia, polycystic kidney disease, medullary cystic disease (medullary sponge kidney and nephronophthisis), acquired (dialysis-associated) cystic disease, localized renal cysts (simple cysts), hereditary malformation syndromes-related cysts (such as tuberous sclerosis), glomerulocystic disease, and extraparenchymal cysts such as hilar lymphangitic cysts.

4. (A) Adult form shows an autosomal-recessive pattern of inheritance.

The specimen shows an enlarged multicystic kidney, with cysts distributed throughout the cortex and medulla, without any identifiable residual parenchyma. The age of the patient and bilateral involvement are consistent with adult polycystic kidney disease. The adult form is inherited as an autosomal-dominant disease, while the childhood polycystic disease shows an autosomal-recessive mode of inheritance. Grossly, the autosomal-recessive form shows smaller cysts with dilated channels that are usually oriented perpendicular to the renal cortical surface. As the cysts initially involve only part of the nephron, the renal function is preserved until the 4th or 5th decade of life. In addition to polycystic liver disease, intracranial

berry aneurysms and mitral valve prolapse are also associated with this condition.

5. (E) Antibodies against NC1 domain of collagen type IV in glomerular basement membrane.

Most glomerular disorders occur as a result of direct immunologic injury and deposition of immune complexes. The two main forms of antibody-associated injury are: 1) injury associated with antibodies reacting to in-situ glomerular antigens or antigens planted within the glomerulus, and 2) injury resulting from deposition of circulating antigen-antibody complexes within the glomerulus. All the choices, except E, result in a granular pattern of immunofluorescence. In Goodpasture syndrome, the linear pattern of immunofluorescence is produced due to antibodies directed against the NC1 domain of the glomerular basement membrane.

6. (A) Acute poststreptococcal glomerulonephritis.

The renal biopsy shows an enlarged, hypercellular glomerulus infiltrated by leukocytes and monocytes, along with proliferation of endothelial cells and mesangial cells. Electron microscopy shows discrete, amorphous electron dense deposits on the epithelial side of the membrane or "subepithelial humps." This pattern of glomerular injury is consistent with acute poststreptococcal glomerulonephritis. Immunofluorescence usually shows granular deposits of IgG, IgM, and C3 in the mesangium and along the basement membranes. Only some strains of beta-hemolytic streptococci (12, 4, and 1) are nephritogenic and the circulating immune complexes are typically deposited on the epithelial side of the membrane. Conservative therapy leads to complete recovery in most patients. Other infections, such as, bacterial infections (staphylococcal endocarditis, pneumococcal pneumonia), viral infections (Hepatitis B, C, HIV), and parasitic infections (malaria, toxoplasmosis) can also show a similar pattern of glomerular injury. *Electron microscopy image*—Courtesy of James McMahon, Ph.D., Department of Anatomic Pathology, Cleveland Clinic.

7. (A) Electron microscopy shows no changes.

The figure shows crescentic glomerulonephritis (rapidly progressive glomerulonephritis) characterized by a crescent-shaped proliferation of parietal cells and leukocytes internal to the Bowman capsule. The cellular layers often show fibrin in between the cells. Electron microscopic examination usually shows rupture and wrinkling of glomerular basement membrane and, therefore, choice A is incorrect. Three groups of disorders can lead to rapidly progressive glomerulonephritis (RPGN)-pattern of injury. Type I form is anti-GBM antibody-induced disease (Goodpasture syndrome). Type II RPGN results from multiple immune complex nephritides, such as, postinfectious, SLE, and Henoch-Schönlein purpura (IgA). Type III RPGN is defined by the lack of anti-GBM antibodies or immune complexes by immunofluorescence or electron microscopy (pauci-immune). This form has antineutrophil cytoplasmic antibodies (ANCA) and is associated with Wegener granulomatosis and microscopic polyangiitis. In nearly 50% of cases, the disorder is idiopathic.

8. **(E) Minimal change disease.**
    In childhood, the most common form of glomerular disease causing nephrotic syndrome in minimal change disease.

9. **(B) Idiopathic.**
    The figure shows a glomerulus with uniform, diffuse, capillary wall thickening without hypercellularity, mesangial sclerosis, or inflammatory cells. Electron microscopy shows characteristic dark electron-dense immune deposits scattered within the thickened basement membrane. These findings are diagnostic of membranous glomerulopathy. The "spikes" seen on a silver stain highlight the basement membrane matrix present between the deposits. Nearly 85% of cases of membranous glomerulopathy are idiopathic in nature. Other cases are associated with drug injury (penicillamine, gold, nonsteroidal anti-inflammatory drugs), malignancy (colon, lung), SLE, infections (chronic hepatitis B, hepatitis C, syphilis, malaria), and autoimmune disorders (thyroiditis). *Electron microscopy image—Courtesy of James McMahon, Ph.D., Department of Anatomic Pathology, Cleveland Clinic.*

10. **(B) Hypercellular glomeruli.**
    Minimal change disease is characterized by diffuse effacement of epithelial foot processes of the glomeruli, which appear unremarkable on light microscopy. The disease usually follows a respiratory infection, or immunization, and typically responds very well to steroid therapy. Clinically, patients present with highly selective proteinuria composed mostly of albumin.

11. **(A) Focal segmental glomerulosclerosis.**
    Focal segmental glomerulosclerosis (FSGS) pattern of injury affects some glomeruli (focal) and involves only a portion of the glomerular capillary tuft (segmental). It presents as nephrotic syndrome and is associated with HIV, heroin addiction, sickle cell disease, and massive obesity. Mutations in genes encoding the nephrin and podocin proteins localized to the slit diaphragm also result in FSGS-pattern of injury. Damage to the visceral epithelium causes leakage of plasma proteins and deposition

of extracellular matrix along with hyalinosis. EM shows effacement of foot processes, similar to minimal change disease. Collapsing glomerulopathy is a specific variant of FSGS that affects HIV patients. In these cases, in addition to FSGS lesions, the entire glomerular tuft shows collapse and sclerosis.

12. **(A) Focal segmental glomerulosclerosis.**
    Although membranous glomerulopathy is common in adults, due to a gradual increase in incidence, focal segmental glomerulosclerosis is now the most common cause of nephrotic syndrome in adults.

13. **(D) Monoclonal deposits of IgA in mesangial region.**
    All the listed choices, except D, are seen in IgA nephropathy, also known as Berger's disease. Glomerulonephritis occurs due to deposition of increased amounts of polymeric IgA produced in patients with celiac disease or due to decreased hepatobiliary clearance of IgA in patients with liver disease (secondary IgA nephropathy). The IgA deposits are polyclonal in nature. On light microscopy, the glomeruli may either appear normal, or may show mesangial expansion and proliferation (m,esangioproliferative glomerulonephritis), focal proliferative glomerulonephritis, or rarely crescentic glomerulonephritis. The disease has an indolent course and progresses to chronic renal failure in 15–40% of cases.

14. **(A) Alport syndrome.**
    The combination of nerve deafness and eye disorder, in a young adult with hematuria, is characteristic of Alport syndrome. The basket-weave appearance of the glomerular basement membrane on electron microscopy is diagnostic. It occurs as a result of abnormality in the type IV collagen layer. Alport syndrome shows an X-linked pattern of inheritance. Thin basement membrane disease is the most common cause of benign familial hematuria. It is characterized by diffuse thinning of the glomerular basement membrane. The lack of ocular and hearing abnormalities are helpful in distinguishing it from Alport syndrome.

15. **(D) Poststreptococcal glomerulonephritis.**
    Of the listed conditions, poststreptococcal glomerulonephritis is least likely to progress towards chronic renal disease. In contrast, rapidly progressive glomerulonephritis has the highest likelihood of progressing towards chronic glomerulonephritis.

16. **(C) Subendothelial.**
    The figure shows the characteristic wire-loop lesions of lupus nephritis associated with class IV disease. Electron microscopy typically shows deposition of extensive and confluent electron-dense immune

complexes within the subendothelial space. The glomerular lesions in SLE are due to deposition of immune complexes in the mesangium or glomerular basement membrane (GBM). The five main histologic patterns of lupus include minimal mesangial (class I), mesangial proliferative (class II), focal proliferative (class III), diffuse proliferative (class IV), and membranous (class V). Classes I and II show mesangial deposits of immune complexes, while class III and beyond show progressively severe involvement of the glomeruli with crescent formation, fibrinoid necrosis, proliferation of endothelial and mesangial cells, infiltrating leukocytes, and eosinophilic deposits, or intracapillary thrombi. Immune complex deposits may be mesangial, intramembranous, subepithelial, and/or subendothelial in location. Class V or membranous form shows subepithelial deposits. Classes III and IV show subendothelial deposits. Extensive subendothelial deposits cause homogenous thickening of the capillary wall, giving rise to the called "wire-loop" lesions. Presence of these lesions indicates active disease.

17. **(A) Diabetic glomerulosclerosis.**
The figure shows nodular deposits of matrix located towards the periphery of the glomerulus, called nodular glomerulosclerosis (also known as intercapillary glomerulosclerosis or Kimmelstiel-Wilson lesion). In addition to these lesions, diabetic nephropathy is characterized by capillary basement membrane thickening, diffuse mesangial sclerosis, and accumulation of hyaline material within capillary loops (fibrin caps) or Bowman's capsule (capsular drops). The early stage of glomerular injury often causes microalbuminuria (defined as urinary albumin excretion of 30–300 mg/day).

18. **(B) Hepatitis C infection.**
Essential mixed cryoglobulinemia is a systemic disorder characterized by deposition of cryoglobulins composed of IgG-IgM complexes that lead to cutaneous vasculitis, synovitis, and proliferative glomerulonephritis. Most cases are associated with Hepatitis C infection.

19. **(C) Mismatched blood transfusion.**
Acute tubular necrosis (ATN) is the most common cause of acute renal failure characterized by destruction of tubular epithelial cells and acute loss of renal function. Ischemia, direct toxic injury, acute tubulointerstitial nephritis, disseminated intravascular coagulation, and urinary obstruction are other causes of ATN. ATN has been categorized into ischemic type and nephrotoxic type. Ischemic

type results from poor blood flow, marked hypotension, and shock. All the agents listed in this question, except choice C, cause nephrotoxic ATN. Ischemic ATN shows tubular epithelial necrosis, tubulorrhexis (rupture of basement membrane), and occlusive casts within tubules. Eosinophilic hyaline casts are common in the distal tubules and collecting ducts. Ischemic ATN most commonly affects straight segments of proximal tubules and ascending limbs of loops of Henle. In contrast, toxic ATN affects proximal convoluted tubules.

20. **(D) Chronic pyelonephritis.**
The gross description of kidneys is characteristic of chronic pyelonephritis. Malignant hypertension causes small pinpoint petechial hemorrhages on the cortical surface ("flea-bitten" kidney). Benign nephrosclerosis results from medial and intimal thickening of arterioles and small arteries along with hyalinization of the walls. Grossly, the kidneys are normal to moderately reduced in size, and show fine granular appearance of the surface. Acute pyelonephritis shows foci of abscess formation. Chronic glomerulonephritis results in symmetrically contracted kidneys with granular surface. On cut section, the cortex is diffusely thinned out, and there is an increase in the amount of peripelvic fat.

21. **(B) Antibiotics.**
All the listed conditions, except antibiotic use, cause renal papillary necrosis. Antibiotics usually result in toxic acute tubular necrosis or tubulointerstitial nephritis pattern of renal injury.

SUGGESTED READING

1. Grantham JJ. Polycystic kidney disease: from the bedside to the gene and back. *Curr Opin Nephrol Hypertens.* 2001;10: 533-542.
2. Matsell DG. Renal dysplasia: new approaches to an old problem. *Am J Kidney Dis.* 1998;32:535-543.
3. Griffin MD, Bergstralhn EJ, Larson TS. Renal papillary necrosis: a sixteen year clinical experience. *J Am Soc Nephrol.* 1995;6:248-256.
4. Wan L, Bellomo R, Di Giantomasso D, Ronco C. The pathogenesis of septic acute renal failure. *Curr Opin Crit Care.* 2003;9:496-502.
5. Arant BS Jr. Vesicoureteric reflux and renal injury. *Am J Kidney Dis.* 1991;17:491-511.
6. Kumar V, Abbas AK, Fausto N, Aster JC. The kidney. In: *Robbins and Cotran Pathologic basis of disease*, 8th ed. Philadelphia, PA: Saunders Elsevier; 2010:905-969. Chapter 20.

CHAPTER 20

NEUROPATHOLOGY

1. The neurons shown in Figure 20-1 are most likely located where in the central nervous system?

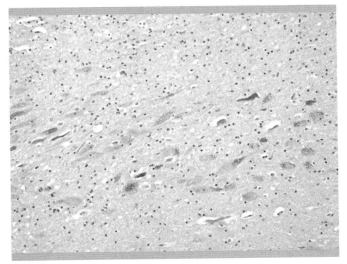

FIGURE 20-1

(A) Anterior horn of spinal cord
(B) Dentate nucleus
(C) Nucleus basalis of Meynert
(D) Red nucleus
(E) Substantia nigra

2. Creutzfeldt cells, a form of reactive astrocytes with abundant cytoplasm and fragmented nuclear material, are most likely to be encountered in which of the following settings?
(A) Demyelinating disease
(B) Diffuse astrocytomas
(C) Elevated ammonia levels

(D) Radiation therapy
(E) Viral encephalitis

3. Microglial cells are best highlighted by which of the following antibodies?
(A) CD3
(B) CD48
(C) CD68
(D) CD138
(E) GFAP

4. Herring bodies in the pituitary gland are filled with neurosecretory granules containing which of the following?
(A) Adrenocorticotropic hormone
(B) Growth hormone
(C) Prolactin
(D) Thyroid stimulating hormone
(E) Vasopressin

5. All of the following are neuronal neuropathologic features of normal aging except
(A) Corpora amylacea
(B) Ferrugination
(C) Lipofuscin accumulation
(D) Marinesco bodies
(E) Neurofibrillary tangles

6. What percent of the total cardiac output circulates to the brain?
(A) 5%
(B) 15%
(C) 25%
(D) 35%
(E) 50%

7. This section (Figure 20-2) was taken from an autopsy in a 72-year-old woman who had stagnant hypoxia for the last 24 hours of her life. A section from which part of the brain would contain neurons that are the most susceptible to anoxic damage?

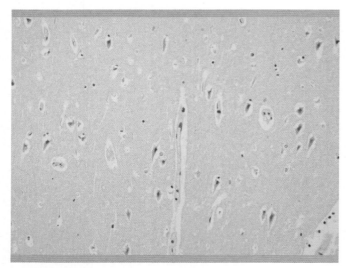

FIGURE 20-2

   (A) Amygdala
   (B) Basal ganglia
   (C) Hippocampus
   (D) Mamillary bodies
   (E) Nucleus basalis of Meynert

8. Which of the following cells are most sensitive to ischemic damage?
   (A) Astrocytes
   (B) Endothelial cells
   (C) Meningothelial (arachnoidal cap) cells
   (D) Neurons
   (E) Oligodendrocytes

9. The earliest light microscopic evidence of acute hypoxic damage is typically observed how many hours after the hypoxic event?
   (A) <2 hours
   (B) 3–4 hours
   (C) 5–7 hours
   (D) 9–11 hours
   (E) 13–15 hours

10. An acute infarct involving the occipital lobe visual cortex would be most likely due to an occlusion in which artery?
   (A) Anterior cerebral artery
   (B) Anterior inferior cerebellar artery
   (C) Middle cerebral artery
   (D) Posterior cerebral artery
   (E) Superior cerebellar artery

11. The most common location for an acute hypertensive hemorrhage is which of the following locations?
   (A) Basal ganglia
   (B) Cerebellum
   (C) Frontal lobe
   (D) Parietal lobe
   (E) Pons

12. The lesion shown in Figure 20-3 was found at autopsy in a 69-year-old man. The lesion was diagnosed as an infarct. The best approximation of the age of this lesion would be which of the following?

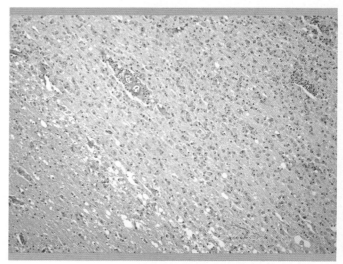

FIGURE 20-3

   (A) 10–12 hours
   (B) 3 days
   (C) 1 week
   (D) 3 weeks
   (E) >3 months

13. The abnormality illustrated (Figure 20-4) in this section from the frontal lobe in a 22-year-old man represents which of the following?

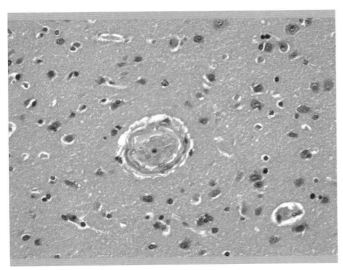

FIGURE 20-4

  (A) Alzheimer type II astrocytes
  (B) Anoxic changes
  (C) Microglial cell proliferation
  (D) No abnormality is present
  (E) Red cell disorder

14. The most common location for the lesion shown in Figure 20-5 is which of the following arterial branch points?

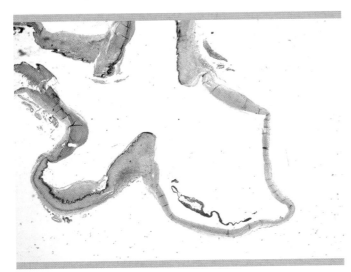

FIGURE 20-5

  (A) Anterior cerebral-anterior communicating arteries
  (B) Basilar-posterior cerebral arteries
  (C) Internal carotid-posterior communicating arteries
  (D) M1-M2 division of the middle cerebral artery
  (E) Vertebral-basilar arteries

15. The most common cause for dolichoectasia is which of the following?
  (A) Amyloid
  (B) Atherosclerosis
  (C) Moyamoya syndrome
  (D) Mycotic aneurysm
  (E) Subarachnoid hemorrhage

16. All of the following lesions are associated with a circle of Willis berry aneurysm except
  (A) Arterial fibromuscular dysplasia
  (B) Coarctation of the aorta
  (C) Hemangioblastoma
  (D) Marfan disease
  (E) Polycystic kidney disease

17. Most arteriovenous malformations occur within which of the following vascular distributions?
  (A) Anterior cerebral artery
  (B) Anterior choroidal artery
  (C) Middle cerebral artery
  (D) Posterior cerebral artery
  (E) Superior cerebellar artery

18. The arteriovenous malformation resected (Figure 20-6) here is located where?

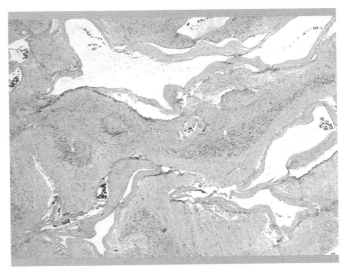

FIGURE 20-6

  (A) Brain stem
  (B) Cannot tell
  (C) Caudate or putamen
  (D) Cerebellum
  (E) Hippocampus

19. All of the following are true regarding the lesion illustrated in Figure 20-7 except

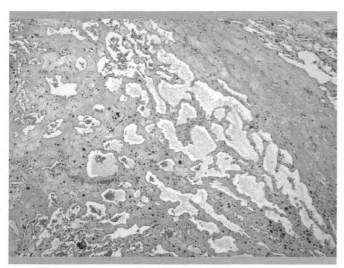

FIGURE 20-7

(A) About one-third of patients present with focal epilepsy
(B) Annual risk of hemorrhage exceeds 5%
(C) More common in men
(D) More common in young versus old adults
(E) Most are supratentorial

20. Familial forms of cavernous angioma are associated with mutations of the CCM1 gene on chromosome 7q 11-21, which encodes for which of the following?
(A) Beta-1-integrin
(B) GTPase
(C) ICAP-1
(D) KRIT1
(E) RAS

21. All of the following proteins are potentially associated with cerebral amyloid angiopathy except
(A) Abeta-amyloid peptide
(B) Beta-2-microglobulin
(C) Cystatin C
(D) Prion protein
(E) Transthyretin

22. A 62-year-old patient presents with a large bleed. Evacuation of the clot with some adjacent brain parenchyma was performed. The blood vessels show thioflavin-S staining. The most likely location of the bleed is which of the following? (Figure 20-8)

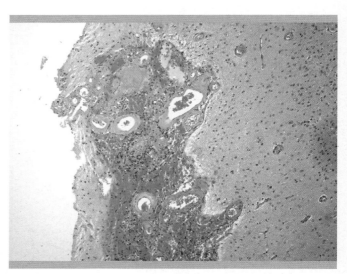

FIGURE 20-8

(A) Basal ganglia
(B) Frontal lobe
(C) Occipital lobe
(D) Parietal lobe
(E) Temporal lobe

23. The vasculitic pattern of injury shown (Figure 20-9) in the brain is most likely associated with which of the following processes?

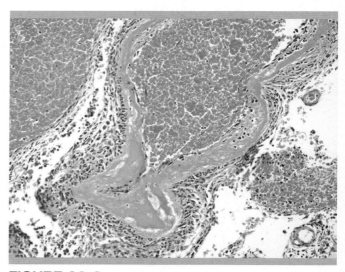

FIGURE 20-9

(A) Amyloid-associated vasculitis
(B) Giant cell arteritis
(C) Lymphoproliferative disorder
(D) Polyarteritis nodosa
(E) Primary angiitis of the central nervous system

24. The changes shown in Figure 20-10 are best diagnosed as which of the following?

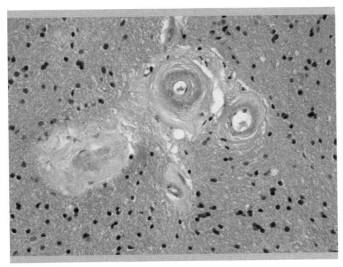

FIGURE 20-10

(A) Amyloid angiopathy
(B) Atherosclerotic disease
(C) Binswanger disease
(D) CADASIL (cerebral autosomal-dominant arteriopathy with subcortical infarcts and leukoencephalopathy)
(E) MELAS (mitochondrial encephalomyopathy with lactic acidosis and stroke-like episodes)

25. All are true regarding CADASIL except
(A) Associated with seizures in most patients
(B) Associated with white matter infarcts
(C) Mean age of onset 40–50 years
(D) NOTCH 3 gene mutations
(E) Systemic disorder

26. The most common source of blood in an epidural hematoma associated with skull fracture is
(A) Bridging vein
(B) Dural sinus
(C) Middle meningeal artery
(D) Middle meningeal vein
(E) None of the above

27. The most likely etiology of the lesion shown in Figure 20-11 in the temporal lobe of a 82-year-old man is which of the following?

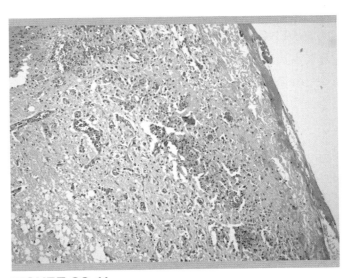

FIGURE 20-11

(A) Carbon monoxide poisoning
(B) Embolism
(C) Infection
(D) Trauma
(E) Tumor

28. Which of the following stains is useful in highlighting dystrophic axons in diffuse axonal injury after about 2 hours survival time?
(A) Beta-amyloid precursor protein
(B) NeuN
(C) S-100 protein
(D) Synaptophysin
(E) Tau protein

29. All of the following are causes of microcephaly except
(A) Achondroplasia
(B) Down syndrome
(C) Maternal alcohol abuse
(D) Prenatal radiation
(E) Prenatal toxoplasmosis infection

30. All of the following are causes of secondary megalencephaly except
(A) Alexander disease
(B) Canavan disease
(C) Maternal anticonvulsant therapy
(D) Mucopolysaccharidoses
(E) Sphingolipidoses

31. Potential risk factors for the development of neural tube closure defects include all of the following except
    (A) Anticonvulsant therapy
    (B) Hypothermia
    (C) Maternal diabetes
    (D) Deletions on chromosome 22q11
    (E) Vitamin deficiency

32. Which of the following is most associated with the development of holoprosencephaly?
    (A) Klinefelter syndrome
    (B) Monosomy 18
    (C) Trisomy 13
    (D) Trisomy 21
    (E) Turner syndrome

33. Which of the following features is not associated with holoprosencephaly?
    (A) Absent ears
    (B) Cleft lip and palate
    (C) Cyclopia
    (D) Hypotelorism
    (E) Proboscis

34. All of the following are gross manifestations of focal cortical dysplasia or malformations of cortical development except
    (A) Cortical tuber
    (B) Alexander disease
    (C) Lissencephaly
    (D) Pachygyria
    (E) Polymicrogyria

35. All of the following are associated with a Dandy–Walker malformation except
    (A) Agenesis of the cerebellar vermis
    (B) Association with congenital heart disease
    (C) Associated with maternal diabetes
    (D) Cystic dilatation of the fourth ventricle
    (E) Hydrocephalus

36. The cerebellar lesion shown in Figure 20-12 was excised in a 22-year-old patient with headaches. This lesion is associated with which of the following?

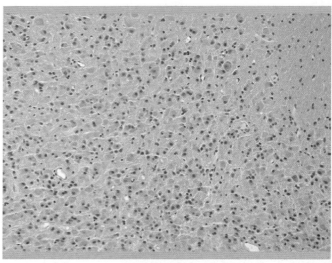

FIGURE 20-12

    (A) Cowden syndrome
    (B) Joubert syndrome
    (C) Neurofibromatosis type 1
    (D) Tuberous sclerosis
    (E) von Hippel–Lindau syndrome

37. Which of the following features is most characteristic of a Chiari type I malformation?
    (A) Cerebellar polymicrogyria
    (B) Cerebellar tonsillar displacement below the foramen magnum
    (C) Hydrocephalus
    (D) Myelomeningocele
    (E) Platybasia

38. The changes seen in ulegyria are usually attributable to which of the following?
    (A) Germinal matrix bleed
    (B) Infection
    (C) Ischemic or hypoxic damage
    (D) Malformation of development
    (E) Trauma

39. The highest risk period for the development of periventricular leukomalacia is in infants delivered at how many weeks postconception?
    (A) 26–30 weeks
    (B) 30–34 weeks
    (C) 34–36 weeks
    (D) 40–44 weeks
    (E) After the 1st month of life

40. A germinal matrix bleed that ruptures into the ventricles without expansion of the ventricles is classified radiologically as which grade?
   (A) Grade I
   (B) Grade II
   (C) Grade III
   (D) Grade IV
   (E) Grade V

41. A 26-year-old woman presents with a 16-year history of medically intractable seizures. The patient undergoes a temporal lobe resection. The findings shown (Figure 20-13) in the hippocampal region suggest which of the following?

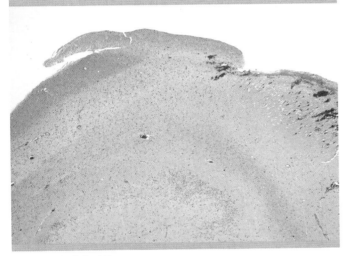

FIGURE 20-13

   (A) Double dentate nucleus
   (B) Focal cortical dysplasia
   (C) Ganglioglioma
   (D) Hippocampal sclerosis
   (E) Trisomy 21

42. All of the following brain findings are associated with Down syndrome except
   (A) An atrophic superior temporal gyrus
   (B) A subependymal giant cell astrocytoma
   (C) Cerebellar atrophy
   (D) Foreshortening of the frontal lobe
   (E) Increased risk of Alzheimer disease

43. All of the features are major pathologic criteria for the diagnosis of neurofibromatosis type 1 except
   (A) Axillary freckling
   (B) Optic nerve glioma
   (C) Plexiform neurofibroma
   (D) Six or more café-au-lait macules
   (E) Two vestibular schwannomas

44. The lesion shown in Figure 20-14 is most commonly associated with which of the following?

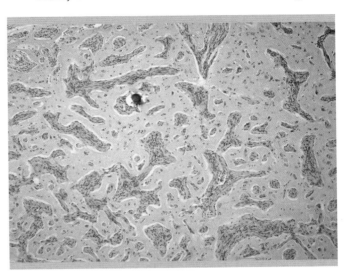

FIGURE 20-14

   (A) Neurofibromatosis type 1
   (B) Neurofibromatosis type 2
   (C) Sturge–Weber syndrome
   (D) Tuberous sclerosis
   (E) von Hippel–Lindau syndrome

45. All of the following are associated with neurofibromatosis type 2 except
   (A) Autosomal-dominant inheritance
   (B) Meningioma
   (C) Mutated merlin protein
   (D) Pheochromocytoma
   (E) Posterior subcapsular lens opacity

46. All of the following features are associated with tuberous sclerosis except
   (A) Renal angiomyolipoma
   (B) Renal cell carcinoma
   (C) Shagreen patch
   (D) Subependymal giant cell astrocytoma
   (E) Subungual fibroma

47. The VHL gene for von Hippel–Lindau disease is located on which of the following chromosomes?
   (A) 1
   (B) 3
   (C) 11
   (D) 17
   (E) 22

48. The lesion illustrated in Figure 20-15 represents a section from the meninges of a 6-year-old patient with refractory seizures. The most likely diagnosis for the patient based on the pathology is which of the following?

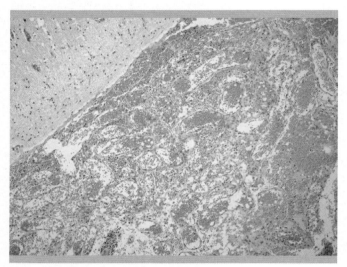

FIGURE 20-15

   (A) Ataxia-telangiectasia
   (B) Neurofibromatosis type 1
   (C) Sturge–Weber syndrome
   (D) Tuberous sclerosis
   (E) von Hippel–Lindau disease

49. A defect in the PTEN/MMAC1 gene on chromosome 10q23 is associated with all of the following lesions except
   (A) Breast carcinoma
   (B) Dysplastic gangliocytoma of the cerebellum
   (C) Pituitary adenoma
   (D) Trichilemmoma
   (E) Thyroid nodules

50. All of the following tumors may be encountered in patients with Li–Fraumeni syndrome except
   (A) Astrocytoma
   (B) Choroid plexus papilloma
   (C) Ganglioglioma
   (D) Medulloblastoma
   (E) Meningioma

51. All of the following central nervous system findings have been noted in Gorlin syndrome except
   (A) Agenesis of the corpus callosum
   (B) Glioblastoma
   (C) Macrocephaly
   (D) Medulloblastoma
   (E) Meningioma

52. Which of the following disorders is X-linked and caused by a defect in the adenosine 5′-triphosphate-binding cassette transporter (ABCD1) gene, resulting in an accumulation of long-chain fatty acids?
   (A) Adrenoleukodystrophy
   (B) Canavan disease
   (C) Krabbe disease
   (D) Metachromatic leukodystrophy
   (E) Pelizaeus–Merzbacher disease

53. All of the following are true regarding metachromatic leukodystrophy except
   (A) Adult form presents with psychiatric changes
   (B) Autosomal-dominant condition
   (C) Deficiency of arylsulfatase A
   (D) Preferentially involves the frontal lobes
   (E) Spares the subcortical U-fibers

54. The lesion shown in Figure 20-16 is from the brain of an 8-month-old girl who presented with hyperirritability, limb stiffness, and weight loss. Imaging shows confluent and symmetrical periventricular lesions. The best diagnosis for this lesion is which of the following?

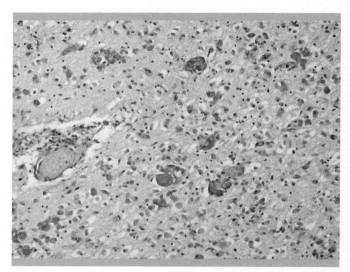

FIGURE 20-16

   (A) Alexander disease
   (B) Krabbe disease
   (C) Metachromatic leukodystrophy
   (D) Multiple infarcts
   (E) Multiple sclerosis

55. The lesion illustrated in Figure 20-17 presented at age 2 with developmental delay, seizures, and psychomotor retardation. Which of the following is the underlying defect in this patient?

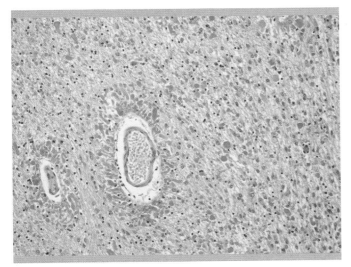

FIGURE 20-17

(A) Deficiency of aspartoacylase
(B) Deficiency of galactosylceramidase
(C) Mutation in the GFAP gene
(D) Mutation in the PLP1 gene
(E) Mutation in the PTEN gene

56. The highest incidence area for multiple sclerosis of the countries listed here is which of the following?
(A) Brazil
(B) Egypt
(C) India
(D) Mexico
(E) United Kingdom

57. Multiple sclerosis is associated with which of the following?
(A) HLA-B3
(B) HLA-B8
(C) HLA-D3
(D) HLA-D5
(E) HLA-DR15

58. All of the following are useful stains in evaluating the lesion shown in Figure 20-18 except

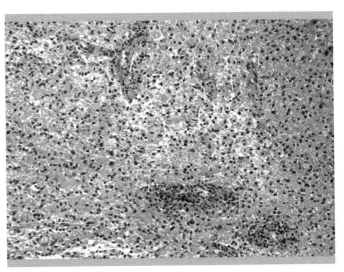

FIGURE 20-18

(A) CD3
(B) CD68
(C) Luxol fast blue
(D) Neurofilament
(E) Reticulin

59. All of the following are true regarding acute disseminated encephalomyelitis except
(A) Can occur after measles
(B) More frequent in children than pediatric multiple sclerosis
(C) Most develop multiphasic disease course
(D) Most present with pyramidal signs or acute hemiplegia
(E) Perivascular demyelination

60. The lesions illustrated in Figure 20-19 represents which of the following?

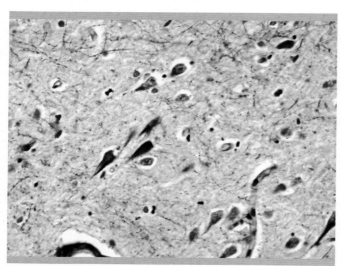

FIGURE 20-19

(A) Granulovacuolar degeneration
(B) Hirano bodies
(C) Neurofibrillary tangles
(D) Pick bodies
(E) Senile plaques

61. All of the following stains are useful in highlighting the lesion shown in Question 60 except
(A) Alpha-synuclein
(B) Bielschowsky
(C) Bodian
(D) Gallyas
(E) Tau

62. All of the following genes are associated with early onset Alzheimer disease except
(A) Alpha-synuclein
(B) Amyloid precursor protein
(C) Apolipoprotein E
(D) Presenilin-1
(E) Presenilin-2

63. The lesion shown (Figure 20-20) in a 76-year-old woman with Alzheimer disease stains with all of the following markers except

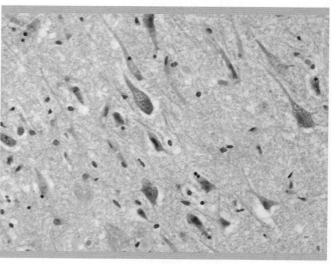

FIGURE 20-20

(A) Neurofilament
(B) Tau
(C) Thioflavin-S
(D) Tubulin
(E) Ubiquitin

64. In neurofibrillary tangle predominant dementia, a high density of neurofibrillary tangles are found in all of the following locations except
(A) Amygdala
(B) Basal ganglia (caudate and putamen)
(C) CA1 region of the hippocampus
(D) Entorhinal cortex
(E) Subiculum

65. Mutations in all of the following genes are associated with familial cases of Parkinson disease except
(A) Alpha-synuclein
(B) Parkin
(C) PINK1
(D) Tau
(E) UCHL1

66. The most sensitive and specific marker for the eosinophilic cytoplasmic inclusions shown in Figure 20-21 is which of the following?

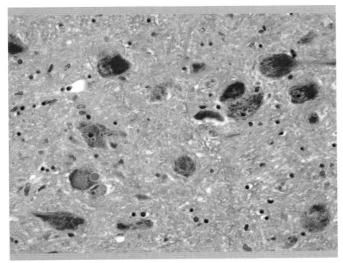

FIGURE 20-21

(A) Alpha-synuclein
(B) GFAP
(C) Neurofilament
(D) Tau
(E) Ubiquitin

67. All of the following are true regarding multiple system atrophy except
(A) Atrophy of the caudate and putamen in parkinsonian predominant type
(B) Cerebellar degeneration with Purkinje cell loss in cerebellar predominant type
(C) Male preponderance
(D) May present with akinesias, dystonia, and rigidity
(E) Neuronal cytoplasmic inclusions

68. All of the following are features of Pick disease except
(A) Argyrophilic intracytoplasmic inclusions
(B) Ballooned neurons
(C) Frontotemporal atrophy
(D) GFAP-positive Pick cells
(E) Spared involvement of the posterior superior temporal gyrus

69. Which of the following is the most common type of frontotemporal lobar degeneration?
(A) FTLD-1F
(B) FTLD-ni
(C) FTLD-tau
(D) FTLD-TDP
(E) FTLD-U

70. All of the following are true regarding frontotemporal lobar atrophy-U except
(A) Alpha-synuclein negative
(B) Association with charged multivesicular body protein mutation 2B gene
(C) Neuron loss and gliosis in frontal and temporal lobes
(D) Patients may develop progressive aphasia
(E) Tau positivity

71. A 62-year-old man is suspected of having amyotrophic lateral sclerosis) All of the following are findings expected at autopsy except
(A) Bunina bodies
(B) Lateral corticospinal tract degeneration
(C) Loss of anterior horn cells
(D) Loss of Betz cells in the primary motor cortex
(E) Loss of neurons in locus ceruleus

72. A 6-month-old boy presents with recent onset areflexia and fasciculations. Over the next few years, he develops contractures and kyphoscoliosis. The best diagnosis is which of the following?
(A) Familial amyotrophic lateral sclerosis
(B) Myotonic dystrophy
(C) Spinal muscular atrophy 1
(D) Spinal muscular atrophy 2
(E) Spinal muscular atrophy 3

73. All of the following are trinucleotide repeat disorders except
(A) Becker muscular dystrophy
(B) Friedreich ataxia
(C) Huntington disease
(D) Myotonic muscular dystrophy
(E) Spinal bulbar muscular atrophy

74. A patient with suspected Huntington disease has neuronal loss and astrocytosis involving most of the caudate and putamen with sparing of the nucleus accumbens. Which Vonsattel grade most accurately describes the findings?
(A) Grade 0
(B) Grade 1
(C) Grade 2
(D) Grade 3
(E) Grade 4

75. All of the following are features of hereditary spinocerebellar ataxia type 3 (Machado–Joseph disease) except
(A) Inferior olivary nuclei relatively preserved
(B) Loss of neurons in the putamen
(C) Neuronal loss in the cerebellar dentate nucleus
(D) Spinocerebellar tract degeneration
(E) Substantia nigra degeneration

76. A patient with Friedreich ataxia might be expected to have all of the following except
    (A) Cataracts
    (B) Gait ataxia
    (C) Hypertrophic cardiomyopathy
    (D) Scoliosis
    (E) Sensorineural hearing loss

77. All of the following are features associated with neurodegeneration with brain iron accumulation (Hallervorden–Spatz disease) except
    (A) Axonal spheroids
    (B) Glial cytoplasmic tau positive inclusions
    (C) Globus pallidus and substantia nigra neuronal loss
    (D) Mutation in pantothenate kinase gene
    (E) X-linked condition

78. In a hospitalized patient, the most likely etiology for the changes shown in Figure 20-22 is which of the following?

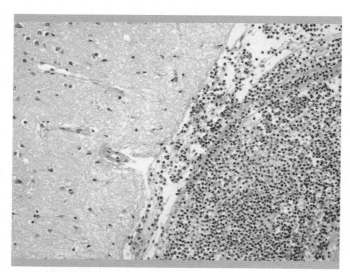

FIGURE 20-22

(A) Gram-negative bacilli
(B) *Listeria monocytogenes*
(C) *Neisseria meningitidis*
(D) *Nocardia asteroides*
(E) *Streptococcus pneumoniae*

79. All of the following are conditions that predispose to the development of the changes shown in Figure 20-23 except

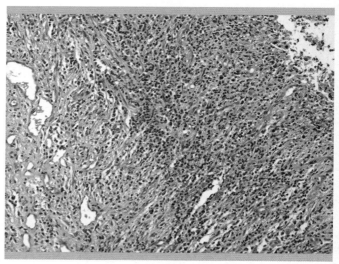

FIGURE 20-23

(A) Bacterial endocarditis
(B) Cardiac disease with left-to-right shunt
(C) Chronic pulmonary disease
(D) Dental infection
(E) Urinary tract infection

80. The most likely etiology of the parietal lobe lesion shown in Figure 20-24 is which of the following?

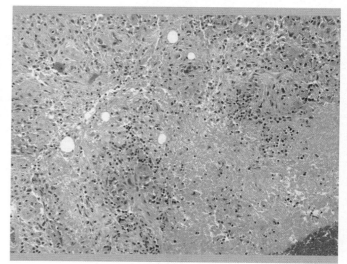

FIGURE 20-24

(A) Actinomycosis
(B) *Candida albicans*
(C) Group B streptococcus
(D) *Mycobacterium leprae*
(E) *Mycobacterium tuberculosis*

81. A 62-year-old cardiac transplant patient develops right parietal lobe abscess. A Gomori methenamine silver (GMS) stain of the lesion is shown in Figure 20-25. The most likely etiology of the abscess is which of the following?

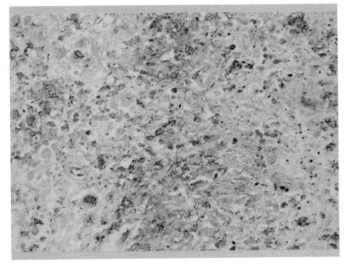

FIGURE 20-25

- (A) *Aspergillus*
- (B) *Fusarium*
- (C) *Mucor*
- (D) *Mycobacterium*
- (E) *Nocardia*

82. The meningitis shown in Figure 20-26 was identified in a 38-year-old immunocompromised man. The most likely etiology is which of the following?

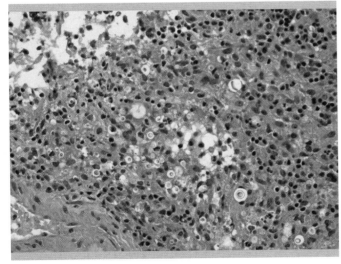

FIGURE 20-26

- (A) Blastomycosis
- (B) Candidiasis
- (C) Cannot tell the etiology
- (D) Coccidioidomycosis
- (E) Cryptococcosis

83. The lesion shown in Figure 20-27 is associated with all of the following conditions except

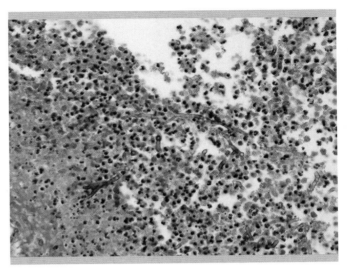

FIGURE 20-27

- (A) Collagen vascular disease
- (B) Corticosteroid therapy
- (C) Diabetes mellitus
- (D) Organ transplantation
- (E) Travel to Southwest United States

84. The best diagnosis for this lesion shown (Figure 20-28) in a biopsy from a 59-year-old man is which of the following?

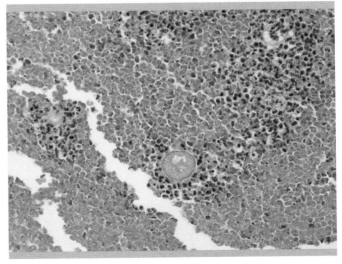

FIGURE 20-28

- (A) Blastomycosis
- (B) Coccidioidomycosis
- (C) Glioblastoma
- (D) Sarcoidosis
- (E) Tuberculosis

85. A patient is diagnosed with histoplasmosis menin-
gitis. He is most likely a resident of which state?
(A) Arizona
(B) Florida
(C) Maine
(D) Ohio
(E) Texas

86. A 12-year-old girl presents with fever, headaches,
and new onset seizures. She is diagnosed with
herpes encephalitis, based on a cerebrospinal fluid
(CSF) polymerase chain reaction (PCR) study.
Where in the brain is she most likely to have
radiographic abnormalities?
(A) Basal ganglia
(B) Cerebellum
(C) Mamillary bodies
(D) Pons
(E) Temporal lobes

87. The changes shown (Figure 20-29) in the optic
nerve most commonly are marked by which of the
following patterns of injury?

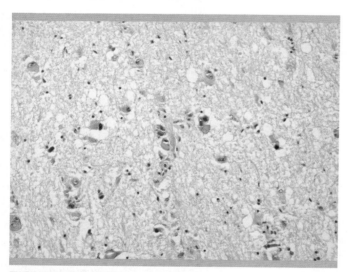

FIGURE 20-29

(A) Abscess
(B) Acute meningitis
(C) Empyema
(D) Inflammatory pseudotumor
(E) Microglial nodules

88. A 68-year-old man with a history of hypertension
and non-Hodgkin lymphoma develops limb weakness and confusion. On imaging, he has multiple
subcortical white matter lesions. One is biopsied
and shown in Figure 20-30. The best diagnosis for
this patient is which of the following?

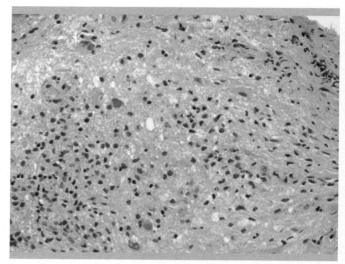

FIGURE 20-30

(A) Cytomegalovirus encephalitis
(B) Metastatic lymphoma
(C) Multiple sclerosis
(D) Progressive multifocal leukoencephalopathy
(E) Subacute sclerosing panencephalitis

89. Tropical spastic paraparesis is caused by which of
the following?
(A) Arbovirus
(B) HIV
(C) HTLV-1
(D) HTLV-2
(E) Syphilis

90. A liver transplant patient develops frontotemporal
lesions on imaging. These abnormalities are due to
which of the following? (Figure 20-31)

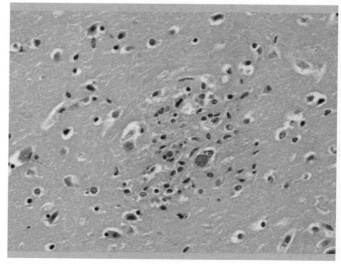

FIGURE 20-31

(A) Ameba
(B) Chagas disease
(C) Histoplasmosis
(D) Leishmaniasis
(E) Toxoplasmosis

91. A 10-year-old boy presents with severe frontal headaches, nausea, vomiting, and stiff neck. (He recently has been playing in a pond in his backyard.) Which of the following is the most likely cause of this presentation?
(A) *Acanthamoeba*
(B) *Balamuthia*
(C) Cysticercosis
(D) *Naegleria*
(E) Toxoplasmosis

92. All of the following are true regarding neuroschistosomiasis except
(A) Eggs may embolize to the brain from the portal mesenteric system
(B) May be associated with granulomatosis inflammation
(C) More common in men
(D) Most cases are asymptomatic
(E) Most commonly due to *Schistosoma haematobium*

93. All of the following are true regarding Creutzfeldt–Jakob disease except
(A) About 10% are familial cases
(B) Associated with a prion protein abnormality
(C) Elevated protein 14-3-3 in CSF
(D) Rapidly progressive dementia
(E) Spongiform changes with microglial nodules

94. Which of the following is least effective in decreasing the risk of transmission of prion disease?
(A) Autoclaving
(B) Bleach
(C) Formalin fixation
(D) Lye
(E) Postfixation with formic acid

95. Which ethnic group or region has a higher incidence of Neimann–Pick disease?
(A) Ashkenazi Jews
(B) Finland
(C) Mexico
(D) Northern Europe
(E) Nova Scotia

96. All of the following are sphingolipidoses that present in the neonatal period except
(A) Fabry disease
(B) Farber disease
(C) Krabbe disease
(D) Niemann–Pick disease type B
(E) Pompe disease

97. All of the following are lysosomal storage diseases that can affect the nervous system except
(A) Alexander disease
(B) Ceroid lipofuscinosis
(C) Gaucher disease
(D) Globoid cell leukodystrophy
(E) Metachromatic leukodystrophy

98. All of the following are associated with Tay–Sachs disease except
(A) Blindness
(B) Cherry red spots
(C) Hepatosplenomegaly
(D) Hexosaminidase A deficiency
(E) Membranous cytoplasmic bodies by electron microscopy

99. Angiokeratoma corporis diffusion or cutaneous telangiectasis in a bathing trunk distribution and renal dysfunction are features associated with which of the following?
(A) Fabry disease
(B) Farber lipogranulomatosis
(C) Gaucher disease
(D) Niemann–Pick disease type A
(E) Sandhoff disease

100. All of the following ultrastructural features are associated with neuronal ceroid lipofuscinoses except
(A) Curvilinear bodies
(B) Fingerprint bodies
(C) Granular osmophilic deposits
(D) Lipofuscin-like deposits
(E) Zebra bodies

101. All of the following represent mitochondrial diseases except
(A) Kearns–Sayre Syndrome
(B) Leigh syndrome
(C) MELAS
(D) Progressive external ophthalmoplegia
(E) Zellweger syndrome

102. All of the following are features of MELAS except
   (A) Age of presentation typically 5th and 6th decades
   (B) Dementia
   (C) Elevated cerebrospinal fluid lactate
   (D) Headaches
   (E) Infarct-like lesions

103. All of the following are true regarding Menkes disease except
   (A) Abnormal hair
   (B) Alzheimer type II astrocytes
   (C) Copper deficiency
   (D) Failure to thrive
   (E) X-linked recessive disorder

104. At autopsy, the mamillary bodies are noted to be brown in discoloration and atrophic. The most likely underlying abnormality is a deficiency in which of the following?
   (A) Copper
   (B) Thiamine
   (C) Vitamin B12
   (D) Vitamin E
   (E) Zinc

105. All of the following are associated with the development of a neuronopathy except
   (A) Aluminum
   (B) Lead
   (C) Mercury
   (D) Methanol
   (E) Toluene

106. All of the following are features used in grading fibrillary or diffuse astrocytomas except
   (A) Cellularity
   (B) Mitoses
   (C) Necrosis
   (D) Secondary structures of Sherer
   (E) Vascular proliferation

107. Which of the following antibodies would be best at differentiating this lesion from gliosis? (Figure 20-32)

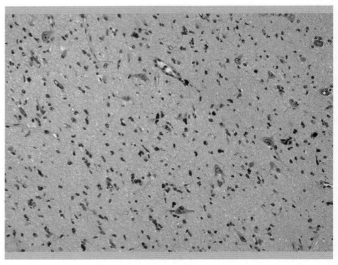

FIGURE 20-32

   (A) EGFR
   (B) GFAP
   (C) IDH-1
   (D) Ki-67
   (E) S-100 protein

108. The best diagnosis for the frontal lobe lesion illustrated (Figure 20-33) in a 62-year-old patient is which of the following?

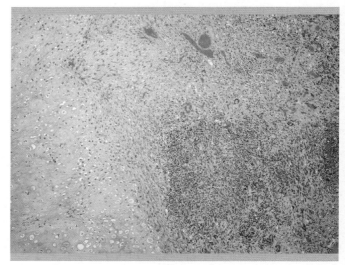

FIGURE 20-33

   (A) Chordoma
   (B) Gliosarcoma
   (C) Malignant meningioma
   (D) Metastatic chondrosarcoma
   (E) Metastatic osteosarcoma

109. Which of the following abnormalities is most consistently found in this glioblastoma variant? (Figure 20-34)

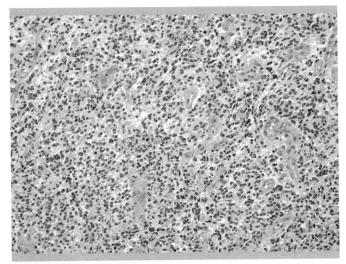

FIGURE 20-34

   (A) Chromosome 1p deletion
   (B) Chromosome 19q deletion
   (C) EGFR overexpression
   (D) IDH-1 mutation
   (E) p53 mutation

110. Which of the following antibodies is least likely to stain the neoplasm shown in Figure 20-35?

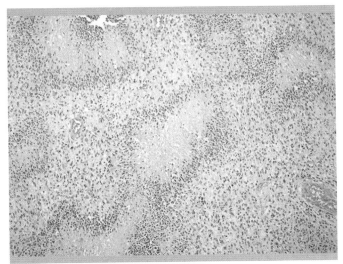

FIGURE 20-35

   (A) CAM 5.2
   (B) Cytokeratins AE1/3
   (C) GFAP
   (D) p53
   (E) S-100 protein

111. The lesion shown in Figure 20-36 presented as a cyst with mural nodules in the cerebellum of a 4-year-old girl. The best diagnosis is which of the following?

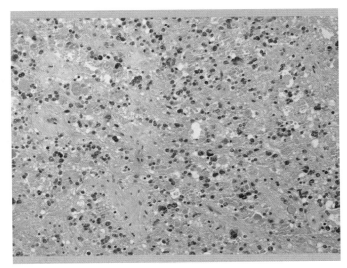

FIGURE 20-36

   (A) Ependymoma
   (B) Ganglioglioma
   (C) Hemangioblastoma
   (D) Medulloblastoma
   (E) Pilocytic astrocytoma

112. The lesion, shown in Figure 20-37, arising in a 12-year-old with tuberous sclerosis is most likely located where in the central nervous system?

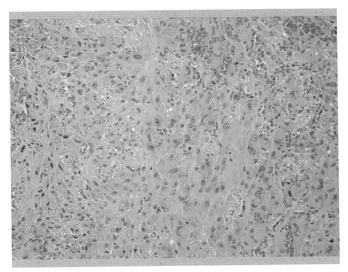

FIGURE 20-37

   (A) Brain stem
   (B) Fourth ventricle
   (C) Lateral ventricle
   (D) Optic nerve
   (E) Temporal lobe

113. All of the following are histologic features commonly associated with pleomorphic xanthoastrocytoma (WHO grade II) except
    (A) Eosinophilic granular bodies
    (B) Increased mitotic figures (>2/10 high-power fields)
    (C) Increased reticulin staining
    (D) Lipidized astrocytes
    (E) Rosenthal fibers

114. All of following are true regarding chordoid glioma except
    (A) Arises in fourth ventricle region
    (B) Lymphoplasmacytic infiltrate with Russell bodies
    (C) Mucin-rich stroma with clusters and cords of epithelial cells
    (D) Typically presents in adults
    (E) WHO grade II neoplasms

115. The lesion shown in Figure 20-38 was resected in a 15-year-old girl with a history of chronic epilepsy and a temporal lobe mass. The best diagnosis is which of the following?

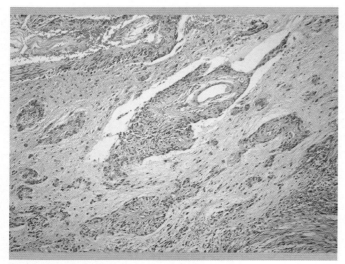

FIGURE 20-38

    (A) Angiocentric glioma
    (B) Dysembryoplastic neuroepithelial tumor
    (C) Ganglioglioma
    (D) Low-grade oligoastrocytoma
    (E) Pilocytic astrocytoma

116. Chromosome deletions on 1p and 19q correlate with chemoresponsiveness in which of the following tumors?
    (A) Atypical teratoid/rhabdoid tumor
    (B) Ependymomas

    (C) Fibrillary astrocytomas
    (D) Medulloblastomas
    (E) Oligodendrogliomas

117. Which of the following is true regarding the "fried egg" appearance in oligodendrogliomas?
    (A) Is exclusively seen in oligodendrogliomas
    (B) Is useful at frozen section to differentiated oligodendroglioma from astrocytoma
    (C) Portends a better prognosis when present
    (D) Represents an artifact of delayed formalin fixation
    (E) Represents the cytoplasm of tumor cells

118. The most common site for this lesion in adults is which of the following? (Figure 20-39)

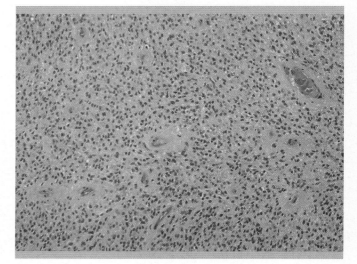

FIGURE 20-39

    (A) Brain stem
    (B) Fourth ventricle
    (C) Lateral ventricles
    (D) Third ventricle
    (E) Spinal cord

119. The most powerful predictor of prognosis in the lesion shown in the last question (118) is which of the following?
    (A) Extent of surgical resection
    (B) Histologic variant (epithelial versus glial)
    (C) Ki-67 labeling index
    (D) Patient age
    (E) Tumor grade

120. The lesion, shown in Figure 20-40, presented in a
28-year-old man. The most common location for
this tumor is which of the following?

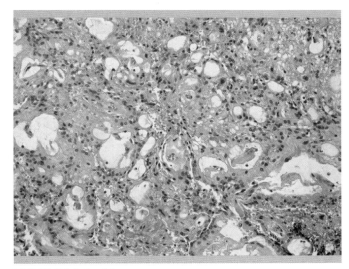

FIGURE 20-40

(A) Cervical cord
(B) Fourth ventricle
(C) Lateral ventricle
(D) Lumbosacral cord
(E) Thoracic cord

121. The lesion shown in Figure 20-41 arose in the
fourth ventricle of a 65-year-old man. The WHO
grade for this lesion is which of the following?

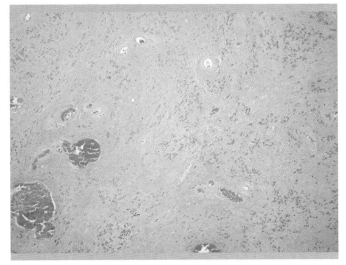

FIGURE 20-41

(A) It does not have a WHO grade designation
(B) WHO grade I
(C) WHO grade II
(D) WHO grade III
(E) WHO grade IV

122. Which of the following tumors is associated with
adjacent cortical architectural disorganization
(focal cortical dysplasia)?
(A) Chordoid glioma
(B) Desmoplastic infantile astrocytoma
(C) Dysembryoplastic neuroepithelial tumor
(D) Low-grade mixed glioma
(E) Pilomyxoid glioma

123. Meningiomas are associated with all of the
following except
(A) Breast carcinoma
(B) Female gender
(C) Neurofibromatosis type 2
(D) Prior history of radiation
(E) Tuberous sclerosis

124. The best diagnosis for the pathology shown in
Figure 20-42 is which of the following?

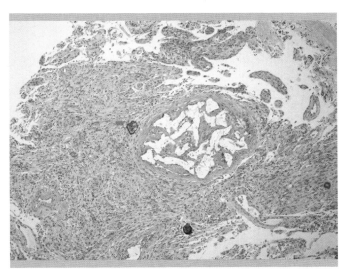

FIGURE 20-42

(A) Atypical meningioma
(B) Atypical meningioma with embolization
(C) Syncytial meningioma
(D) Syncytial meningioma with embolization
(E) Transitional meningioma

125. The lesion shown in Figure 20-43 was excised from the frontal convexity of a 72-year-old woman. The best diagnosis is which of the following?

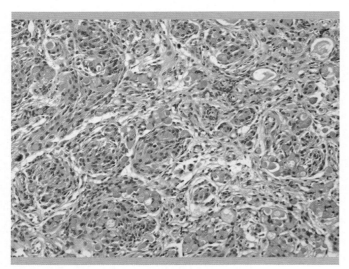

FIGURE 20-43

   (A) Metastatic adenocarcinoma
   (B) Metastatic squamous cell carcinoma
   (C) None of the above
   (D) Secretory meningioma
   (E) Syncytial meningioma

126. All of the following variants of meningioma are associated with increased risk of recurrence except
   (A) Chordoid
   (B) Clear cell
   (C) Metaplastic
   (D) Papillary
   (E) Rhabdoid

127. All of the following features are used in grading hemangiopericytoma of the central nervous system except
   (A) Glomeruloid vascular proliferation
   (B) Hemorrhage
   (C) Hypercellularity
   (D) Mitotic figures
   (E) Necrosis

128. The best diagnosis for this inhibin positive cerebellar mass (Figure 20-44) is which of the following?

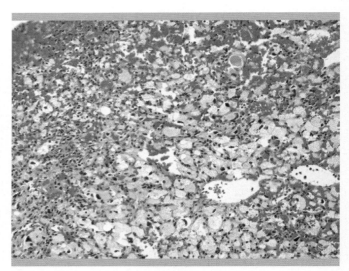

FIGURE 20-44

   (A) Angiomatous meningioma
   (B) Hemangioblastoma
   (C) Hemangiopericytoma
   (D) Metastatic renal cell carcinoma
   (E) Schwannoma

129. Which panel of antibodies would be most useful in working up this neoplasm? (Figure 20-45)

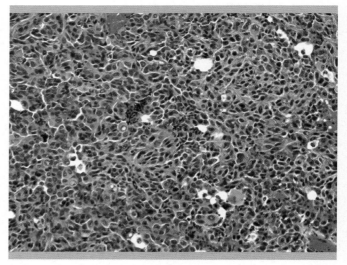

FIGURE 20-45

   (A) CLA (CD45RB), GFAP, cytokeratins AE1/3, CD99
   (B) GFAP, S-100, melan A, CAM 5.2
   (C) GFAP, S-100, melan A, cytokeratins AE1/3
   (D) Vimentin, GFAP, CAM 5.2, neurofilament
   (E) Vimentin, GFAP, cytokeratins AE1/3, neurofilament

130. The intraventricular lesion shown in Figure 20-46 may stain with all of the antibodies listed except

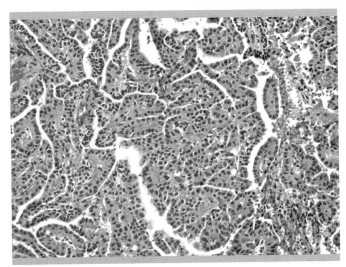

FIGURE 20-46

(A) Cytokeratins AE1/3
(B) GFAP
(C) S-100 protein
(D) Synaptophysin
(E) Transthyretin

131. The lesion, shown in Figure 20-47, presented as a lateral ventricular mass in a 30-year-old man. The lesion stains diffusely with antibodies to synaptophysin and MAP2. The best diagnosis for this tumor is which of the following?

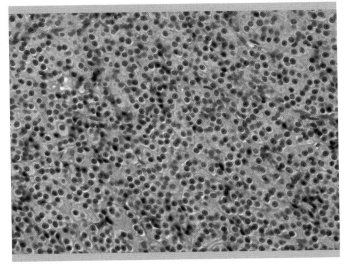

FIGURE 20-47

(A) Central neurocytoma
(B) Clear cell ependymoma

(C) Dysembryoplastic neuroepithelial tumor
(D) Liponeurocytoma
(E) Oligodendroglioma

132. The most common tumor arising in the pineal gland is which of the following?
(A) Germinoma
(B) Pineal parenchymal tumor of intermediate differentiation
(C) Pineoblastoma
(D) Pineocytoma
(E) Teratoma (mature)

133. Distinction of this cerebellar lesion (Figure 20-48) arising in a 8-year-old patient from an atypical teratoid/rhabdoid tumor is best done with which of the following?

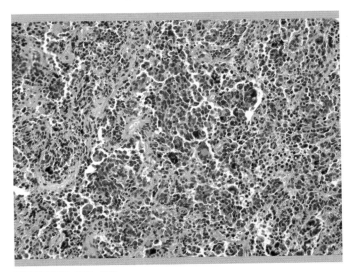

FIGURE 20-48

(A) EGFR amplification by FISH
(B) FISH test for chromosome 22 deletion
(C) GFAP stain
(D) Ki-67 stain
(E) Synaptophysin stain

134. Poor prognosis in medulloblastoma is associated with all of the following features except
(A) Age <3 years
(B) Desmoplastic variant
(C) GFAP expression
(D) MYC gene amplification
(E) Subtotal resection

135. All of the following are true regarding the lesion shown in Figure 20-49 except

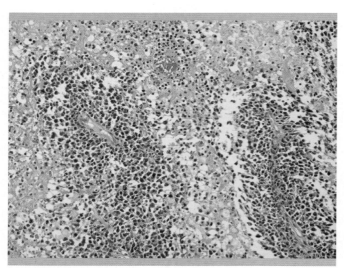

FIGURE 20-49

(A) Associated with AIDS
(B) Associated with EBV infection
(C) Increased risk following transplantation
(D) Majority of cells stain with CD79a antibody
(E) Temporal lobe most common site of origin

136. The cystic lesion shown in Figure 20-50 was excised from the surface of the right temporal lobe of a 37-year-old woman. The best diagnosis is which of the following?

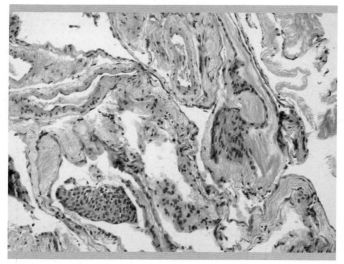

FIGURE 20-50

(A) Arachnoid cyst
(B) Colloid cyst
(C) Endodermal cyst

(D) Epidermoid cyst
(E) Rathke cleft cyst

137. The lesion shown in Figure 20-51 represents the most common tumor that arises in the posterior pituitary gland. The lesion is most likely secreting which of the following?

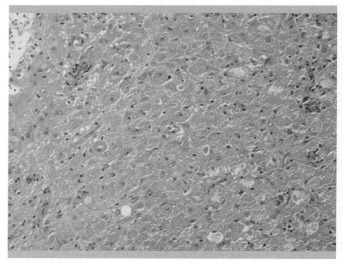

FIGURE 20-51

(A) ACTH
(B) Growth hormone
(C) It is nonsecretory
(D) Prolactin
(E) TSH

138. A postpartum 32-year-old woman has a biopsy of the pituitary gland done for insufficiency. The most likely diagnosis is which of the following? (Figure 20-52)

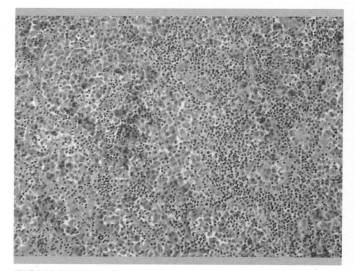

FIGURE 20-52

(A) Abscess
(B) Lymphocytic hypophysitis
(C) Pituicytoma
(D) Pituitary adenoma
(E) Pituitary carcinoma

139. A 14-year-old boy presents with a midline mass
arising in the pineal gland. The lesion is biopsied
and shown in Figure 20-53. The best diagnosis for
this lesion is which of the following?

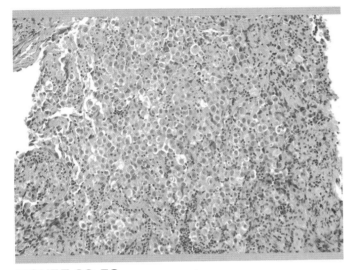

FIGURE 20-53

(A) Embryonal carcinoma
(B) Germinoma
(C) Pineoblastoma
(D) Pineocytoma
(E) Yolk sac tumor

140. This sellar mass (Figure 20-54) presented in a
50-year-old man with visual disturbances. The best
diagnosis for this lesion is which of the following?

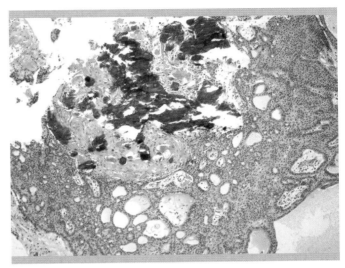

FIGURE 20-54

(A) Craniopharyngioma
(B) Epidermoid cyst
(C) Metastatic squamous cell carcinoma
(D) Pituicytoma
(E) Rathke cleft cyst

141. Which of the following tumors represents the least
common brain metastasis?
(A) Breast carcinoma
(B) Colon carcinoma
(C) Lung carcinoma
(D) Melanoma
(E) Renal cell carcinoma

142. The best stain to highlight ragged red fibers in a
mitochondrial myopathy is which of the following?
(A) Cytochrome oxidase
(B) Nicotinamide adenine dinucleotide (NADH)
(C) Periodic acid-Schiff (PAS)
(D) Succinate dehydrogenase (SDH)
(E) Trichrome

143. The findings in this muscle biopsy (Figure 20-55) are consistent with which of the following?

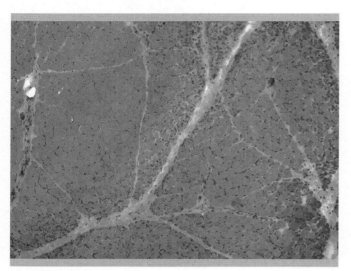

FIGURE 20-55

    (A) Dermatomyositis
    (B) Focal myositis
    (C) Inclusion body myositis
    (D) Polymyositis
    (E) Viral myositis

144. All of the following are features seen on a muscle biopsy with denervation atrophy except
    (A) Angular atrophic esterase positive fibers
    (B) Fiber type grouping
    (C) Myonecrosis
    (D) Nuclear bags
    (E) Target fibers

145. Fascicular atrophy on a muscle biopsy is most likely to be encountered in which of the following conditions?
    (A) Chloroquine toxicity
    (B) Dermatomyositis
    (C) Diabetic neuropathy
    (D) Multiple sclerosis
    (E) Werdnig–Hoffman disease

146. An absence of dystrophin staining on a muscle biopsy would be indicative of which of the following conditions?
    (A) Congenital muscular dystrophy
    (B) Duchenne muscular dystrophy
    (C) Hypokalemic periodic paralysis
    (D) Limb-girdle muscular dystrophy 1B
    (E) Myotonic muscular dystrophy

147. A 66-year-old man presents with muscle weakness and difficulty in weaning from a ventilator. A muscle biopsy is taken and shown in Figure 20-56. The vacuoles demonstrate positive staining with acid phosphatase. Which of the following is the most likely diagnosis?

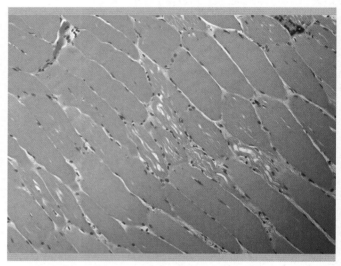

FIGURE 20-56

    (A) Acid maltase deficiency
    (B) Carnitine deficiency
    (C) Carnitine palmitoyltransferase II deficiency
    (D) Myophosphorylase deficiency
    (E) Phosphofructokinase deficiency

148. A 18-year-old man presents with slowly progressive distal weakness, hammer toes, and pes cavus. The sural nerve is noted to be palpably enlarged at the time of biopsy. The biopsy shows numerous onion bulb formations. The best diagnosis is which of the following?
    (A) Charcot–Marie–Tooth disease
    (B) Dejerine–Sottas syndrome
    (C) Guillain–Barré syndrome
    (D) Paraproteinemic neuropathy
    (E) Schwannoma

149. Most familial amyloid polyneuropathies result from mutations in which of the following proteins?
    (A) Abeta-amyloid
    (B) Gelsolin
    (C) Haptoglobin
    (D) Prion
    (E) Transthyretin

150. A 38-year-old HIV-positive patient presents with a new onset neuropathy. A biopsy of the right sural nerve is taken and shown in Figure 20-57. The best diagnosis is which of the following?

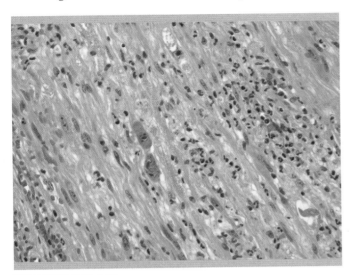

FIGURE 20-57

(A) Chronic inflammatory demyelinating polyradiculoneuropathy
(B) Cytomegalovirus neuritis
(C) Guillain–Barré Syndrome
(D) HIV-associated distal sensory polyneuropathy
(E) Vasculitis

ANSWERS

1. **(E) Substantia nigra.**
The figure shows a cluster of neurons (nucleus) that contains brown granular pigment in their cytoplasm, consistent with neuromelanin. Three nuclei in the central nervous system contain neuromelanin pigment in the cytoplasm of their neurons: substantia nigra, locus ceruleus, and the dorsal motor nucleus of the vagus nerve.

2. **(A) Demyelinating disease.**
Creutzfeldt cells, which represent a form of reactive astrocyte with abundant cytoplasm and fragmented nuclear material, are most likely encountered in demyelinating diseases such as multiple sclerosis. Alzheimer type II astrocytes are associated with elevated ammonia levels. Astrocytomas are marked by atypical neoplastic astrocytic cells with high nuclear to cytoplastic ratios and irregular nuclear contours. Encephalitis and radiation therapy may be associated with reactive astrocytes that have abundant eosinophilic cytoplasm and enlarged, eccentrically placed nucleus.

3. **(C) CD68.**
Microglia represent cells in the central nervous system that are of macrophage lineage and stain with macrophage markers such as CD68 and/or HAM 56. CD138 is a plasma cell marker. GFAP stains astrocytic cells. CD3 and CD45 are lymphoid markers.

4. **(E) Vasopressin.**
Herring bodies represent eosinophilic structures that are filled with neurosecretory granules containing vasopressin. Herring bodies are found in the posterior portion of the pituitary gland or neurohypophysis.

5. **(A) Corpora amylacea.**
Increased corpora amylacea are not reliably associated with any particular pathologic process. All of the other findings listed here are associated with normal aging. Corpora amylacea, when present, are associated with astrocytic cell processes.

6. **(B) 15%.**
The brain receives approximately 15% of the total cardiac output, which accounts for approximately 20% of the body's oxygen consumption.

7. **(C) Hippocampus.**
The figure shown here is marked by the presence of ischemic neurons in the Sommer sector of the hippocampus. These ischemic neurons are marked by cell shrinkage with increased eosinophilic staining of the cytoplasm and nuclear shrinking and hyperchromasia. The area of the brain that is most sensitive to anoxic damage is the Sommer sector of hippocampus. Other neurons that are particularly susceptible to ischemic damage include the Purkinje of the cerebellum and the large cortical neurons in layers 3 and 5 of the cortex.

8. **(D) Neurons.**
Of the cells listed here, the neurons are the most susceptible to ischemic damage. In decreasing order of susceptibility, oligodendrocytes, astrocytes, and endothelial cells are also vulnerable. Meningothelial cells are relatively resistant to anoxic damage.

9. **(E) 13–15 hours.**
Alterations associated with acute hypoxic or ischemic injury are usually observable within 12–24 hours of the initiating event. Organelle changes may be observable earlier, if an electron microscopic evaluation is used.

10. **(D) Posterior cerebral artery.**
An infarct located in the visual cortex of the occipital lobe would be most likely due to an occlusion in the posterior cerebral artery. Uncal herniation is particularly associated with compression of the posterior cerebral artery and infarcts in this location.

11. **(A) Basal ganglia.**
The most common location for an acute hypertensive bleed, of the sites listed here, is the basal ganglia. Other less common sites include the thalamus, lobar region of the cerebrum (a more common site for amyloid-associated bleeds), cerebellum, and pons.

12. **(B) 3 days.**
The lesion illustrated in the figure represents changes consistent with an acute infarct and is marked by the presence of macrophages. Macrophages appear as early as 24 hours after onset of the infarct. Vascular epithelial reactive changes and edema and vascular congestion are also common features of acute infarct. Reactive astrocytosis or gliosis around the perimeter of the infarct usually develops at 1 week to 10 days, marking the subacute phase of the infarct. Cavitary changes, marking a remote infarct, often develop a few months after the onset of anoxic or ischemic damage.

13. **(E) Red cell disorder.**
This histologic section shows sickled red blood cells consistent with a red cell disorder. The surrounding parenchyma looks fairly unremarkable.

14. **(A) Anterior cerebral-anterior communicating arteries.**
The lesion illustrated in the figure represents an example of a berry or congenital aneurysm. These lesions are defined by an absence of the media and frequently internal elastic lamina of the arterial blood vessel. The most common locations for aneurysms of the central nervous system are at bifurcation or branching points within the circle of Willis. The single most common location is the anterior cerebral-anterior communicating artery intersection.

15. **(B) Atherosclerosis.**
Dolichoectasia refers to a widening and increased tortuosity of blood vessels. This condition is most commonly associated with atherosclerosis.

16. **(C) Hemangioblastoma.**
Of the lesions listed as options, hemangioblastoma is not known to be associated with berry aneurysm. Hemangioblastoma is known to be associated with von Hippel–Lindau syndrome and secondary polycythemia vera.

17. **(C) Middle cerebral artery.**
Most arteriovenous malformations are supratentorial in location and most commonly arise in the middle cerebral artery distribution.

18. **(B) Cerebellum.**
The arteriovenous malformation, shown in the figure, is marked by the presence of intervening neural parenchyma. Focal hypercellular areas, marked by small round cells, suggest that the location of the lesion is the cerebellum. These hypercellular areas correspond to the granular cell layer of the cerebellum.

19. **(B) Annual risk of hemorrhage exceeds 5%.**
The lesion illustrated in the figure represents a vascular malformation marked by the back-to-back arrangement of venous type blood vessels, consistent with a cavernous angioma or cavernoma. These lesions may occur anywhere in the brain but typically involve a cerebral cortex, with 80% of them being located in the supratentorial compartment. The lesion shows a slight male predominance and most commonly affects young adults. The single most common presentation is focal epilepsy. The annual risk of acute hemorrhage is approximately 1%.

20. **(D) KRIT1.**
A small percentage of cavernous angiomas are associated with mutations of the CCM1 gene on chromosome 7q11-21. This gene encodes for KRIT1, which interacts with proteins of the RAS family. These mutations are more common in Hispanic populations.

21. **(B) Beta-2-microglobulin.**
A variety of proteins may be responsible for the development of amyloid in the central nervous system. Abeta-amyloid peptide is the primary culprit. Less commonly, amyloid accumulation in the central nervous system may be due to cystatin C, transthyretin, prion, and gelsolin proteins. Beta-2-microglobulin is more commonly associated with renal failure and dialysis-associated amyloid accumulation outside the central nervous system.

22. **(B) Frontal lobe.**
The lesion, shown in the figure, is marked by an abnormal thickening of blood vessels by an amorphous eosinophilic material, suggestive of amyloid, as indicated by the thioflavin-S staining. The most likely location for an amyloid associated hemorrhage is the frontal lobe.

23. **(D) Polyarteritis nodosa.**
The figure illustrates blood vessels showing inflammation in the vessel wall with associated fibrinoid necrosis of the vessel wall. These findings are suggestive of a necrotizing vasculitic process such as one might see in polyarteritis nodosa.

24. **(D) CADASIL.**
The figure shows an abnormally thickened blood vessel wall with granular basophilic material within the vessel. This change is highly suggestive of CADASIL. By electron microscopy, the granularity corresponds to the accumulation of granular osmiophilic material within the vessel wall. This

disorder is systemic and similar vessel changes may be seen in other organ systems.

25. **(A) Associated with seizures in most patients.**
CADASIL affects both genders equally and typically presents in the 5th and 6th decades of life. Patients may present with cognitive decline, migraines, altered mental status, and seizures. The vascular changes are often associated with ischemic and infarct lesions involving the white matter and deep cerebral nuclei. The disorder is systemic and associated with point mutations or small deletions on the NOTCH 3 gene, located on chromosome 19p13.

26. **(C) Middle meningeal artery.**
Most epidural hemorrhages are associated with skull fractures and are related to trauma. The most common etiology is tearing of the middle meningeal artery. Bleeding from the bridging veins is usually associated with subdural hematomas.

27. **(D) Trauma.**
The lesion illustrated in the figure shows changes consistent with a contusion. A contusion represents an infarct that is trauma related. In contrast to many vascular infarcts, contusional damage is maximum at the surface of the cortex. Evidence of infarct damage is shown in this figure with involvement of the molecular layer of the cortex. In vascular-related infarcts, the molecular layer of the cortex is often spared.

28. **(A) Beta-amyloid precursor protein.**
In diffuse axonal injury, a rotational pattern of motion results in a shearing of axons. At the point of tearing, dystrophic axons or axonal balls are observed. Approximately 2 hours after survival, these axonal swellings may stain with antibody to beta-amyloid precursor protein.

29. **(A) Achondroplasia.**
The term microcephaly refers to a head circumference that is <2 standard deviations below the mean for age and gender. A variety of conditions may be associated with microcephaly. All of the conditions listed as options for this question have been implicated as potential causes with the exception of achondroplasia, which is usually associated with megalencephaly, a term used to describe an enlarged head >2.5 standard deviations above the mean for age and gender.

30. **(C) Maternal anticonvulsant therapy.**
The use of maternal anticonvulsant therapy is more commonly a cause of secondary microcephaly. The other conditions here are all potential causes of secondary megalencephaly.

31. **(B) Hypothermia.**
Neural tube defects may be caused by a variety of abnormalities including diabetes, hypothermia,

vitamin deficiency, and anticonvulsive therapies. Genetic factors may also increase risk including chromosomal abnormalities on chromosomes 13 and 18 and deletions on chromosome 22q11. Hypothermia is not known to be particularly associated with the development of neural tube defects.

32. **(C) Trisomy 13.**
Holoprosencephaly, which is failure of normal forebrain induction/patterning, resulting in a spectrum of abnormalities and midline facial defects, is most commonly associated with trisomy 13 and trisomy 18.

33. **(A) Absent ears.**
Holoprosencephaly is known to be associated with a variety of midline facial defects including hypotelorism, cyclopia, cleft lip, cleft palate, and proboscis formation. Absent ears are generally not a common finding in holoprosencephaly.

34. **(B) Alexander disease.**
All of the lesions, with the exception of Alexander disease, represent gross manifestations of focal cortical dysplasia or malformations of cortical development. Cortical tubers are most commonly seen in the setting of tuberous sclerosis. Polymicrogyria is characterized by numerous microconvolutions. Pachygyria refers to a condition marked by a few abnormally broad gyri. Agyria or lissencephaly is characterized by an absence of gyral formations. Alexander disease represents a dysmyelinating disorder of white matter due to a mutation in the GFAP (glial fibrillary acidic protein) gene.

35. **(C) Associated with maternal diabetes.**
The Dandy–Walker malformation is marked by an absence or partial agenesis of the cerebellar vermis with cystic dilatation of the fourth ventricle. It is often associated with hydrocephalus and may be seen in association with certain cardiac defects. Maternal diabetes is not known to afford an increased risk for the development of a Dandy–Walker malformation.

36. **(A) Cowden syndrome.**
The lesion illustrated in the figure represents an abnormal collection of neuronal cells representing a dysplastic cerebellar gangliocytoma. This lesion, known as Lhermitte–Duclos disease, is associated with Cowden syndrome.

37. **(B) Cerebellar tonsillar displacement below the foramen magnum.**
A Chiari type 1 malformation is marked by displacement of cerebellar tonsillar tissue into or below the foramen magnum. A Chiari type 2 malformation, in addition to displacement of the tonsils and cerebellum downward, is often associated with other malformations such as hydrocephalus and myelomeningocele.

38. **(C) Ischemic or hypoxic damage.**
Ulegyria is a term used to refer to a local hypoxic or ischemic injury to the cortex that results in neuronal loss, cortical atrophy, and gliosis at the depths of the sulci with a relative sparing of the crests of the gyri.

39. **(A) 26–30 weeks.**
For premature infants, the greatest risk for the development of periventricular leukomalacia is during the 24–32 weeks of gestational age. This time is also a period of increased risk for the development of germinal matrix bleeds.

40. **(B) Grade II.**
Germinal matrix bleeds arise from the periventricular germinal matrix zone. The highest incidence of these lesions is in infants born at <34 weeks of gestational age. A radiologic grading schema for germinal matrix hemorrhages has been developed. In grade I lesions, the hemorrhage is limited to the germinal matrix zone. Grade II lesions are marked by a rupture of blood from the germinal matrix into the ventricles, without ventricular expansion, as described in this question. Grade III lesions are marked by intraventricular hemorrhage with ventricular enlargement. Grade IV lesions are marked by intraventricular hemorrhage and hemorrhage into the hemispheric parenchyma. Grade V lesions are not defined in this approach.

41. **(D) Hippocampal sclerosis.**
The figure shows focal loss and gliosis in the hippocampal region. Along with the classic history of a young patient with medically intractable seizures, a diagnosis of hippocampal sclerosis is most likely.

42. **(B) A subependymal giant cell astrocytoma.**
Subependymal giant cell astrocytoma is most commonly associated with tuberous sclerosis. All of the other options here represent findings associated with Down syndrome or trisomy 21.

43. **(E) Two vestibular schwannomas.**
The diagnosis of bilateral vestibular schwannomas is definitional for neurofibromatosis type 2, not type 1. All of the other features listed as options are major criteria for the diagnosis of neurofibromatosis type 1.

44. **(B) Neurofibromatosis type 2.**
The lesion illustrated in the figure is marked by a proliferation of meningothelial cells surrounding blood vessels within the brain parenchyma. This finding represents an entity referred to as meningioangiomatosis, which is most commonly seen in association with neurofibromatosis type 2.

45. **(D) Pheochromocytoma.**
Of the options listed here, all of them are associated with neurofibromatosis type 2 with the exception of pheochromocytomas, which are more commonly seen in neurofibromatosis type 1 and in von Hippel–Lindau syndrome.

46. **(B) Renal cell carcinoma.**
All of the lesions listed here are associated with tuberous sclerosis except renal cell carcinoma, which is more commonly associated with von Hippel–Lindau syndrome.

47. **(B) 3.**
The VHL gene responsible for von Hippel–Lindau disease is located on chromosome 3p, similar to the location of the major gene associated with the development of many renal cell carcinomas.

48. **(C) Sturge–Weber syndrome.**
The lesion illustrated in the figure is marked by a proliferation of venous vessels within the meninges. This finding is most typical of Sturge–Weber syndrome. This entity usually arises in young patients with medically intractable seizures. The underlying cortex often shows gliosis and calcifications.

49. **(C) Pituitary adenoma.**
The defect in the PTEN/MMAC1 gene on chromosome 10q23 is associated with Cowden disease. All of the lesions listed here are associated with Cowden disease except pituitary adenoma.

50. **(C) Ganglioglioma.**
Li–Fraumeni syndrome is associated with a variety of neoplasms in both childhood and early adult life including astrocytomas, medulloblastomas, cerebral primitive neuroectodermal tumors, choroid plexus tumors, ependymal neoplasms, meningiomas, schwannomas, soft tissue and bone sarcomas, breast cancer, leukemias, adrenal cortical carcinoma, and visceral epithelial malignancies. Gangliogliomas are not known to be associated with Li–Fraumeni syndrome.

51. **(B) Glioblastoma.**
Gorlin syndrome, also called nevoid basal cell carcinoma syndrome, is marked by the development of medulloblastoma, agenesis of the corpus callosum, meningioma, congenital hydrocephalus, and macrocephaly. Glioblastoma is not known to be associated with Gorlin syndrome.

52. **(A) Adrenoleukodystrophy.**
Adrenoleukodystrophy is an X-linked peroxisomal disorder of myelin and myelin-producing cells associated with a defect in the ABCD1 gene, resulting in an accumulation of long-chain fatty acids.

53. **(B) Autosomal-dominant condition.**
Metachromatic leukodystrophy represents an autosomal-recessive, not dominant, condition resulting in abnormal accumulation of sulfatide due to a deficiency of the lysosomal enzyme arylsulfatase A.

The disorder results in a loss of myelin and axonal degeneration. A variety of presentations have been described. The adult form usually presents in patients who are in their 20s and 30s with psychiatric and behavioral changes or psychosis. The lesions are usually bilateral, symmetrically distributed, and generally spare the subcortical U-fibers. The frontal lobes are preferentially involved by the disorder in contrast to adrenoleukodystrophy, where there is a relative sparing of the frontal lobes.

54. **(B) Krabbe disease.**
The lesion, illustrated in the figure, is composed of clusters of large globoid cells and is marked by an accumulation of psychosine material within phagocytes. The clinical presentations in these histologic findings are most consistent with Krabbe disease, an autosomal-recessive condition marked by a deficiency of the lysosomal enzyme galactosylceramidase.

55. **(C) Mutation in the GFAP gene.**
The lesion illustrated in the figure is marked by the presence of numerous markedly eosinophilic Rosenthal fibers. In the setting of a white matter abnormality, this finding is suggestive of Alexander disease, which is due to a mutation in the GFAP gene.

56. **(E) United Kingdom.**
The incidence of multiple sclerosis is more common in countries that are located far from the equator. Of the countries listed here, the United Kingdom would be the country with the highest incidence of multiple sclerosis. Other high-incidence locations include Canada, Australia, and United States.

57. **(E) HLA-DR15.**
In most populations, multiple sclerosis is associated with HLA-DR15.

58. **(E) Reticulin.**
The findings shown in this biopsy are marked by increased numbers of white matter macrophages, reactive astrocytes, and benign-appearing perivascular lymphocytes. A CD68 immunostain would highlight the macrophages. A CD3 stain highlights the presence of T lymphocytes, which is the phenotype of most of the lymphocytes seen in multiple sclerosis. A Luxol fast blue stain would be useful in highlighting white matter loss, and a neurofilament stain would highlight a relative preservation of axons. Reticulin staining would be least useful in the assessment of a multiple sclerosis lesion or plaque.

59. **(C) Most develop multiphasic disease course.**
Acute disseminated encephalomyelitis is a monophasic acute demyelinating disorder marked by perivascular demyelination. The disorder is associated with vaccinations as well as a variety of viral infections. The entity is more frequently seen in children than pediatric multiple sclerosis. Patients most frequently present with bilateral pyramidal signs, acute hemiplegia, ataxia, and cranial nerve palsies.

60. **(C) Neurofibrillary tangles.**
The lesions illustrated in the figure on silver staining represent neurofibrillary tangles. These are cytoplasmic neuronal inclusions associated with an abnormally phosphorylated tau protein. Senile plaques are extracellular collections of neurites and amyloid material. Hirano bodies are intracytoplasmic eosinophilic inclusions composed of actin material. Granulovacuolar degeneration is marked by small cytoplasmic vacuoles with a dark cytoplasmic granule. Pick bodies are silver positive, round inclusions associated with frontotemporal dementia.

61. **(A) Alpha-synuclein.**
The lesion shown in Question 60 represents a neurofibrillary tangle. Tangles are best highlighted on silver stains, such as Bielschowsky or Bodian. Tangles may also stain positively with antibody to tau and a Gallyas stain. Alpha-synuclein is better for highlighting Lewy bodies.

62. **(A) Alpha-synuclein.**
All of the genes listed here, with the exception of alpha-synuclein, are associated with early onset Alzheimer disease.

63. **(C) Thioflavin-S.**
Thioflavin-S is an immunofluorescent stain useful for identifying amyloid material. The lesion illustrated in the figure represents an example of granulovacuolar degeneration within hippocampal neurons. Granulovacuolar degeneration may be highlighted with antibodies to neurofilament, ubiquitin, tau, and tubulin.

64. **(B) Basal ganglia (caudate and putamen).**
In neurofibrillary tangle predominant dementia, a high density of neurofibrillary tangles is found in all of the locations listed with the exception of the basal ganglia region. This form of dementia presents with memory impairment in the elderly and is characterized by numerous neurofibrillary tangles at autopsy. There are relatively few or no amyloid deposits in contrast with Alzheimer disease.

65. **(D) Tau.**
There are a variety of mutations that have been described in cases of familial Parkinson disease. The most common of these involves the alpha-synuclein gene. Other responsible genes include parkin, UCHL1, PINK1, DJ-1, LRRK2, ATP13A2, and

Omi/HtrA2. Tau mutations are associated with certain forms of frontotemporal dementia (FTDP-17).

66. **(A) Alpha-synuclein.**
The most sensitive and specific marker for Lewy bodies, which are the eosinophilic cytoplasmic inclusions surrounded by a clear halo, shown here in substantia nigra pigmented neurons, is alpha-synuclein. Lewy bodies may also stain with ubiquitin and neurofilament antibodies, although these antibodies are less sensitive and specific for this lesion.

67. **(E) Neuronal cytoplasmic inclusions.**
Multiple system atrophy is a sporadic, progressive adult-onset disease marked by the presence of alpha-synuclein positive glial cytoplasmic inclusions. Patients with the parkinsonian predominant type often present with akinesia, rigidity, dysesthesia, and dystonia. Patients who have the cerebellar predominant type tend to present with gait and limb ataxia, oculomotor disturbances, and dysarthria. Dysautonomia is a common feature of both types. The disease typically presents in adults and shows a male predominance. Pathologically, the parkinsonian type shows atrophy of the caudate nucleus and putamen. The cerebellar type shows atrophy of the cerebellum, middle cerebellar peduncle, and pons. The cerebellar type histologically is marked by Purkinje cell loss. The inclusions one sees are usually glial and not neuronal.

68. **(D) GFAP-positive Pick cells.**
Pick cells demonstrate positive staining with neurofilament antibody and not GFAP. Pick disease is marked by ballooned neurons or Pick cells, as well as cells that contain silver positive staining cytoplasmic inclusions within neurons. Classically, Pick disease results in frontotemporal atrophy with a relative sparing of the posterior superior temporal gyrus.

69. **(E) FTLD-U.**
The most common type of frontotemporal lobe degeneration is the FTLD-U type. This type is characterized by ubiquitin immunoreactive structures that are tau, neurofilament, alpha-synuclein, and prion negative. A subset of patients demonstrates a mutation in CHMP2B.

70. **(E) Tau positivity.**
The lesions shown in FTLD-U do not stain with antibody to tau or alpha-synuclein. The entity is associated with neuron loss and gliosis in the frontal and temporal lobes. The entity is associated with a mutation in the charged multivesicular body protein 2B gene. Patients often present with behavioral and personality changes, progressive aphasia, akinetic rigidity, and dystonia.

71. **(E) Loss of neurons in locus ceruleus.**
Amyotrophic lateral sclerosis or ALS is marked by a loss of anterior horn cells as well as Betz cells in the primary motor cortex. There is a loss of myelinated axons in the lateral and anterior cortical spinal tracts. Small round eosinophilic neuronal cytoplasmic inclusions involving anterior horn cells, called Bunina bodies, are also a feature of this disorder. Neuronal loss in locus ceruleus is not a common finding in ALS.

72. **(D) Spinal muscular atrophy 2.**
Spinal muscular atrophy 1 or Werdnig–Hoffmann disease typically has onset at infancy. Onset before 18 months is typical of spinal muscular atrophy 2 and onset after 18 months is a feature of spinal muscular atrophy 3. Clinical features described in this patient are typical of the spinal muscular atrophies.

73. **(A) Becker muscular dystrophy.**
Of all the entities listed here, Becker muscular dystrophy is not a trinucleotide repeat disorder. Becker muscular dystrophy represents an abnormality of the dystrophin protein.

74. **(D) Grade 3.**
The Vonsattel grading schema has been used to assess the degree of pathology both grossly and microscopically in patients with Huntington disease. Grade 0 lesions indicate no gross or microscopic changes and are defined by either a clinical or family history of the disease or DNA analysis suggesting the disease. Grade 1 lesions show no gross abnormalities of the neostriatum, but show microscopic evidence of neuron loss and gliosis in the dorsomedial caudate, tail of the caudate, and dorsal putamen. Grade 2 lesions show gross atrophy of the neostriatum with extension of the neuronal loss in the ventrolateral direction. Grade 3 lesions, as described in the current case, are defined by atrophy of most of the putamen and caudate nuclei. Grade 4 lesions show severe neuronal loss and gliosis involving all the caudate and putamen with extension into the nucleus accumbens.

75. **(B) Loss of neurons in the putamen.**
Hereditary spinocerebellar ataxias represent a group of inherited ataxias (mostly dominant inheritance pattern) related to trinucleotide repeats. Machado–Joseph disease represents type 3, which usually has an onset between the 4th and 6th decades of life. This type is marked by a severe neuronal loss in the cerebellar dentate nucleus with a relative preservation of the cerebellar cortex and inferior olivary nuclei. Degeneration of the superior peduncle and spinocerebellar tracts are often seen. Degeneration of the basis pontis gray

matter, neurons of Clarke column, lower motor neurons, and substantia nigra may also be present. Putamen neuronal loss is not a feature of this disorder.

76. **(A) Cataracts.**
All of the features listed here are associated with Friedreich ataxia except cataracts. Additionally, patients may have diabetes mellitus.

77. **(E) X-linked condition.**
Neurodegeneration with brain iron accumulation or Hallervorden–Spatz disease is a group of rare disorders resulting in prominent iron accumulation in the brain, particularly in the basal ganglia region. Most are associated with a mutation in the PANK2 gene on chromosome 20 (pantothenate kinase 2). The lesion is not inherited as an X-linked condition. The entity is marked by axonal spheroids, neuronal loss, and gliosis predominantly in the medial globus pallidus and substantia nigra. Glial cytoplasmic inclusions, which are tau and alpha-synuclein positive, may be seen in involved areas.

78. **(E) *Streptococcus pneumoniae*.**
The figure represents acute inflammation in the leptomeninges constituting acute meningitis. In a hospitalized patient, the most likely etiology of nosocomial meningitis is *Streptococcus pneumoniae*.

79. **(B) Cardiac disease with left-to-right shunt.**
The lesion illustrated in the figure represents part of an abscess. A variety of conditions predispose one to the development of abscess including acute bacterial endocarditis, congenital heart disease with right-to-left shunts, chronic pulmonary disease, intraabdominal abscesses, urinary tract infections, and dental infections.

80. **(E) *Mycobacterium tuberculosis*.**
The figure shown here is marked by the presents of necrotizing granulomatous inflammation, which is most consistent with infection by *Mycobacterium tuberculosis*. Certain fungal organisms may also result in necrotizing granulomatous inflammation. Leprosy, due to infection by *Mycobacterium leprae*, more commonly involves the peripheral rather than the central nervous system.

81. **(E) *Nocardia*.**
The lesion, shown in the figure, stained with a Gomori methenamine silver (GMS) stain highlights the presents of a thin delicate filamentous structures most consistent with *Nocardia*.

82. **(E) Cryptococcosis.**
The lesion illustrated in the figure is marked by budding yeast forms. The yeast contains a capsule that may be highlighted with mucicarmine or

PAS staining. The organism ranges from 5 to 15 microns in diameter. The background inflammatory response is often marked by chronic inflammation, consisting of macrophages, small granulomas, lymphocytes, and plasma cells.

83. **(E) Travel to Southwest United States.**
The lesion shown in the figure is characterized by the presence of septated hyphae that branch at acute angles, most consistent with *Aspergillus*. *Aspergillus* may be associated with all of the conditions listed except travel to the Southwest United States, which is more commonly associated with *Coccidioides* infection.

84. **(B) Coccidioidomycosis.**
The lesion, shown in the figure, shows evidence of a cyst associated with a granulomatous response. This is most consistent with a diagnosis of *Coccidioides* infection.

85. **(D) Ohio.**
Histoplasmosis has a worldwide distribution but in the United States occurs most commonly in the Ohio, Mississippi, and St. Lawrence River valleys. In the central nervous system, it is responsible for either meningitis or an abscess lesion, usually with a granulomatous inflammatory infiltrate. Organisms may be seen within the cytoplasm of macrophages.

86. **(E) Temporal lobes.**
In patients with herpes encephalitis, the temporal and frontal lobes preferentially are involved. These areas may demonstrate edema with hemorrhagic necrosis and a mixture of acute and chronic inflammation.

87. **(E) Microglial nodules.**
The large intranuclear and cytoplasmic inclusions seen in cells of this optic nerve biopsy are suggestive of cytomegalovirus infection. Most commonly, cytomegalovirus is associated with chronic perivascular inflammation and microglial nodule formations.

88. **(D) Progressive multifocal leukoencephalopathy.**
The lesion, shown in the figure, is marked by the presence of white matter macrophages with intranuclear viral inclusions within oligodendrocytes. Given the background of an immunocompromised individual and the presence of subcortical white matter lesions, the most likely diagnosis is progressive multifocal leukoencephalopathy.

89. **(C) HTLV-1.**
Tropical spastic paraparesis is associated with HTLV-1 infection. This retrovirus is endemic to Southern Japan, Africa, South America, and the Caribbean. It is also associated with the development of T-cell leukemia.

90. **(E) Toxoplasmosis.**
The figure shown is marked by the presence of microglial nodule associated cysts of *Toxoplasma gondii*. Most commonly, toxoplasmosis manifests as a necrotic abscess, but occasionally microglial nodule associated encephalitis may occur with this organism.

91. **(D)** *Naegleria.*
The development of meningoencephalitic picture in someone exposed to contaminated freshwater raised the possibility of amebic encephalitis caused by *Naegleria*. *Acanthamoeba* and *Balamuthia* represent other forms of amebic infection.

92. **(E) Most commonly due to *Schistosoma haematobium*.**
Neuroschistosomiasis is caused by infection from trematodes. Cerebral involvement most commonly occurs in association with *Schistosoma japonicum*. The eggs may embolize to the brain from the portal mesenteric system. Infection in the brain is more common in men. Most patients are asymptomatic. Histologically, a granulomatous inflammatory response may be seen. Eggs may be seen in inflamed areas, as well as away from regions of inflammation.

93. **(E) Spongiform changes with microglial nodules.**
Creutzfeldt–Jakob disease represents a prion protein abnormality marked by rapidly progressive dementia and myoclonus. Approximately 10% of cases are familial. Patients frequently have an elevated protein 14-3-3 in the cerebrospinal fluid. Spongiform changes with neuron loss and gliosis are a frequent finding of Creutzfeldt–Jakob disease. Microglial nodules and acute or chronic inflammation are not typical features of prion diseases.

94. **(C) Formalin fixation.**
All of the options listed here decrease the admission of prion disease with the exception of formalin fixation, which does not appear to have a significant impact on transmission.

95. **(E) Nova Scotia.**
Niemann–Pick disease represents a form of lysosomal storage disease that is particularly prevalent in Nova Scotia. Tay-Sachs disease and Gaucher disease are common in the Ashkenazi Jewish population. Some forms of infantile and juvenile neuronal ceroid lipofuscinosis are common in Scandinavian and Northern European populations.

96. **(E) Pompe disease.**
All of the entities listed here represent sphingolipidoses, which are forms of lysosomal storage diseases presenting in the neonatal period, except Pompe disease. Pompe disease represents lysosomal storage disease that is not classified as a sphingolipidosis; it is a glycogen storage disease.

97. **(A) Alexander disease.**
All of the entities listed here represent lysosomal storage diseases that can affect the nervous system except Alexander disease, which is a dysmyelinating abnormality associated with a mutations in the GFAP gene.

98. **(C) Hepatosplenomegaly.**
Tay–Sachs disease is an autosomal-recessive disorder caused by a deficiency in hexosaminidase A. Patients may present with blindness, cherry red spots, and accumulation of GM2 ganglioside material within neurons. Ultrastructurally, membranous cytoplasmic bodies may be seen. Hepatosplenomegaly is generally not a feature of this disorder and is more commonly seen in other metabolic diseases such as Niemann–Pick disease.

99. **(A) Fabry disease.**
Fabry disease is due to a deficiency in alpha-galactosidase, resulting in accumulation of trihexosylceramide. Angiokeratoma corporis diffusum or cutaneous telangiectasias in a bathing trunk distribution and renal dysfunction are features associated with Fabry disease. Additionally, corneal opacities, hypertension, and heart disease may also be encountered.

100. **(E) Zebra bodies.**
The ultrastructural features listed here are all present in various forms of neuronal ceroid lipofuscinosis with the exception of zebra bodies, which are characteristic of certain other metabolic abnormalities.

101. **(E) Zellweger syndrome.**
Zellweger syndrome represents a peroxisomal abnormality characterized by dysmorphic features, calcific stippling of the patella, liver disease, neuronal migration abnormalities, and white matter changes. All of the other entities listed represent a form of mitochondrial disease.

102. **(A) Age of presentation typically 5th and 6th decades.**
MELAS, which represents mitochondrial encephalomyopathy with lactic acidosis and stroke-like episodes, usually presents in young age patients (childhood or young adulthood). Patients develop infarct-like lesions with dementia, headaches, and an elevated cerebrospinal fluid lactate level. The abnormalities are caused by a mitochondrial DNA mutation and are maternally inherited.

103. **(B) Alzheimer type II astrocytes.**
Menkes disease is an X-linked recessive disorder of copper metabolism resulting in a failure to thrive, hypothermia, hypotonia, seizures, and psychomotor retardation, eventually resulting in

death. Affected children often have a characteristic cherubic facial appearance with hair alterations. Alzheimer type II astrocytes are not a feature of this disorder and are usually seen in conditions that result in increased ammonia levels.

104. **(B) Thiamine.**
The findings described here are consistent with Wernicke–Korsakoff syndrome, which is due to a thiamine deficiency. This most commonly arises in the setting of a malnourished alcoholic.

105. **(E) Toluene.**
Toluene is associated with a peripheral neuropathy that is primarily demyelinating. All of the other substances listed here result in a neuronopathy.

106. **(D) Secondary structures of Sherer.**
The grading of fibrillary diffuse astrocytomas is predicated on assessment of degree of cellularity, mitotic activity, vascular proliferative changes, and necrosis. The formation of secondary structures of Sherer, which represent infiltrating tumor cells satelliting around preexisting structures like neurons or blood vessels, is not a feature useful in grading these tumors.

107. **(C) IDH-1.**
IDH-1 antibody has been shown to stain the majority of low-grade fibrillary astrocytomas, mixed gliomas, and oligodendrogliomas but does not stain conditions resulting in gliosis. Ki-67 may be useful in certain cases, when a high labeling index is noted; this would be suggestive of a tumor. One can see Ki-67 immunostaining in reactive processes and care should be taken not to misinterpret inflammatory cells or microglial cell staining as tumor cell staining. The lesion illustrated in the figure represents a low-grade astrocytoma, WHO grade II.

108. **(B) Gliosarcoma.**
The lesion shown in the figure is marked by a proliferation of atypical glial cells and atypical cartilaginous tissue. This combination of tissue types is most characteristic of gliosarcoma. Gliosarcoma represents a form of glioblastoma, WHO grade IV.

109. **(C) EGFR overexpression.**
The majority of small cell glioblastoma, shown in the figure, characteristically show overexpression of epidermal growth factor receptor (EGFR). 1p and 19q deletions are more commonly associated with oligodendrogliomas. IDH-1 mutations are not specific for this variant of a glioblastoma. p53 mutations may be seen in some but not all cases of small cell glioblastoma.

110. **(A) CAM 5.2.**
The lesion, shown in the figure, represents a glioblastoma. Glioblastoma may demonstrate positive staining with antibodies to GFAP and S-100 protein. Cross-immunoreactivity with certain cytokeratin markers such as cytokeratins AE1/3 has been well described in glioblastoma. A subset of these lesions, which may have arisen from a lower grade astrocytoma (secondary glioblastoma), may demonstrate p53 immunoreactivity associated with p53 mutations. Only rare cases of glioblastoma stain with cytokeratin CAM 5.2.

111. **(E) Pilocytic astrocytoma.**
The lesion shown in the figure is marked by the presence of numerous eosinophilic granular bodies. In the context of a cyst with a mural nodule tumor arising in the cerebellum of a child, the best diagnosis is pilocytic astrocytoma.

112. **(C) Lateral ventricle.**
The lesion shown in the figure is marked by the presence of large astrocytic cells. In the setting of tuberous sclerosis, this finding is most consistent with a subependymal giant cell astrocytoma, WHO grade I. This lesion typically arises in the lateral ventricles.

113. **(B) Increased mitotic figures (>2/10 high-power fields).**
Pleomorphic xanthoastrocytomas are typically seen in the temporal lobe of younger patients. Patients usually present with a history of chronic epilepsy. Morphologically, the tumors are marked by prominent cellularity with atypical appearing astrocytic cells, some of which may be lipidized. Increased reticulin deposition between tumor cells is noted. Eosinophilic granular bodies and Rosenthal fibers are also commonly encountered in this tumor. Increased mitotic activity and necrosis are not usual features of pleomorphic xanthoastrocytoma but may be seen in the rare anaplastic pleomorphic xanthoastrocytoma (WHO grade III), and may be used in establishing the differential diagnosis with glioblastoma.

114. **(A) Arises in the fourth ventricle.**
Chordoid gliomas represent a rare glioma arising in the third ventricle, not the fourth ventricle. Tumor typically presents in adults over the age of 30 years and shows a female predominance. Histologically, the neoplasm is marked by cores and clusters of epithelioid cells embedded in a mucin-rich stroma. Vacuolation in the stroma may be seen, as well as a lymphoplasmacytic infiltrate with Russell bodies. The neoplasm represents a WHO grade II lesion.

115. **(A) Angiocentric glioma.**
The lesion, shown in the figure, is marked by perivascular pseudorosette structures, which are characteristic of angiocentric glioma. Most of these lesions arise in children or young adults

with a history of chronic epilepsy; it preferentially involves the temporal lobe. The tumor represents a WHO grade I neoplasm.

116. **(E) Oligodendrogliomas.**
Large deletions on chromosomes 1p and 19q have been associated with chemoresponsiveness and a better outcome in oligodendrogliomas and mixed gliomas (oligoastrocytomas). Similar changes have been observed in a smaller percentage of astrocytomas, and the literature appears divided as to the prognostic significance in that setting. Approximately 60–80% of oligodendrogliomas demonstrate the deletions.

117. **(D) Represents an artifact of delayed formalin fixation.**
The "fried egg" appearance, which is classically associated with oligodendrogliomas, is a result of a delay in formalin fixation. This change will therefore not be evident at frozen section. In rapidly fixed tissue, the alteration will also not be as evident. Although a salient feature of many oligodendrogliomas, this finding is not exclusively seen in these tumors and may be seen in other glial neoplasms, particularly some astrocytomas (so, not everything with a fried egg appearance is an oligodendroglioma).

118. **(E) Spinal cord.**
The lesion shown in the figure represents a low-grade ependymoma with perivascular pseudorosettes. The most common site for this lesion in adults is the spinal cord. In children, the most common location for this tumor is the posterior fossa.

119. **(A) Extent of surgical resection.**
The extent of surgical resection is the most important prognostic factor in ependymal neoplasms. A worse prognosis has been associated with young age at diagnosis, intracranial location versus spinal cord location, and higher grade (WHO grade III).

120. **(D) Lumbosacral cord.**
The lesion shown in the figure represents a myxopapillary ependymoma, WHO grade I. Myxopapillary ependymomas are marked by architecture in which there is a central vessel surrounded by mucin positive stroma and ependymal cells around the perimeter. The lesion may or may not have an obviously papillary architecture. Most myxopapillary ependymomas arise in the lumbosacral region of the spinal cord. Occasional cases may arise elsewhere in the spinal cord and rare intracranial cases have been documented. Subcutaneous tumors have also been reported, particularly in the lower back region.

121. **(B) WHO grade I.**
The lesion shown in the figure represents a subependymoma. Subependymomas are marked by clusters of ependymoma-like cells arranged against a fibrillary background. The cells are often loosely clustered in nests. Microcystic changes are frequently evident. Mitotic activity, vascular proliferative changes, and necrosis are not salient features of this tumor. Subependymomas are low-grade lesions, corresponding to WHO grade I neoplasms.

122. **(C) Dysembryoplastic neuroepithelial tumor.**
Of the tumors listed here, the dysembryoplastic neuroepithelial tumor is classically associated with adjacent cortical architectural abnormalities, known as focal cortical dysplasia or malformations of focal cortical development. This coexistence suggests a possible developmental origin to this tumor. Other lesions in which adjacent cortical dysplasia have been reported include ganglioglioma, pleomorphic xanthoastrocytoma, and angiocentric glioma.

123. **(E) Tuberous sclerosis.**
Meningiomas are well-known to be associated with neurofibromatosis type II, a prior history of radiation therapy, breast and uterine cancers, and female gender. Meningiomas are not known to be associated with tuberous sclerosis. In tuberous sclerosis, the main central nervous system-related pathologies include the subependymal giant cell astrocytoma, ventricular hamartomas, and the cortical tuber (a gross manifestation of focal cortical dysplasia).

124. **(D) Syncytial meningiomas with embolization.**
The lesion illustrated in the figure represents a syncytial or meningothelial meningioma with evidence of intravascular embolization. Tumors are sometimes embolized prior to surgery in order to reduce the amount of bleeding sustained during the surgical procedure. Atypical meningiomas would be marked by increased mitotic activity (4 or more mitoses per 10 high-power fields, but <20), evidence of brain invasion or the presence of three or more atypical or unusual features such as disordered architecture, hypercellularity, small cell change, prominent nucleation, or necrosis. In the setting of embolization, necrosis needs to be interpreted with caution, in that it may be related to the embolization. A transitional meningioma is most commonly marked by a mixture of syncytial and fibrous patterns.

125. **(D) Secretory meningioma.**
The lesion, shown in the figure, is marked by eosinophilic round structures, which are characteristic of the secretory or pseudopsammomatous meningioma. These eosinophilic structures can be highlighted with a PAS stain. Secretory meningiomas are typically WHO grade I neoplasms.

126. **(C) Metaplastic.**
     Clear cell and chordoid meningiomas represent WHO grade II variants with an increased risk of recurrence. Papillary and rhabdoid meningiomas represent WHO grade II neoplasms with an increased risk of recurrence and metastasis. Metaplastic meningiomas are generally considered WHO grade I tumors and are marked by the presence of benign-appearing bone, cartilage, or adipose tissue.

127. **(A) Glomeruloid vascular proliferation.**
     Hemangiopericytomas are generally graded as WHO grade II or III lesions. Anaplastic or grade III lesions are marked by at least 5 mitoses per 10 high-power fields and/or necrosis or a tumor with 2 or more worrisome features including hemorrhage, moderate-to-high nuclear atypia, and hypercellularity. Vascular proliferation is not a feature used in grading these tumors. Glomeruloid vascular proliferation is a feature used in grading fibrillary astrocytomas and denotes a WHO grade IV tumor (glioblastoma).

128. **(B) Hemangioblastoma.**
     The lesion illustrated in the figure is marked by the presence of vacuolated stromal cells with an admixture of capillary and venous vessels. In the cerebellum, this should raise the possibility of a hemangioblastoma. Hemangioblastomas stain with antibody to inhibin and generally do not stain with markers such as EMA (epithelial membrane antigen), which stains many metastatic clear cell renal cell carcinomas. Metastatic clear cell renal cell carcinomas are in the differential diagnosis of hemangioblastoma, particularly in patients with von Hippel–Lindau syndrome.

129. **(B) GFAP, S-100, melan A, CAM 5.2.**
     The lesion shown in the figure represents poorly differentiated neoplasm with large nucleolated cells. Major differential diagnostic considerations include metastatic melanoma, epithelioid glioblastoma, and metastatic large cell carcinoma. GFAP staining would be helpful in highlighting the glioblastoma. S-100 and melan A will stain melanoma. S-100 will also stain glioblastoma. CAM 5.2 is a better marker than cytokeratins AE1/3 in highlighting metastatic carcinoma in that cytokeratins AE1/3 frequently cross-immunoreactive with high-grade astrocytomas. The lesion shown in the figure represented a metastatic malignant melanoma.

130. **(D) Synaptophysin.**
     The lesion shown in the figure represents an intraventricular mass and is consistent with a choroid plexus papilloma. Choroid plexus papillomas stain with all of the immunomarkers listed as options for this question except synaptophysin.

131. **(A) Central neurocytoma.**
     Central neurocytomas classically arise in the lateral ventricles in young adults. The lesions resemble oligodendrogliomas in that they are characterized by a proliferation of generally rounded cells with scant cytoplasm. The nuclei often have a speckled or salt-and-pepper chromatin pattern. Central neurocytomas will demonstrate evidence of neural differentiation and will mark with antibodies such as synaptophysin and MAP2. Clear cell ependymomas may rarely have rounded nuclei and resemble oligodendroglioma or central neurocytoma, but will not stain with neural markers. Dysembryoplastic neuroepithelial tumors are usually intraparenchymal, cortical based lesions, and do not present as intraventricular masses. Liponeurocytomas usually arise in the cerebellum and are admixed with adipose tissue.

132. **(A) Germinoma.**
     The most common tumor arising in the pineal gland is the germinoma, which accounts for more than half of pineal neoplasms.

133. **(B) FISH test for chromosome 22 deletions.**
     The lesion shown in the figure represents a large cell medulloblastoma. Medulloblastomas should be differentiated from atypical teratoid/rhabdoid tumors, which have a worse prognosis. Atypical teratoid/rhabdoid tumors demonstrate deletions on chromosomes 22 (the hSNF5/INI1 genes).

134. **(B) Desmoplastic variant.**
     The prognosis in embryonal tumors is dependent on the tumor type. Poor prognostic features associated with medulloblastomas include young age at diagnosis (<3 years), the presence of metastasis at the time of diagnosis, subtotal surgical resection, large cell variant, GFAP immunoreactivity, and MYC gene amplification. The desmoplastic variant, although historically in the literature was suggested to have a worse prognosis, is now generally not thought of as an adverse prognostic variant.

135. **(E) Temporal lobe most common site of origin.**
     The lesion shown in the figure is characterized by a proliferation of discohesive cells, typical of a primary central nervous system lymphoma. These lesions are well-known to be associated with HIV and EBV infection. There is also an increased risk of this lesion developing following transplantation (posttransplant lymphoproliferative disorder). Tumors usually present as an intraparenchymal mass, in contrast to metastatic lymphomas that are more commonly meningeal based. The frontal lobe is the most common site of origin. The majority of

these tumors represents diffuse large B-cell lymphomas and therefore stains with B-cell markers such as CD20 and CD79a.

136. **(A) Arachnoid cyst.**
The lesion shown in the figure is marked by a rare nest of meningothelial cells and is suggestive of a benign arachnoid cyst. The temporal lobe is a fairly common location for this lesion.

137. **(C) It is nonsecretory.**
The lesion illustrated in the figure is marked by a proliferation of large cells with abundant granular eosinophilic cytoplasm suggestive of a granular cell tumor. These lesions most commonly arise in the posterior pituitary gland or neurohypophysis and do not secrete pituitary hormones. Granular cell differentiation may also be occasionally encountered in a glioblastoma.

138. **(B) Lymphocytic hypophysitis.**
In a pituitary gland from a postpartum woman that is marked by prominent lymphocytic infiltrate, a diagnosis of lymphocytic hypophysitis should be entertained. This lesion is probably an immune-mediated process, which results in destruction of the anterior portion of the gland. Patients often present with pituitary insufficiency.

139. **(B) Germinoma.**
The lesion shown in the figure is marked by large germ cells with prominent nucleolation and an intermixed population of benign-appearing lymphocytes. Given the age of presentation and pineal gland location, a germinoma diagnosis should be entertained. Occasionally, nonnecrotizing granulomatous inflammation may be associated with this tumor.

140. **(A) Craniopharyngioma.**
The lesion shown in the figure arising in the sellar area is marked by a squamoid type epithelium with a peripheral basaloid cell layer. This lesion is consistent with a diagnosis of craniopharyngioma. These often present as cystic lesions. The most common variant, shown in the figure, is the adamantinomatous variant, which is often accompanied by fibrosis, dystrophic mineralization, and lipid and cholesterol formation. Keratin type material, which is also evident here, is characteristic of many of these lesions. Occasionally, craniopharyngiomas may be cystic. Differentiation from epidermoid cyst may be a differential diagnostic consideration. Epidermoid cysts usually contain a granular cell layer, which is absent in craniopharyngioma.

141. **(B) Colon carcinoma.**
Tumors that are most likely to metastasize to the central nervous system include lung carcinomas, breast carcinomas, melanomas, and renal cell carcinomas. Colon cancers, although fairly common metastases, are the least common of the tumors entities listed as options to this question.

142. **(E) Trichrome.**
Ragged red fibers are suggestive of mitochondrial cytopathy. Ragged red fibers are best highlighted on trichrome stain, where the mitochondria accumulate, particularly in a subsarcolemmal region, stain red on the Gomori trichrome stain. Mitochondria may also be highlighted on a succinate dehydrogenase (SDH) stain, where they appear as ragged blue fibers.

143. **(A) Dermatomyositis.**
The biopsy shown in the figure is marked by a prominent pattern of perifascicular atrophy. The presence of perifascicular atrophy in the background of an inflammatory myopathy is highly suggestive of dermatomyositis. Inflammatory myopathies are generally marked by the presence of chronic inflammation, in the case of dermatomyositis, usually perivascular in distribution, muscle fiber degeneration, and muscle fiber regeneration.

144. **(C) Myonecrosis.**
Denervation atrophy on a muscle biopsy is due to pathology in the peripheral nervous system resulting in secondary changes in the skeletal muscle. Angular atrophic esterase positive staining fibers are indicative of acute denervation atrophy. Nuclear bag formations, in which cells become atrophic and the amount of cytoplasm is significantly decreased, are suggestive of atrophy and may be seen frequently in the denervation atrophy setting. Target fibers, best highlighted on a NADH stain, are also commonly observed in denervation atrophy. Fiber type grouping is best highlighted on the ATPase stains where there is loss of the normal checkerboard pattern of fiber type distribution. Fiber type grouping is usually the result of denervation with reinnervation. Mild necrosis is usually seen in myopathic processes such as inflammatory myopathies and muscular dystrophy.

145. **(E) Werdnig–Hoffman disease.**
The presence of fascicular atrophy, in which entire muscle fascicles are atrophic, raises a rather limited differential diagnosis, which includes the spinal muscular atrophies, such as Werdnig–Hoffman disease, nerve infarct, such as one might see with vasculitis, and Charcot–Marie–Tooth disease.

146. **(B) Duchenne muscular dystrophy.**
Duchenne muscular dystrophy is associated with an absence of dystrophin protein or the presence of a dystrophin protein that may be only partially formed but is functionally inactive. Becker muscular dystrophy is also a dystrophin-associated

abnormality in which there is a partial absence or partially functional protein present. Duchenne muscular dystrophy is an X-linked condition, usually presenting in childhood.

147. **(A) Acid maltase deficiency.**
The biopsy shown in the figure is marked by scattered muscle fibers showing large vacuoles. Acid phosphatase positive staining in association with the vacuoles is suggestive of acid maltase deficiency. A PAS stain would highlight the presence of glycogen accumulation within these vacuoles. Difficulty in weaning an adult patient from a ventilator is typical scenario associated with adult patients presenting with this abnormality.

148. **(A) Charcot–Marie–Tooth disease.**
The clinical presentation given is very suggestive of Charcot–Marie–Tooth disease. These patients have palpably enlarged nerves and show numerous onion bulb formations on biopsy. Onion bulb formation is a marker of repeated patterns of demyelination and remyelination.

149. **(E) Transthyretin.**
In familial amyloid neuropathies, the most common protein responsible for the amyloid accumulation is transthyretin.

150. **(B) Cytomegalovirus neuritis.**
The biopsy shown in the figure is taken from a sural nerve and shows large intranuclear inclusions suggestive of cytomegalovirus infection.

SUGGESTED READING

1. Adams D. Hereditary and acquired amyloid neuropathies. *J Neurol*. 2001;248:647-657.
2. Anthony DC, Crain BJ. Peripheral nerve biopsies. *Arch Pathol Lab Med*. 1996;120:26-34.
3. Biggio EH. Update on recent molecular and genetic advances in frontotemporal lobar degeneration. *J Neuropathol Exp Neurol*. 2008;67:635-648.
4. Bornemann A, Goebel HH. Congenital myopathies. *Brain Pathol*. 2001;11:206-217.
5. Braak H, Braak E. Neuropathological staging of Alzheimer-related changes. *Acta Neuropathol (Berl)*. 1991;82:239-259.
6. Brat DJ, Scheithauer BW, Staugaitis SM, et al. Third ventricular chordoid glioma: a distinct clinicopathologic entity. *J Neuropathol Exp Neurol*. 1998;57:283-290.
7. Brown HG, Kepner JL, Perlman EJ, et al. 'Large cell/anaplastic' medulloblastomas: a Pediatric Oncology Group Study. *J Neuropathol Exp Neurol*. 2000;59:857-865.
8. Cairns NG, Biggio EH, Mackenzie IR, et al. Neuropathologic diagnostic and nosologic criteria for frontotemporal lobar degeneration: consensus of the consortium for frontotemporal lobar degeneration. *Acta Neuropathol*. 2007;114:5-22.
9. Carpenter S. Inclusion body myositis, a review. *J Neuropathol Exp Neurol*. 1996;55:1105-1114.
10. Chabriat H, Joutel A, Dichgans M, et al. CADASIL. *Lancet Neurol*. 2009;8:643-653.
11. Challa V, Moody DM, Brown W. Vascular malformations of the central nervous system. *J Neuropathol Exp Neurol*. 1995; 54:609-621.
12. Chimelli L, Mahler-Araújo MB. Fungal infections. *Brain Pathol*. 1997;7:613-627.
13. Conway JE, Chou D, Clatterbuck RE, et al. Hemangioblastomas of the central nervous system in von Hippel-Lindau syndrome and sporadic disease. *Neurosurgery*. 2001;48:55-63.
14. Dalakas MC. Advances in chronic inflammatory demyelinating polyneuropathy: disease variants and inflammatory response mediators and modifiers. *Curr Opin Neurol*. 1999; 12:403-409.
15. Daumas-Duport C, Scheithauer BW, Chodkiewicz JP, et al. Dysembryoplastic neuroepithelial tumor: a surgically curable tumor of young patients with intractable partial seizures. Reports of thirty-nine cases. *Neurosurgery*. 1988;23: 545-556.
16. Davies S, Ramsden D. Huntington's disease. *Mol Pathol*. 2001;54:409-413.
17. DeArmond SJ, Prusiner SB. Perspectives on prion biology, prion disease pathogenesis and pharmacologic approaches to treatment. *Clin Lab Med*. 2003;23:1-41.
18. Dyck PJ, Giannini C. Pathologic alterations in the diabetic neuropathies of humans: a review. *N J Neuropathol Exp Neurol*. 1996;55:1181-1193.
19. Eberhart CG, Kepner JL, Goldthwaite PT, et al. Histopathologic grading of medulloblastomas: a Pediatric Oncology Group Study. *Cancer*. 2002;94:552-560.
20. Edgar MA, Rosenblum MK. Mixed glioneuronal tumors. *Arch Pathol Lab Med*. 2007;131:228-233.
21. Franklin RJM, Cotter MR. The biology of CNS remyelination. The key to therapeutic advances. *J Neurol*. 2008;255 Suppl 1:19-25.
22. Furnari FB, Fenton T, Bachoo RM et al. Malignant astrocytic glioma: genetics, biology, and pathways to treatment. *Genes Dev*. 2007;21:2683-2710.
23. Giannini CM, Scheithauer BW, Burger PC, et al. Pleomorphic xanthoastrocytoma: what do we really know about it? *Cancer*. 1999;85:2033-2045.
24. Gleckman A, Evans RJ, Bell MD, et al. Optic nerve damage in shaken baby syndrome: detection by beta-amyloid precursor protein immunohistochemistry. *Arch Pathol Lab Med*. 2000;124:251-256.
25. Graham D, Adams JH, Nicoll JA, et al. The nature, distribution and causes of traumatic brain injury. *Brain Pathol*. 1995;5:397-406.
26. Gray F, Keohane C. The neuropathology of HIV infection in the era of highly active antiretroviral therapy (HAART). *Brain Pathol*. 2003;13;79-83.
27. Gupta M, Djalilvand A, Brat DJ. Clarifying the diffuse gliomas. An update on the morphologic features and markers that discriminate oligodendroglioma from astrocytoma. *Am J Clin Pathol*. 2005;124:755-768.
28. Guzzetta F, Rodriguez J, Deodato M, et al. Demyelinating hereditary neuropathies in children: a morphometric and ultrastructural study. *Histol Histopathol*. 1995;10:91-104.

29. Heffner RR. Inflammatory myopathies. A review. *J Neuropathol Exp Neurol*. 1993;52:339-350.
30. Hirose T, Scheithauer BW, Lopes MB, et al. Tuber and subependymal giant cell astrocytoma associated with tuberous sclerosis: an immunohistochemical, ultrastructural, and immunoelectron and microscopic study. *Acta Neuropathol (Berl)*. 1995;90:287-399.
31. Kalimo H, Ruchoux M-M, Viitanen M, et al. CADASIL: a common form of hereditary arteriopathy causing brain infarcts and dementia. *Brain Pathol*. 2002;12:371-384.
32. Kepes JJ. Large focal tumor-like demyelinating lesions of the brain: intermediate entity between multiple sclerosis and acute disseminated encephalomyelitis? A study of 31 patients. *Ann Neurol*. 1993;33:18-27.
33. Kiechle FL, Kaul KL, Farkas DH. Mitochondrial disorders. Methods and specimen selection for diagnostic molecular pathology. *Arch Pathol Lab Med*. 1996;120:597-603.
34. Kleinschmidt-Demasters BK, Gilden DH. The expanding spectrum of herpesvirus infections of the nervous system. *Brain Pathol*. 2001;11:440-451.
35. Latronico N, Fenzi F, Recupero D, et al. Critical illness myopathy and neuropathy. *Lancet*. 1996;347:1579-1582.
36. Leonard J, Schapira A. Mitochondrial respiratory chain disorders Part I: mitochondrial DNA defects. *Lancet*. 2000; 355: 299-304.
37. Leonard J, Schapira A. Mitochondrial respiratory chain disorders Part II: neurodegenerative disorders and nuclear gene defects. *Lancet*. 2000;355:389-394.
38. Louis DN, Ohgaki H, Wiestler OK, et al, eds. *World Health Organization Classification of Tumours of the Central Nervous System*. Lyon, France: IARC Press; 2007.
39. Ludwin SK. Pathogenesis of multiple sclerosis. *J Neuropathol Exp Neurol*. 2006;65:305-318.
40. Mackenzie IR, Feldman HH. Ubiquitin immunohistochemistry suggests classic motor neuron disease, motor neuron disease with dementia, and frontotemporal dementia of the motor neuron disease type represent a clinicopathologic spectrum. *J Neuropathol Exp Neurol*. 2005;64:730-739.
41. Maritnez AJ, Visvesvara GS. Free-living, amphizoic and opportunistic amebas. *Brain Pathol*. 1997;7:583-598.
42. Matsutani M, Sano K, Takakura K, et al. Primary intracranial germ cell tumors, a clinical analysis of 153 histologically verified cases. *J Neurosurg*. 1997;86:446-455.
43. Mena H, Ribas JL, Pezeshkpou GH, et al. Hemangiopericytoma of the central nervous system: a review of 94 cases. *Hum Pathol*. 1991;22:84-91.
44. Miller CR, Perry A. Glioblastoma. Morphologic and molecular genetic diversity. *Arch Pathol Lab Med*. 2007;131:397-406.
45. Morgello S. Pathogenesis and classification of primary central nervous system lymphoma: an update. *Brain Pathol*. 1995;5:383-393.
46. Mrak RE, Young L. Rabies encephalitis in humans: pathology, pathogenesis and pathophysiology. *J Neuropathol Exp Neurol*. 1994;53:1-10.
47. Packer RJ, Biegel JA, Blaney S, et al. Atypical teratoid/rhabdoid tumor of the central nervous system: report on workshop. *J Pediatr Hematol Oncol*. 2002;24:337-342.
48. Perry A, Aldape KD, George DH, et al. Small cell astrocytoma: an aggressive variant that is clinicopathologically and genetically distinct from anaplastic oligodendroglioma. *Cancer*. 2004;101:2318-2326.
49. Perry A, Scheithauer BW, Nascimento AG. The immunophenotypic spectrum of meningeal hemangiopericytoma: a comparison with fibrous meningioma and solitary fibrous tumor of the meninges. *Am J Surg Pathol*. 1997;21:1354-1360.
50. Perry A, Scheithauer BW, Stafford SL, et al. 'Malignancy' in meningiomas: a clinicopathologic study of 116 patients, with grading implications. *Cancer*. 1999;85:2046-2056.
51. Perry A, Stafford SL, Scheithauer BW, et al. Meningioma grading: an analysis of histologic parameters. *Am J Surg Pathol*. 1997;21:1455-1465.
52. Perry A. Oligodendroglial neoplasms: current concepts, misconceptions, and folklore. *Adv Anat Pathol*. 2001;8: 183-199.
53. Perry AM, Scheithauer BW, Stafford SL, et al. 'Rhabdoid' meningioma: an aggressive variant. *Am J Surg Pathol*. 1998; 22:1482-1490.
54. Pirko I, Lucchinetti CF, Sriram S, et al. Gray matter involvement in multiple sclerosis. *Neurology*. 2007;68:634-642.
55. Prayson RA. Cell proliferation and tumors of the central nervous system, part II: radiolabeling, cytometric, and immunohistochemical techniques. *J Neuropathol Exp Neurol*. 2002;61:663-672.
56. Prayson RA. Skeletal muscle vasculitis exclusive of inflammatory myopathic conditions: a clinicopathologic study of 40 patients. *Hum Pathol*. 2002;33:989-995.
57. Prayson RA (ed.). *Neuropathology. Foundations in Diagnostic Pathology*. 2nd ed. Philadelphia, PA: Elsevier Saunders; 2012.
58. Prayson RA, Suh JH. Subependymomas: clinicopathologic study of 14 tumors, including comparative MIB-1 immunohistochemical analysis with other ependymal neoplasms. *Arch Pathol Lab Med*. 1999;123:306-309.
59. Raben N, Nichols RC, Boerkoel C, et al. Genetic defects in patients with glycogenosis type II (acid maltase deficiency). *Muscle Nerve*. 1995;3:S70-S74.
60. Rhodes RH, Madelaire NC, Petrelli M, et al. Primary angiitis and angiopathy of the central nervous system and their relationship to systemic giant cell arteritis. *Arch Pathol Lab Med*. 1995;119:334-349.
61. Robitaille Y, Lopes-Cendes I, Becher M, et al. The neuropathology of CAG repeat diseases: review and update of genetic and molecular features. *Brain Pathol*. 1997;7:901-926.
62. Ross ME, Walsh CA. Human brain malformations and their lessons for neuronal migration. *Annu Rev Neurosci*. 2001;24: 1041-1070.
63. Schmalbruch H, Haase G. Spinal muscular atrophy: present state. *Brain Pathol*. 2001;11:231-247.
64. Scolding NJ, Joseph F, Kirby PA, et al. Aβ-related angiitis: primary angiitis of the central nervous system associated with cerebral amyloid angiopathy. *Brain*. 2005;128:500-515.
65. Sonneland PRL, Scheithauer BW, Onofrio BM. Myxopapillary ependymoma. A clinicopathologic and immunocytochemical study of 77 cases. *Cancer*. 1985;56:883.
66. Tomita T, Gates E. Pituitary adenomas and granular cell tumors: incidence, cell type, and location of tumor in 1000 pituitary glands at autopsy. *AM J Clin Pathol*. 1999;111: 817-825.

67. Uno K, Takita J, Yokomori K, et al. Aberrations of the hSNF5/INI1 gene are restricted to malignant rhabdoid tumors of atypical teratoid/rhabdoid tumors in pediatric solid tumors. *Genes Chromosomes Cancer.* 2002;34: 33-41.

68. Van den Bent MJ, Kros JM. Predictive and prognostic markers in neuro-oncology. *J Neuropathol Exp Neurol.* 2007;66: 1074-1081.

69. Yachnis AT. Intraoperative consultation for nervous system lesions. *Semin Diagn Pathol.* 2002;19:192-206.

70. Yasargil MG, von Ammon K, von Deimling A, et al. Central neurocytoma: histopathologic variants and therapeutic approaches. *J Neurosurg.* 1992;76:32-37.

71. Yip S, Iafrate AJ, Louis DN. Molecular diagnostic testing in malignant gliomas. *J Neuropathol Exp Neurol.* 2008;67: 1-15.

72. Zorludemir S, Scheithauer BW, Hirose T, et al. Clear cell meningioma: a clinicopathologic study of a potentially aggressive variant of meningioma. *Am J Surg Pathol.* 1995; 19:493-505.

CHAPTER 21

PEDIATRIC AND GENETIC DISORDERS

1. All of the following are true regarding single-nucleotide polymorphisms except
   (A) May be found within either exons or introns
   (B) May serve as a marker that is co-inherited with a disease-associated gene
   (C) Most are associated with gene-coding sequences
   (D) Represent a variation at single nucleotide positions
   (E) They are almost always biallelic

2. What percent of newborn infants are thought to possess a gross chromosomal abnormality?
   (A) 0.02%
   (B) 0.1%
   (C) 1%
   (D) 3%
   (E) 5–7%

3. A 32-year-old man is diagnosed with sickle cell anemia. His condition is caused by which of the following?
   (A) Deletion involving a coding sequence
   (B) Insertion involving a coding sequence
   (C) Point mutation within a coding sequence
   (D) Point mutation within a noncoding sequence
   (E) Trinucleotide repeat mutation

4. Which of the following represents an autosomal-recessive condition?
   (A) Cystic fibrosis
   (B) Huntington disease
   (C) Lesch–Nyhan syndrome
   (D) Polycystic kidney disease
   (E) Wiskott–Aldrich syndrome

5. Which of the following conditions is transmitted by an affected heterozygous female to half her sons and half her daughters and by an affected male patient to all his daughters but none of his sons, if the female parent is unaffected?
   (A) Autosomal dominant
   (B) Autosomal recessive
   (C) X-linked dominant
   (D) X-linked recessive
   (E) None of the above

6. Which of the following conditions is due to missense mutations?
   (A) Beta-thalassemia
   (B) Duchenne muscular dystrophy
   (C) Marfan syndrome
   (D) Tay–Sachs disease
   (E) Vitamin-D-resistant rickets

7. A 16-year-old male presents with bilateral subluxation of the lens. On exam, he is noted to be dolichocephalic with long extremities and long tapering fingers and toes. All of the following are true regarding this patient's condition except
   (A) Associated with kyphosis and scoliosis
   (B) Associated with mitral valve prolapse
   (C) Due to a defect in the synthesis of fibrillar collagen
   (D) May be due to mutations in genes for TGF-beta receptors
   (E) Most are due to mutations on chromosome 15q

8. A 3-year-old patient presents with severe skin fragility, bruising, and cutis laxa. A gene defect in procollagen N-peptidase is discovered. The most accurate diagnosis for the patient is which of the following?
   (A) Ehlers–Danlos type I (classical)
   (B) Ehlers–Danlos type III (hypermobility)
   (C) Ehlers–Danlos type IV (vascular)
   (D) Ehlers–Danlos type VIIa (arthrochalasia)
   (E) Ehlers–Danlos type VIIc (dermatosparaxis)

9. Familial hypercholesterolemia is the result of a mutation in the gene encoding for the receptor for which of the following?
    (A) Apo C
    (B) Apo E
    (C) IDL
    (D) LDL
    (E) VLDL

10. Which of the following is least likely to be associated with familial hypercholesterolemia?
    (A) Acute tubular necrosis in the kidney
    (B) Myocardial infarction
    (C) Peripheral vascular atherosclerosis
    (D) Skin xanthomas
    (E) Stroke

11. Cholesterol is involved with all of the following processes except
    (A) Activates acyl-coenzyme A: cholesterol acyltransferase
    (B) Disrupts coated pit function
    (C) Inhibits 3-hydroxy-3-methylglutaryl coenzyme A reductase
    (D) Suppresses LDL receptor synthesis
    (E) Used for lysosomal membrane synthesis

12. There are 5 classes of LDL receptor mutations that have been described. Those that disrupt transport to the Golgi complex by encoding receptor proteins that accumulate in the endoplasmic reticulum because of folding defects represent which mutation class?
    (A) Class I
    (B) Class II
    (C) Class III
    (D) Class IV
    (E) Class V

13. All of the following represent lysosomal storage diseases except
    (A) Gaucher disease
    (B) Krabbe disease
    (C) McArdle syndrome
    (D) Pompe disease
    (E) Tay–Sachs disease

14. A 3-month-old infant of Ashkenazi Jewish heritage develops motor and mental deterioration and blindness. A cherry-red spot is noted in the right eye. The most likely diagnosis is which of the following?
    (A) Gaucher disease
    (B) Metachromatic leukodystrophy
    (C) Niemann–Pick disease type A
    (D) Pompe disease
    (E) Tay–Sachs disease

15. A bone marrow biopsy was performed in a 28-year-old man and is shown in Figure 21-1. All of the following are true regarding this patient's condition except

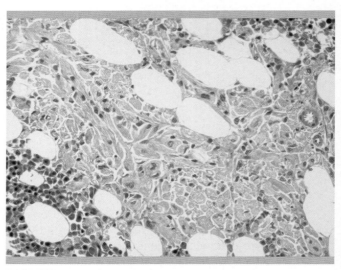

FIGURE 21-1

    (A) Autosomal-dominant disorder.
    (B) Defect in glucocerebrosidase.
    (C) Increased cytokines IL-1 and IL-6 secreted by macrophages.
    (D) Patients often are thrombocytopenic.
    (E) Splenomegaly is a common finding.

16. The muscle biopsy seen in Figure 21-2 in a 42-year-old woman shows scattered fibers with vacuoles filled with PAS-positive material. The vacuoles also show positive staining with acid phosphatase. The best diagnosis for this patient is a deficiency in which of the following?

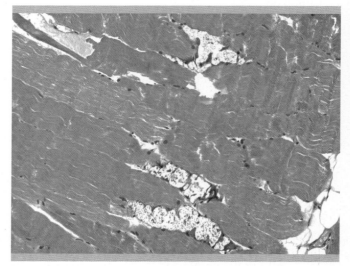

FIGURE 21-2

(A) Acid maltase
(B) Debranching enzyme
(C) Glucose-6-phophatase
(D) Myophosphorylase
(E) Phosphofructokinase

17. A 26-year-old man presents with painful muscle cramps associated with strenuous exercise and myoglobinuria. The patient has an elevated serum creatine level and a normal serum lactate level with exercise. The patient has a deficiency in which of the following?
(A) Acid maltase
(B) Debranching enzyme
(C) Glucose-6-phosphatase
(D) Myophosphorylase
(E) Phosphofructokinase

18. In studying chromosomes by karyotyping, chromosomes are typically examined in which phase?
(A) Anaphase
(B) Interphase
(C) Metaphase
(D) Prophase
(E) Telophase

19. A 2-year-old male has a karyotype performed. The result of his karyotype was 46,XY/47,XY, +21. Which of the following is the best assessment of this child's condition?
(A) Down syndrome
(B) Down syndrome mosaic
(C) Edwards syndrome
(D) Edwards syndrome mosaic
(E) Patau syndrome

20. Which of the following is least likely to be associated with Edwards syndrome?
(A) Cleft lip and palate
(B) Congenital heart defects
(C) Micrognathia
(D) Prominent occiput
(E) Rocker bottom feet

21. All of the following features are commonly encountered in a patient who has a karyotype of 46,XX+13,der (13;14) (q10;q10) except
(A) Microcephaly with mental retardation
(B) Polydactyly
(C) Rocker bottom feet
(D) Simian crease
(E) Umbilical hernia

22. In examining the placenta of a 38-week gestational age newborn, atypical cells are noted in the fetal

circulation as seen in Figure 21-3. You recommend that a bone marrow biopsy be done. Which of the following conditions is the patient most likely to have?

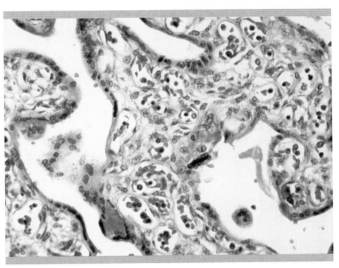

FIGURE 21-3

(A) Klinefelter syndrome
(B) Trisomy 13
(C) Trisomy 18
(D) Trisomy 21
(E) Turner syndrome

23. A 17-year-old male presents with delayed sexual development and a diagnosis of Klinefelter syndrome is being entertained. All of the following are associated with this condition except
(A) Higher risk for breast cancer
(B) Higher risk for coarctation of the aorta
(C) Higher risk for mitral valve prolapse
(D) Higher risk for systemic lupus erythematosus
(E) Higher risk for type 2 diabetes

24. All of the following conditions are examples of trinucleotide repeat disorders except
(A) Fragile-X syndrome
(B) Friedreich ataxia
(C) Huntington disease
(D) Myotonic dystrophy
(E) Spinal muscular atrophy

25. Mitochondrial DNA encodes for enzymes that are involved with oxidative phosphorylation. Which of the following organs is least dependent on oxidative phosphorylation for functioning?
(A) Brain
(B) Cardiac muscle
(C) Liver
(D) Skeletal muscle
(E) Spleen

26. All of the following are true regarding Prader–Willi syndrome except
(A) Chromosome 15 deletion
(B) Hypotonia
(C) Inappropriate laughter
(D) Obesity
(E) Short stature

27. All of the following are indications for prenatal genetic analysis except
(A) Abnormal alpha-fetoprotein (AFP) and estriol levels
(B) Fetus with ultrasound abnormality
(C) Maternal age 37 years
(D) Parent who is a carrier of an autosomal-recessive disorder
(E) Parent who is a carrier of a Robertsonian translocation

28. Postnatal genetic analysis in a patient with multiple congenital anomalies is usually performed on which of the following specimens?
(A) Bone marrow tissue
(B) Peripheral blood lymphocytes
(C) Peripheral blood red cells
(D) Skin
(E) Umbilical cord/placental tissue

29. A sensitivity control is required with which of the following molecular tests?
(A) Chromogenic in situ hybridization
(B) Fluorescence in situ hybridization
(C) Gene rearrangement Southern blots
(D) Quantitative polymerase chain reaction
(E) Sanger DNA sequencing

30. All of the following are acceptable routes for laboratory proficiency testing for molecular assays except
(A) "Chart review" or another clinical correlation with test results
(B) College of American Pathologists program
(C) Performance of at least 100 tests before "going live"
(D) Splitting of samples with another laboratory
(E) Testing of samples against another in-house method

31. All of the following methods of cell lysis in preparing specimens for molecular testing are effective except
(A) Alcohol
(B) Boiling
(C) Chaotropic salt solution
(D) Detergent
(E) Thio reduction

32. Maximal spectrophotometric absorbance for nucleotides occurs at which wavelength
(A) 180 nm
(B) 200 nm
(C) 240 nm
(D) 260 nm
(E) 280 nm

33. Reverse transcription-polymerase chain reaction uses which of the following as starting material for in vitro nucleic acid amplification?
(A) Complementary DNA (cDNA)
(B) Double-stranded DNA
(C) Protein
(D) RNA
(E) Single-stranded DNA

34. All of the following are advantages of real-time polymerase chain reaction (PCR) over conventional PCR except
(A) Ability to perform melting curve analysis
(B) A narrow dynamic range
(C) More reproducible
(D) No need for postamplification processing
(E) Reaction tubes remain closed, decreasing risk of amplicon contamination

35. All of the following are true regarding polymerase chain reaction (PCR) and its diagnostic use except
(A) Limit to the maximum length of the PCR product that can be synthesized
(B) Testing for large chromosomal deletions or additions works well (better than fluorescence in situ hybridization testing)
(C) The DNA target sequence of interest needs to be known
(D) The primer-annealing sequence in the target DNA needs to be conserved among individuals
(E) The primer sequence needs to be unique

36. All of the following tumor suppression gene–syndrome paired matches is correct except
(A) APC–familial adenomatous polyposis
(B) BRCA2–familial breast cancer
(C) DCC–Wilms tumor syndrome
(D) p53–Li–Fraumeni syndrome
(E) PTEN–Cowden syndrome

37. All of the following are potential disadvantages of loss of heterozygosity analysis except
(A) Contaminated tumor samples
(B) Poor markers
(C) Lack of normal comparison sample
(D) Low DNA concentration
(E) Will not work without microdissection

38. All of the following are necessary components of DNA sequencing by the Sanger method except
    (A) Four dNTPs
    (B) One ddNTP
    (C) Primer
    (D) RNA polymerase
    (E) Single-stranded DNA template

39. Fluorescence in situ hybridization may be appropriately used in evaluating for all of the following except
    (A) Deletion of chromosome 1p in oligodendroglioma
    (B) HER2/neu amplification in invasive breast carcinoma
    (C) MGMT promoter methylation in glioblastoma
    (D) t(9;22)(q34;q11) BCR/ABL in chronic myeloid leukemia
    (E) Trisomy 12 in B-cell chronic lymphocytic leukemia

40. Gene rearrangement testing to demonstrate monoclonality is a useful tool in evaluating and diagnosing lymphomas. A number of lymphoid disorders are known to be clonal but not necessarily malignant. All of the following are examples of such lesions except
    (A) Castleman disease
    (B) Idiopathic thrombocytopenic purpura
    (C) Large granular lymphocytosis
    (D) Primary angiitis of the central nervous system
    (E) Refractory sprue

41. The most common cause of death in children in the age group of 4–15 years is which of the following?
    (A) Accidents
    (B) Heart disease
    (C) Homicide
    (D) Malignant neoplasms
    (E) Suicide

42. Which of the following is the most common underlying factor responsible for deformations?
    (A) Abnormal fetal presentation
    (B) Bicornuate uterus
    (C) Multiple fetuses
    (D) Oligohydramnios
    (E) Small uterine size

43. Which of the following is the most common birth defect?
    (A) Anencephaly
    (B) Cleft lip and/or palate
    (C) Gastroschisis
    (D) Tetralogy of Fallot
    (E) Trisomy 13

44. A 6-week-old infant presents with microcephaly, an atrial septal defect, short palpebral fissures, and maxillary hypoplasia. The most likely cause of this constellation of findings is related to maternal use of which of the following?
    (A) 13-cis-retinoic acid
    (B) Alcohol
    (C) Folate antagonist
    (D) Thalidomide
    (E) Warfarin

45. All of the following have been identified as risk factors for preterm premature rupture of placental membranes except
    (A) Maternal smoking
    (B) Poor maternal nutrition
    (C) Preterm vaginal bleeding
    (D) Prior history of preterm labor
    (E) Twins

46. Prematurity is associated with an increased risk for the development of all of the following conditions except
    (A) Germinal matrix hemorrhage
    (B) Hyaline membrane disease
    (C) Necrotizing enterocolitis
    (D) Omphalocele
    (E) Sepsis

47. All of the following play a role in the development of neonatal respiratory distress syndrome except
    (A) Acidosis
    (B) Atelectasis
    (C) Decreased alveolar surfactant
    (D) Hyaline membranes
    (E) Pulmonary vasodilation

48. The image shown here (Figure 21-4) is from a 39-week gestational age infant who developed neonatal respiratory distress syndrome requiring oxygen therapy for 2 months. A diagnosis of bronchopulmonary dysplasia is made. All of the following factors contribute to the development of this disorder except

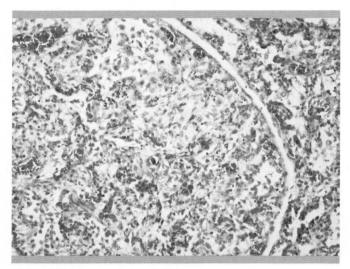

FIGURE 21-4

(A) Decreased interleukin-6
(B) Hyperoxemia
(C) Hyperventilation
(D) Increased tumor necrosis factor
(E) Inflammatory cytokines

49. A newborn, full-term infant is diagnosed with hydrops fetalis. A histologic section from the placenta is illustrated in Figure 21-5. The presence of increased nucleated red blood cells in the fetal circulation is consistent with all of the following etiologies except

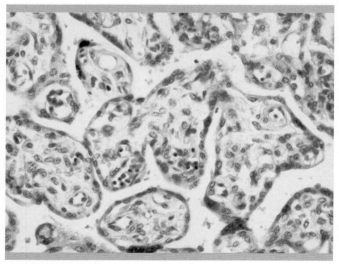

FIGURE 21-5

(A) ABO incompatibility
(B) Homozygous alpha-thalassemia
(C) Parvovirus B19 infection
(D) Rh incompatibility
(E) Trisomy 21

50. All of the following findings are expected in a patient with phenylketonuria except
(A) Deficiency in phenylalanine hydroxylase
(B) Lens defects in the eyes
(C) Mental retardation
(D) Musty smelling sweat
(E) Seizures

51. The abnormality shown in this lung section from a 7-year-old patient in Figure 21-6 may be accompanied by all of the following findings elsewhere in the body except

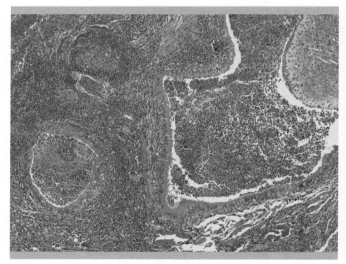

FIGURE 21-6

(A) Hepatic cirrhosis
(B) Kernicterus
(C) Male infertility
(D) Pancreatic insufficiency
(E) Steatorrhea

52. The gene for cystic fibrosis (cystic fibrosis transmembrane conductance regulator gene) has been localized to which of the following chromosomes?
(A) Chromosome 1
(B) Chromosome 7
(C) Chromosome 17
(D) Chromosome X
(E) Chromosome Y

53. All of the following are parental risk factors associated with sudden infant death syndrome except
    (A) Long intergestational intervals
    (B) Maternal age 15 years
    (C) Maternal opiate use
    (D) Maternal smoking
    (E) No prenatal care

54. Which of the following is the most common autopsy finding in infants who have died of sudden infant death syndrome (SIDS)?
    (A) Frontal lobe gliosis
    (B) Increased brown fat
    (C) Persistent extramedullary hematopoiesis
    (D) Petechiae
    (E) Pulmonary edema

55. Which of the following is the most common tumor of infancy?
    (A) Fibroma
    (B) Hemangioma
    (C) Leiomyoma
    (D) Lymphangioma
    (E) Teratoma

56. Which of the following malignant tumors of childhood is the most common tumor in children less than 10 years of age?
    (A) Ependymoma
    (B) Hepatocellular carcinoma
    (C) Leukemia
    (D) Neuroblastoma
    (E) Rhabdomyosarcoma

57. All of the following are favorable prognostic features in the adrenal tumor shown in Figure 21-7 except

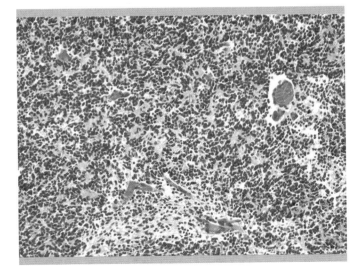

FIGURE 21-7

    (A) Absent chromosome 1p loss
    (B) Age <18 months
    (C) Gangliocytic differentiation
    (D) Hyperdiploid
    (E) N-MYC amplified

58. A 3-year-old male is diagnosed with a neuroblastoma. The tumor is localized. Ipsilateral nonadherent lymph nodes are positive for tumor. Three enlarged contralateral lymph nodes are sampled and are all found to be negative for tumor. Using the International Neuroblastoma Staging System, the tumor is which stage?
    (A) Stage 1
    (B) Stage 2
    (C) Stage 3
    (D) Stage 4
    (E) Stage 4S

59. A 6-year-old patient is diagnosed with Denys–Drash syndrome. The patient is at increased risk of developing which of the following tumors?
    (A) Ewing sarcoma
    (B) Neuroblastoma
    (C) Pheochromocytoma
    (D) Retinoblastoma
    (E) Wilms tumor

60. All of the following are true regarding anaplastic Wilms tumors except
    (A) Accounts for almost all cases of bilateral Wilms tumors
    (B) Associated with p53 mutations
    (C) Associated with resistance to chemotherapy
    (D) Comprises about 5% of Wilms tumor
    (E) Defined by cells with large pleomorphic nuclei

61. All of the following are characteristic features of eosinophilic esophagitis except
    (A) At least 10 eosinophils per high-power field
    (B) Dysphagia or food impaction
    (C) History of atopic disease
    (D) No response to a high-dose proton pump inhibition
    (E) Normal results on pH monitoring of the distal esophagus

62. Which of the following antibodies is most useful in the evaluation of biopsies in Hirschsprung disease?
    (A) Calretinin
    (B) Glial fibrillary acidic protein
    (C) Neu N
    (D) Neuron-specific enolase
    (E) Synaptophysin

63. Which of the following antibodies may be most useful in distinguishing a complete hydatidiform mole from a partial hydatidiform mole?
    (A) Beta-HCG
    (B) Calretinin
    (C) Cytokeratin 5/6
    (D) p57 (KIP 2)
    (E) p63

64. Fetal thrombotic vasculopathy is a placental lesion characterized by regionally distributed avascular villi and is often accompanied by upstream thrombosis in placental fetal vessels. Which of the following is generally not associated with this placental finding?
    (A) Preeclampsia
    (B) Fetal cardiac abnormalities
    (C) Intrauterine growth restriction
    (D) Oligohydramnios
    (E) Stillbirth

65. Abnormalities of which of the following neurotransmitters have been recognized in the medulla oblongata in patients with sudden infant death syndrome?
    (A) Acetylcholine
    (B) Dopamine
    (C) Epinephrine
    (D) GABAA
    (E) Serotonin

ANSWERS

1. **(C) Most are associated with gene-coding sequences.**
   Single-nucleotide polymorphisms represent variations at single isolated nucleotide positions and are almost always biallelic. Over 6 million single-nucleotide polymorphisms have been identified in the human population, many of which show a wide variation in frequency in different populations. These polymorphisms may occur anywhere in the genome, that is, within exons, introns, or intergenic regions, with less than 1% of them occurring in coding regions. They also serve as markers that may be co-inherited with a disease-associated gene, due to their physical proximity to the gene. In contrast, copy number variations consist of different numbers of large contiguous stretches of DNA. Approximately half of copy number variations involve gene-coding sequences.

2. **(C) 1%.**
   Approximately 1% of all newborn infants possess a gross chromosomal abnormality, and approximately 5% of individuals under age 25 years develop a serious disease with a significant genetic component. Approximately half of spontaneous abortuses

during early months of gestation have a demonstrable chromosomal abnormality.

3. **(C) Point mutation within a coding sequence.**
   Sickle cell disease represents a disorder in which a point mutation occurs within a coding sequence. In sickle cell anemia, the nucleotide triplet CTC, which encodes glutamic acid, is changed to a CAC, which encodes for valine.

4. **(A) Cystic fibrosis.**
   Of the conditions listed as options for this question, cystic fibrosis is the only one that represents an autosomal-recessive condition. Polycystic kidney disease and Huntington disease represent autosomal-dominant disorders. Wiskott–Aldrich syndrome and Lesch–Nyhan syndrome represent X-linked-recessive disorders.

5. **(C) X-linked dominant.**
   X-linked-dominant conditions are relatively rare disorders that are caused by dominant disease-associated alleles on the X chromosome. These disorders are transmitted by an affected heterozygous female to half her sons and half her daughters and by an affected male parent to all his daughters but none of his sons. Vitamin D-resistant rickets represents an example of a disease with this type of inheritance pattern.

6. **(C) Marfan syndrome.**
   Of the conditions listed as options for this question, Marfan syndrome results from missense mutations. Tay–Sachs disease may result from splice-site mutations or frame shift mutations with stop codon. Vitamin D-resistant rickets may result from point mutations, resulting in a failure of normal signaling. Duchenne muscular dystrophy results from an abnormality in the dystrophin gene, resulting in its deletion with complete absence or markedly reduced synthesis of the protein. Beta-thalassemia may result from defective mRNA processing, resulting in a reduced amount of hemoglobin.

7. **(C) Due to a defect in the synthesis of fibrillar collagen.**
   The clinical features described in the presentation of this patient are suggestive of Marfan syndrome. Marfan syndrome results from an inherited defect in extracellular glycoprotein fibrillin-1, the gene for which is located on chromosome 15q. In a small number of patients with clinical features of Marfan syndrome, mutations in genes that encode TGF-beta receptors have been described. In addition to the features listed in the clinical presentation, patients with Marfan syndrome may have a variety of spinal deformities including kyphosis, scoliosis, rotation of the dorsal or lumbar vertebrae, pectus excavatum, ocular changes including bilateral subluxation or

dislocation of the lens (ectopia lentis), mitral valve prolapse, dilatation of the ascending aorta and aortic valve incompetence. Ehlers–Danlos syndrome is associated with a defect in the synthesis or structure of fibrillar collagen.

8. **(E) Ehlers–Danlos type VIIc (dermatosparaxis).**
The clinical features of the patient presented in this question and a documented gene defect in procollagen N-peptidase are consistent with a diagnosis of Ehlers–Danlos type VIIc. This condition is inherited as an autosomal-recessive type. The other major autosomal-recessive type is type VI (kyphoscoliosis), which is marked by hypertonia, joint laxity, ocular fragility, and congenital scoliosis. The other types listed as options in this question are inherited as autosomal-dominant conditions and are variously marked by skin and joint abnormalities.

9. **(D) LDL.**
Familial hypercholesterolemia is the result of a mutation in the gene encoding the receptor for low-density lipoprotein (LDL), which is involved in the transport and metabolism of cholesterol.

10. **(A) Acute tubular necrosis in the kidney.**
Patients with familial hypercholesterolemia have an increased risk of developing tendinous xanthomas, skin xanthomas, vascular atherosclerosis involving coronary cerebral and peripheral blood vessels, myocardial infarction, and cerebral infarction or stroke. Acute tubular necrosis in the kidney is least likely to be seen in association with familial hypercholesterolemia.

11. **(B) Disrupts coated pit function.**
All of the options listed as answers to this question are functions of cholesterol except Answer B. Coated pits are involved with the binding of LDL to cell surface receptors, particularly in the liver. These receptors are clustered in specialized regions of the plasma membrane, referred to as coated pits. Cholesterol is generally not thought to cause disruption of these pits.

12. **(B) Class II.**
One classification of LDL receptor mutations is based on various abnormal functions of the mutant protein. Those that involve disruption of the transport to the Golgi complex by encoding receptor proteins that accumulate in the endoplasmic reticulum because of folding defects represent mutation class II lesions. Class I mutations disrupt receptor synthesis in the endoplasmic reticulum. Mutation class III lesions disrupt binding of LDL protein ligands. Class IV mutations disrupt clustering in coated pits. Class V mutations disrupt recycling in endosomes.

13. **(C) McArdle syndrome.**
All of the conditions listed as options to this question represent lysosomal storage diseases except McArdle syndrome. McArdle syndrome represents type V glycogenosis and is due to a defect in muscle myophosphorylase.

14. **(E) Tay–Sachs disease.**
The clinical presentation of this patient is most consistent with that of Tay–Sachs disease, a lysosomal storage disease that belongs to the sphingolipidoses group. The abnormality is due to an enzyme deficiency in hexosaminidase alpha-subunit, resulting in an accumulation of ganglioside material. Pompe disease results in accumulation of glycogen material. Metachromatic leukodystrophy results in an accumulation of sulfatide material. Niemann–Pick disease represents a sulfatidosis, which results in an accumulation of sphingomyelin. Gaucher disease is also a member of the sulfatidosis group and results in an accumulation of glucocerebroside.

15. **(A) Autosomal-dominant disorder.**
The bone marrow biopsy shown here is marked by the presence of macrophages filled with glucocerebroside material, which has an appearance resembling "crumpled tissue paper." This finding is suggestive of Gaucher disease. All of the options listed as answers to this question are associated with Gaucher disease except Answer A; Gaucher disease is an autosomal-recessive disorder.

16. **(A) Acid maltase.**
The muscle biopsy shown here shows scattered fibers with large vacuoles. Vacuoles filled with PAS-positive material and associated with acid phosphatase (a lysosomal enzyme) are suggestive of acid maltase deficiency or Pompe disease. None of the other glycogen pathway-associated enzyme deficiencies is associated with acid phosphatase staining.

17. **(D) Myophosphorylase.**
The clinical history given in this patient is suggestive of McArdle disease or myophosphorylase deficiency. On biopsy, glycogen accumulation may be frequently seen in scattered muscle fibers, particularly in the subsarcolemmal region.

18. **(C) Metaphase.**
In a routine chromosome karyotype, chromosomes are usually examined in arrested, dividing cells in a metaphase with mitotic spindle inhibitors.

19. **(B) Down syndrome mosaic.**
The karyotype indicates a mixed population of cells with normal 46XY and a population of cells with trisomy 21, consistent with a Down syndrome mosaic. Edwards syndrome represents trisomy 18, and Patau syndrome represents trisomy 13.

20. **(A) Cleft lip and palate.**
Cleft lip and palate is a more common feature encountered in the setting Patau syndrome. All of the other features listed here are found in Edwards syndrome. Additionally, patients with Edwards syndrome may demonstrate mental retardation, low set ears, a short neck, overlapping fingers, renal malformations, and limited hip abduction.

21. **(D) Simian crease.**
The karyotype represents the translocation type of Patau syndrome. All of the features listed here are typical of Patau syndrome except simian creases, which are more classically a feature of Down syndrome. Additionally, patients with Patau syndrome may demonstrate microphthalmia, cleft lip and palate, renal defects, and cardiac defects.

22. **(D) Trisomy 21.**
Careful examination of the placental section shows atypical cells located within fetal blood vessels in the placental villi. These cells, in the congenital setting, most likely represent a possible fetal leukemia, which would warrant a bone marrow biopsy to confirm the diagnosis. There is a well-known association of congenital leukemia with trisomy 21.

23. **(B) Higher risk for coarctation of the aorta.**
All of the options listed here are associated with Klinefelter syndrome, except a higher risk of coarctation of the aorta. Coarctation of the aorta is more typically associated with Turner syndrome. Patients with Klinefelter syndrome are characterized by having 2 or more X chromosomes and 1 or more Y chromosome(s).

24. **(E) Spinal muscular atrophy.**
Spinal muscular atrophy represents an autosomal-recessive condition. Spinal muscular atrophy is usually not associated with a trinucleotide repeat abnormality. All of the other conditions listed as answer options in this question are well-known trinucleotide repeat disorders.

25. **(E) Spleen.**
Mitochondrial DNA mutations typically impact oxidative phosphorylation activity in cells. Of the organs listed as options to this question, the spleen has the least demand for oxidative phosphorylation functioning.

26. **(C) Inappropriate laughter.**
Prader–Willi syndrome is characterized by mental retardation, hypotonia, short stature, hyperphagia, obesity, hypogonadism, and small hands and feet. Most cases are the result of a deletion on chromosome 15. A presentation of inappropriate laughter is more commonly seen in patients with Angelman syndrome, which may also result from abnormalities on chromosome 15.

27. **(D) Parent who is a carrier of an autosomal-recessive disorder.**
There are a variety of indications for prenatal genetic testing or analysis. Among these indications are increased maternal age of over 35 years (due to increased risk of trisomies); a parent who is the carrier of a balanced reciprocal translocation; Robertsonian translocation or inversion and fetus with ultrasound-detected abnormalities; a parent with a previous child with a chromosome abnormality; a parent who is a carrier of an X-linked genetic disorder, or abnormal levels AFP, beta-HCG, or estriol performed as part of the triple test.

28. **(B) Peripheral blood lymphocytes.**
Postnatal genetic analysis or testing in patients with multiple congenital anomalies can often be performed using peripheral blood lymphocytes.

29. **(C) Gene rearrangement Southern blots.**
A sensitivity control is required in performing gene rearrangement Southern blots.

30. **(C) Performance of at least 100 tests before "going live."**
In establishing proficiency training for molecular assays in the laboratory, a number of acceptable routes may be utilized. If a formal College of American Pathologists (CAP) program is available for the analyte of interest, that can be used. An alternative proficiency testing provider program can also be employed. When such proficiency testing programs are not available, splitting of samples with another laboratory, testing of samples against another in-house method, or correlation of test results with chart review and clinical information can be utilized.

31. **(A) Alcohol.**
A variety of methods can be used to facilitate cell lysis. Chemical disruption using detergents, chaotropic salt solutions, thio reduction, or enzymatic digestion, and mechanical disruption (boiling, sonication, or homogenization) can be utilized. Alcohol is not typically used for this purpose.

32. **(D) 260 nm.**
Maximal spectrophotometric absorbance for nucleotides occurs at a wavelength of 260 nm. Protein absorption is maximal at 280 nm.

33. **(D) RNA.**
Reverse transcription-polymerase chain reaction uses RNA as a starting material for in vitro nucleic acid amplification. Reverse transcriptase enzyme is used to catalyze DNA synthesis, using RNA as the template.

34. **(B) A narrow dynamic range.**
There are a variety of advantages of real-time PCR versus conventional PCR. All of the options listed as answers to this question are advantages to real-time PCR with the exception of option B. Real-time PCR methods have a wide dynamic range, as-high-as 10 logs.

35. **(B) Testing for large chromosomal deletions or addition works well (better than fluorescence in situ hybridization testing).**
All of the options listed as answers to this question are true regarding polymerase chain reaction except option B. When testing for large chromosomal deletions or additions, fluorescence in situ hybridization testing is often a better methodology to employ.

36. **(C) DCC–Wilms tumor syndrome.**
All of the listed tumor suppressor gene–syndrome paired matches are correct except option C. The DCC tumor suppressor gene is associated with colon cancer. Wilms tumor syndrome is associated with the WT1 tumor suppressor gene.

37. **(E) Will not work without microdissection.**
All of the following options listed as answers to this question are potential disadvantages of a loss of heterozygosity analysis except option E. As long as there is an adequate amount of abnormal tissue present in the sample provided for testing, there is no need to microdissect tumor cells from contaminant normal tissues.

38. **(D) RNA polymerase.**
All of the following components listed as options for this question are required for DNA sequencing by the Sanger method except RNA polymerase; a DNA polymerase is required instead.

39. **(C) MGMT promoter methylation in glioblastoma.**
Fluorescence in situ hybridization testing in routine clinical practice can be used to identify several types of genetic abnormalities including genomic gains at specific loci or for entire chromosomes, gene amplification, loss of specific loci or entire chromosomes, and the presence of translocations. All of the examples listed as options for this question represent appropriate uses for this methodology except MGMT promoter methylation in glioblastoma, which is better accomplished by a polymerase chain-reaction methodology.

40. **(D) Primary angiitis of the central nervous system.**
There are a variety of lymphoid disorders that may be clonal but not necessarily malignant. All of the conditions listed as options to this question represent such entities, except primary angiitis of the central nervous system. Additional lesions that fit this profile include myoepithelial sialadenitis; immunodeficiency-related lymphoproliferations; monoclonal gammopathy of undetermined significance; clonal lymphocytosis of undetermined significance; viremia due to viruses such as cytomegalovirus or Epstein–Barr virus; and certain dermatologic lesions, such as lymphomatoid papulosis, parapsoriasis, vulvar lichen sclerosis, and pityriasis lichenoides varioliformis acuta.

41. **(A) Accidents.**
The most common cause of death in children in the age group of 4–15 years is accidents and adverse effects related to accidents. This was also the leading cause of death in the age group of 1–4 years and 15–24 years. In children under 1 year of age, congenital malformations, deformations, and chromosomal anomalies are the most common cause of death.

42. **(E) Small uterine size.**
The most common underlying factor responsible for deformations is uterine constraint related to small size. All of the other factors may also result in disruptions in development causing deformations, but are less common.

43. **(B) Cleft lip and/or palate.**
Of the birth defects listed as options in this question, cleft lip and/or palate is the most commonly encountered group with a national prevalence of approximately 10.5 per 10,000 live births in the United States.

44. **(B) Alcohol.**
The clinical presentation described in this infant is most consistent with fetal alcohol spectrum disorder. All of the other drugs listed as optional answers here are potentially teratogenic as well.

45. **(E) Twins.**
Approximately 3% of all pregnancies are complicated by preterm premature rupture of placental membranes. All of the conditions listed as optional answers to this question represent identified risk factors for preterm premature rupture of placental membranes except twins. Other risk factors include a prior history of preterm delivery, preterm labor, and low socioeconomic status.

46. **(D) Omphalocele.**
All of the listed options to this question represent conditions that may result from prematurity, except omphalocele, which represents a musculoskeletal birth defect.

47. **(E) Pulmonary vasodilation.**
All of the answers listed as options represent components involved in the development of neonatal respiratory distress syndrome, except pulmonary vasodilation. Acidosis resulting from

hypoxemia and carbon dioxide retention usually results in pulmonary vasoconstriction and pulmonary hypoperfusion, in this clinical setting

48. **(A) Decreased interleukin-6.**
The picture shown here represents bronchopulmonary dysplasia, which is morphologically marked by airway epithelial hyperplasia and squamous metaplasia, alveolar thickening, and peribronchial and interstitial fibrosis. Dysmorphic capillary configurations and a decrease in alveolar septation may be also present. A variety of factors may promote injury in the setting of bronchopulmonary dysplasia. All of the answers listed as options here function in this capacity except decreased interleukin-6; often in this setting, interleukin-6 levels are elevated.

49. **(E) Trisomy 21.**
The presence of prominent number of nucleated red blood cells in the fetal circulation in a full-term placenta is abnormal and suggests an anemic condition. All of the options listed as answers to this question are potential causes of nonimmune fetal hydrops and may cause persistence of nucleated red blood cells in the fetal circulation except trisomy 21.

50. **(B) Lens defects in the eyes.**
Phenylketonuria is due to an abnormality in phenylalanine metabolism, resulting in hyperphenylalaninemia. The condition is inherited in an autosomal-recessive fashion, with the majority of cases caused by biallelic mutations of the gene encoding for phenylalanine hydroxylase. The patients may present with musty smelling sweat, mental retardation, and seizures. Decreased pigmentation of hair and skin and eczema may also develop. Lens defects in the eyes are typically not associated with this condition.

51. **(B) Kernicterus.**
The section of lung shown here shows markedly distended airways, and filled with mucus and inflammatory material. These findings in a child are suggestive of cystic fibrosis. All of the options listed as potential answers to this question are associated with cystic fibrosis, with the exception of kernicterus.

52. **(B) Chromosome 7.**
The gene for cystic fibrosis has been localized to chromosome 7q31.2.

53. **(A) Long intergestational intervals.**
The parental risk factors associated with the development of sudden infant death syndrome include young maternal age of less that 20 years, maternal smoking during pregnancy, drug abuse in either parent, short intergestational intervals, minimal or no prenatal care, and socioeconomic factors.

54. **(D) Petechiae.**
The most common finding, in approximately 80% of cases of sudden infant death syndrome-related deaths, is multiple petechiae, usually present on the visceral and parietal pleura and epicardium. Additional frequent findings include vascular congestion and edema in the lungs, evidence of infection in the upper respiratory system, gliosis in the brain stem and cerebellum, hypoplasia of the arcuate nucleus and certain brain stem neuronal populations, persistent hepatic extramedullary hematopoiesis, and a persistent periadrenal brown fat.

55. **(B) Hemangioma.**
Hemangiomas represent the most common tumors of infancy. The majority of these in children are located in the skin, particularly in the face and scalp region.

56. **(C) Leukemia.**
In a child less than 10 years of age, the most common malignant neoplasm is leukemia.

57. **(E) N-MYC amplified.**
The lesion shown here represents a neuroblastoma, arising in the adrenal gland region. Favorable prognostic factors in neuroblastomas include low stage of tumor (stages 1, 2A, 2B, and 4S are favorable), age less than 18 months, schwannian stroma and gangliocytic differentiation, a low mitosis-karyorrhexis index, hyperdiploidy or near triploidy, absence of N-MYC amplification, low or absent telomerase, and low or absent telomerase expression. TRKA expression, if present, is considered favorable in some studies. An absence of TRKB expression is also considered a favorable prognostic finding.

58. **(B) Stage 2.**
Findings described in this case are consistent with a stage 2 neoplasm. In the setting of an ipsilateral nonadherent lymph node negative for tumor microscopically, a designation of stage 2a is used. In the current case where the ipsilateral nonadherent lymph nodes are positive for tumor, a designation of stage 2b is used.

59. **(E) Wilms tumor.**
Patients with Denys–Drash syndrome have a higher risk of developing Wilms tumor. This syndrome is characterized by gonadal dysgenesis and early onset nephropathy, leading to renal failure. The glomerular lesions in these patients are marked by diffuse mesangial sclerosis.

60. **(A) Accounts for almost all cases of bilateral Wilms tumors.**
All of the answers provided as options to this question are true regarding anaplastic Wilms tumors, except option A. A strong association of the anaplastic Wilms tumor phenotype with bilaterality is

not well documented. Approximately 10% of all Wilms tumors may be bilateral or multicentric at the time of diagnosis.

61. **(A) At least 10 eosinophils per high-power field.**
Although eosinophilic esophagitis predominantly affects males in the age group of 20–40 years, cases in women and in younger patients also have been reported. In one study involving children, the incidence was estimated at 10 per 1,00000 children per year. Up to 80% of patients with eosinophilic esophagitis have a history of atopic disease, such as asthma, allergies to food or medicine, or allergic rhinitis. Up to half of patients have a peripheral eosinophilia. In children, presenting symptoms vary with age and may include feeding disorders, vomiting, abdominal pain, dysphagia, and food impaction. On biopsy, at least 15 eosinophils per high-power field need to be seen. Frequently, basal zone hyperplasia, edema, and papillary elongation are also present. Patients do not respond to high-dose proton pump inhibiters and demonstrate normal results on pH monitoring of the distal esophagus.

62. **(A) Calretinin.**
A number of recent studies have shown calretinin to be a useful antibody in evaluating biopsies taken in patients suspected to have Hirschsprung disease. An absence of staining supports the diagnosis. False positive rates are negligible. Staining with calretinin appears to be more useful than traditional acetylcholinesterase histochemistry.

63. **(D) p57 (KIP2).**
Traditionally, DNA ploidy studies have been used to help differentiate a triploid partial mole from a diploid complete mole. The p57 gene is strongly paternally imprinted and expressed from the maternal allele. Because complete moles lack a maternal genome, p57 immunostaining is absent, whereas hydropic abortuses and partial moles show positive staining.

64. **(A) Preeclampsia.**
Fetal thrombotic vasculopathy is a placental lesion characterized by regionally distributed avascular villi. The abnormalities are often accompanied by upstream thrombosis of placental fetal vessels. A recent study showed an increased incidence of stillbirths, intrauterine growth restriction, oligohydramnios, and fetal cardiac abnormalities in cases where fetal thrombotic vasculopathy was identified in the placenta. The study did not show a significant increase in pregnancy-induced hypertension or preeclampsia, when adjusted for maternal and gestational age.

65. **(E) Serotonin.**
A number of recent studies have shown an association of sudden infant death syndrome with abnormalities related to the neurotransmitter serotonin in the medulla oblongata. Serotonin neurons in the medulla play a role in the regulation of multiple aspects of respiratory and autonomic function. Subsets of infants with sudden infant death syndrome have abnormalities in medullary markers for serotonin function.

SUGGESTED READING

1. Abrams ME, Meredith KS, Kinnard P, et al. Hydrops fetalis: a retrospective review of cases reported to a large national database and identification of risk factors associated with death. *Pediatrics*. 2007;120:84-89.
2. Al-Adnani M, Williams S, Rampling D, et al. Histopathological reporting of pediatric cutaneous vascular anomalies in relation to proposed multidisciplinary classification system. *J Clin Pathol*. 2006;49:1278-1282.
3. American Academy of Pediatrics Task Force on Sudden Infant Death Syndrome. The changing concepts of sudden infant death syndrome: diagnostic coding shifts, controversies regarding the sleeping environment, and new variables to consider in reducing risk. *Pediatrics*. 2005;116:1245-1256.
4. Bancalari E, Claure N. Definitions and diagnostic criteria for bronchopulmonary dysplasia. *Semin Perinatol*. 2006;30:164-170.
5. Bojesen A, Gravholt CH. Klinefelter syndrome in clinical practice. *Nat Clin Pract Urol*. 2007;4:192-204.
6. Chen C, Visootsak J, Dills S, et al. Prader-Willi syndrome: an update and review for the primary pediatrician. *Clin Pediatr*. 2007;46:580-591.
7. Chess PR, D'Angio CT, Pryhuber GS, et al. Pathogenesis of bronchopulmonary dysplasia. *Semin Perinatol*. 2006;30:171-178.
8. Dome JS, Cotton CA, Perlman EJ, et al. Treatment of anaplastic histology Wilms Tumor: results from the fifth National Wilms Tumor Study. *J Clin Oncol*. 2006;24:2352-2358.
9. Esteller M. Epigenetics and cancer. *N Engl J Med*. 2008;358:1148-1159.
10. Furuta GT, Liacouras CA, Collins MH, et al. Eosinophilic esophagitis in children and adults: a systematic review and consensus recommendations for diagnosis and treatment. *Gastroenterology*. 2007;133:1342-1363.
11. Hjerrild BE, Mortensen KH, Gravholt CH. Turner syndrome and clinical treatment. *Br Med Bull*. 2008;86:77-93.
12. Hoot AC, Russo P, Judkins AR, et al. Immunohistochemical analysis of hSNF5/INI1 distinguishes renal and extrarenal malignant rhabdoid tumors from other pediatric soft tissue tumors. *Am J Surg Pathol*. 2004;28:1485-1491.
13. Kaplan CG. Fetal and maternal vascular lesions. *Semin Diagn Pathol*. 2007;24:14-22.
14. Kapur RP, Reed RC, Finn LS, et al. Calretinin immunohistochemistry versus acetylcholinesterase histochemistry in the evaluation of suction rectal biopsies for Hirschsprung disease. *Pediatr Dev Pathol*. 2009;12:6-15.
15. Kinney HC, Richerson GB, Dymecki SM, et al. The brainstem and serotonin in the sudden infant death syndrome. *Annu Rev Pathol*. 2009;4:517-550.

16. Kumar V, Abbas AK, Fausto N, Aster JC (eds.). Genetic disorders. In: *Robbins and Cotran Pathologic Basis of Disease.* 8th ed. Philadelphia, PA: Saunders Elsevier; 2010:135-182.

17. Langston C, Patterson K, Dishop MK, et al. A protocol for the handling of tissue obtained by operative lung biopsy: recommendations of the chILD pathology co-operative group. *Pediatr Dev Pathol.* 2006;9:173-180.

18. Lutz RE. Trinucleotide repeat disorders. *Semin Pediatr Neurol.* 2007;14:26-33.

19. Maitra A. Diseases of infancy and childhood. In: Kumar V, Abbas AK, Fausto N, Aster JC, eds. *Robbins and Cotran Pathologic Basis of Disease.* 8th ed. Philadelphia, PA: Saunders Elsevier; 2010:447-483.

20. Mao JR, Bristow J. The Ehlers-Danlos syndrome: on beyond collagens. *J Clin Invest.* 2001;107:1062-1069.

21. Maris JM, Hogarty MD, Bagatell R, et al. Neuroblastoma. *Lancet* 2007;369:2106-2120.

22. Miura K, Yoshiura K, Miura S, et al. Clinical outcome of infants with confined placental mosaicism and intrauterine growth restriction of unknown cause. *Am J Med Genet A.* 2006;140A:1827-1833.

23. Moon RY, Horne RS, Hauck FR. Sudden infant death syndrome. *Lancet.* 2007;370:1578-1587.

24. Nesin M. Genetic basis of preterm birth. *Front Biosci.* 2007; 12:115-124.

25. Nonevski IT, Downs-Kelly E, Falk GW. Eosinophilic esophagitis: an increasingly recognized cause of dysplasia, food impaction, and refractory heartburn. *Cleve Clin J Med.* 2008; 75:623-633.

26. Perlman EJ. Pediatric renal tumors: practical updates for the pathologist. *Pediatr Dev Pathol.* 2005;8:320-328.

27. Ramirez F, Dietz HC. Marfan syndrome: from molecular pathogenesis to clinical treatment. *Curr Opin Genet Dev.* 2007; 17:252-258.

28. Ramphal R, Pappo A, Zielendska M, et al. Pediatric renal cell carcinoma: clinical, pathologic, and molecular abnormalities associated with the members of the mit transcription factor family. *Am J Vlin Pathol.* 2006;126: 349-364.

29. Redline RW. Disorders of placental circulation and the fetal brain. *Clin Perinatol.* 2009;36:549-559.

30. Redline RW. Villitis of unknown etiology: noninfectious chronic villitis in the placenta. *Hum Pathol.* 2007;36: 1439-1446.

31. Roizen NJ, Patterson D. Down's syndrome. *Lancet.* 2003; 361:1281-1289.

32. Saleemuddin A, Tantbirojn P, Sirois K, et al. Obstetric and perinatal complications in placentas with fetal thrombotic vasculopathy. *Pediatr Dev Pathol.* 2010;13:459-464.

33. Schapira AH. Mitochondrial disease. *Lancet.* 2006;368: 70-82.

34. Scriver CR. The PAH gene, phenylketonuria, and a paradigm shift. *Hum Mutat.* 2007;28:831-845.

35. Sebire NJ, Lindsay I. p57KIP2 immunostaining in the diagnosis of complete versus partial hydatidiform moles. *Histopathology.* 2006;48:873-874.

36. Shin YS. Glycogen storage disease: clinical biochemical, and molecular heterogeneity. *Semin Pediatr Neurol.* 2006;13: 115-120.

37. Tubbs RR, Stoler MH (eds.). *Cell and Tissue Based Molecular Pathology.* Philadelphia, PA: Churchill Livingstone Elsevier; 2009.

CHAPTER 22

PULMONARY AND MEDIASTINAL PATHOLOGY

1. All the following are examples of processes that diffusely involve the lung airspaces, except
   (A) Eosinophilic pneumonia
   (B) *Pneumocystis jiroveci* pneumonia
   (C) Pulmonary alveolar proteinosis
   (D) Pulmonary hemorrhage
   (E) Sarcoidosis

2. Which of the following structures, depicted in Figure 22-1, is commonly found in the sinusoidal spaces of peribronchial and mediastinal lymph nodes involved by sarcoidosis?

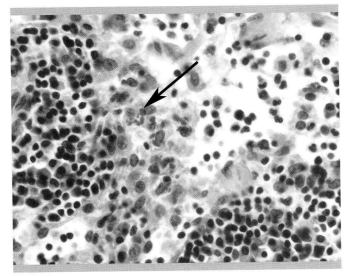

FIGURE 22-1

   (A) Blastomyces
   (B) Corpora amylacea
   (C) Hamazaki-Wesenberg bodies
   (D) Hemosiderin granules
   (E) Histoplasma organisms

3. A specimen from a patient who died of septicemia is shown here. The approximate age of the form of lung injury depicted in Figure 22-2 is

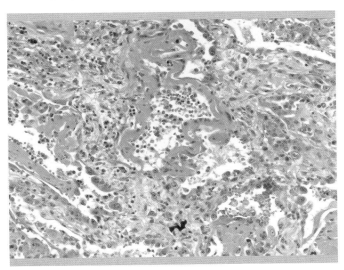

FIGURE 22-2

   (A) 12 hours
   (B) 2 days
   (C) 3–5 days
   (D) 1 month
   (E) 3 months

4. Which form of lung injury is similar to diffuse alveolar damage, is localized to the peribronchiolar parenchyma, and is characterized by fibroblastic plugs?
   (A) Acute interstitial pneumonia
   (B) Bronchiolitis obliterans-organizing pneumonia
   (C) Lymphocytic interstitial pneumonia
   (D) Non-specific interstitial pneumonia
   (E) Pulmonary alveolar proteinosis

5. A 70-year-old man presents with dyspnea and progressive worsening of symptoms over the past few months. High-resolution CT scan shows bilateral, interstitial, reticular markings prominent at the bases and periphery of the lungs. Based on Figure 22-3, what is the most likely diagnosis?

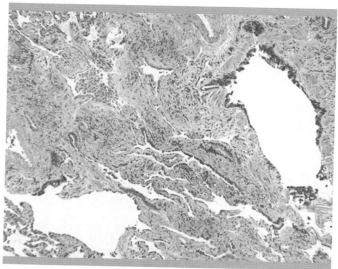

FIGURE 22-3

(A) Acute interstitial pneumonia
(B) Bronchiolitis obliterans-organizing pneumonia
(C) Desquamative interstitial pneumonia
(D) Non-specific interstitial pneumonia
(E) Usual interstitial pneumonia

6. A wedge biopsy from a patient with interstitial lung disease is shown here (Figure 22-4). Based on the histologic features, what is the best diagnosis?

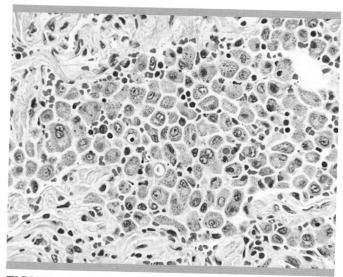

FIGURE 22-4

(A) Acute interstitial pneumonia
(B) Bronchiolitis obliterans-organizing pneumonia
(C) Desquamative interstitial pneumonia/Respiratory bronchiolitis interstitial lung disease
(D) Non-specific interstitial pneumonia
(E) Usual interstitial pneumonia

7. The gross appearance of lung shown in Figure 22-5 may be associated with all the following conditions, except

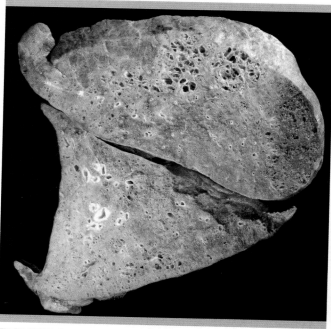

FIGURE 22-5

(A) Diffuse alveolar damage
(B) Eosinophilic pneumonia
(C) Idiopathic interstitial pneumonia
(D) Inorganic dust exposure
(E) Lymphoma

8. Which of the following histologic reactions/findings is least likely to be encountered in a quarry worker?
(A) Concentric hyaline nodules
(B) Dust macule
(C) Diffuse interstitial fibrosis
(D) Pulmonary alveolar proteinosis
(E) Stellate interstitial fibrosis

9. Which of the following statements about asbestos fibers is incorrect?
(A) By definition, their length is three times their diameter
(B) Heavy exposure may lead to development of carcinoma and mesothelioma

(C) Serpentine and amphibole groups are the commonly encountered classes

(D) They are composed of silica plus iron, magnesium, sodium, and other metals

(E) They cause a more localized reaction compared to silicosis

10. Coating with which of the following particles leads to formation of an asbestos body?
(A) Cadmium
(B) Calcium
(C) Copper
(D) Iron
(E) Lead

11. In contrast to simple coal worker's pneumoconiosis, complicated coal worker's pneumoconiosis is usually associated with which of the following features?
(A) Dust-filled macrophages in the interstitium surrounding respiratory bronchioles
(B) Hyalinized and collagenous stroma
(C) Minimal radiographic changes
(D) Progressive massive fibrosis
(E) Reaction to inhaled coal dust particles

12. The finding of giant cell interstitial pneumonia is most likely associated with which of the following conditions?
(A) Berylliosis
(B) Coal workers' pneumoconiosis
(C) Hard metal pneumoconiosis
(D) Siderosis
(E) Silicosis

13. The pathologic triad of temporally uniform chronic interstitial pneumonia with peribronchiolar accentuation, non-necrotizing granulomas in peribronchiolar interstitium, and foci of bronchiolitis obliterans is diagnostic of which of the following pathologic entities?
(A) Diffuse alveolar damage
(B) Hypersensitivity pneumonia
(C) Lymphoid interstitial pneumonia
(D) Sarcoidosis
(E) Usual interstitial pneumonia

14. A 25-year-old man presents with acute onset hemoptysis, anemia, azotemia, and diffuse pulmonary infiltrates. A kidney biopsy shows membranoproliferative glomerulonephritis with linear IgG deposits. What is the most likely cause of this patient's symptoms?
(A) Cocaine intoxication
(B) Drug reaction
(C) Goodpasture's syndrome
(D) Heart failure
(E) Idiopathic pulmonary hypertension

15. A 35-year-old woman of African descent presents with dyspnea and cough. She is found to have extensive hilar adenopathy. Infectious processes and neoplasms have been clinically excluded. All of the following are associated with this condition, except
(A) Asteroid bodies
(B) Granulomatous vasculitis
(C) Granulomas within airspaces
(D) Hyalinized fibrosis
(E) Well-formed epithelioid granulomas

16. A 45-year-old man presents with history of fever, weight loss, hemoptysis, and sinusitis. Preliminary investigation reveals elevated serum antineutrophil cytoplasmic antibodies (ANCA) targeted against proteinase-3 and cavitary pulmonary nodules. Which of the following clinicopathologic features is not associated with this condition?
(A) Can be fatal if not treated promptly
(B) Geographic areas of parenchymal necrosis bound by epithelioid histiocytes
(C) Glomerulonephritis
(D) Necrotizing vasculitis
(E) Blood eosinophilia

17. Churg-Strauss syndrome is characterized by all of the following clinicopathologic features, except
(A) Asthma
(B) Blood eosinophil count of <500/μL
(C) Elevated p-ANCA
(D) Mild segmental glomerulonephritis
(E) Necrotizing vasculitis

18. A 75-year-old man presents with hemoptysis and is found to have a 4.5 cm nodular lesion in the left lobe of the lung (see Figure 22-6). The cells of interest in the lesion are diffusely positive for CD20 and coexpress CD43. They are negative for CD5 and CD10. These findings are diagnostic of

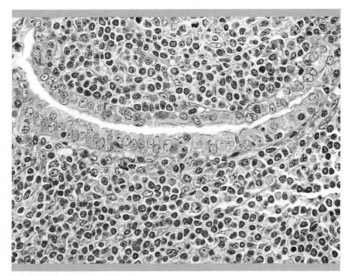

FIGURE 22-6

   (A) Follicular bronchiolitis
   (B) Low-grade B-cell lymphoma
   (C) Lymphoid interstitial pneumonia
   (D) Lymphomatoid granulomatosis
   (E) Nodular lymphoid hyperplasia

19. A 57-year-old man presents with hemoptysis and is found to have bilateral necrotizing nodules in the lung. Histologically, they are composed of small lymphocytes, histiocytes, plasma cells, and large atypical lymphocytes with prominent vascular involvement. The large lymphoid cells are CD20-positive and the background cells are CD3-positive. What is the most likely diagnosis?
   (A) Hodgkin disease
   (B) Lymphomatoid granulomatosis
   (C) Lymphoid interstitial pneumonia
   (D) Tuberculosis
   (E) Wegener's granulomatosis

20. All the following viruses cause organizing pneumonia with multinucleated giant cells, except
   (A) Adenovirus
   (B) Measles virus
   (C) Parainfluenza virus
   (D) Respiratory-syncytial virus
   (E) Varicella-zoster virus

21. Which of the following fungal organisms causes a "target-like lesion" characterized by hemorrhagic infarction with a dark rim surrounding a central yellow-gray area?
   (A) *Aspergillus*
   (B) *Candida*
   (C) *Fusarium*
   (D) *Pseudoallescheria boydii*
   (E) Mucor

22. All the following morphologic features favor the presence of mucormycosis over *Aspergillosis*, except
   (A) Haphazard tissue distribution
   (B) 90° branching
   (C) Non-septate hyphae
   (D) Regular branching points
   (E) Wide hyphae

23. Which of the following types of crystals is *Aspergillus niger* mycetoma associated with?
   (A) Calcium oxalate
   (B) Calcium phosphate
   (C) Calcium silicate
   (D) Triple phosphate
   (E) Tyrosine

24. A 25-year-old young man with a history of renal transplantation develops a pulmonary abscess. Histologic evaluation shows poorly formed granulomas surrounding necrotic debris. A modified Ziehl-Neelsen preparation is shown here (Figure 22-7). What is the etiology of his pulmonary abscess?

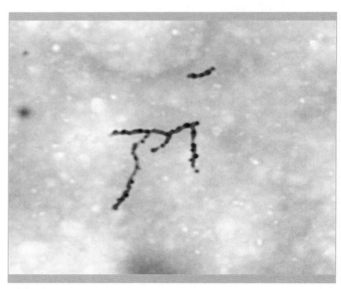

FIGURE 22-7

   (A) Actinomycosis
   (B) Botryomycosis
   (C) Sporotrichosis

(D) Nocardiosis
(E) Tuberculosis

25. A 45-year-old woman with a history of systemic lupus erythematosus presents with fever and dyspnea. The histologic changes in her lung biopsy (Figure 22-8) are pathognomonic of which of the following entities?

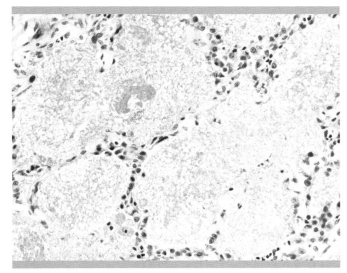

FIGURE 22-8

(A) Bronchopneumonia
(B) Diffuse alveolar damage
(C) Pulmonary alveolar proteinosis
(D) Pulmonary edema
(E) *Pneumocystis jiroveci* infection

26. A farmer from Southwest region of United States is found to have a 2.5 cm lung nodule. The wedge biopsy findings shown in Figure 22-9 are diagnostic of

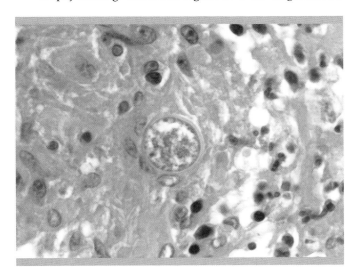

FIGURE 22-9

(A) Blastomycosis
(B) Coccidioidomycosis
(C) Cryptococcosis
(D) Histoplasmosis
(E) Paracoccidioidomycosis

27. The pulmonary infection depicted in Figure 22-10 is associated with all of the following features, except

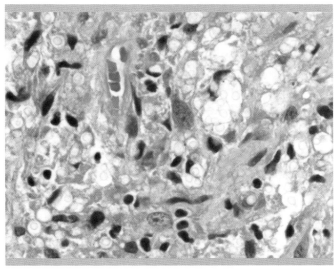

FIGURE 22-10

(A) Approximately a third of patients are asymptomatic
(B) Hilar lymph node enlargement is common
(C) Non-necrotizing granulomas
(D) Oval yeasts without a capsule
(E) Pigeon breeders

28. A biopsy from a patient exposed to hot tub water shows a combination of well-formed non-necrotizing granulomas and organizing pneumonia. What is the most likely cause of patient's lung injury?
(A) *Mycobacterium avium-intracellulare complex*
(B) *Mycobacterium chelonei*
(C) *Mycobacterium fortuitum*
(D) *Mycobacterium kansasii*
(E) *Mycobacterium tuberculosis*

29. The filariform larval form of which of the following intestinal nematodes is associated with hyperinfection syndrome and bronchopneumonia?
(A) *Ascaris lumbricoides*
(B) *Ankylostoma duodenale*
(C) *Enterobius vermicularis*
(D) *Trichuris trichiura*
(E) *Strongyloides stercoralis*

30. A pneumonectomy specimen from a 36-year-old woman with long-standing history of exertional dyspnea and pulmonary hypertension shows this lesion (Figure 22-11). What is the best diagnosis?

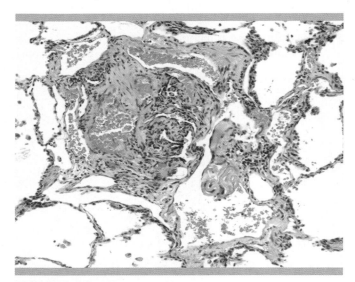

FIGURE 22-11

   (A) Concentric laminar fibrosis
   (B) Medial hypertrophy of arteries
   (C) Muscularization of arteries
   (D) Necrotizing arteritis
   (E) Plexiform lesion

31. Pulmonary sequestration is characterized by all the following pathologic findings, except
   (A) Lacks communication with the tracheobronchial tree
   (B) May rarely have a connection to the esophagus or stomach
   (C) May occur within or outside of the visceral pleural lining
   (D) Most commonly occurs in the right lobe
   (E) Receives blood supply from one or more anomalous systemic arteries

32. Which of the following statements does not apply to congenital cystic adenomatoid malformation (CCAM)?
   (A) It has features of immaturity and malformation of small airways and distal lung parenchyma
   (B) It is most commonly seen in stillborn or premature infants with anasarca
   (C) It is often associated with spontaneous pneumothorax
   (D) It is sometimes associated with elevated maternal serum alpha-fetoprotein
   (E) Most CCAMs communicate with the normal tracheobronchial tree

33. A wedge biopsy from a nodular lesion in a 50-year-old man with history of smoking is shown in Figure 22-12. Which immunohistochemical stain is most useful in highlighting the cells of interest?

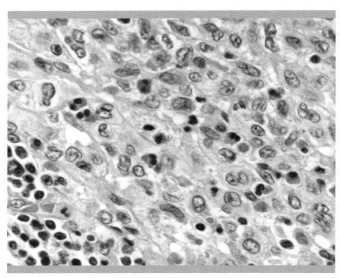

FIGURE 22-12

   (A) CD1a
   (B) CD4
   (C) CD10
   (D) Smooth muscle actin
   (E) Chromogranin

34. The lesion depicted in Figure 22-13 is associated with which of the following gene mutations?

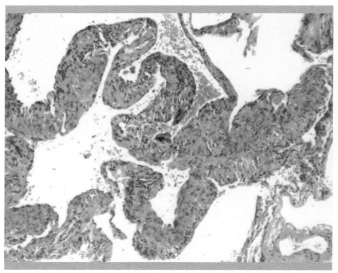

FIGURE 22-13

(A) *APC*
(B) β-*catenin*
(C) *KIT*
(D) *NF1*
(E) *TSC1*

35. A 50-year-old woman has a history of autoimmune pancreatitis and is found to have a nodular lesion in the lung. All the following features would confirm a diagnosis of IgG4-related sclerosing lesion, except
(A) Fibrosis
(B) Increased numbers of IgG4-positive plasma cells
(C) Intimal and mural inflammation involving the pulmonary arteries
(D) Lymphoplasmacytic infiltrate
(E) Serum IgG4 <10 mg/dL

36. Which is the most common organism isolated from cystic fibrosis patients presenting with recurrent pulmonary infections?
(A) *Chlamydia pneumoniae*
(B) *Haemophilus influenzae*
(C) *Mycoplasma pneumoniae*
(D) *Pseudomonas aeruginosa*
(E) *Streptococcus pneumoniae*

37. A wedge biopsy of lung shows a small lesion composed of ovoid cells with stippled chromatin pattern, arranged as nests within the alveolar septa and around pulmonary veins. Additional work-up shows that the cells are strongly positive for EMA and vimentin, and do not express cytokeratin, chromogranin, S-100, and actin. What is the best diagnosis for this lesion?
(A) Carcinoid tumorlet
(B) Granuloma
(C) Minute meningothelial-like lesion
(D) Paraganglioma
(E) Sclerosing hemangioma

38. A lobectomy specimen from a 45-year-old woman with a lung mass is shown in Figure 22-14. What is the most likely diagnosis?

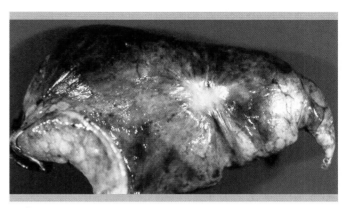

FIGURE 22-14

(A) Adenocarcinoma
(B) Bronchioloalveolar carcinoma
(C) Carcinoid tumor
(D) Large cell carcinoma
(E) Squamous cell carcinoma

39. Per the 2011 International Association for the Study of Lung Cancer (IASLC)/American Thoracic Society (ATS)/European Respiratory Society (ERS) international multidisciplinary classification of lung adenocarcinoma, which of these patterns is not categorized as a distinct histologic pattern of invasive adenocarcinoma?
(A) Acinar
(B) Micropapillary
(C) Mucinous
(D) Papillary
(E) Solid

40. A 65-year-old man with a significant smoking history is found to have an exophytic, cavitary mass obstructing the main bronchus. Based on this information, what is the most likely diagnosis?
(A) Adenocarcinoma
(B) Carcinoid tumor
(C) Large cell carcinoma
(D) Small cell carcinoma
(E) Squamous cell carcinoma

41. A transbronchial lung biopsy of a perihilar mass in a 55-year-old man with significant smoking history is depicted in Figure 22-15. Which of these morphologic findings is not typical of this entity?

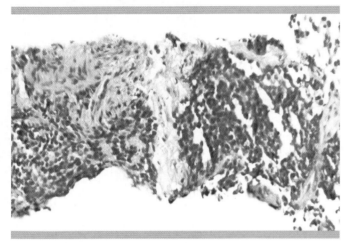

FIGURE 22-15

(A) Coarse nuclear chromatin with prominent nucleoli
(B) Crush artifact
(C) High nuclear-to-cytoplasmic ratio
(D) High mitotic rate
(E) Nuclear molding

42. A 47-year-old woman with history of hemoptysis, cough, and wheezing is found to have this peribronchial lesion (see Figure 22-16). The most likely diagnosis is

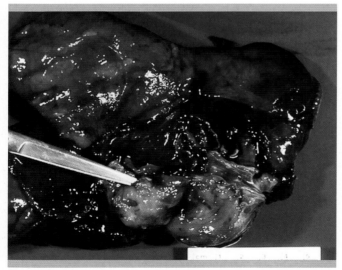

FIGURE 22-16

(A) Adenocarcinoma
(B) Carcinoid tumor
(C) Large cell carcinoma

(D) Small cell carcinoma
(E) Squamous cell carcinoma

43. A 75-year-old man undergoes wedge resection of a solitary pulmonary nodule which is shown in Figure 22-17. The tumor cells express CD10 and vimentin and are negative for cytokeratin 7. What is the most likely diagnosis?

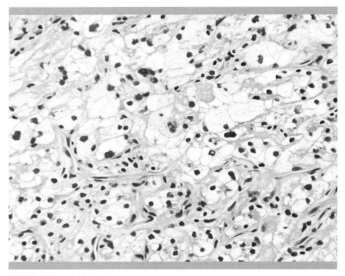

FIGURE 22-17

(A) Invasive mucinous pulmonary adenocarcinoma
(B) Clear cell "sugar" tumor
(C) Metastatic clear cell sarcoma
(D) Metastatic clear cell renal cell carcinoma
(E) Squamous cell carcinoma with clear cell features

44. This endobronchial lesion from a 64-year-old man is characterized by all of the following clinicopathologic findings, except (Figure 22-18)

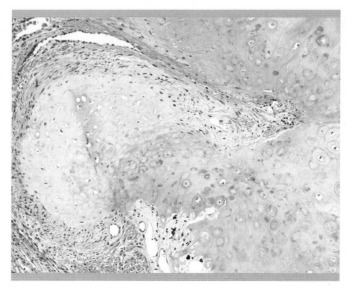

FIGURE 22-18

(A) Benign neoplasm
(B) "Popcorn" calcifications are diagnostic
(C) The lesion may show variable amount of adipose tissue, smooth muscle, bone, and fibrovascular tissue
(D) The lesion usually measures >5.0 cm
(E) Usually asymptomatic

45. Which of the following stains is expressed by pulmonary adenocarcinoma and helps in distinguishing it from an epithelioid malignant mesothelioma?
(A) Ber-EP4
(B) Calretinin
(C) Cytokeratin 5/6
(D) D2-40
(E) WT-1

46. A 70-year-old man is found to have digital clubbing and pulmonary hypertrophic osteoarthropathy. Further investigation reveals a 5.5 cm lesion in the upper lobe, depicted in Figure 22-19. All the following statements regarding this lesion are true, except

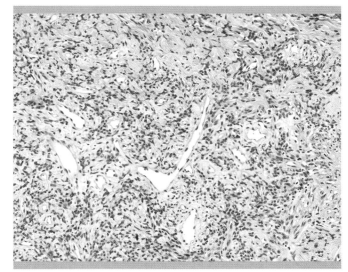

FIGURE 22-19

(A) Does not express CD34
(B) Incomplete resection can lead to local recurrence
(C) Often attached to the pleural surface by a vascular pedicle
(D) Often shows a "patternless" growth pattern
(E) Typically demonstrates a whorled, gray-white cut surface

47. A 70-year-old man with a history of myasthenia gravis undergoes resection of a mediastinal mass shown in Figure 22-20. The lesional cells are positive for cytokeratin AE1/AE3. Which of the following is not considered to be a poor prognostic factor associated with this tumor?

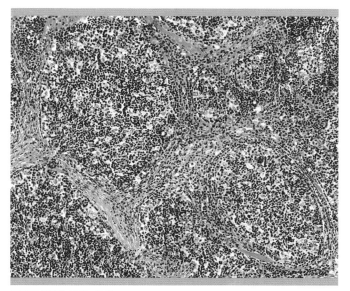

FIGURE 22-20

(A) High stage
(B) Histologic type
(C) Invasion of capsule
(D) Necrosis and hemorrhage
(E) Positive margin

48. An 11-year-old boy is presents with cough and chest pain and is found to have a 6 cm lung mass (see Figure 22-21). Which of the following statements about this lesion is true?

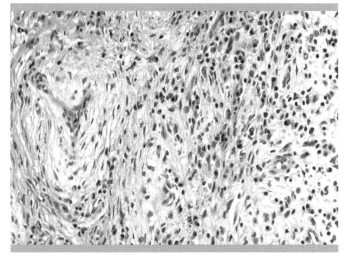

FIGURE 22-21

(A) Commonly occurs in children and young adults
(B) Corticosteroid therapy is the treatment of choice
(C) Majority of the cases show marked cytologic atypia, ganglion-like cells, and necrosis
(D) Metastasis to liver is very common
(E) The lesional cells are diffusely positive for CD34

49. Centrilobular emphysema is most closely associated with which of the following etiologies?
    (A) α-1 antitrypsin deficiency
    (B) Aspiration
    (C) Focal lesions
    (D) Large scars
    (E) Long-standing tobacco use

50. Primary effusion lymphoma has been causally linked to which of the following viral infection?
    (A) Adenovirus
    (B) Cytomegalovirus
    (C) HTLV-1
    (D) Human herpes virus-8
    (E) Human papilloma virus

ANSWERS

1. **(E) Sarcoidosis.**
   Sarcoidosis typically presents as a patchy, interstitial pattern of lung injury that follows the distribution of lymphatics. All the other diseases are examples that diffusely involve the airspaces.

2. **(C) Hamazaki-Wesenberg bodies.**
   The figure shows Hamazaki-Wesenberg bodies, which are small, oval, brown structures located within sinusoidal spaces that stain strongly with Giemsa stain. Their only clinical significance is that they can be confused with budding yeast forms. Ultrastructurally, they correspond to giant lysosomes and residual bodies. Hemosiderin granules are a close differential. However, hemosiderin granules are refractile in nature.

3. **(C) 3–5 days.**
   The figure hyaline membranes associated with acute, early, or exudative phase of diffuse alveolar damage (DAD). The acute phase occurs in the first week after injury and is characterized by the presence of edema and hyaline membranes. The membranes are composed of proteinaceous exudate and cellular debris. They appear as homogeneous, amorphous eosinophilic structures lining the alveolar spaces. The organizing phase of DAD is characterized by fibroblast proliferation within the interstitium. This finding is most prominent after 2 weeks of lung injury.

4. **(B) Bronchiolitis obliterans-organizing pneumonia (BOOP).**
   BOOP is a pattern of injury that may be encountered as a focal finding in several diseases such as eosinophilic pneumonia, nonspecific interstitial pneumonia, hypersensitivity pneumonia, or as a reaction to prior infection, drug reactions (gold, amiodarone, bleomycin), radiation of breast, aspiration, or collagen vascular diseases. Organizing DAD can be distinguished from BOOP by the interstitial location of fibroblast proliferation in DAD.

5. **(E) Usual interstitial pneumonia (UIP).**
   UIP is the most common idiopathic interstitial pneumonia and is typically seen in older patients. Men are affected twice more commonly than women. The disease is usually progressive and ultimately fatal in most patients. Spatial (nonuniform interstitial fibrosis with scarred areas located adjacent to normal parenchyma) and temporal heterogeneity (areas of active, ongoing fibrosis adjacent to inactive collagen-type fibrosis) are the classic features of UIP. The end stage is characterized by honeycomb lung typified by bronchiolar metaplasia of alveoli.

6. **(C) Desquamative interstitial pneumonia/ Respiratory bronchiolitis interstitial lung disease.**
   The biopsy shows extensive and diffuse intraalveolar accumulation of macrophages with lightly pigmented cytoplasm. These features are characteristic of desquamative interstitial pneumonia/respiratory bronchiolitis interstitial lung disease (DIP/RBILD). This form of interstitial lung disease usually affects middle-aged men and is commonly associated with smoking. The most common CT findings are bilateral ground glass opacities and centrilobular nodules. Most patients respond to corticosteroid therapy.

7. **(E) Lymphoma.**
   The lung specimen shows relatively uniformly sized cysts with intervening fibrosis characteristic of honeycomb lung. The extensive scarring and reparative activity is associated with an increased risk of developing lung carcinomas, not lymphoma.

8. **(B) Dust macule.**
   It is typically associated with exposure to coal dust or iron/iron oxides. The rest of the reactions are pulmonary reactions to silicosis. Silica occurs in crystalline and amorphous forms. The crystalline form of silica (quartz is a major source) is associated with a fibrogenic response. Stonecutting, quarry mining, and sandblasting are some occupations that may lead to silica exposure. Formation of hyaline and collagenous nodules is the classic response to crystalline silica.

9. **(E) They cause a more localized reaction compared to silicosis.**
   There are two general classes of asbestos fibers: serpentine (chrysotile is the major type) and amphibole (amosite and crocidolite are the major types). Chrysotile is the most frequently encountered asbestos fiber. In general, asbestos fibers are

usually associated with a more diffuse parenchymal reaction compared to compact silica particles.

10. **(D) Iron.**
The endogenous ferritin coats asbestos fibers to form asbestos bodies (also known as ferruginous bodies). On H&E stain, they are characterized by a central, clear core surrounded by golden yellow coating with terminal bulbs or knobs. They can also be highlighted by iron stain.

11. **(D) Progressive massive fibrosis.**
Large, bilateral areas of fibrosis (progressive massive fibrosis, PMF) may be a feature of several different types of pneumoconioses. Nodules >1 cm are designated as PMF. In coal worker's pneumoconiosis, the lesions are composed of large, black masses, which often contain a central cavity. They lead to pulmonary function abnormalities, such as obstructive defects, abnormal diffusing capacity, and restrictive defects.

12. **(C) Hard metal pneumoconiosis.**
Individuals working in diamond polishing and tool grinding industries are exposed to hard metals such as tungsten carbide and cobalt, which are associated with a form of chronic interstitial pneumonia known as giant cell interstitial pneumonia. The striking feature is accumulation of intra-alveolar multinucleated giant cells that often contain ingested inflammatory cells (emperipolesis).

13. **(B) Hypersensitivity pneumonia.**
Hypersensitivity pneumonia (also known as extrinsic allergic alveolitis) is an immunologic reaction to inhaled antigens. Some of the common etiologic agents include thermophilic bacteria (farmer's lung, humidifier lung), fungi (maple bark stripper's lung), and animal proteins (pigeon breeder's lung). Diffuse alveolar damage typically affects the alveolar spaces rather than airways. Lymphoid interstitial pneumonia is a diffuse parenchymal disease that shows a random pattern of distribution. It is composed of lymphoid aggregates with germinal centers. Although sarcoidosis is characterized by non-caseating granulomas, it usually does not present as an interstitial pneumonia. Lastly, usual interstitial pneumonia is characterized by temporal heterogeneity without granulomas or foci of bronchiolitis obliterans.

14. **(C) Goodpasture's syndrome.**
All the listed conditions are included in the differential diagnosis of pulmonary hemorrhage. Pulmonary hemorrhage is classified into three categories: alveolar hemorrhagic syndromes (Goodpasture's syndrome, idiopathic pulmonary hemosiderosis, capillaritis syndrome, drug reactions, cocaine injury, etc.), secondary alveolar hemorrhage (infections,

renal failure with volume overload, coagulopathies, venous congestion), and localized pulmonary hemorrhage (parenchymal lesion such as neoplasms, airway lesions such as bronchiectasis/bronchitis). Goodpasture's syndrome typically affects young adults (males>females). It is manifestation of an immunologic reaction resulting form antibodies to glomerular basement membranes that cross-react with pulmonary basement membranes. Linear staining for immunoglobulins (usually IgG) can be demonstrated along alveolar septae, and is helpful in establishing the diagnosis.

15. **(C) Granulomas within airspaces.**
The patient most likely has sarcoidosis. Sarcoidosis frequently affects young to middle-aged women and individuals of African descent. Granulomas predominantly involve the interstitium, rather than the airspaces, and usually follow the lymphatic distribution. Hyalinized fibrous tissue often replaces portions of granulomas. Numerous non-specific cytoplasmic inclusions (asteroid bodies, Schaumann bodies, and conchoid bodies), composed of calcium oxalate and calcium carbonate, are found within the granulomas.

16. **(E) Blood eosinophilia.**
The condition described is Wegener's granulomatosis. The classic form is manifested by a triad of upper respiratory tract and lung involvement along with glomerulonephritis. Histologically, this form is associated with necrotizing granulomas and vasculitis. BOOP-like variant and alveolar hemorrhage and capillaritis, are other manifestations of this disease. Serum cytoplasmic-ANCA levels are usually elevated. Peripheral eosinophilia is not a feature of this disease. Cyclophosphamide accompanied by corticosteroids is the treatment of choice. Without treatment, generalized Wegener's granulomatosis follows a fulminant course and is almost always fatal.

17. **(B) Blood eosinophil count of <500/μL.**
The clinical diagnostic criteria for Churg-Strauss syndrome includes asthma, high blood eosinophil count (>1500/μL), and evidence of vasculitis involving two or more extrapulmonary sites. Nearly 50–70% patients have elevated p-ANCA levels. Histologically, a combination of eosinophilic pneumonia, granulomatous inflammation and necrotizing vasculitis is considered to be pathognomonic of this entity.

18. **(B) Low-grade B-cell lymphoma.**
Low-grade B-cell lymphoma of mucosa-associated lymphoid tissue (MALT) is the most common primary lymphoma of the lung. It presents as an interstitial mass composed of monomorphic small

lymphoid cells with variable numbers of plasma cells, immunoblasts, and histiocytes. Lymphoepithelial lesions, characterized by infiltration of the bronchiolar epithelium by neoplastic lymphocytes (CD20-positive B lymphocytes with aberrant expression of CD43, a T-cell marker), are a common finding. The lymphangitic distribution along the bronchovascular tree and interlobular septa is a helpful feature. Unlike follicular bronchiolitis, nodular lymphoid hyperplasia, and lymphoid interstitial pneumonia, well-formed lymphoid follicles are not typical of this lesion.

19. **(B) Lymphomatoid granulomatosis.**
Lymphomatoid granulomatosis is an angiocentric T-cell rich EBV-associated B-cell lymphoproliferative disorder that usually presents as multiple necrotic nodules. Due to the presence of necrosis, tuberculosis and Wegener's granulomatosis are of clinical consideration, and can be distinguished by the lack of large atypical CD20-positive B lymphocytes. Hodgkin disease in lung usually presents as contiguous involvement of mediastinal disease. Presence of eosinophils, Reed-Sternberg cells, CD15-postivity and lack of CD20 expression are helpful in distinguishing lymphomatoid granulomatosis from Hodgkin disease. Lymphoid interstitial pneumonia shows a diffuse pattern of distribution and is composed of lymphoid follicles with germinal centers.

20. **(A) Adenovirus.**
Measles, parainfluenza, respiratory-syncytial virus (RSV), and varicella-zoster virus cause pneumonia with multinucleated giant cells. Measles virus additionally demonstrates both intranuclear and intracytoplasmic eosinophilic inclusions. Varicella-zoster virus shows intranuclear inclusions, while RSV and parainfluenza virus demonstrate intracytoplasmic inclusions. Sometimes pneumonias secondary to these viral infections are referred to as giant cell pneumonia, although this term is more commonly used for measles pneumonia. Adenovirus infection is characterized by homogeneous, intranuclear basophilic inclusions within the bronchiolar epithelium, or alveolar lining cells.

21. **(A) *Aspergillus*.**
Aspergillus pneumonia is the most common form of invasive aspergillosis. The other forms are necrotizing tracheobronchitis, necrotizing granulomatous inflammation, and chronic necrotizing aspergillosis. The classic tissue reaction is that of a hemorrhagic infarct with sparse inflammatory infiltrate. Fungal hyphae are often found infiltrating the walls of blood vessels. While mucormycosis may also show extensive parenchymal and vascular invasion, "target lesions" are characteristic of aspergillosis.

Candidiasis presents as miliary lung nodules and *Pseudoallescheria boydii* causes lung abscesses.

22. **(D) Regular branching points.**
Mucormycosis usually shows irregular branching points as opposed to regular, dichotomous, 45° branching of *Aspergillus* hyphae.

23. **(A) Calcium oxalate.**
Deposits of birefringent calcium oxalate crystals are commonly found at the edge of an *Aspergillus niger* mycetoma. The oxalic acid produced by the organism damages blood vessels and causes hemoptysis.

24. **(D) Nocardiosis.**
The lung is the most common primary site of involvement by Nocardiosis. Most patients are immunocompromised, and hematogenous dissemination, especially to the brain, is common. The organisms are gram-positive filamentous rods that have a characteristic beaded appearance. They are weakly acid fast, and therefore the Kinyoun modification of Ziehl-Neelsen stain should be employed to demonstrate these organisms in tissue sections. Actinomycosis presents as a suppurative infection containing long, branching, filamentous rods that are associated with granules. This organism does not stain with Ziehl-Neelsen stain. Botryomycosis is a suppurative infection caused by bacterial organisms, such as *Staphylococcus* and *Pseudomonas*. Sporothrix infection produces granules, but this fungus is not acid fast. Mycobacteria appear as thinner and shorter rods that do not show evidence of branching.

25. **(E) *Pneumocystis jiroveci* infection.**
The figure demonstrates frothy, foamy/honeycomb exudate within alveolar spaces that is diagnostic of *Pneumocystis* infection. Although commonly associated with AIDS infection, it has emerged as an important infection in patients receiving immunosuppressive therapy for malignant or autoimmune diseases or in organ transplant recipients. Diffuse alveolar damage with hyaline membranes is the next most common histologic pattern of *Pneumocystis* pneumonia. GMS stain highlights cysts measuring 4–6 μm in size. In contrast, Giemsa stain highlights the 1–2 μm intracystic sporozoites or trophozoites, but not stain the cyst walls.

26. **(B) Coccidioidomycosis.**
The biopsy shows an area of necrosis with large round spherules measuring 30–60 μm in diameter. The cysts exhibit refractile walls, and contain basophilic endospheres, characteristic of coccidioidomycosis. Eosinophils are a major component of the inflammatory infiltrate. Most cases are diagnosed by positive cultures and serologic tests. A solitary nodule may mimic a neoplastic process.

27. **(D) Oval yeasts without a capsule.**
Cryptococci typically show rounded yeast forms with a thick mucinous capsule that stains bright red on mucicarmine stain. Rarely, some species may lack this mucinous capsule. The yeast forms of blastomyces are oval and lack a mucinous capsule. The cryptococcal yeast forms are found in the soil contaminated with pigeon droppings. A non-necrotizing granulomatous reaction often accompanies this infection.

28. **(A) *Mycobacterium avium-intracellulare complex.***
Except *Mycobacterium tuberculosis*, all of the listed choices are examples of non-tuberculous or atypical mycobacteria. Their staining characteristics are similar to *Mycobacterium tuberculosis. Mycobacterium avium-intracellulare complex-* infected hot tub water has been linked to a specific lung infection known as "hot tub lung" that is characterized by non-necrotizing granulomas and organizing pneumonia.

29. **(E) *Strongyloides stercoralis.***
In immunocompromised individuals, strongyloidosis has been associated with superinfection, wherein large numbers of parasitic organisms proliferate, and involve extraintestinal organs, such as lungs. Patients present with cough, wheezing, and interstitial lung infiltrates. The diagnosis is usually made by identifying the parasites in sputum or bronchoalveolar lavage specimens.

30. **(E) Plexiform lesion.**
The lesion depicted in this figure shows a muscular artery with complex, interlacing, slit-like channels arising from the artery, along with intimal, and medial hypertrophy. This lesion is associated with severe pulmonary hypertension. Plexiform lesions form as a result of vascular necrosis, followed by secondary thrombosis, associated with organization and recanalization of blood vessels.

31. **(D) Most commonly occurs in the right lobe.**
Pulmonary sequestration occurs most commonly in the left lobe and may occur within the visceral pleural lining (intralobar sequestration) or outside this pleural investment (extralobar sequestration). Systemic arteries arising from thoracic aorta supply both types of sequestrations. Majority of them arise in the left lobe. Due to the lack of communication with the tracheobronchial tree, they are often accompanied by inflammation, infection, and cyst formation due to retained secretions.

32. **(C) It is often associated with spontaneous pneumothorax.**
All the above choices are features of congenital cystic adenomatoid malformation (CCAM), except answer C. Spontaneous pneumothorax is an unusual presenting feature. CCAMs are classified into five subtypes based on the gross and histologic features. Type 1 lesions are the most common, and are composed of large cysts (3–10 cm) lined by pseudostratified, ciliated columnar epithelium. Type 2 CCAM lesions show multiple, evenly spaced cysts that are <2 cm, and are lined by cuboidal to ciliated columnar epithelium. Type 3 lesions almost exclusively occur in males and have a spongy gross appearance without evidence of macroscopic cysts. Histologically, they are composed of dilated, irregularly branching channels resembling primitive airspaces that are lined by cuboidal epithelium. Type 0 CCAM is incompatible with life. Grossly, the lungs appear solid. Histologically, they are composed of bronchial-like structures that contain smooth muscle, cartilage, and glands within the wall. These structures are lined by respiratory epithelium. Type 4 CCAM is considered to be a malformation of the distal acinus and shows thin-walled cysts lined by type 1 pneumocytes and low cuboidal cells.

33. **(A) CD1a.**
The lesion depicted in this figure is pulmonary Langerhans cell histiocytosis, which almost exclusively occurs in smokers. Patients may present with multiple, bilateral lung nodules that are most prominent in the upper lobes . The hallmarks of this entity include nodular interstitial infiltrates of Langerhans cells that are CD1a and S-100-positive, peribronchial location, stellate-shaped lesions, and desquamative-interstitial pneumonia-like pattern with intra-alveolar macrophage accumulation. The inflammatory infiltrate is rich in eosinophils; hence the earlier name pulmonary eosinophilic granuloma. By electron microscopy, characteristic rod- to racquet-shaped pentalaminar inclusions, known as Birbeck granules, can be found within the cytoplasm of Langerhans cells.

34. **(E) *TSC1.***
Lymphangioleiomyomatosis is an important pulmonary manifestation of tuberous sclerosis in women. It is characterized by random, disorderly proliferation of bland smooth muscle bundles within the interstitium, which may be arranged around bronchioles, arteries, veins, or lymphatic spaces. A helpful histologic finding is the presence of an air-filled cyst within the lesion. The cyst occurs as a result of air trapping due to bronchiolar narrowing. The smooth muscle cells express HMB-45, smooth muscle actin, and in some cases, estrogen and progesterone receptor. This lesion has been associated with tuberous sclerosis and can show mutations involving the *TSC1* gene.

35. **(E) Serum IgG4 <10 mg/dL.**
IgG4-related sclerosing disease is characterized by elevated serum IgG4 levels and a distinct inflammatory

process composed of lymphoplasmacytic infiltrate, increased IgG4-positive plasma cells, fibrosis, and phlebitis. In contrast to the findings in IgG4-associated autoimmune pancreatitis, which is usually associated with sparing of the arteries, both pulmonary arteries and veins are involved by intimal and mural inflammation. Pulmonary involvement may be in the form of nodular opacities, interstitial lung disease, pleural nodules, pleural effusion, tracheobronchial stenosis, mediastinal lymphadenopathy, and fibrosing mediastinitis.

36. **(D) *Pseudomonas aeruginosa*.**
Patients with cystic fibrosis suffer from recurrent pulmonary infections. Mucoid strains of *Pseudomonas aeruginosa* and *Staphylococcus aureus* are the most commonly isolated organisms in this setting. The main pathologic manifestation is widespread bronchiectasis.

37. **(C) Minute meningothelial-like lesion.**
These are incidental lesions found in nearly 1% of autopsy lungs. They are also referred to as chemodectoma-like bodies. They may be found in the setting of emphysema, congestive heart failure, and thromboembolic disease. Carcinoid tumorlets are distinguished by their location (usually peribronchial) and immunoreactivity with neuroendocrine markers. Sclerosing hemangiomas are much larger lesions that express TTF-1. Paragangliomas show a "zellballen" or nested architecture, and the cells usually express neuroendocrine markers.

38. **(A) Adenocarcinoma.**
The figure shows an area of pleural puckering or scar. Pulmonary adenocarcinoma accounts for nearly 35% of all lung tumors and is the most frequent type of lung cancer in women and non-smokers. It commonly presents as a peripheral lung lesion. The tumor may also be found in association with fibrosis and pleural puckering, and occasionally mimics mesothelioma by presenting as a rind-like area of pleural thickening.

39. **(C) Mucinous.**
Acinar, micropapillary, papillary, solid, and lepidic (formerly non-mucinous bronchioloalveolar carcinoma pattern with >5 mm invasion) patterns are the five histologic patterns of invasive adenocarcinoma. Invasive mucinous adenocarcinoma is now considered as a histologic variant of invasive adenocarcinoma (formerly known as mucinous bronchioloalveolar carcinoma); the other variants being colloid, fetal (low and high grade), and enteric adenocarcinoma.

40. **(E) Squamous cell carcinoma.**
Most squamous cell carcinomas arise in the proximal airways, frequently causing post-obstructive pneumonia. The lesion often shows areas of necrosis and central cavitation. Squamous cell carcinoma is strongly associated with cigarette smoking. Its histologic variants include papillary, clear cell, small cell, and basaloid types.

41. **(A) Coarse nuclear chromatin with prominent nucleoli.**
The biopsy shows a sheet-like growth pattern of small cell lung carcinoma. The lesion is composed of sheets of small cells (usually less than the size of 3 small lymphocytes) that have round, or oval to spindle-shaped nuclei. The nuclear chromatin is fine or granular ("salt and pepper"), and nucleoli are usually absent or inconspicuous. The differential diagnosis includes crushed lymphoid cells, carcinoid tumor, basaloid squamous cell carcinoma, and large cell neuroendocrine carcinoma. Small cell carcinoma has a very poor prognosis.

42. **(B) Carcinoid tumor.**
The specimen shows a well-defined tumor with a homogeneous, tan-gray cut-surface occluding one of the branches of the main-stem bronchus. This is a common presentation of carcinoids. Despite their low metastatic potential, typical and atypical carcinoids are considered as true malignant lesions, since up to 15% of typical carcinoids (no necrosis and mitotic activity <2 per 10 high-power field) and up to 50% of atypical carcinoids (2–10 mitoses per 10 high-power field and/or foci of necrosis) metastasize. Some tumors may harbor *MEN1* gene mutations.

43. **(D) Metastatic clear cell renal cell carcinoma.**
The morphologic features of nests of clear cells intermixed with delicate vasculature, in conjunction with immunohistochemical findings, are most consistent with metastatic clear cell renal cell carcinoma. Metastasis is the most common malignancy in the lung. According to an autopsy series, the tumors that most commonly metastasize to the lung include tumors arising from the breast, colon, kidney, uterus, and head and neck region. Pulmonary adenocarcinoma usually expresses CK7 and TTF-1. Clear cell sarcoma and "sugar tumor" express melanocytic markers HMB-45 and Melan-A. Squamous cell carcinoma is usually negative for vimentin and CD10.

44. **(D) They usually measure >5.0 cm.**
The lesion depicted in this figure is a pulmonary hamartoma that is composed of nodules of cartilaginous tissue along with entrapped respiratory epithelium. This lesion needs to be distinguished from a true chondroma and chondrosarcoma. Chondromas typically do not contain other mesenchymal elements and usually

occur in young women. They are known to arise in the setting of Carney triad (pulmonary chondroma, gastrointestinal stromal tumor, and extra-adrenal paraganglioma). Chondrosarcomas can be readily distinguished by their cytological details such as binucleation, nuclear membrane irregularities, hyperchromasia, and presence of nucleoli.

45. **(A) Ber-EP4.**
Epithelioid malignant mesotheliomas express all the above markers, except Ber-EP4 (also known as epithelial cell adhesion molecule), an antibody that targets the cell membrane glycoproteins. Other markers that are positive in adenocarcinoma and negative in mesothelioma are CEA, MOC-31, and TTF-1.

46. **(A) Does not express CD34.**
The figure shows a cellular proliferation of uniform, bland spindle cells in a densely collagenous background, characteristic of solitary fibrous tumor (SFT). Other growth patterns that can be seen in this tumor include fascicular, storiform, and hemangiopericytic pattern. Lesional cells usually express CD34, vimentin, and bcl-2 and lack immunoreactivity with cytokeratin, EMA, calretinin, S-100, desmin, and actin. This immunoprofile helps in distinguishing SFT from sarcomatoid and desmoplastic mesothelioma (calretinin and cytokeratin positive), desmoid tumor (actin positive), and monophasic synovial sarcoma (usually at least focally positive for cytokeratin and EMA). The proposed histologic criteria for malignancy include mitotic activity >4 per 10 high-power field, increased pleomorphism, and necrosis.

47. **(D) Necrosis and hemorrhage.**
The tumor depicted in the figure is thymoma, a biphasic tumor composed of bland epithelial cells and lymphocytes. Necrosis and hemorrhage have no bearing on the prognosis of this tumor.

48. **(A) Commonly occurs in children and young adults.**
The lesion depicted in this figure is an inflammatory myofibroblastic tumor composed of bland spindle cells arranged in a vague storiform pattern accompanied by numerous plasma cells and lymphocytes. The tumor is relatively frequent in this age group. Cytologic atypia, mitotic activity, and necrosis are uncommon. The tumor cells express vimentin, smooth muscle actin, and calponin. Translocation involving the ALK locus at 2p23 is frequently associated with this lesion. Surgical resection is associated with an excellent outcome. Metastatic disease is rare.

49. **(E) Long-standing tobacco use.**
Emphysema is defined as an abnormal, permanent enlargement of air spaces distal to the terminal bronchiole due to destruction of the alveolar walls, without accompanying fibrosis. There are 4 four variants of emphysema: centrilobular emphysema, panacinar emphysema, paraseptal emphysema, and irregular emphysema. Centrilobular emphysema is most closely associated with long-standing tobacco use. Panacinar emphysema is associated with α-1antitrypsin deficiency. Irregular emphysema occurs at the periphery of large scars and focal lesions.

50. **(D) Human herpes virus-8.**
Primary effusion lymphoma usually affects immunocompromised hosts. Patients typically present with a lymphomatous effusion without evidence of lymphadenopathy or organomegaly. Immunohistochemically, the neoplastic cells are positive for CD45, CD138, and CD30, and are negative for CD20, CD19, and CD79a. Immunohistochemical staining for HHV-8 is helpful for confirming the diagnosis. The prognosis as well as response to chemotherapy are poor.

SUGGESTED READING

1. Chalabreysse L, Roy P, Cordier JF, et al. Correlation of the WHO schema for the classification of thymic epithelial neoplasms with prognosis: a retrospective study of 90 tumors. *Am J Surg Pathol*. 2002;26:1605-1611.

2. Gjevre JA, Myers JL, Prakash UB. Pulmonary hamartomas. *Mayo Clin Proc*. 1996;71:14-20.

3. Glassberg MK. Lymphangioleiomyomatosis. *Clin Chest Med*. 2004;25:573-582.

4. Granville L, Laga AC, Allen TC, et al. Review and update of uncommon primary pleural tumors: a practical approach to diagnosis. *Arch Pathol Lab Med*. 2005;129:1428-1443.

5. Hamutcu R, Rowland JM, Horn MV, et al. Clinical findings and lung pathology in children with cystic fibrosis. *Am J Respir Crit Care Med*. 2002;165:1172-1175.

6. Ionescu DN, Sasatomi E, Aldeeb D, et al. Pulmonary meningothelial-like nodules: a genotypic comparison with meningiomas. *Am J Surg Pathol*. 2004;28:207-214.

7. Jaffe ES, Wilson WH. Lymphomatoid granulomatosis: pathogenesis, pathology and clinical implications. *Cancer Surv*. 1997;30:233-248.

8. Jamison BM, Michel RP. Different distribution of plexiform lesions in primary and secondary pulmonary hypertension. *Hum Pathol*. 1995;26:987-993.

9. Katzenstein, A-AL. Acute lung injury patterns: diffuse alveolar damage and bronchiolitis obliterans-organizing pneumonia. In: Katzenstein A-L, ed. *Katzenstein and Askin's Surgical Pathology of Non-Neoplastic Lung Disease: Major Problems in Pathology*. Philadelphia, PA: Saunders Elsevier;2006:17-50.

10. Katzenstein A-AL. Idiopathic interstitial pneumonia. In: Katzenstein A-L, ed. *Katzenstein and Askin's Surgical*

Pathology of Non-Neoplastic Lung Disease: Major Problems in Pathology. Philadelphia, PA: Saunders Elsevier;2006:51-84.

11. Katzenstein A-AL. Pneumoconiosis. In: Katzenstein A-L, ed. *Katzenstein and Askin's Surgical Pathology of Non-Neoplastic Lung Disease: Major Problems in Pathology*. Philadelphia, PA: Saunders Elsevier;2006:127-150.

12. Katzenstein A-AL. Pulmonary vasculitis. In: Katzenstein A-L, ed. *Katzenstein and Askin's Surgical Pathology of Non-Neoplastic Lung Disease: Major Problems in Pathology*. Philadelphia, PA: Saunders Elsevier; 2006: 217-236.

13. Katzenstein A-AL. Primary lymphoid lung lesions. In: Katzenstein A-L, ed. *Katzenstein and Askin's Surgical Pathology of Non-Neoplastic Lung Disease: Major Problems in Pathology*. Philadelphia, PA: Saunders Elsevier; 2006: 237-260.

14. Katzenstein A-AL. Infection II—granulomatous infections. In: Katzenstein A-L, ed. *Katzenstein and Askin's Surgical Pathology of Non-Neoplastic Lung Disease: Major Problems in Pathology*. Philadelphia, PA: Saunders Elsevier; 2006:305-328.

15. Katzenstein, A-AL. Pulmonary hypertension and other vascular disorders. In: Katzenstein A-L, ed. *Katzenstein and Askin's Surgical Pathology of Non-Neoplastic Lung Disease: Major Problems in Pathology*. Philadelphia, PA: Saunders Elsevier; 2006:351-384.

16. Katzenstein A-AL. Pediatric disorders. In: Katzenstein A-L, ed. *Katzenstein and Askin's Surgical Pathology of Non-Neoplastic Lung Disease: Major Problems in Pathology*. Philadelphia, PA: Saunders Elsevier;2006:385-414.

17. Libshitz HI, North LB. Pulmonary metastases. *Radiol Clin North Am*. 1982;20:437-451.

18. Mukhopadhyay S. Role of histology in the diagnosis of infectious causes of granulomatous lung disease. *Curr Opin Pulm Med*. 2011;17:189-196.

19. Ordonez NG. Immunohistochemical diagnosis of epithelioid mesothelioma: an update. *Arch Pathol Lab Med*. 2005; 129:1407-1414.

20. Orr DP, Myerowitz RL, Dubois PJ. Patho-radiologic correlation of invasive pulmonary aspergillosis in the compromised host. *Cancer*. 1978;41:2028-2039.

21. Ryu JH, Sekiguchi H, Yi ES. Pulmonary manifestations of immunoglobulin G4-related sclerosing disease. *Eur Respir J*. 2012;39:180-186.

22. Stocker JT. Cystic lung disease in infants and children. *Fetal Pediatr Pathol*. 2009;28:155-184.

23. Stocker JT. Sequestrations of the lung. *Semin Diagn Pathol*. 1986;3:106-121.

24. Sullivan DC, Chapman SW. Bacteria that masquerade as fungi: actinomycosis/nocardia. *Proc Am Thorac Soc*. 2010; 7:216-221.

25. Travis WD. Update on small cell carcinoma and its differentiation from squamous cell carcinoma and other non-small cell carcinomas. *Mod Pathol*. 2012;25(Suppl 1):S18-S30.

26. Travis WD, Brambilla E, Noguchi M, et al. International Association for the Study of Lung Cancer/American Thoracic Society/European Respiratory Society international multidisciplinary classification of lung adenocarcinoma. *J Thorac Oncol*. 2011;6:244-285.

27. Vassallo R, Ryu JH, Colby TV, et al. Pulmonary Langerhans'-cell histiocytosis. *N Engl J Med*. 2000;342:1969-1978.

28. Coffin CM, Dehner LP, Meis-Kindblom JM. Inflammatory myofibroblastic tumor, inflammatory fibrosarcoma, and related lesions: an historical review with differential diagnostic considerations. *Semin Diagn Pathol*. 1998;15:102-110.

29. Karcher DS, Alkan S. Human herpesvirus-8-associated body cavity-based lymphoma in human immunodeficiency virus-infected patients: a unique B-cell neoplasm. *Hum Pathol*. 1997;28:801-808.

CHAPTER 23

TRANSPLANTATION PATHOLOGY

1. A 25-year-old man with hemophilia is undergoing renal transplantation. Following anastomosis of the graft and recipient vasculature, the surgeon notices that the kidney rapidly becomes cyanotic, mottled, and flaccid. A biopsy from this kidney will most likely to show
   - (A) Arterial obliterative intimal fibrosis
   - (B) Endotheliitis
   - (C) Lymphocytic tubulitis
   - (D) Numerous fibrin thrombi within the glomeruli and vasculitis
   - (E) Tubular atrophy

2. Which of the following histologic findings is not associated with acute cellular rejection in renal transplantation?
   - (A) Fibrinoid necrosis of vessels
   - (B) >6 mononuclear cells per tubular cross-section
   - (C) >10 neutrophils in a single glomerulus
   - (D) >25% parenchyma involved by mononuclear cell inflammation
   - (E) Transmural arteritis

3. Chronic/sclerosing allograft nephropathy is characterized by all of the following features, except
   - (A) Arterial hyalinosis
   - (B) "Double contours" of capillary basement membranes
   - (C) Interstitial fibrosis
   - (D) Tubular atrophy
   - (E) Vasculitis

4. The striped pattern of renal interstitial fibrosis is characteristically associated with

   - (A) Chronic rejection
   - (B) Cyclosporine/tacrolimus toxicity
   - (C) Glomerulonephritis
   - (D) Persistent urinary tract obstruction
   - (E) Renal artery stenosis

5. All the following histologic changes can be associated with this finding in a renal allograft biopsy (see Figure 23-1), except

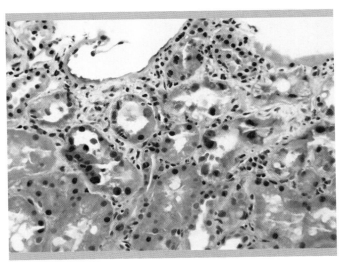

FIGURE 23-1

   - (A) Interstitial fibrosis
   - (B) Ischemic and transplant glomerulopathy
   - (C) Parenchymal hemorrhage
   - (D) Tubular atrophy
   - (E) Tubular microcalcifications

6. A 52-year-old man undergoes cardiac transplantation for end-stage congestive cardiac failure. The findings in this endomyocardial biopsy (see Figure 23-2) are associated with all of the following, except

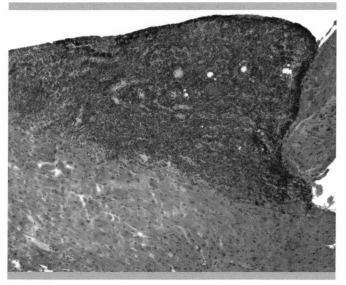

FIGURE 23-2

(A) Acute cellular rejection
(B) Endocardial or myocardial infiltrates
(C) Predominantly CD4+ T-lymphocytic infiltrate
(D) Prolonged cyclosporine use
(E) Vascular proliferation and stromal fibrosis

7. A posttransplantation cardiac biopsy obtained from a 56-year-old woman is depicted in Figure 23-3. The histologic features are consistent with

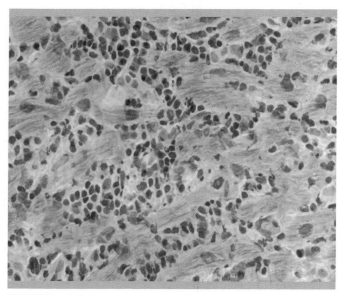

FIGURE 23-3

(A) Acute cellular rejection
(B) Antibody-mediated rejection
(C) Chronic rejection
(D) Hyperacute rejection
(E) Quilty effect

8. Post-transplant recurrent hepatitis C is characterized by all of the following features, except
(A) Focal bile duct damage
(B) Hepatitis C viral titer of 69000000 IU/mL
(C) Macrovesicular steatosis
(D) Numerous acidophil bodies
(E) Portal inflammation with activated lymphocytes

9. A 47-year-old man with a history of liver transplantation for Hepatitis C-induced cirrhosis presents to the emergency room with severe jaundice and altered sensorium. He is found to have a viral load of 47000000 IU/mL, prolonged prothrombin time, and a moderate increase in serum transaminases. Based on his post-transplant liver biopsy findings (see Figure 23-4), the most likely diagnosis is

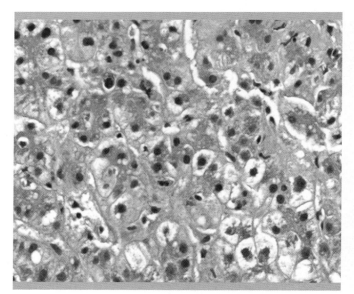

FIGURE 23-4

(A) Bile duct obstruction
(B) Drug toxicity
(C) Fibrosing cholestatic hepatitis
(D) Ischemic cholangiopathy
(E) Severe acute cellular rejection

10. In a transbronchial biopsy sample, which of the following features is least diagnostic of acute cellular rejection?
(A) Endotheliitis
(B) Hyaline membranes

(C) Intra-alveolar macrophages with brown/black material
(D) Lymphocytic bronchiolitis
(E) Perivascular mononuclear inflammation

11. A 43-year-old man, who is 6 months post-simultaneous pancreas-kidney transplant for type I diabetes mellitus, presents with abdominal pain and increased serum lipase level. He has been non-compliant with his medications and is clinically suspected to have acute rejection. His pancreas biopsy is least likely to show
(A) Acinar damage
(B) Arteritis
(C) Islet cell injury
(D) Lobular septal inflammation
(E) Venous endotheliitis

12. In a small-bowel allograft biopsy obtained 5 months following transplantation that shows minimal villous blunting and expansion of the lamina propria by activated lymphocytes, the number of apoptotic figures per 10 consecutive crypts that is indicative of mild acute cellular rejection is
(A) 2
(B) 3
(C) 4
(D) 5
(E) 6

13. A 20-year-old patient undergoes bone marrow transplantation and presents with severe diarrhea. Based on the findings in his colon biopsy is shown in Figure 23-5, the most likely diagnosis is

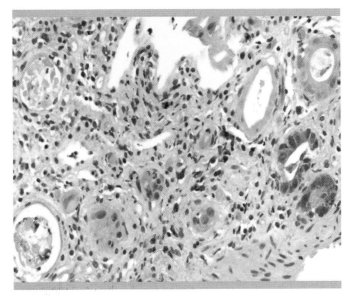

FIGURE 23-5

(A) Cytomegalovirus colitis
(B) Drug-induced colitis
(C) Mild graft-versus-host disease
(D) Moderate graft-versus-host-disease
(E) Severe graft-versus-host-disease

14. In the appropriate clinical setting, all the following histologic findings are seen in cutaneous graft-versus-host disease, except
(A) Apoptosis in the superficial keratinocytes
(B) Epidermal compact orthokeratosis, hypergranulosis, and acanthosis with lichenoid changes
(C) Fibrous thickening of the fascia with inflammation
(D) Lymphocyte satellitosis
(E) Sclerosis of papillary or reticular dermis

15. In a patient with bone marrow transplantation, which of the following endoscopic findings in esophagus is diagnostic of chronic graft-versus-host disease?
(A) Hiatal hernia
(B) Irregular Z-line
(C) Ulcers
(D) Upper esophageal webs
(E) Salmon-colored mucosa

16. The split products of which of the following complement protein is considered to be a marker of antibody-mediated rejection?
(A) C4
(B) C5
(C) C6
(D) C7
(E) C9

ANSWERS

1. **(D) Numerous fibrin thrombi within the glomeruli and vasculitis.**
The gross description of the kidney is highly suggestive of hyperacute rejection, which occurs when preformed antibodies in the recipient mount a response against the donor organ. Multiparous women and patients who have a history of multiple blood transfusions are exposed to several HLA antigens, and therefore, are at risk for developing this form of rejection. Antigen-antibody reaction targets the vascular endothelium and causes thrombotic occlusion of the capillaries, fibrinoid necrosis of arteries, and infarction. Endotheliitis and lymphocytic tubulitis are hallmarks of acute cellular rejection, while arterial obliterative intimal fibrosis and tubular atrophy are features of chronic rejection.

2. **(C) >10 neutrophils in a single glomerulus.**
Tubulitis and arteritis are the hallmarks of acute cellular rejection. Tubulitis score or "t" score refers to the number of mononuclear cells per tubular cross section. If the tubule is cut longitudinally, the results are expressed as number of mononuclear cells per 10 tubular cells. Interstitial inflammation involving >10% of unscarred parenchyma is significant and contributes to the "i" score. Any intimal arteritis contributes to the "v" score. A minimum of 4 cells per tubular cross-section with interstitial inflammation is required for a diagnosis of mild acute cellular rejection.

3. **(E) Vasculitis.**
All of the above choices except vasculitis are histologic features of chronic/sclerosing allograft nephropathy. Vasculitis is a feature of acute rejection.

4. **(B) Cyclosporine/tacrolimus toxicity.**
Cyclosporine/tacrolimus toxicity is an important cause of renal allograft dysfunction and can lead to acute tubular necrosis, vacuolar change of tubular epithelium, as well as microvascular injury with vascular thrombosis. Prolonged administration is manifested by a specific striped pattern of interstitial fibrosis. This pattern of fibrosis is associated with arteriolopathy, and is therefore, thought to be ischemic in origin.

5. **(C) Parenchymal hemorrhage.**
The figure shows an example of BK virus nephropathy. JC virus, BK virus, and SV40 viruses are the three types of polyoma viruses (DNA virus) that infect humans. The characteristic findings on histology include intranuclear basophilic and gelatinous inclusions within the epithelial cells. All the histologic changes listed in the question, except parenchymal hemorrhage, can be associated with BK virus infection. The degree of inflammatory changes can be confused with acute cellular rejection, acute tubular necrosis, and interstitial nephritis. In urine cytology preparation, BK virus inclusion-bearing cells are referred to as "Decoy cells." An immunohistochemical stain for BK virus or cross-reacting SV40 large T antigen may be employed to highlight these inclusions.

6. **(A) Acute cellular rejection.**
The endomyocardial biopsy shows endocardial lymphocytic infiltrates, also known as Quilty effect. These are collections of T-lymphocytes admixed with macrophages, plasma cells, and B-lymphocytes. The lesion was first described by Billingham and was named after the patient in whom it was first observed. The exact pathogenesis is uncertain and the lesions have been associated with cyclosporine use. They have been classified as type A (noninvasive), restricted to the endocardium, and type B (invasive), extending into the myocardium. The subclassification has no clinical significance. It is important to recognize this lesion, as it is often misdiagnosed as acute cellular rejection. Lack of myocyte damage, presence of prominent vascularity, and stromal fibrosis are helpful is diagnosing Quilty effect.

7. **(A) Acute cellular rejection.**
The biopsy shows acute cellular rejection that is characterized by perivascular or interstitial mononuclear inflammatory infiltrate with myocyte damage. Accurate interpretation of myocyte damage is key to the diagnosis. Myocyte injury is accompanied by vacuolization, perinuclear halos, ruffling of cytoplasmic membranes, irregular myocyte borders, hypereosinophilia, nuclear pyknosis, clearing of sarcoplasm, nuclear enlargement, and occasional prominent nucleoli. Myocyte necrosis, edema, vasculitis, and leukocyte infiltrates (especially eosinophils) are features of moderate-to-severe acute cellular rejection.

8. **(E) Portal inflammation with activated lymphocytes.**
Lobular hepatitis with acidophil bodies, portal lymphoid aggregates with small mature-appearing lymphocytes, and focal bile duct damage favor a diagnosis of recurrent hepatitis C. A biopsy diagnosis of acute rejection is based on three main features: (1) polymorphous, but predominantly mononuclear portal inflammation, containing activated lymphocytes, neutrophils, and eosinophils; (2) portal and/or terminal hepatic vein endotheliitis; and (3) bile duct inflammation and damage. The minimal findings needed to establish the diagnosis of acute rejection include the presence of at least two of the above histopathologic features along with biochemical evidence of liver damage.

9. **(C) Fibrosing cholestatic hepatitis.**
The figure shows marked cholestasis and hepatocyte swelling. Clinically, fibrosing cholestatic hepatitis (FCH) is characterized by rapidly deteriorating graft function with jaundice, coagulopathy, encephalopathy, and death within 4–6 weeks of onset of symptoms. Histologically, the presence of marked hepatocyte ballooning, cholestasis, and periportal and/or perisinusoidal collagen deposition, in an acutely ill patient with an increased HCV viral load, should prompt a diagnosis of FCH. Bile duct obstruction is usually accompanied by lamellar portal edema and ductular reaction. The histologic features of FCH were first described in patients with Hepatitis B infection.

10. **(C) Intra-alveolar macrophages with brown/black material.**

    Acute rejection is characterized by perivascular and interstitial mononuclear cell inflammation, which may be accompanied by endotheliitis, lymphocytic bronchitis, and bronchiolitis. It is graded as A0-A4 (none, minimal, mild, moderate, and severe rejection). Airway inflammation is graded as B0, B1R (low grade), B2R, and BX (ungradable). Hyaline membranes can be associated with marked alveolar pneumocyte damage and is usually a feature of severe acute rejection. The presence of alveolar macrophages with brown/black pigment indicates smokers'-type respiratory bronchiolitis. This finding is increasingly recognized in transplant biopsies due to the expansion of donor pool to include organs from patients with history of smoking.

11. **(C) Islet cell injury.**

    Acute rejection in pancreas biopsies is characterized by a mixed inflammatory infiltrate composed of activated lymphocytes, eosinophils, plasma cells, and occasional neutrophils. The inflammation involves the exocrine compartment of pancreas (ducts, acini, and lobular septae), as well as the arteries, nerves and veins. Islets of Langerhans are usually spared in acute cellular rejection.

12. **(E) 6.**

    The histologic diagnosis of acute small bowel rejection is based on a combination of three main features: (1) infiltration by a mixed but primarily mononuclear inflammatory population including activated lymphocytes, (2) crypt injury and inflammation, and (3) increase in crypt apoptotic bodies. Although crypt apoptosis can be identified in normal mucosa (usually <2 per 10 crypts), in the presence of other features, a cut-off of ≥6 apoptotic bodies per 10 consecutive crypts, is considered to be diagnostic of mild acute cellular rejection.

13. **(A) Cytomegalovirus colitis.**

    Graft-versus-host disease (GVHD) usually occurs in the setting of bone marrow transplantation and the target organs include epithelium of the skin, liver, and intestines. Patients usually present with profuse diarrhea, and biopsies from the tubular gastrointestinal tract typically show crypt apoptosis. The grading of GVHD depends on the extent of crypt injury and mucosal involvement. Crypt apoptosis can also be present in other conditions such as cytomegalovirus colitis and drug-induced colitis (especially mycophenolate mofetil).

14. **(A) Apoptosis in the superficial keratinocytes.**

    Apoptoses in the basal epidermal layer (not the superficial keratinocytes), vacuolar change in basilar layer, lichenoid inflammation, and lymphocyte satellitosis can be present in all stages of graft-versus-host disease (GVHD). Chronic GVHD can manifest in various forms: lichen planus-like (choice B), fasciitis-like (choice C), or sclerotic or morpheic (choice E).

15. **(D) Upper esophageal webs.**

    Upper esophageal webs are considered to be a diagnostic clinical feature of chronic graft-versus-host disease (GVHD). No other endoscopic finding in the gastrointestinal tract is specific for GVHD.

16. **(A) C4.**

    Complement activation product C4d is considered to be a histologic marker of humoral or antibody-mediated rejection in solid organ transplantation.

SUGGESTED READING

1. Bohl DL, Brennan DC. BK virus nephropathy and kidney transplantation. *Clin J Am Soc Nephrol.* 2007;2(suppl 1): S36-S46.
2. Dell'Antonio G, Randhawa PS. "Striped" pattern of medullary ray fibrosis in allograft biopsies from kidney transplant recipients maintained on tacrolimus. *Transplantation.* 1999;67:484-486.
3. Demetris AJ. Evolution of hepatitis C virus in liver allografts. *Liver Transpl.* 2009;15(suppl 2):S35-S41.
4. Filipovich AH, Weisdorf D, Pavletic S, et al. National Institutes of Health consensus development project on criteria for clinical trials in chronic graft-versus-host disease: I. Diagnosis and staging working group report. *Biol Blood Marrow Transplant.* 2005;11:945-956.
5. Nankivell BJ, Alexander SI. Rejection of the kidney allograft. *N Engl J Med.* 2010;363:1451-1462.
6. Patil DT, Yerian LM. Pancreas transplant: recent advances and spectrum of features in pancreas allograft pathology. *Adv Anat Pathol.* 2010;17:202-208.
7. Racusen LC, Solez K, Colvin RB, et al. The Banff 97 working classification of renal allograft pathology. *Kidney Int.* 1999; 55:713-723.
8. Shulman HM, Kleiner D, Lee SJ, et al. Histopathologic diagnosis of chronic graft-versus-host disease: National Institutes of Health Consensus Development Project on Criteria for Clinical Trials in Chronic Graft-versus-Host Disease: II. Pathology Working Group Report. *Biol Blood Marrow Transplant.* 2006;12:31-47.
9. Stewart S, Fishbein MC, Snell GI, et al. Revision of the 1996 working formulation for the standardization of nomenclature in the diagnosis of lung rejection. *J Heart Lung Transplant.* 2007;26:1229-1242.
10. Tan CD, Baldwin WM, 3rd, Rodriguez ER. Update on cardiac transplantation pathology. *Arch Pathol Lab Med.* 2007; 131:1169-1191.
11. Wu T, Abu-Elmagd K, Bond G, et al. A schema for histologic grading of small intestine allograft acute rejection. *Transplantation.* 2003;75:1241-1248.
12. Xiao SY, Lu L, Wang HL. Fibrosing cholestatic hepatitis: clinicopathologic spectrum, diagnosis and pathogenesis. *Int J Clin Exp Pathol.* 2008;1:396-402.

INDEX

Note: Page number followed by f indicates figure only.